Natural Therapeutics Pocket Guide

2000-2001

Natural
Therapeutics
Pocket Guide

2000-2001

Natural Therapeutics Pocket Guide

2000-2001

James B. LaValle, RPh, DHM, NMD, CCN
President, Natural Health Resources
Cincinnati, Ohio
Adjunct Associate Professor
University of Cincinnati, College of Pharmacy
Professor of Pharmacology
Central States College of Health Sciences School for Naturopathy

Daniel L. Krinsky, RPh, MS
Director of Patient Care Services and Pharmacy Practices
Ritzman Pharmacies, Inc
Wadsworth, Ohio

Ernest B. Hawkins, RPh, MS
Technology Specialist
Natural Health Resources
Riddle Farm, North Carolina

Ross Pelton, RPh, PhD, CCN
Director of Education
Natural Health Resources
San Diego, California

Nancy Ashbrook Willis, BA, JD
Attorney at Law
Terrace Park, Ohio

LEXI-COMP, INC
Hudson, OH

NATURAL HEALTH RESOURCES
Cincinnati, OH

AMERICAN PHARMACEUTICAL ASSOCIATION APhA

NOTICE

This handbook is intended to serve the user as a handy quick reference and not as a complete herb information resource. It does not include information on every product available. The publication is specifically designed to present certain important aspects of herb/nutraceutical/natural product data in a more concise format than is generally found in other publications or product information supplied by manufacturers.

While great care has been taken to ensure the accuracy of the information presented, the reader is advised that the authors, editors, reviewers, contributors, and publishers cannot be responsible for the continued currency of the information or for any errors, omissions, or the application of this information, or for any consequences arising therefrom. There-fore, the author(s) and/or the publisher shall have no liability to any person or entity with regard to claims, loss, or damage caused, or alleged to be caused, directly or indirectly, by the use of information contained herein. Because of the dynamic nature of natural product information, readers are advised that decisions regarding therapy must be based on the independent judgment of the healthcare provider, changing information (as reflected in literature), and changing medical practices. The editors are not responsible for any inaccuracy of quotation or for any false or misleading implication that may arise due to the text or formulas as used or due to the quotation of revisions no longer official. Further, the *Natural Therapeutics Pocket Guide* is not offered as a guide to dosing. The reader, herewith, is advised that information relating to dosing is provided only as an indication of the amount typically given or taken during therapy. Actual dosing amount should be based on an in-depth evaluation of the individual's therapy requirement and strong consideration given to such issues as contraindications, warnings, precautions, adverse reactions, along with the interaction of other herbs/drugs. The manufacturers most current product information or other standard recognized references should always be consulted for such detailed information prior to drug/natural product/nutraceutical use.

The editors and contributors have written this book in their private capacities. No official support or endorsement by any federal agency, pharmaceutical company, or natural product manufacturer is intended or inferred.

If you have any suggestions or questions regarding any information presented in this handbook, please contact Lexi-Comp at

1-877-837-LEXI (5394)

This manual was produced using the FormuLex™ Program —
a complete publishing service of Lexi-Comp, Inc.

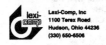

Lexi-Comp, Inc
1100 Terex Road
Hudson, Ohio 44236
(330) 650-6506

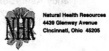

Natural Health Resources
4439 Glenway Avenue
Cincinnati, Ohio 45205

ISBN 0-916589-80-3

NATURAL THERAPEUTICS
POCKET GUIDE
TABLE OF CONTENTS

INTRODUCTION
   About the Authors 2
   Acknowledgments 4

PART I. INTRODUCTION TO NATURAL THERAPEUTICS
   Using the Natural Therapeutics Pocket Guide 5
   Introduction to Natural Medicine 9
   Introduction to Herbs 11
   Introduction to Nutrition 19
   Introduction to Homeopathy 31
   Introduction to Glandular Extracts 36

PART II. CONDITIONS
   Table of Contents 39
   Introduction to Conditions 41
   Conditions / Decision Trees / Considerations 44

PART III. ALPHABETICAL LISTING
  OF NATURAL PRODUCTS 379

PART IV. CHARTS AND LISTS
   Herb Quick Reference Chart 538
   Nutraceutical Chart 573
   Homeopathic Quick Reference Chart for Common
      Complaints 587
   Vitamins / Minerals / Trace Elements / Amino Acids 604
   Drug-Induced Nutrient Depletions 625
   Nutrient Depletion and Cancer Chemotherapy 637
   Herbal Medicine Use In Pediatrics 641
   Herb/Drug Potential Interactions 642
   Unsafe Herbs 654
   Common Herbal Supplements Contraindicated During
      Pregnancy 656
   Pregnancy & Lactation Nutritional Chart 657
   Organ System Support Using Natural Products 660

PART V. GLOSSARY OF NATURAL MEDICINE TERMS 663

NATURAL PRODUCT CATEGORY INDEX 669

ALPHABETICAL INDEX 673

ABOUT THE AUTHORS

James B. LaValle, RPh, DHM, NMD, CCN

James B. LaValle has been involved with natural medicine for the past fifteen years and is a nationally recognized figure in the field of natural therapeutics. He is currently President and founder of Natural Health Resources, Inc. Dr LaValle's experience ranges from extensive clinical practice, product design and formulation, and technology transfer, to author educator, and media personality. He maintains a practice at Good Samaritan Hospital's Tri-Health Integrative Medicine Center and is currently Adjunct Associate Professor at the University of Cincinnati College of Pharmacy and Professor of Pharmacology at Central States College of Health Sciences School for Naturopathy. Dr LaValle is on the Advisory Boards of the Better Life Institute and New Hope Communications. He is featured on "Healthwell.com Ask the Experts". Dr LaValle has educated the pharmacy industry as Associate Editor for natural products for *Drug Store News* and *Retail Pharmacy News*. He also has a featured column, the "Prescription Pad," in *Natural Pharmacy* magazine. Dr LaValle is independent counsel for The Rite Aid Vitamin Institute, and through his company, NHR, has developed educational programs for McKesson (Nutri-Station Program), CVS, Longs Drugs, and others. He has trained hundreds of independent pharmacists about integrating natural medicine into pharmacy practice. Dr LaValle was named one of the "50 Most Influential Druggists" by *American Druggist* in 1998 for his work in natural medicine. Current book titles include **Smart Medicine for Healthier Living** (Avery Publishing), **Drug-Induced Nutrient Depletion Handbook** (Lexi-Comp, Inc, 1999), **The Black Cohosh Book** (Avery Publishing), and **The Cholestin Breakthrough** (Prima), with several other titles on the way.

Daniel L. Krinsky, MS, RPh

Daniel L. Krinsky received both his BS in Pharmacy and MS in Hospital Pharmacy from the University of Toledo. He was the Coordinator of the Clinical Pharmacokinetic Consult Service at the University of Alabama Hospital in Birmingham, Alabama from 1985 to 1991. More recently, he was a Clinical Information Specialist with the Ohio Region of Kaiser Permanente from 1991 to 1994. Mr Krinsky is currently the Vice President of Professional Services with Ritzman Pharmacies, Inc, in Wadsworth, Ohio, and Assistant Clinical Professor, Raabe College of Pharmacy, Ohio Northern University. His primary responsibilities include overseeing the EduCare Division, establishing disease management programs, developing and delivering internal and external educational programs, overseeing quality assurance activities, answering drug information questions, and educating graduate pharmacy students. Professional interests include research in the community pharmacy setting, development of disease-state management programs, clinical pharmacokinetics, patient outcome assessments, quality assurance and improvement activities, and payment for cognitive services. He recently co-authored the **Drug-Induced Nutrient Depletion Handbook** (Lexi-Comp, Inc, 1999).

Ernest B. Hawkins, MS, RPh

Ernest B. Hawkins has over 10 years of experience in hospital and retail pharmacy, as well as pharmaceutical research. He has worked extensively in the herbal supplement industry, focusing on the manufacturing and quality control of herbal ingredients. He is a consultant, author, and educator in the dietary supplement arena, authoring and coauthoring numerous articles, continuing education programs, books, and other educational materials. Mr Hawkins is a featured columnist for *Natural Pharmacy* magazine, and his work has appeared in other national pharmacy magazines such as *Drug Store News, Retail Pharmacy News,* and *Chain Drug Review*. Current book titles include **Drug-Induced Nutrient Depletion Handbook** (Lexi-Comp, Inc, 1999) and **The Black Cohosh Book** (Avery Publishing), with several other titles in process. He is currently a principal author, lecturer, and technology specialist for Natural Health Resources.

Ross Pelton, RPh, PhD, CCN

Ross Pelton received a pharmacy degree from the University of Wisconsin in 1966 and a PhD in psychology with an emphasis in Holistic Health from the University for Humanistic Studies in San Diego, California, in 1984. In 1994, he became a Certified Clinical Nutritionist (CCN) through the International and American Association of Clinical Nutritionists (IAACN). In 1982-83, Dr Pelton conducted cancer research at the University of California, San Diego (UCSD). Working with the world-renowned scientist, Dr Gerhard Schrauzer, Pelton's research involved studying the relationship between the trace mineral selenium and breast cancer. This research was instrumental in shifting the focus of Dr Pelton's professional interests into the direction of nutrition and natural therapies. In 1985-86, Dr Pelton worked as a consultant to The Gerson Institute, one of the oldest and most successful alternative, nontoxic cancer therapies. In 1988, Dr Pelton moved to Baja, Mexico where he became the administrator of one of the largest hospitals in the world specializing in alternative, nontoxic cancer therapies. For five and one-half years, Dr Pelton directed the inpatient and outpatient therapies for all patients. *Alternatives in Cancer Therapy*, one of four books by Dr Pelton, was based on his experiences with alternative cancer therapies in Mexico. From 1994 to 1998, Dr Pelton worked as a pharmacist and also developed a practice in clinical nutrition. In 1997, Dr Pelton wrote **The Guide to Drug-Induced Nutritional Depletion**. His continued research on this topic has recently resulted in the publication of a reference book for health professionals titled the **Drug-Induced Nutrient Depletion Handbook**, (Lexi-Comp, Inc, 1999). Dr Pelton is the author of three other books, which include **Mind Food & Smart Pills** (Doubleday, 1988), **Alternatives in Cancer Therapy** (Simon & Schuster, 1994), and **How To Prevent Breast Cancer** (Simon & Schuster, 1995). Dr Pelton also writes a regular column on clinical nutrition for *American Druggist* magazine and he was named by *American Druggist* as one of the "50 Most Influential Pharmacists of 1999" for his educational efforts and contributions to natural medicine. He is currently the Director of Education for Natural Health Resources, Inc.

Nancy Ashbrook Willis, BA, JD

Nancy Ashbrook Willis is an attorney with experience in various state agencies, including the Ohio Attorney General and the Ohio Department of Commerce. She has drafted legislation and testified before Ohio legislative committees. A former Assistant Dean at the Ohio State University College of Law, she has a background in legal research and public interest law. As the former Vice President of Natural Health Resources, Inc, she provided legal and management services to the corporation. Her long-time interest in natural approaches to health provided a framework for her to edit articles, continuing education courses, and various media presentations on numerous aspects of natural medicine for NHR. These articles have appeared in such publications as *Drug Store News, Retail Pharmacy News, Natural Pharmacy*, and *The Rite Aid Vitamin Institute Newsletter*. Nancy is currently in private practice, with an emphasis on dietary supplement law, a topic on which she has lectured.

ACKNOWLEDGMENTS

The *Natural Therapeutics Pocket Guide* exists in its present form as the result of the concerted efforts of the following individuals: Robert D. Kerscher, publisher and president of Lexi-Comp, Inc; Lynn D. Coppinger, managing editor; Mark F. Bonfiglio, BS, PharmD, RPh, director of pharmacotherapy resources; Barbara F. Kerscher, production manager; Leslie J. Ruggles, project manager; David C. Marcus, director of information systems; and Julian I. Graubart, American Pharmaceutical Association (APhA), Director of Books and Electronic Products.

Other members of the Lexi-Comp staff whose contributions deserve special mention include Jeanne E. Wilson, production/systems liaison; Ginger S. Conner and Kathleen E. Schleicher, reference publishing project managers; Stacey L. Hurd, Tonya Parsley, Jennifer L. Rocky, and Linda L. Taylor, custom publishing project managers; Alexandra J. Hart, composition specialist; Kathy Smith and Stacy S. Robinson, production assistants; Tracey J. Reinecke, graphic designer; Leonard L. Lance, BSPharm, RPh, pharmaceutical database specialist; Liz Tomsik, PharmD, pharmacotherapy specialist; Cynthia A. Bell, CPhT, drug identification database manager; Edmund A. Harbart, vice-president, custom publishing division; Jack L. Stones, vice-president, reference publishing division; Jay L. Katzen, director of marketing and business development; Jerry M. Reeves, Marc L. Long, and Patrick T. Grubb, regional sales managers; Brad F. Bolinski, Kristin M. Thompson, Matthew C. Kerscher, Tina L. Collins, and Kelene A. Gluntz, sales and marketing representatives; Paul A. Rhine and Jason M. Buchwald, academic account managers; Kenneth J. Hughes, manager of authoring systems; Sean M. Conrad, James M. Stacey, and Matthew J. Houser, system analysts; Thury L. O'Connor, vice-president of technology; David J. Wasserbauer, vice-president, finance and administration; Elizabeth M. Conlon, Rebecca A. Dryhurst, and Leslie G. Rodia, accounting; Marta Pacur and Mary Jane Podesta, receptionists; and Frederick C. Kerscher, inventory and fulfillment manager.

Natural Health Resources, Inc.

Natural Health Resources was founded by James B. LaValle with the mission to increase the awareness and promote to healthcare professionals, corporations and the lay public the value of natural therapeutics. The NHR team has conducted seminars for some of the largest corporations in America. Thousands of professionals each month are reached through various media (T.V., radio, live, written, tape) in coordination with manufacturers, education certification boards, and various schools. To contact NHR on available services, please call (513) 244-2200 or email nhr@one.net.

USING THE NATURAL THERAPEUTICS POCKET GUIDE

The *Natural Therapeutics Pocket Guide* is designed to offer the healthcare provider with a comprehensive guide to using natural products for many common medical conditions. The authors have included information on many of the most commonly used natural products. These natural products can be used for prevention, health enhancement, or as a complement to drug therapy. These agents may also be considered for individuals who, for whatever reason, elect **not** to use traditional medicine. This book should be used as a guide to integrating natural products into one's health and wellness program. This *Pocket Guide* is meant to be a handy reference that will offer the healthcare provider a logical first step for suggesting natural therapeutics as a part of health management. The suggestions made in this book are intended to improve health, and the natural products discussed are not intended as a cure for any disease and should not be construed as curative or healing.

This book is divided into five parts, with each presenting a different aspect of natural therapeutics. Information from each part of the book is designed to complement information in other sections.

Part I: Introduction to Natural Therapeutics

Part I of the *Natural Therapeutics Pocket Guide* offers the healthcare provider with introductory information on the field of natural medicine and some of the most common types of natural therapies available.

- **Introduction to Natural Medicine** provides an overview of natural medicine, including emphasis on food intake and nutrient status, stress management, and the importance of determining underlying disturbances to an individual's biochemistry. This section provides suggestions for integrating natural medicine with traditional allopathic therapy.

- **Introduction to Herbs** covers the history of herbs, contemporary uses of herbs, their manufacturing and standardization, and quality assurance issues. This section also discusses the legal status of herbs and potential herb/drug interactions.

- **Introduction to Nutrition** provides an overview of vitamins, minerals, amino acids, essential fatty acids, antioxidants, and nutraceuticals. This section discusses the role of each of these agents in good health, their availability through food sources and dietary supplements, current nutritional status in the United States, and a recommendation for basic daily nutritional supplement intake.

- **Introduction to Homeopathy** reviews the history of homeopathy, its basic tenets, and the main approaches for the use of homeopathic remedies. The manufacturing of homeopathic remedies and their legal status are also discussed, along with clinical studies on homeopathy, and its possible mechanisms of action.

- **Introduction to Glandular Extracts** deals with the composition and use of glandulars, their manufacturing and quality, and research on their effectiveness.

Part II: Conditions

Part II of the *Natural Therapeutics Pocket Guide* is the core of the book. More than 80 common health conditions are covered in this section. Each condition

USING THE NATURAL THERAPEUTICS POCKET GUIDE
(Continued)

includes Condition Overview, Lifestyle Recommendations, Decision Tree, Table of Natural Product suggestions, and Special Considerations.

- **Condition Overview**: A general overview of the condition, with basic information on its etiology, typical symptoms, who may be affected, associated disorders, common interventions to provide relief, general complications, and the predicted duration of the condition.

- **Lifestyle Recommendations**: Suggestions are offered for lifestyle changes for each condition. Most of these recommendations revolve around certain behavioral modifications that are likely to provide benefit. General lifestyle recommendations are provided as options that may provide benefit to an individual with the specific condition.

- **Decision Tree**: A decision tree is provided for each condition to help identify when to apply natural products. Each decision tree covers a series of questions that help determine situation complexity. Decision points are identified in the trees to assist in deciding how to proceed based on an individual's particular situation.

- **Table of Natural Product Suggestions**: This table lists common natural products used to support each medical condition. Every table includes a classification system, which was developed by the authors, for each natural product. Classification is based on the type and amount of scientific support that exists for using that product for the specific condition.

- **Special Considerations**: The information in this section is extracted from the monographs on individual herbs, nutritionals, and nutraceuticals. It is included in the Conditions section to provide a quick reference to important risk issues for each product. This section offers information that is important to consider when deciding how to apply natural products to a specific condition. The information is customized for each medical condition.

A more detailed description of the information in this section is included in the Introduction to Conditions *on page 41.*

Part III: Monographs

Part III of the *Natural Therapeutics Pocket Guide* contains individual monographs for each herb, vitamin, mineral, amino acid, nutraceutical, and glandular extract discussed in the *Pocket Guide*. The information in the monographs includes dosage ranges, reported uses, a summary of the agent, a description of its pharmacology, and any warnings, cautions, toxicities, or contraindications related to its use. Besides listing the Recommended Dietary Intake (RDI), the monographs for each vitamin, mineral, and amino acid specify a dosage titled ODA (Optimal Daily Allowance). ODA is a term coined by the authors to describe the suggested daily dietary intake of a nutrient that will assist the individual in achieving optimal health. The vitamin, mineral, amino acid, and nutraceutical monographs also list the active forms of each agent, deficiency symptoms, and reported interactions.

MONOGRAPH FORMAT OVERVIEW

Field Label	Field Description
Name	Common name with acronym or Latin binomial when appropriate
Category	Identifies the natural product as an herb, nutraceutical, glandular, vitamin, mineral, or amino acid
Synonym	Other names or accepted abbreviations
Plant Part (herbs only)	Most commonly used plant part with medicinal value
Dosage (all products except herbs)	Amount of the natural product typically taken for common uses
Dosage and Standardization (herbs only)	Standardized herbs are necessary to ensure consistent results. Dosages are based on currently accepted practice and clinical efficacy. As with all medicinal substances, dosages can be altered based on clinical presentation, including age, weight, health status, and other pertinent factors. Standardization numbers may also vary slightly, as more companies enter the market with clinical research. Ask the manufacturer for documented efficacy of its product.
Active Forms (all products except herbs)	Lists primary active chemical constituents of the commercially available natural products
Reported Uses	Reported uses are based on clinical efficacy in human and animal studies. These uses are not all-inclusive for each plant, but are the most widely recommended and currently accepted in the medical community.
Summary	A brief summary of the individual plant and its use as a therapeutic agent
Pharmacology	Documented pharmacology based on reported studies. Some studies are reported on isolated chemical constituents in the herbs and extrapolated to the whole plant when standardized.
Toxicities, Warnings, and Interactions (all products except herbs)	These warnings are categorized and based on (1) human clinical trials; (2) animal and/or in vitro studies; (3) case reports; (4) potential interaction based on pharmacology. Again, any individual taking pharmaceutical medications should use dietary supplements with caution.
Theoretical Cautions and Contraindications (herbs only)	See Toxicities, Warnings, and Interactions
General Warnings (herbs only)	Warnings which apply to all herbal supplements, including general warnings about the potential for interactions with traditional medications and clinical situations in which herbal therapies must be approached with caution; occasionally, these warnings are superceded by information which may be listed in the Theoretical Cautions and Contraindications field and which is specific to the herb in question
Symptoms of Deficiency (all products except herbs)	List of symptoms caused by deficiency of the particular natural product
Reported Interactions	List of potentially interacting medicines and/or nutrients based on either literature support, product pharmacology, or theoretical considerations
Theoretical Interactions	
References	Sources used to verify included information

USING THE NATURAL THERAPEUTICS POCKET GUIDE
(Continued)

Part IV: Charts and Lists

Part IV of the *Natural Therapeutics Pocket Guide* contains numerous charts that can be used for quick reference.

- **Herb Quick Reference Chart** provides basic information on more than 80 herbs, including plant part used, dosage and standardization, reported uses, whether the herb has any complementary effect with drug therapy, cautions and contraindications, and any interactive drug or drug category.

- **Nutraceutical Chart** provides basic information on more than 50 nutraceutical agents, including dosage ranges, reported uses, functions in the body, deficiency symptoms, and warnings and interactions.

- **Homeopathic Quick Reference Chart for Common Complaints** includes a listing of more than 90 common conditions and the homeopathic remedies that are useful for those conditions based on symptomatology.

- **Vitamins/Minerals/Trace Elements/Amino Acids Chart** provides basic information on more than 35 vitamins, minerals, trace elements, and amino acids. The chart includes dosages, reported uses, functions in the body, food sources, deficiency symptoms, and toxicity.

- **Drug-Induced Nutrient Depletions Chart** lists various prescription and nonprescription drugs that deplete specific nutrients in the body.

- **Nutrient Depletion and Cancer Chemotherapy Chart** discusses the depletion of nutrients by this broad group of chemical agents. The processes which contribute to nutrient depletion during cancer chemotherapy are reviewed in the introduction. The chemotherapy tables include ratings of individual agents in terms of their emetogenic potential and their effects on the integrity of an individual's gastrointestinal mucosa. Additional notes concerning their nutritional impact are also included in the tables.

- **Herbal Medicine Use in Pediatrics List** explains how to calculate herbal doses for children and guidelines for using herbal products for childhood illnesses.

- **Herb/Drug Potential Interactions Chart** classifies herbs, based on their chemical constituents and pharmacological properties. Their potential or theoretical interactions with pharmaceutical drugs are listed.

- **Unsafe Herbs List** details herbs that should not be used due to reported toxicity.

- **Common Herbal Supplements Contraindicated During Pregnancy List** is an alphabetical listing of herbs that should not be taken during pregnancy.

- **Pregnancy & Lactation Nutritional Chart** lists vitamins, minerals, and trace elements, with specific dosage guidelines to be followed during pregnancy and lactation. Functions in the body and any cautions or contraindications are also listed for each agent.

- **Organ System Support Using Natural Products Chart** lists herbal, nutritional, and homeopathic products that support the major organ systems in the body.

Part V: Glossary of Natural Medicine Terms

Part V of the *Natural Therapeutics Pocket Guide* contains a glossary of natural medicine terms to assist the healthcare provider who may not be familiar with the terminology in this field.

INTRODUCTION TO
NATURAL MEDICINE

Natural medicine has been in existence as long as man has walked the earth. There is an inseparable connection between man and the healing ability of nature. For us to divorce ourselves from the use of natural medicine is to deny the heritage of the evolving healing arts. As science and medicine progressed, the inclusion of natural medicine diverged from the forum of the day at times. However, a model of health and disease has clearly evolved into a model that believes bioenergetic and biochemical complexities are intertwined. The inter-relationship among spiritual, emotional, and physical human experiences and the interplay with the environment create our human experience and contribute to the continuum of health. To look at disease as only a set of symptoms to be blocked by the action of a certain drug or herb limits our ability to understand the nature of disease. As the biochemistry of a person becomes disrupted over time (through various factors such as emotional stress, poor nutrition, environ-mental toxicity, drug use, and viral, bacterial, fungal or parasitic load), chaos within the homeostatic system creates a symptom picture. Over the last few decades, people have developed varying symptoms, conditions, and diseases with no apparent related or connected causes when viewed from the allopathic perspective.

In a world where medicine has become very specialized, we often fail to take into account the whole individual and not just a diseased liver, a cancer case, or clogged arteries. Contemporary natural therapeutics has begun to consider nutrient status, structural integrity, functional enzymatic activity, detoxification pathways, and biochemical messengers along with psycho-neuro-endocrine function as factors that create the symptom picture. Determining underlying disturbances (such as the role of bacteria in cardiovascular disease), evaluating the Syndrome X patient, and addressing functional errors in metabolism that create symptoms can be a challenge. In any case, supporting organ structure and function and repleting nutrient status can make the individual more resis-tant to illness, improve quality of life and, hopefully, reduce or eliminate life-limiting symptoms. At times, recommendations in natural medicine are intended to strengthen health and vitality and not necessarily based on a direct cause and effect relationship.

Although a more complex approach, acknowledging this expanded view allows for a broader spectrum of therapeutic tools. Modern drug therapy has saved millions of lives. Yet a study published in the April 1998 issue of the *Journal of the American Medical Association* reported that the **correct** use of medications in hospitals accounted for an estimated 106,000 deaths, which makes it one of the leading causes of death in the United States.[1] People are looking for safer first options to reduce potential risks and side effects. They are also seeking information and guidance in the use of natural products. It is not a matter of becoming an advocate for natural health. It is a simple fact that natural thera-pies can often provide benefit and may be recommended by a healthcare professional or requested by a patient. In either case, healthcare professionals need to be able to inform and guide their patients on the safe use of natural agents. Personal biases should be removed and we must open ourselves to the possibility of new answers using time-honored solutions.

There are a variety of ways to consider applying natural therapies into practice. Consider how the antibiotic resistant bacteria problem we are facing would be reduced if natural agents that improve immune competence were used as a first line of defense more frequently. As professionals, we also need to be concerned about whether the overuse of antibiotics might actually weaken immune resiliency. This is just one area that could have a tremendous impact on the health of many people, especially children and the elderly. In the list which follows are some of the most common situations where natural therapeu-tics might apply.

INTRODUCTION TO
NATURAL MEDICINE *(Continued)*

- Natural therapeutics can be utilized as a first line of defense for common OTC complaints and conditions for people who prefer a natural agent or for the "at risk" population, which cannot use traditional OTC medicines. One example would be an individual with a kidney disorder who is looking for arthritis relief could consider using an agent like glucosamine. A pilot who is seeking cold and flu support, but who is not allowed to take an antihistamine or decongestant, could consider elderberry, echinacea, or vitamin C. There are numerous other situations where this new flexibility with recommendations might apply.

- Natural therapeutics can be used as a part of disease state management to improve quality of life or to improve the status of a given condition. A clear example of this would be the use of various natural agents that can improve glucose regulation and, thereby, decrease insulin resistance, or using an herb to improve microcirculation to the eyes and, thus, reduce the risk of diabetic retinopathy. These suggestions are not a cure for diabetes; however, they can reduce risks associated with the disease.

- Natural therapeutics can be used to complement traditional medical care. Examples include the use of standardized ginkgo biloba and cordyceps sinensis to counteract the decrease in sexual libido that occurs with antidepressant medication. Compliance might easily improve from this type of complementary suggestion. Another example would be the use of milk thistle to protect the liver when people are taking drugs that elevate liver enzymes and stress liver detoxification pathways.

- Natural therapeutics may be used to replete nutrients that are depleted during drug therapy. For example, oral contraceptives can deplete nutrients such as magnesium, folic acid, vitamin B_6, vitamin B_{12}, and others. Nutrient depletion from prescription and OTC medications can be a contributing factor to side effects and disease state induction.

- Natural therapeutics can be used for anti-aging, prevention, and performance enhancement. Common examples include vitamin E for cardiovascular health, creatine to improve athletic performance, and calcium and magnesium intake to help prevent osteoporosis.

This book was created as a resource guide to assist healthcare professionals in counseling patients about the appropriate use of natural products and therapies. It is designed to provide information quickly to facilitate a dialogue with the client about a specific natural product. For most professionals, the first step will be a conservative one. Over time, by making suggestions and giving advice, the professional will evolve into a resource for natural care. Bear in mind that there are a variety of disciplines in natural therapeutics that are not discussed in this book, but which have historical and validated evidence of use. Ayurvedic medicine, traditional Chinese medicine, massage, chiropractic, and many other disciplines have their place in the healing process.

Footnote
1. Lazarou J, Pomeranz BH, and Corey PN, "Incidence of Adverse Drug Reactions in Hospitalized Patients: A Meta-Analysis of Prospective Studies," *JAMA*, 1998, 279(15):1200-5.

INTRODUCTION TO HERBS

Herbal supplements once lined the shelves of every community pharmacy in this country, waiting to be compounded into various "remedies" prescribed by the local physician. These preparations dominated the early practices of medicine and pharmacy in the United States. Herbal supplements were the hallmark of the pharmaceutical industry during the late 1800s and early 1900s. At that time, crude botanical drugs were still sold in the apothecary as leaves and roots for teas, powders, and liquid extracts. Herbs are a rich part of our medicinal heritage. The first edition of the United States Pharmacopoeia (USP), which was published in 1820, contained 425 botanical entries, representing 67% of all items. This is in contrast with the 22nd edition (the latest), which contains monographs for only 58 botanical substances or 2% of all entries.[1]

Definition of Herbal Supplements

The World Health Organization (WHO) defines herbal supplements as:

> Finished, labeled medicinal products that contain as active ingredients aerial or underground parts of plants, or other plant material, or combinations thereof, whether crude state or as plant preparations. Plant material includes juices, gums, fatty oils, essential oils, and any other substances of this nature. Herbal supplements may contain excipients in addition to the active ingredients. Medicine containing plant material combined with chemically defined substances, including chemically defined, isolated constituents of plants, are not considered to be herbal supplements. Exceptionally, in some countries, herbal supplements may also contain, by tradition, natural organic or inorganic active ingredients which are not of plant origin.[2]

For the past 25 years, well over half of modern U.S. pharmaceuticals: (1) have been derived from natural sources (plant, animal, and microbial); (2) are synthetic analogs of natural products; or (3) were developed based on structural leads gained from natural products. Herbal supplements became overshadowed after World War II, when isolated chemicals began to be synthesized in laboratories. Acceptance of herbal supplements waned, in part due to these scientific advances, but also because of the economic potential of patentable, isolated chemical entities.

Examples of Plant-Derived Pharmaceuticals

Aspirin	White willow bark (*Salix alba*)
Caffeine	Coffee shrub (*Caffea arabica*)
Colchicine	Autumn crocus (*Crocus sativus*)
Cromolyn	Khella (*Amni visnagu*)
Cyclosporine	Cordyceps (*Cordyceps sinensis*)
Digoxin	Foxglove (*Digitalis purpurea*)
Morphine	Opium poppy (*Papaver somniferum*)
Quinine	Cinchona bark (*Cinchona* spp)
Taxol	Pacific yew (*Taxus* spp)
Theophylline	Tea shrub (*Camellia sinensis*)
Vincristine	Periwinkle (*Vinca* spp)

Current Environment

Recently, there has been a tremendous renewed interest in the healing properties of herbal supplements. They have again surfaced in the mainstream American marketplace. The sale of herbal supplements has risen steadily over the past few years, as more and more consumers have begun purchasing these health-related agents. Herbal supplements are used to help relieve various

INTRODUCTION TO HERBS *(Continued)*

symptoms and to support individuals with certain diseases and health-related problems. In a survey, nearly 33% of American adults have used herbal supplements in the past year.[3] That means that almost 60 million people over the age of 18 have used herbs for such problems as colds, headaches, burns, allergies, PMS, and mild depression.

Herbal supplements are now sold in health food stores, grocery stores, chain retail stores, convenience stores, on the internet, and in just about any other retail outlet imaginable. Herb sales have been the fastest growing segment of dietary supplements. Sales have gone from $570 million in 1992 to over $3.87 billion in 1998.[4] Of note are the top reported sources of information on herbal supplements: Friends and family (41%); health food store clerks (13%); physicians (9%); and pharmacists (4%). Sales of herbs in pharmacies continue to rise, indicating that professionals have a better understanding of the positive impact herbal supplements can have on the healthcare of our population.

Leading Uses of Herbal Supplements

The most common self-limiting health problems for which people seek over-the-counter (OTC) relief[5] are listed in the following table.

Health Problem	Percentage Using OTC Product
Colds	59
Burns	45
Headaches	22
Allergies	21
Rashes	18
Insomnia	18
PMS	17
Depression	7
Diarrhea	7
Menopause	4

Legal Status of Herbal Supplements

Under current law, herbal supplements are classified as dietary supplements in the United States and fall under the regulations for the food service industry, including the manufacturing practices imposed by the local agriculture departments for food manufacturers. Good Manufacturing Practices (GMPs) for herbal manufacturers are not currently required by the Food and Drug Administration (FDA), the arm of the government that regulates dietary supplements. However, some progressive manufacturers have joined together to create and follow self-imposed GMPs. Establishment of industry-wide GMPs will be an important and welcomed step in the progress of the herbal supplement arena. The quality and efficacy of herbal supplements for the consumer depends on the regulations imposed in the manufacturing of these products. GMPs for herbal supplements should include at least the following:

- Proper plant identification
- Quantitative assays of marker constituents
- Purity limits involving negative markers and analytical parameters, including ash content and loss on drying
- Heavy metal and pesticide content
- Microbial content
- Processing requirements
- Labeling

The Dietary Supplement Health and Education Act of 1994 (DSHEA) established the legal status of dietary supplements. The burden of proof regarding the safety of herbs and other supplements was shifted to the FDA. DSHEA also redefined dietary supplements to include herbs, vitamins, minerals, and amino acids. The act also stated that new ingredients introduced after October 15, 1994 must be shown to be safe by the manufacturer. DSHEA contains the following provisions:

- Third party information can be used to support the sale of an herbal supplement; however, it cannot promote a specific product or manufacturer and it cannot be false or misleading.

- The information must be reprinted in its entirety, unless it is an abstract of a peer-reviewed scientific journal that was prepared by the author(s) or editor(s).

- Drug or health claims may not be used; no reference can be made to the treatment of a disease or condition.

- Product labeling may include structure/function claims or statements about well-being. (For example, a structure/function claim for hawthorn would be: "Used for a healthy heart.")

- The manufacturer must substantiate any claim stated on the label and notify the Secretary of Health and Human Services within 30 days of making the claim.

- The term "dietary supplement" and a list of ingredient amounts are required on all labels.

- A disclaimer on the label must state, "This statement has not been evaluated by the Food and Drug Administration. This product is not intended to diagnose, treat, cure, or prevent any disease."

Quality of Herbal Supplements

Herbs are natural products, but nature does not always supply its products with a consistent, standardized composition. We know from experience that there are differences in nature: the vintages of wines, different qualities of black and green teas, high-acid and low-acid coffees, and sweet or hot peppers, to name a few. Similarly, the constituents of medicinal herbs can vary greatly as a result of genetic factors, climate, soil quality, and other external factors. Interestingly, approximately 90% of the plants used by one European manufacturer are cultivated rather than collected in the wild. This is the opposite of typical practices in the United States, where many of the plants used in herbal supplements are still wild-crafted, causing more final product variability if not standardized to constituent content. Poor quality raw materials may not only be subtherapeutic when processed into herbal supplements, they may contain adulterants, such as other plant species, and contaminants such as bacteria, fungus, radiation, heavy metals, or pesticide residues.

The quality of herbal supplements is a major concern in today's marketplace. In the past decade, the American herbal industry has been transformed from "Mom and Pop" businesses into an organized group of manufacturers that are beginning to appear more like their pharmaceutical cousins. However, not all manufacturers adhere to quality control. Subquality products may not only be useless to a patient, but may also be adulterated and cause potential health problems. At this point in time, herbal supplements may vary from company to company, and also from batch to batch within a company. Many manufacturers in the marketplace prepare herbal supplements based only on economic gain, meaning as "cheaply as possible." Some supplement manufacturers will compromise the final product in order to meet a deadline in manufacturing or for various other business reasons. Healthcare professionals who use herbal supplements need to choose a product wisely, assuring that its quality is the best available.

INTRODUCTION TO HERBS *(Continued)*

Herbal supplements, along with other dietary supplements, are healthcare products and should always be manufactured according to the highest standards possible. This means complete compliance with manufacturing standards and strict adherence to Good Manufacturing Practices (GMPs), whether self-imposed at this point in time or governmentally regulated in the future. As stated, herbal manufacturers only have to adhere to food service GMPs, so it is important to ensure that the company chosen has furthered its quality assurance by providing a certificate of analysis and clinical documentation of the product (or product ingredients) when requested.

The essentials for determining a quality herb product include:

1. A product that is a standardized herbal extract (if standardization has been established for the specific herb), which has been reported to be effective for a given application (eg, St John's wort, standardized to contain 0.3% to 0.5% hypericin per dose for mild depression). **Note:** A common problem is that many herb products on the market are standardized to the weight of the capsule, not to the percentage of the active constituents. For example: A ginger label reads: Standardized to contain 300 mg ginger root powder per capsule, instead of true standardization, which would state: Each capsule contains 300 mg ginger, standardized to contain 5% gingerols. This directly misleads the consumer.

2. The dosage recommendation on the label is within a therapeutic dosage range. For example: St John's wort, take 300 mg, 3 times/day. Any dosage less than this would not provide the expected effect. Consumers commonly go shopping for a product, buy it, and never realize that the dosage is not adequate for their needs.

3. A product that is stable and screened for contaminants (the manufacturer can provide a certificate of analysis upon request). Contamination is a common problem with imported herbs, and unless they are checked, they could pose a potential health risk.

4. The product meets the label claim for potency (the product actually contains a certain known level of constituent(s) within a range of ±10%). There are some products on the market that simply don't match label claim.

In educating consumers, suggest only herbal supplements from a reputable manufacturer, which produces quality finished products. Remember "Therapeutic efficacy begins with choosing a quality product." More and more clinical studies are being performed using herbal supplements. This requires quality and consistently manufactured products. If a study uses an herbal supplement that was pulled off a retail shelf and has not been assayed, the product may in fact be below label claim or potentially contaminated, leading to erroneous test results. Clinical studies with reported negative results may be due to poor quality products. Another issue of concern is that the herbal supplements used in clinical trials, which serve as the basis for structure/function claims, are often not the actual products that end up on the shelf. The "gold standard" for any herbal supplement is that human clinical trials have been performed on the particular extract that is for sale on the shelf.

Herb Buying Tips for Consumers

- Rely on established, authoritative books on herbs that are based on factual information and written by qualified healthcare professionals.

- Find a retailer whose product selection meets your needs and whose staff is knowledgeable.

- Find a physician or other healthcare professional who is knowledgeable about herbs to avoid potentially dangerous side effects and interactions.

- Herbal supplements may interact with prescription medications – inform your pharmacist and physician of their use.

- Ask a pharmacist or other healthcare provider for product information – recommended doses, interactions, side effects, and effectiveness.

- Look for labels that state the product is "standardized."

- Do not use supplements during pregnancy and lactation except with the advice of a physician.

- Individuals with serious health conditions should **NOT** use herbal supplements except with the advice and supervision of a qualified healthcare provider.

- Be aware that there are subtherapeutic products on the shelf and misleading the consumer is a common occurrence.

Standardization of Herbs

Standardization for constituent content is an important consideration. Standardization, or guaranteed potency, means that the botanical extract has been assayed for and contains a certain known level of constituents (within a range of ±10%). These constituent levels help the healthcare provider have confidence that the product chosen for the patient will have at least a baseline for effectiveness and quality. Decreasing product variability is essential in realizing herbal supplements' full potential as therapeutic agents. Until mandatory U.S. standards are set for all manufacturers of herbal supplements, it is wise to use standardized products whenever possible. Nonstandardized products or teas may have variable quality and limited laboratory investigation as to the quality of the final product. Advances in extraction technology and analytical methods have allowed many herbal manufacturers in the United States to begin standardizing their herbal supplements for known constituents, and several companies are developing standard testing for the top herbs that are gaining industry-wide acceptance.

Need for Education

Here is a typical scenario, circa 1999.

> Mrs Jones has heard some interesting reports in the media regarding the use of hawthorn for heart problems. She has hypertension and is taking an ACE inhibitor along with a beta-blocker for her condition. So, off she goes to the local outlet that sells the herbal supplement, hawthorn. Mrs Jones asks appropriate questions: "Which hawthorn product should I choose? Should it be standardized or not? Can I take this herb with my heart medications?" Mrs Jones expects professional and accurate advice.

Mrs Jones' situation identifies the need for educating healthcare professionals about herbal supplements. It's crucial that Mrs Jones be able to obtain appropriate information from a trained healthcare professional, especially since she is on prescription medications and has a pre-existing medical condition. In Mrs Jones' case, the problem is that hawthorn has been reported to have ACE-inhibiting activity and may potentiate the effects of her current ACE inhibitor.

Competent healthcare practice involves advising individuals on the proper use of over-the-counter supplements and how they can choose safe and appropriate therapies for various self-limiting conditions – and also knowing when to seek medical attention. Healthcare providers must be educated on the proper use and potential side effects of dietary supplements, including herbs. These agents are fast becoming part of a safe and effective approach to healthcare in the 21st century. Herbs are once again becoming part of the healthcare professional's arsenal of therapeutic approaches. Healthcare professionals can help disseminate sound, accurate advice on the use of dietary supplements versus exotic claims and unsound uses.

INTRODUCTION TO HERBS *(Continued)*

Herbs in This Book

Both physician-diagnosed conditions and self-limiting conditions may be supported with nutritional therapies, including herbs. This book presents suggested herbal supplements for various conditions. It also includes monographs of individual herbs that contain dosages, reported uses, pharmacology, contraindications, and other scientifically-related material. There are also numerous charts including pediatric herbal use, potential herb interactions, unsafe herbs, and herbs that are contraindicated during pregnancy.

The herb monographs in this book are divided into:

- **Name** – includes common name used and Latin binomial. All species of a particular herb genus are not listed; only the most commonly used in botanical medicine.

- **Plant Part** – most commonly used plant part with medicinal value.

- **Dosage and Standardization** – as stated previously, standardized herbs are necessary to ensure consistent results. Dosages are based on currently accepted practice and clinical efficacy. As with all medicinal substances, dosages can be altered based on clinical presentation, including age, weight, health status, and other pertinent factors. Standardization numbers may also vary slightly, as more companies enter the market with clinical research. Ask the manufacturer for documented efficacy of its product.

- **Reported Uses** – reported uses are based on clinical efficacy in human and animal studies. These uses are not all-inclusive for each plant, but are the most widely recommended and currently accepted in the medical community.

- **Summary** – a brief summary of the individual plant and its use as a therapeutic agent.

- **Pharmacology** – documented pharmacology based on reported studies. Some studies are reported on isolated chemical constituents in the herbs and extrapolated to the whole plant when standardized.

- **Theoretical, Cautions, and Contraindications** – these warnings are categorized and based on (1) human clinical trials; (2) animal and/or *in vitro* studies; (3) case reports; (4) potential interaction based on pharmacology. Again, any individual taking pharmaceutical medications should use dietary supplements with caution.

Herb/Drug Interactions (HDIs)

It is becoming increasingly important for the healthcare provider to be aware of herb/drug interactions. Recent reports show that 18% of adults in the United States use prescription drugs concurrently with herbal or vitamin products, placing an estimated 15 million Americans at risk of potential drug-dietary supplement interactions. Despite this widespread concurrent use of conventional medicines and dietary supplements, documented HDIs are sparse. Herbs are not isolated pharmaceutical chemicals and are unlikely to be linked to widespread adverse effects. However, with over 80 million Americans taking prescription medications (many of these being geriatric patients on multiple prescriptions), the growing popularity of herbs increases the possibility of HDIs. As professionals writing this book, we need to present the theoretical or possible interactions between herbal supplements and a pharmaceutical drug, based on pharmacological relationships. There have been some documented interactions in humans and these are reported as such.

It cannot be stressed enough that herbal supplements are not pharmaceutical drugs and do not act pharmacologically on the body as isolated chemical constituents do. When potential HDIs are discussed in this book and carry the warning "use with caution", we, the authors, are trying to relay the message to monitor these individuals for any adverse effects. Herbal supplements have been used in Europe for years without many reports of adverse events. Most of the potential interactions listed are based on animal studies, where they were exposed to very high doses of a particular herb. Often in clinical studies it is an isolated chemical constituent that is the culprit of the interaction. The normal plethora of chemical constituents that are found in herbal supplements are not in these isolated chemicals given to laboratory animals. For example, tubocurarine, isolated from the curare plant, is a potent nondepolarizing neuromuscular-blocking agent used in almost every hospital in the country. However, South American shaman have used the whole curare plant for many generations for a variety of health reasons, including as a tonic. If a clinician deems an herbal supplement not useful based on potential interactions, some individuals that present with disease states such as diabetes or hypertension may not be effectively supported with herbal supplements, due to a theoretical interaction based on pharmacological principles.

In summary, the practitioner should always use caution if an individual presents with other medications and/or clinical disease and wants to take a dietary supplement. Appropriate monitoring of patients is essential. Use your professional judgment in advising these individuals. Proper documentation and reporting of adverse events should be observed as with all supplements and drugs used as healthcare products.

> Report adverse events to Medwatch at 1-800-FDA-1088. You can print a reporting form by connecting to the internet at the following address: http://web1.po.com/html/medwatch/form.shtml

General Cautions When Using Herbal Supplements

- Use herbs with extreme caution in children younger than 2 years of age.
- Always use herbs with caution in pregnant or lactating women; some herbs are contraindicated in pregnancy – make sure to observe warnings.
- Use herbs with caution in all individuals on pharmaceutical medications – always review for potential herb-drug interactions (HDIs).
- Large and prolonged doses of herbs increase the potential for adverse effects.
- Many herbs, due to a variety of chemical constituents, may cause transient adverse effects such as nausea, vomiting, and GI distress.

Questions to Consider When Advising on Herb Use

- What prescription and nonprescription medications is this individual taking?
- What other dietary supplements is this individual taking?
- Are there any potential interactions when using this supplement, either with drugs or other supplements?
- What is the appropriate dosage form of this product?
- What is the appropriate dosage amount and length of therapy for the product?
- What are the contraindications of using this particular dietary supplement?
- Can this supplement be used during pregnancy and lactation?
- What is the appropriate children's dosage when applicable?

Determining what drugs (prescription and nonprescription) and dietary supplements an individual is currently taking is critical. Contraindications for specific herbal supplements need to be considered. There are relatively few reported adverse reactions associated with herbal supplements when compared to prescription drugs, but herbs must be used appropriately to achieve a positive clinical effect. When used appropriately, herbal supplements can provide the healthcare professional with an extra tool in the war against disease and poor health.

INTRODUCTION TO HERBS *(Continued)*

Selected Reference Materials

Listed below are reference materials that discuss pharmacy principles and use of herbal supplements. Included in this list are contraindications and herb/drug interactions (HDIs), herb/nutrient depletion, clinical utility, and scientific studies.

Bradley PR, ed, *British Herbal Compendium*, Vol 1, Bournemouth, England: British Herbal Medicine Association, 1992.

Brinker FJ, *Herb Contraindications and Drug Interactions*, Sandy, OR: Eclectic Medical Publications, 1997.

Leung AY and Foster S, *Encyclopedia of Common Natural Ingredients Used in Food, Drugs, and Cosmetics*, 2nd ed, New York, NY: John Wiley and Sons, Inc, 1996.

McGuffin M et al, eds, *American Herbal Products Association's Botanical Safety Handbook*, Boca Raton, FL: CRC Press, 1997.

Newall CA, Anderson LA, and Phillipson D, *Herbal Medicines: A Guide for Healthcare Professionals*, London, England: The Pharmaceutical Press, 1996.

Pelton R, LaValle J, Hawkins E, et al, *Drug-Induced Nutrient Depletion Handbook*, Hudson, OH: Lexi-Comp, Inc, 1999.

Schilcher H, *Phytotherapy in Pediatrics: Handbook for Physicians and Pharmacists*, Stuttgart, Germany: Medpharm Scientific Publications, 1997.

Schulz V, Hansel R, and Tyler VE, *Rational Phytotherapy: A Physician's Guide to Herbal Medicine*, New York; NY: Springer-Verlag, 1998.

Wichtl M and Bissett NG, eds, *Herbal Drugs and Phytopharmaceuticals: A Handbook for the Practice on a Scientific Basis*, Boca Raton, FL: CRC Press, 1994.

Footnotes

1. Williamson JM and Wyandt CM, "An Herbal Update," *Drug Topics*, 1998, 66-73.
2. World Health Organization Programme on Traditional Medicines, "Guideline for the Assessment of Herbal Medicines," Geneva, Switzerland: 1991.
3. *Prevention*, 1997.
4. *Natural Foods Merchandiser*, 1998.
5. Brevoort P, "The Booming U.S. Botanical Market: A New Overview," *Herbal Gram*, 1998, 44:33-46.

INTRODUCTION TO NUTRITION

VITAMINS, MINERALS, AMINO ACIDS, ESSENTIAL FATTY ACIDS, ANTIOXIDANTS, AND NUTRACEUTICALS

Nutrition

Nutrition is the process of taking in and utilizing food. Nutrients are the substances, obtained primarily from foods, which support all life processes in the body. Nutrients provide the building blocks for cell formation and energy production. Nutrients are categorized as macronutrients and micronutrients. Essential nutrients are nutrients that the body must have on a regular basis, but cannot make on its own.

Macronutrients

The basic nutrients – proteins, carbohydrates, and fats – are considered macronutrients. The body uses water to help process these. Choosing nutrient dense forms of each of these in a good balance helps the body function properly.

- **Water** intake is a key component to good health. Water is involved in every function of the body. It serves as the medium that transports all nutrients in the body, which is composed of 65% to 75% water. The body needs water to remove waste products and process toxins efficiently. If the body retains waste products and metabolites, normal metabolic function becomes disrupted. Adequate water intake is essential to a healthy body.

  Water Quality today is a significant issue in the United States. Recognizing this, President Clinton highlighted water in his State of the Union Address in 1998, calling for a new Clean Water Initiative.[1] At least 50 million Americans are drinking water that is contaminated with lead,[2] herbicides and pesticides,[3] feces,[4] or other contaminants.[5] In view of this, quality bottled or filtered water is recommended. Experts recommend drinking at least eight 8-ounce glasses of quality water daily.

- **Proteins** are a class of nitrogen-containing compounds that are comprised of amino acids. Proteins are essential for anabolic growth and repair processes throughout the body. All tissues in the body are made up of protein – muscle cells, skin cells, collagen, elastin, keratin (hair and nails), and red and white blood cells. Enzymes in the body are composed of protein, as are hormones and antibodies. Certain amino acids are needed for production of the different neurotransmitters in the brain. Lean protein is considered an excellent source of fuel. Many experts recommend that the diet consist of approximately 25% protein.

- **Carbohydrates** are divided into three categories – simple carbohydrates (single or simple sugars), complex carbohydrates (multiple chains of sugars called starches), and fiber (the indigestible part of plant foods that plays an important role in human health). Cereals, grains, beans, bread, pasta, potatoes, corn, and other vegetables are examples of complex carbohydrates. Fruits primarily contain simple sugars and fiber and are examples of simple carbohydrates. Unprocessed and unrefined carbohydrates contain fiber. Refined sugars (candies, desserts, and many prepackaged food items) are carbohydrates, but are largely devoid of nutrient value. Over-consumption of refined sugar is one of the biggest dietary issues in the U. S. The average American consumes 153 pounds of sugar per year.

  Dietary Carbohydrate and Fiber Intake – Experts recommend eating at least five servings of fruits and vegetables daily to reduce cancer risk and add fiber for healthy bowel function. Carbohydrate intake should be 40% to 60% of the daily diet. Dietary fiber provides roughage, which aids in proper elimination, an important factor for colon health. Fiber provides a feeling of fullness, thereby helping to keep appetite in check, and helps regulate the

INTRODUCTION TO NUTRITION *(Continued)*

breakdown and release of glucose into the bloodstream. Experts recommend consuming a minimum of 25 grams of fiber daily.

- **Fats** play numerous important roles in the human body: 1) as structural components of cell walls, 2) as insulation for the body, 3) as a stored form of energy, 4) as precursors for prostaglandins, which perform important regulatory functions in the body, and 5) as a carrier for the fat-soluble vitamins A, D, E, and K.

  Dietary Fat Sources – Sources of fat in the diet include saturated fats (coconut oil, lard, beef tallow, and hydrogenated vegetable oil) and unsaturated fats. Unsaturated fats are further categorized into polyunsaturated fats (corn oil, safflower oil, sunflower seed oil, and soybean oil) and monounsaturated oils (olive oil, canola oil, and peanut oil). Of the monounsaturated fats, olive oil contains the highest percent of monounsaturated fats (82%), then canola oil (60%), followed by peanut oil (51%).

  Dietary Fat Intake – The general guideline is to limit total dietary fat intake to 20% to 30% of daily calories. Saturated fat intake should be limited to 10% of this, because diets high in saturated fats, especially hydrogenated oils (trans-fatty acids) have been associated with heart disease and an increased incidence of certain types of cancer.[6] Using monounsaturated fats as the primary source of fat in the diet is preferable.

Micronutrients

Vitamins, minerals, amino acids, and essential fatty acids (EFAs) are essential to life. They are categorized as micronutrients because they are needed in small amounts compared with the macronutrients – protein, carbohydrates, and fats – and water. Vitamins and minerals serve as structural components of tissues. Both function as coenzymes that facilitate thousands of biochemical reactions in the body. Over one-third of all enzymes in the body require a mineral as a cofactor for their activity. Minerals are also important for nerve transmission and muscle contraction. They play a role in regulating fluid levels and maintaining acid-base balance in the body.

The body breaks down dietary protein into its amino acid components. The body then uses these amino acids to build the specific proteins it needs. Thus, the proteins that make up the human body are not obtained directly from the diet, but are produced by the body from amino acids. This is why amino acids are characterized as the building blocks for proteins, which are a part of every living cell in the body.

Contrary to popular belief, fat is essential to proper biological function in the body. However, it must be the right kind of fat. Essential fatty acids are the fats necessary for health. EFAs cannot be manufactured by the body, but must be obtained in the diet through foods or dietary supplementation. Every living cell in the body needs essential fatty acids for rebuilding and producing new cells.

Essential Micronutrients

There are 45 essential micronutrients for humans: 15 vitamins, 20 minerals, 8 essential amino acids, and 2 essential fatty acids. All of these must be obtained from either food or dietary supplements because the body cannot manufacture them.

Chart of Essential Nutrients

Vitamins	
Vitamin A (retinol) or	Biotin
beta-carotene (vitamin A precursor)	Choline
Vitamin B$_1$ (thiamine)	Vitamin C
Vitamin B$_2$ (riboflavin)	Vitamin D
Vitamin B$_3$ (niacin)	Vitamin E
Vitamin B$_5$ (pantothenic acid)	Folic acid
Vitamin B$_6$ (pyridoxine)	Inositol
Vitamin B$_{12}$ (cobalamin)	Vitamin K

Minerals and Trace Elements	
Boron	Manganese
Calcium	Molybdenum
Chloride	Phosphorus
Chromium	Potassium
Cobalt	Selenium
Copper	Silicon
Fluoride	Sodium
Iodine	Sulfur
Iron	Vanadium
Magnesium	Zinc

Essential Amino Acids	
L-Isoleucine	L-Phenylalanine
L-Leucine	L-Threonine
L-Lysine	L-Tryptophan
L-Methionine	L-Valine

Essential Fatty Acids	
Omega-3	Omega-6

- **Fat-Soluble Vitamins**

  Vitamins are divided into either fat-soluble or water-soluble vitamins. Fat-soluble vitamins are stored in fatty tissue in the body, primarily the liver. They are absorbed into the lymphatic system and travel in the blood with the aid of protein carriers. Vitamins A, D, E, and K are fat-soluble vitamins. Because fat-soluble vitamins are stored in the body, toxic levels of these micronutrients can develop.

  Vitamin A is essential for bone and tooth growth, strengthens the eyes and skin, and aids proper immune function. Some vitamins are ingested in their precursor form and are then converted to the active form of the vitamin in the body. Beta-carotene is the precursor to vitamin A.

  Vitamin D is necessary for proper absorption of calcium and phosphorus, both essential for bone formation. Vitamin D is synthesized in the body when the sunlight shines on human skin.

  Vitamin E is essential for normal cell structure and helps protect tissues from damage by pollutants.

  Vitamin K is essential for blood clotting.

- **Water-Soluble Vitamins**

  Water-soluble vitamins are excreted by the body and, therefore, need to be replenished daily. They are absorbed directly into the bloodstream for delivery to the cells. The B vitamins and vitamin C are water-soluble vitamins.

  B vitamins play a role in converting food to metabolic energy. **Vitamin B$_1$** helps the body break down carbohydrates to produce energy. It also supports healthy functioning of the heart, muscles, and nerves. **Vitamin B$_2$**

INTRODUCTION TO NUTRITION *(Continued)*

also plays a role in cell energy production and supports adrenal function. **Vitamin B₃** helps maintain healthy skin and proper nerve and digestive function. **Vitamin B₅** is important for normal growth and development and, like the other B vitamins, plays a role in converting carbohydrates to energy. It also supports the sinuses. **Vitamin B₆** is involved in antibody and red blood cell production. It helps maintain healthy skin and promotes proper nerve and digestive function. **Vitamin B₁₂** helps the body utilize folic acid and support healthy functioning of the nervous system. It is also involved in growth and development and the production of red blood cells.

Vitamin C plays a role in collagen formation. It promotes wound healing and strengthens blood vessels. Vitamin C is needed for proper immune response and helps the body absorb and utilize iron.

- **Minerals**

  Minerals are considered essential micronutrients because they cannot be manufactured by the body. They are naturally-occurring elements that are absorbed by plants and become part of our food supply. **Macrominerals** (calcium, chloride, magnesium, phosphorus, potassium, sodium, and sulfur) are needed in larger quantities by the body. **Microminerals** (boron, chromium, cobalt, copper, fluoride, iodine, iron, manganese, molybdenum, selenium, silicon, vanadium, and zinc) are referred to as **trace minerals**, because of the small amount required by the body.

  Some minerals compete for absorption in the body, and a high dietary intake of one mineral can induce a deficiency of another. For example, calcium and iron compete for absorption, as do calcium and phosphorus. A high intake of zinc can precipitate a copper deficiency.[7] Therefore, excessively high doses of individual mineral supplements should be avoided or taken only under the supervision of a qualified healthcare professional.

- **Essential Amino Acids**

  There are eight essential amino acids – isoleucine, leucine, lysine, methionine, phenylalanine, threonine, tryptophan, and valine. Because the body cannot manufacture these eight amino acids, they must be obtained from food or dietary supplements. Amino acids are the building blocks for proteins in the body. Amino acids have the following functions: to build and maintain body tissues; to regulate growth, digestion, and reproduction; and to act as neurotransmitters or precursors to neurotransmitters. Amino acids that are normally nonessential can become conditionally essential under certain conditions or disease states, or with certain metabolic demands. Biochemical individuality could also influence specific amino acid needs.

- **Essential Fatty Acids (EFAs)**

  Omega-3 (alpha-linolenic acid) and omega-6 (linoleic acid) are classified as essential fatty acids. They are polyunsaturated fats that cannot be manufactured by the body and must, therefore, be obtained through food or dietary supplements. EFAs play a role in maintaining cell membrane integrity. The EFAs, linoleic acid (omega-6) and alpha-linolenic acid (omega-3) are precursors for prostaglandins. Prostaglandins regulate inflammatory response, immune response, blood pressure, blood clotting, and cholesterol levels. A deficiency of EFAs has been linked to cancer, heart disease, allergies, and arthritis. It is important to maintain a proper balance between omega-6 fatty acid and omega-3 fatty acid. Currently, the suggested ratio is 4 (omega-6) to 1 (omega-3). The typical American diet consists of plenty of omega-6 fatty acid (such as beef fat and vegetable oils), but an inadequate amount of omega-3 fatty acid (such as fish oils, flaxseed oil, and wild game). It is estimated that only about 20% of the population consume sufficient EFAs.[8]

Food Supply as Source of Macronutrients/Micronutrients

Agricultural practices in the United States have changed significantly over the past fifty years. Prior to the 1950s, farmers spread manure on their fields and rotated crops, which returned a broad range of nutrients to the soil. Now, the use of synthetic fertilizer is widespread. Most fertilizers consist of only three minerals – nitrogen, phosphorus, and potassium. Other important minerals and trace elements, such as selenium, are not being replaced in the soil. As a result, much of the food grown in the United States today is not as nutritious as it was in the past. Consequently, even if fruits and vegetables are a significant part of their diet, many people may not be getting adequate nutrients from the foods they eat.

Soil Quality

An early study conducted at Rutgers University concluded that the mineral content of certain vegetables differed based on the nutritional content of the soil where the food was grown.[9] Snap peas, cabbage, lettuce, tomatoes, and spinach were evaluated from ten different states. The foods' mineral content, including phosphorus, calcium, magnesium, potassium, sodium, boron, manganese, iron, copper, and cobalt was analyzed. For example, the calcium content of lettuce varied from a low of 6 mEq/100 g to a high of 71 mEq/100 g. The iron content in lettuce varied from a low of 9 ppm to a high of 516 ppm. This study demonstrates that the nutrient content in foods varies widely depending upon the nutrient content of the soil in which it is grown.

Pesticides and Herbicide

Widespread use of pesticides and herbicides has also created problems in our food supply. Besides killing weeds and insects, insecticides kill earthworms and bacteria in the soil. Earthworms perform the valuable function of aerating the soil, and bacteria in the soil facilitate nutrient uptake in plant roots. Traces of these pesticides and herbicides are found in food and water supplies. Many of these chemicals have been studied individually and linked to various forms of cancer. According to the Environmental Protection Agency's latest Toxics Release Inventory (TRI), there were over 2 billion environmental releases of chemicals (air emissions, surface water discharges, underground injection, and on-site land releases) in 1997.[10] This figure encompasses over 127 million pounds of known carcinogens that were released into the atmosphere and over 1 million pounds that were released into the water supply. In addition, there were over 1.3 billion pounds of chemicals released into the air and over 217 million pounds released into the water supply that have suspected negative health effects.[10] The combination effects of these agents could be seen as metabolically disruptive.

Organic Produce

An important study compared organically grown foods with foods grown using standard commercial methods. Foods were picked at random in grocery stores and health food grocery stores. Laboratory analysis revealed that the organically grown foods contained almost twice as much nutritional value as the commercially grown foods.[11] Because organic foods may not be available or desirable to everyone, nutrient supplementation to support health becomes even more important.

Current Nutrient Status in the United States

Adequate nutrient intake is essential for optimum health and well-being, yet many individuals are deficient in essential nutrients. Nutrients play an important role in disease prevention, as well as providing disease state management support. According to a U.S. Department of Agriculture study,[12] most Americans are deficient in one or more essential nutrients. This study concluded that:

- 80% consumed less than the RDA for vitamin B_6
- 75% consumed less than the RDA for magnesium
- 68% consumed less than the RDA for calcium
- 50% consumed less than the RDA for vitamin A

INTRODUCTION TO NUTRITION *(Continued)*

- 45% consumed less than the RDA for vitamin B_1
- 45% consumed less than the RDA for vitamin C
- 34% consumed less than the RDA for vitamins B_2, B_3, and B_{12}

The National Health and Nutrition Examination Survey, Part II (NHANES-II) reported that 91% of Americans do not eat the recommended 3 servings of vegetables and 2 servings of fruit daily.[13] Over a decade ago, the Surgeon General of the United States concluded that: "Approximately two-thirds of all deaths are associated with imbalances in diet and nutrition."[14]

Dietary Supplements as Sources of Macronutrients/Micronutrients

Although outright nutritional diseases such as scurvy, beriberi, and pellagra are rare, studies such as those discussed above indicate that marginal nutritional deficiencies are widespread in the United States. These marginal deficiencies can contribute to altered metabolic functioning of the body, potentially reducing the efficiency of homeostasis. Some of the conditions contributing to this problem include a decline in the mineral content of America's croplands, poor food choices, an increased reliance on processed and/or fast foods, environmental pollution, drug-induced nutrient depletion, and a stressful lifestyle. This has prompted many health professionals to suggest that the health of most Americans could be improved by taking nutritional supplements on a regular basis. At a minimum, a well-designed multivitamin/multimineral formula that contains a wide range of micronutrients would help ensure adequate intake of important vitamins and minerals.

Recommended Dietary Allowances for Vitamins, Minerals, and Trace Elements

Recommended dietary allowances (RDAs) for vitamins, minerals, and trace elements were first established in 1943 by the Food and Nutrition Board, which is a division of the National Research Council of the National Academy of Sciences. Since then, RDAs have been promoted as nutrient guidelines that will meet the needs of most healthy individuals and prevent nutritional deficiency diseases such as scurvy, beriberi, and pellagra. It is important to realize that RDAs do not equate with optimal health and wellness. In most cases, nutrient intake for optimal health is substantially greater than the RDA. Articles in professional journals are now questioning the appropriateness of RDAs. In an article titled, "The RDA Concept: Time for a Change?" the authors state the following, "In their current form, RDAs do not address functions of nutrients other than the prevention of deficiency and are not intended to represent optimal intakes."[15] Many health professionals now believe that a high level of health and wellness is more likely to be achieved if individuals consume daily amounts of nutrients that are somewhat greater than the Recommended Dietary Allowances (RDAs) and the newer standards are known as the Recommended Dietary Intakes (RDIs). RDAs are under review and changes that reflect current research will probably be made over the next few years.

Some express concern that taking quantities of nutrients larger than the RDA is dangerous. It is, of course, possible that excessive amounts of some nutrients could cause harm. However, there is an ever increasing body of scientific evidence which suggests that levels of nutrients greater than the RDA have significant health benefits for different health conditions, as well as for prevention and performance enhancement.

Relative Safety of Dietary Supplements

In April 1998, a study in the *Journal of the American Medical Association* reported that adverse drug reactions in U.S. hospitals were estimated to cause approximately 106,000 deaths per year.[16] It should be emphasized that these deaths were not due to errors in drug administration, noncompliance, overdose, or drug abuse. These deaths happened during the correct use of drugs as prescribed by the patient's physicians, and these figures only reflect deaths tracked by hospitals.

It is interesting to compare the relative safety of dietary supplements with those of prescription and over-the-counter drugs. The American Association of Poison Control Centers track and record fatalities around the United States that occur from the use of prescription drugs, nonprescription drugs, and nutrients. During the eight-year period from 1987 through 1994, the combined statistics from these centers throughout the United States reported a total of 4,065 deaths from drugs (OTC + prescription drugs), compared to only 5 deaths from nutrients.[17] Studies like these emphasize the overall safety of nutritional supplements.

Nutraceuticals

Nutraceuticals are dietary supplements that deliver a concentrated amount of a bioactive substance from food (plant or animal source), which offers medical or health benefits related to the prevention and treatment of disease. One example is the use of lutein (a carotenoid found in dark green leafy vegetables) as a dietary supplement that helps prevent macular degeneration. Lycopene (a substance found in tomatoes) is commonly suggested for enlarged prostate. Soy isoflavones (substances found in soybean products) help with hormonal regulation when taken as dietary supplements. Advances in science and technology are allowing researchers to better identify and extract these active ingredients. These advances enable the development of thousands of new products with a wide variety of biological and physiological functions. In general, nutraceutical dosages are substantially more concentrated than the amount that could be obtained from eating their normal food sources.

Free Radicals and Antioxidant Nutrients

Today, it is widely acknowledged that free radicals are a primary cause of aging. A free radical is a molecule that contains a single, unpaired electron. One of the electrons in an electron pair has been dislodged, leaving behind a free unpaired electron which spins out of control, ripping away an electron wherever it can find one. If a free radical takes an electron away from a cell wall, the cell may die or be damaged. If it takes an electron away from DNA, the genetic blueprint can be damaged over time, hindering the body's ability to efficiently duplicate new cells. One unchecked free radical is capable of causing thousands of damaging incidences at the cellular level. Over time, this destruction contributes to the aging process. However, when there is an optimal level of oxygen present at the cellular level, few free radicals are produced. Too much or insufficient oxygen at the cellular level substantially increases free radical production and subsequent damage.

Some Causes of Free Radical Formation

- Nuclear radiation
- Smoking
- Sunburn
- Lipid peroxidation (when oxygen reacts with unsaturated fats in cell walls and membranes)
- Heavy metal toxins
- Pesticides and other pollutants
- Stress

Antioxidant Nutrients

Antioxidant nutrients neutralize or "kill" free radicals by giving up one of their electrons to the free radical. The antioxidant nutrient itself then becomes a free radical, but much weaker than the free radical it neutralized. Other antioxidants in the body are capable of diffusing this weaker free radical. The body's supply of antioxidant nutrients is continually being depleted because of this process. Higher stress levels, greater exposure to pollutants, or other causes of free radical formation deplete antioxidant nutrients at a faster rate. Therefore, it is important to have antioxidant nutrients available in the system.

INTRODUCTION TO NUTRITION *(Continued)*

Important Antioxidants

- **Vitamin C** (ascorbic acid) is an important water-soluble antioxidant. It also acts as an antiviral agent and improves resistance to stress and infections. In a meta-analysis of vitamin C's effectiveness against the common cold, five studies reported that taking 70-200 mg of vitamin C daily resulted in a 31% reduction in symptoms and severity of colds. In eleven of the studies, a daily dosage of 1000 mg or more resulted in a 40% reduction in symptoms and severity of colds.[18] A meta-analysis of over 90 studies, evaluating vitamin C's role in cancer, reported that in a large majority of the studies vitamin C provided significant protective effects against cancer.[19] Studies have also reported that vitamin C, besides being an antioxidant itself, is capable of regenerating vitamin E to active antioxidant status.[20] This makes vitamins C and E a powerful antioxidant combination.

- **Vitamin E** (alpha tocopherol) is the primary fat-soluble antioxidant. Its major role is to protect cellular membranes. The results of recent research indicate that natural vitamin E (d-alpha tocopherol) is approximately two times more bioavailable and stays in the tissues much longer than synthetic vitamin E (dl-alpha tocopherol).[21] Vitamin E reduces platelet stickiness and is protective against cardiovascular disease, cataracts, and some forms of cancer.

  Two studies published in the *New England Journal of Medicine* reported that both women[22] and men[23] who took daily dosages of 100 int. units of vitamin E for two years, had a 37% to 41% decrease in the risk of developing cardiovascular disease. Also, the Cambridge Heart Antioxidant Study (CHAOS) reported that individuals taking 400-800 int. units of vitamin E daily, had a 77% reduction in nonfatal heart attacks.[24] In another study, subjects 65 years of age and older were divided into groups consuming 60, 200, or 800 mg of vitamin E daily. All three dosages produce significant improvement in immune system function.[25]

- **Vitamin A and Beta-Carotene.** Vitamin A is a fat-soluble antioxidant essential for growth and reproduction. It enhances the immune system and strengthens mucous membranes. Beta-carotene can be converted in the body to vitamin A. It also functions as an antioxidant. In studies, both vitamin A[26] and beta-carotene[27] are protective against a variety of cancers.

- **Selenium.** Selenium's primary function is to inhibit the oxidation of fats (lipids). It protects the immune system by preventing free radical formation. It has also been reported to have antiviral activity and to aid in heavy metal detoxification. A four-year, double-blind, placebo-controlled cancer study reported that patients taking 200 mcg of selenium daily had a 45% reduction in lung cancer, 58% reduction in colorectal cancer, and a 63% reduction in prostate cancer.[28]

- **Coenzyme Q$_{10}$** is a crucial antioxidant nutrient that protects against the oxidation of LDL cholesterol. CoQ$_{10}$ is also capable of crossing cellular membranes, which enables it to provide antioxidant protection inside cells. This is especially important within the mitochondria where the majority of free radicals are generated during the process of mitochondrial energy production. Another important CoQ$_{10}$ attribute is its ability to potentiate and regenerate vitamin E. It is now thought that a deficiency of coenzyme Q$_{10}$ increases an individual's risk for many forms of cardiovascular disease.

- **Alpha-Lipoic Acid** has been called the "pivotal antioxidant" by leading antioxidant researcher Dr Lester Packer. Alpha-lipoic acid has gained this level of distinction because it not only recycles and regenerates all of the other key antioxidants, it is also capable of regenerating itself. Another important feature of alpha-lipoic acid is the fact that it is both water- and fat-soluble, so it is able to provide antioxidant protection in both water and lipid environments throughout the body. Although our bodies can synthesize alpha-lipoic acid, production diminishes with age. Alpha-lipoic acid supplementation increases the activity of the entire antioxidant network in the body and helps retard the aging process.

- **Herbal Antioxidants**. A variety of herbs, which are high in flavonoid content, are generally associated with antioxidant activity. Scientific studies report that standardized extracts of agents such as bilberry, green tea, grape seed, ginkgo biloba, milk thistle, hawthorn berry, lutein, lycopene, and pycnogenol can provide important antioxidant support. Herbal antioxidants are increasingly being used synergistically with nutritional antioxidants in the prevention and treatment of a wide range of health conditions.

Suggested Daily Intake of Nutritional Supplements

Good health requires optimal daily intake of a wide range of nutrients. Several health professionals have collaborated to create the following suggested dosage recommendations for nutritional supplementation. This is not an exact formulation that anyone should try to duplicate or follow. Instead, these suggestions are meant to be a guideline. Although they are still moderate, dosage ranges similar to these will enable most people to achieve greater levels of health.

The suggested nutritional guidelines for a daily multivitamin / mineral supplement, additional antioxidants, and essential fatty acid supplementation are as follows:

Daily Multivitamin / Mineral Supplement

Beta-carotene	5000 int. units
Calcium	1000 mg
Chromium	200 mcg
Copper	2 mg
Folic Acid	800 mcg
Magnesium	600 mg
Manganese	5 mg
Potassium	99 mg
Selenium	100 mcg
Vitamin A	5000 int. units*
Vitamin B$_1$	10 mg
Vitamin B$_2$	10 mg
Vitamin B$_3$	25 mg
Vitamin B$_5$	10 mg
Vitamin B$_6$	20 mg
Vitamin B$_{12}$	500 mcg
Vitamin C	1000 mg
Vitamin D	400 int. units
Vitamin E (natural)	400 int. units
Zinc	15 mg

*Unless pregnant or planning pregnancy

Other nutrients that might be found in some products include biotin, inositol, bioflavonoids, PABA, iodine, molybdenum, phosphatidyl choline, coenzyme Q$_{10}$, alpha-lipoic acid, lutein, various amino acids, and herbal extracts.

In addition to the recommended daily multivitamin / mineral supplements, extra antioxidants can be taken. The following antioxidants will help boost the immune system and provide additional protection against free radical damage.

INTRODUCTION TO NUTRITION *(Continued)*

Alpha-lipoic acid	100 mg
Beta-carotene	10,000 int. units
Coenzyme Q_{10}	30 mg
Selenium	100 mcg
Vitamin A	2500 int. units
Vitamin C	1000 mg
Vitamin E	400 int. units

Essential Fatty Acids

Most Americans do not consume adequate levels of the omega-3 fatty acids. Flaxseed oil is the best source of the omega-3 fatty acid known as alpha-linolenic acid (ALA), containing approximately 58%. Many people, especially individuals with diabetes, do not effectively convert ALA into the longer-chain omega-3 fatty acids known as eicosapentaenoic acid (EPA) and docosahexaenoic acid (DHA). Fish oils, or marine lipids, are the best source of these fats.

Gamma-linolenic acid (GLA) is a member of the omega-6 fatty acids. It is synthesized from the parent omega-6 fatty acid known as linoleic acid. Many people also do not effectively convert linoleic acid into GLA. This can cause a wide variety of health problems, which respond to GLA supplementation. Borage oil and evening primrose oil are good sources of GLA.

Many healthcare professionals feel it is advisable to take the following:

Flaxseed oil: 1 tablespoonful daily provides omega-3 and omega-6 in a 3:1 ratio

Fish oils: 2 capsules daily provide the longer-chain omega-3 fatty acids DHA and EPA

Evening primrose oil or borage oil: Provides gamma-linolenic acid (GLA)

Summary

Essential nutrients and nutraceuticals have been reviewed in this text in order to provide healthcare professionals with the most essential information regarding their use. Essential nutrients include vitamins, minerals, amino acids, and essential fatty acids. These cannot be produced by the body and, therefore, must either come from diet or supplementation. Over the last few years, new laboratory assessments have become available that assess nutrient status and utilization in the body. The healthcare professional's role in suggesting essential nutrients will continue to expand over the next decade.

Specific nutrients play a role in improving health outcomes and quality of life. As professionals, it is essential that we assure adequate nutrient status before looking at other natural therapeutic options. This includes such basics as adequate calcium intake for strong bones, adequate vitamin E intake to reduce cardiovascular risk, adequate vitamin C for proper immune function, and adequate folate to prevent birth defects. These are just several examples of the literally hundreds of health risks associated with poor nutrient status.

Nutraceuticals are a rapidly emerging class of dietary supplements. Although they are not considered to be essential for biological processes, there is tremendous potential for using this class of agents to support, redirect, and enhance functional cellular metabolism. For example, N-acetyl cysteine is used for stimulating glutathione peroxidase and coenzyme Q_{10} is used for cardiovascular and cellular energetics. Nutraceuticals are quickly gaining use in prevention, in performance enhancement, and for disease state and condition management.

Vitamins, Minerals, Amino Acids, Essential Fatty Acids, and Nutraceuticals in This Book

This book contains information on vitamins, minerals, amino acids, essential fatty acids, and nutraceuticals. The following information is provided for each agent:

- Recommended dietary intakes (RDIs), if established, and dosage ranges
- Active forms (for example, vitamin A as retinol acetate or retinol palmitate)
- Primary uses or functions
- Pharmacology
- Warnings and toxicity symptoms
- Deficiency symptoms
- Potential drug/nutrient interactions
- Potential nutrient/nutrient interactions

This book presents suggestions for various conditions using vitamins, minerals, amino acids, essential fatty acids, and nutraceuticals as therapeutic agents.

Footnotes

1. Clinton WJ, "State of the Union Address," United States Capitol, Washington, DC: January 27, 1998.
2. Potula V, Serrano, Sparrow D, et al, "Relationship of Lead in Drinking Water to Bone Lead Levels Twenty Years Later in Boston Men: The Normative Aging Study, *J Occup Environ Med*, 1999, 41(5):349-55.
3. U.S. Geological Survey Circular 1225, "The Quality of Our Nation's Waters: Nutrients and Pesticides," August 6, 1999. Online. Available: <http://water.usgs.gov/pubs/circ/circ1225/html/pesticides.html>.
4. Rose JB, Atlas RM, Gerba CP, et al, "Microbial Pollutants in Our Nation's Water: Environmental and Public Health Issues", Washington, DC: American Society for Microbiology. Online. Available: <www.asmusa.org/pasrc/pdfs/waterreport.pdf>.
5. "Is It Safe to Drink the Water? Report: Drinking Water's Hidden Dangers," *USA Today*, Fall/Winter 1998. Online. Available: <http://www.usatoday.com/news/special/water.001.htm>.
6. Erasmus U, *Fats That Heal, Fats That Kill: The Complete Guide to Fats, Oils, Cholesterol, and Human Health*, Burnaby, BC, Canada: Alive Books, 1993, 31, 54-7.
7. Garrison RH Jr and Somers E, *The Nutrition Desk Reference*, 3rd ed, New Canaan, CT: Keats Publishing, 1995, 246.
8. Murray MT, *Encyclopedia of Nutritional Supplements: The Essential Guide for Improving Your Health Naturally*, Rocklin, CA: Prima Publishing, 1996, 249.
9. Bear FE, et al, "Variation in Mineral Composition of Vegetables," *Soil Sci Soc Am*, 1948, 13:380-4.
10. "1997 Toxics Release Inventory Fact Sheets", Washington, DC: U.S. Environmental Protection Agency, Office of Prevention and Toxics (7408), April 1999.
11. Smith B, "Organic Foods vs Supermarket Foods: Element Levels," *J Appl Nutr*, 1993, 45(1):35-9.
12. Pao EM and Mickle SJ, "Problem Nutrients in the United States," *Food Technol*, 1981, 35:58-62.
13. Patterson BH, Block G, Rosenberger WF, et al, "Fruits and Vegetables in the American Diet: Data from the NANES II Survey," *Am J Public Health*, 1990, 80(12):1443-9.
14. "The Surgeon General's Report on Nutrition and Health", Washington, DC: Department of Health and Human Services, Publication No. 88-50211.
15. Lachance P and Langseth L, "The RDA Concept: Time for a Change?" *Nutr Rev*, 1994, 52(8 Pt 1):266-70.
16. Lazarou J, Pomeranz BH, and Corey PN, "Incidence of Adverse Drug Reactions in Hospitalized Patients: A Meta-analysis of Prospective Studies," *JAMA*, 1998, 279(15):1200-5.
17. Loomis D, "Fatalities From Prescription Drugs, Non-prescription Drugs, and Nutrients," *Townsend Letter for Doctors and Patients*, 1992, 78:41 (with updated information from personal communication to authors in April 1999).
18. Pauling L, *How to Live Longer and Feel Better*, New York, NY: WH Freeman and Company, 1986, 120.
19. Block G, "Epidemiologic Evidence Regarding Vitamin C and Cancer," *Am J Clin Nutr*, 1991, 54(6 Suppl):1310S-14S.

INTRODUCTION TO NUTRITION *(Continued)*

20. Beyer RE, "The Role of Ascorbate in Antioxidant Protection of Biomembranes: Interaction With Vitamin E and Coenzyme Q," *J Bioenerg Biomembr*, 1994, 26(4):349-58.
21. Burton GW, Traber MG, Acuff RV, et al, "Human Plasma and Tissue Alpha-tocopherol Concentrations in Response to Supplementation With Deuterated Natural and Synthetic Vitamin E," *Am J Clin Nutr*, 1998, 67(4):669-84.
22. Stampfer MJ, Hennekens CH, Manson JE, et al, "Vitamin E Consumption and the Risk of Coronary Disease in Women," *N Engl J Med*, 1993, 328(20):1444-9.
23. Rimm EB, Stampfer MJ, Ascherio A, et al, "Vitamin E Consumption and the Risk of Coronary Heart Disease in Men," *N Engl J Med*, 1993, 328(20):1450-6.
24. Stephens NG, Parsons A, Schofield PM, et al, "Randomized Controlled Trial of Vitamin E in Patients With Coronary Disease: Cambridge Heart Antioxidant Study," *Lancet*, 1996, 347(9004):781-6.
25. Meydani SN, Meydani M, Blumberg JB, et al, "Vitamin E Supplementation and *In Vivo* Immune Response in Healthy Elderly Subjects. A Randomized Controlled Trial," *JAMA*, 1997, 277(17):1380-6.
26. Basu TK, "Vitamin A and Cancer of Epithelial Origin," *J Hum Nutr*, 1979, 33(1):24-31.
27. van Poppel G, "Epidemiological Evidence for Beta-Carotene in Prevention of Cancer and Cardiovascular Disease," *Eur J Clin Nutr*, 1996, 50(Suppl 3):S57-61.
28. Clark LC, Combs GF Jr, Turnbull BW, et al, "Effects of Selenium Supplementation for Cancer Prevention in Patients With Carcinoma of the Skin. A Randomized Controlled Trial. Nutritional Prevention of Cancer Study Group" *JAMA*, 1996, 276(24):1957-63.

INTRODUCTION TO HOMEOPATHY

Origins of Homeopathy

The German physician and chemist, Samuel Hahnemann (1755-1843), coined the word "homeopathy" by combining the Greek words "homoios" (meaning similar) with the word "pathos" (meaning suffering). The word refers to the main pharmacological tenet, the law of similars, which serves as the basis for the system of medicine known as homeopathy. This principle was described by Hippocrates, the "Father of Medicine," but the concept has been used by many cultures throughout history, including the Chinese, the Indians, the Mayans, and Native American Indians.[1] Hahnemann, however, was the first to codify and systematize the law of similars.

The Law of Similars

Hahnemann had become disillusioned with many of the medical practices of his day, such as bloodletting and the use of toxic substances to treat illness. While translating a book by Dr William Cullen, a prominent physician during Hahnemann's era, Hahnemann read about using cinchona bark with its bitter and astringent properties as a treatment for malaria. This prompted Hahnemann to begin experimenting with other astringent herbs to see if they would have a similar result. However, they did not relieve the symptoms of malaria. So, Hahnemann began to experiment upon himself, and eventually others, with cinchona. He carefully detailed the body's response to repeated doses of cinchona, and noted the dosage at which fever, chills, and other symptoms similar to malaria appeared. Hahnemann then began to systematically dilute cinchona and administer it to individuals with malaria. He discovered that even a diluted remedy of cinchona was effective in alleviating malaria's symptoms. Hahnemann concluded that cinchona was effective in treating malaria because it caused symptoms similar to those of the disease malaria. He called this phenomenon "*Similia similibus curantur*" or "Likes are cured by likes." This is commonly referred to as the Law of Similars.

Coincidentally, in 1798, Dr Edward Jenner discovered the value of giving an individual a small dose of cowpox in an attempt to immunize that individual against smallpox. Modern pharmacology contains numerous examples of the Law of Similars.

- Aspirin lowers fever, but has fever as one of its toxicologic signs.

- Nitroglycerin is used to treat angina, but causes angina in toxicologic doses.

- Digoxin is used to treat cardiac arrhythmias, but causes fatal arrhythmias in toxic doses.

It is recognized today that some homeopathic applications may not follow this similarity principle and may in fact follow direct pharmacologic principles.

Classical, Clinical, and Complex Homeopathy

During years of experimentation, Hahnemann noted the toxicological effects of a large number of plants on healthy individuals. He called this process of testing the effects of a substance on a healthy individual a "proving." In 1810, Hahnemann recorded his findings in the first homeopathic *Materia Medica*, a book that lists various substances and the symptoms produced by ingesting them. Hahnemann believed in giving a physical examination and conducting a thorough interview of each patient that included questions about general health, symptoms, outlook on life, and any other factors that might be influencing their condition. He wrote about the impact of genetics on health, and he believed that a good diet, proper hygiene, and exercise were all important for good health. Hahnemann also understood the role environmental factors and stress play in health.

INTRODUCTION TO HOMEOPATHY (Continued)

Hahnemann's approach was to match a patient's symptoms to the provings or toxicological profiles of substances that he had recorded. He would then administer a dilution of this compound, following the principle that "Likes are cured by likes," to provoke a positive healing response. This approach is termed **classical homeopathy**, the practice of identifying the correct remedy and giving one dose of one remedy at one potency or strength. A **Repertory** is a book that indexes the body by categories and lists the symptoms associated with each grouping. Category headings include such things as mind, head, eye, ear, nose, mouth, stomach, chest, and extremities. Repertorizing is the process of listing a patient's significant symptoms, locating each symptom in the Repertory, and scoring the various remedies identified to determine the one remedy that has the most similar picture to the patient. The Repertory (listing of symptoms by body grouping) and the *Materia Medica*[2] (listing of substances and the symptoms they produce) are used in conjunction with one another in this process.

Clinical homeopathy developed in Europe as an alternative method for suggesting homeopathic remedies. In this symptom-specific approach, remedies that have a known action on a particular complaint or symptom are used, instead of looking at the totality of the patient's symptoms. The more specific the symptom, the more accurate the remedy selection. An example of this would be to use *Apis mellifica* for a stinging sore throat, without looking at any other symptoms the individual may have.

Over the last 40 years, the practice known as complex homeopathy, or mixing several different homeopathic remedies together for a specific symptom or condition, has evolved. An example of this would be to use a combination homeopathic remedy for sinusitis that might contain *Hepar sulphuris calcareum*, *Kali bichromicum*, and *Silicea*, all remedies that have a known action on the sinuses.

Homeopathic Dilutions

Hahnemann knew that ingesting even small doses of a toxic substance could have deleterious effects, so he developed a system of dilution that is still used today. The most common forms of homeopathic dilution are either X or C dilutions. An X dilution is a 1:10 or decimal dilution. To make a 1X dilution, one part of the mother tincture is mixed with nine parts of diluent (alcohol and water or glycerin). This solution is shaken (a process called succussion) to create a 1X dilution. Taking one part of a 1X dilution, mixing it with nine parts of diluent, and again shaking it, makes a 2X dilution. C dilutions are 1:100 dilutions. A 2X dilution is the approximate equivalent of a 1C dilution.

A homeopathic remedy that is a 6X dilution would be a one part per million dilution, which is still in the physical substance dose range. A dilution that is above a 24X or 12C would be beyond Avogadro's number, meaning that there is no physical substance left in the dilution. While there is evidence in double-blind randomized placebo controlled studies that homeopathic dilutions do in fact work past this dilution point, this area has raised skepticism about homeopathy among many health professionals.[3] It should be emphasized that the overwhelming majority of over-the-counter homeopathic remedies are in a dilution below 24X or 12C. One common misconception about dilutions should be noted. It is not true that the more dilute a remedy, the more potent it is. This is an erroneous concept that has been labeled "the law of infinitesimals." Homeopathic remedies are available for acute and chronic conditions, as well as for self-care complaints, in all of the typical dosage forms, from tablets and pills to creams and suppositories.

History of Homeopathy in the United States

Homeopathy's use grew in Europe, and it was introduced into the United States in the early 1820s. Most pharmacists in the mid-1800s and early 1900s were trained in compounding homeopathic remedies. In the early 1900s, at least 20%

of the physicians trained in the United States were homeopathic physicians. At one time, this number was as high as 14,000 U.S. physicians. At the end of the 19th century, twenty-two medical schools primarily trained doctors in homeopathy and there were over 1000 homeopathic pharmacies.[4] American homeopathic physicians organized the American Institute of Homeopathy in 1844, which became the United States' first national medical society. In 1846, the American Medical Association (AMA) was founded, partially in response to the growth of homeopathy.[5] Its members were not permitted to practice homeopathy or consult with homeopaths. The growth of the AMA, coupled with disagreements on treatment philosophy among homeopaths, led to the decline of homeopathy in the United States in the early 1900s.

Worldwide Use of Homeopathy

Homeopathy remained very popular in Europe. The British Royal Family has received homeopathic care since the 1830s. One-third of the physicians in France recommend homeopathic remedies. In Germany, 20% of physicians prescribe homeopathic remedies. There are 120 homeopathic medical schools in India.[6] Europe's top-selling cold and flu remedy is a homeopathic product, and the majority of European pharmacies stock homeopathic remedies.

Homeopathy in the United States Today

Today, homeopathy is experiencing a resurgence in the United States. By the mid-1980s, there were over 1000 physicians specializing in homeopathy. In addition, other health professionals, such as dentists, veterinarians, chiropractors, naturopaths, nurses, and psychologists use homeopathic remedies.[7] Over 2.5 million Americans have used homeopathic remedies. A variety of chain and independent pharmacies stock homeopathic remedies in their stores. In addition, ongoing research in hospitals and universities is taking place.

Clinical Studies Confirm Effectiveness

A meta-analysis of 107 clinical trials of homeopathy appeared in the *British Medical Journal* in 1991. It reported that 68% of the highest quality studies showed positive results in treating influenza, hay fever, gastritis, migraine headache, trauma, and length of labor.[8] The *Lancet* reported in December, 1994, that asthma patients who were treated with homeopathy showed significantly greater improvement in their symptoms than the placebo group.[9] In May of 1994, a peer-reviewed double-blind study reported the effectiveness of homeopathy in the treatment of acute childhood diarrhea.[10]

A 1997 meta-analysis of placebo-controlled trials on homeopathy concluded that the clinical effects of homeopathy were not completely due to placebo, but found insufficient evidence to substantiate homeopathy's efficacy for any single clinical condition.[11] Subsequent articles have argued that the placebo question is not resolved, claiming that the design of the meta-analysis was flawed, and they have cited results from later unsuccessful trials.[12] Some claim that the effectiveness of homeopathic remedies is not supported by rigorous clinical trials.[9,13] However, there are several OTC drugs that were approved prior to 1962 (when double-blind randomized placebo controlled studies proving effectiveness began to be required) whose effectiveness has not been proven by double-blind studies.

A 1998 study on the clinical efficacy of homeopathy concluded that, although the evidence is not convincing due to methodological shortcomings and inconsistencies, available randomized trials suggest that homeopathy has an effect over placebo.[14] Some have suggested that new methodologies and research paradigms are necessary to adequately and objectively evaluate the efficacy of homeopathic remedies.[15,16,17]

INTRODUCTION TO HOMEOPATHY *(Continued)*

Possible Mechanisms of Action

There is no consensus on how homeopathy works, because it cannot be fully explained by existing pharmacological concepts. However, some principles may provide a partial explanation. One principle is **hormesis**, the process of diluting toxins in parts per million or greater in order to stimulate the body's ability to cope with toxins more efficiently and to improve enzyme function. In fact, the **Arndt-Schulz law of pharmacology**, a well-accepted tenet, states that small doses stimulate enzyme function over time; moderate doses inhibit enzyme function over time; and large doses block enzyme function over time.

Some believe that homeopathic remedies work in a manner similar to vaccines, but this could only be true for certain agents. Others hypothesize that each remedy possesses a specific energy pattern or electromagnetic resonance that is transmitted to sensitized biosystems.[3] Current thinking by some is that low dilutions (1X to 12X) are generally used in acute conditions or for drainage (to enhance an organ's ability to detoxify). Intermediate potencies (12X to 30X) act in a regulatory fashion. High potencies (above 30X or 30C) are generally used for mental and emotional symptoms, to work on an individual's constitutional nature, or for symptom pictures that are highly matched.[18] The book, *Homeopathy: A Frontier in Medical Science*,[19] summarizes the most contemporary viewpoints of potential homeopathic mechanisms of action within pharmacological models. One of the main approaches discussed in this book emphasizes "physiological homeostasis and the exchanges of biological information that regulate it."[19] A homeostatic system is made up of a "set of anatomical, biochemical, and functional elements designed to maintain a physiological variable within minimum and maximum oscillation limits."[19] The regulation center of the homeostatic system receives signals via its receptors. By some process not yet understood, the control system determines whether a stimulatory or inhibitory effect is needed to maintain homeostasis. Through this process, equilibrium is maintained.[19] Homeopathy may play a role in signaling auto-regulatory homeostatic mechanisms to reestablish normal output signals in the body. In sum, the exact mechanism of action in homeopathy remains unknown, just as many allopathic drugs have unknown mechanisms of action. Homeopathy has been used as a valid therapeutic tool by health professionals worldwide for over two centuries.

Legal Status of Homeopathic Remedies

The Food and Drug Administration (FDA) regulates the manufacture and sale of homeopathic remedies as drugs. However, homeopathic remedies are not regulated in the same way as allopathic drugs. Manufacturers of allopathic drugs must submit a new drug application (NDA) or an Abbreviated New Drug Application (ANDA) that supports a drug's safety and efficacy before it can be marketed in the United States. The "Compliance Policy Guide" outlines the FDA's policies and methods for regulating homeopathic remedies. Homeopathic remedies are exempt from the NDA process, because they have a long history of safety in use. In addition, each agent has been reviewed for homeopathic efficacy, toxicology, adverse effects, and clinical use prior to inclusion into the Homeopathic Pharmacopoeia of the United States (HPUS), which is discussed in more detail below.

Homeopathic remedies have both over-the-counter and prescription drug status. OTC homeopathics must have a claim for self-limiting conditions on their labels. This is in contrast to herbal and nutritional supplements, which fall under the Dietary Supplement Health and Education Act of 1994 (DSHEA). Currently, dietary supplements can make structure/function claims on their labels, but can only include a health claim if it has been pre-approved by the FDA.

The Homeopathic Pharmacopoeia of the United States (HPUS) is the official compendium that defines the OTC or Rx status of specific homeopathic remedies. It also provides manufacturing requirements for each of the agents in the formulary. Homeopathic remedies are made in FDA-drug licensed laboratories that follow drug Good Manufacturing Practices (GMP). About 60% of HPUS remedies are derived from plant sources. Animal sources (honeybees, cuttlefish ink, snake and spider venoms) are the source of other homeopathic remedies. Mineral sources for homeopathic remedies include calcium, graphite, iodine, potassium, selenium, silica, sodium, and sulfur. Chemicals that are considered toxic in crude drug form, such as mercury, can be used in a homeopathic dilution process. Some modern homeopathic agents are made from synthetic sources.

Homeopathy in This Book

Homeopathic remedies are available as either single remedies or combination formulas. This book contains suggestions for some of the most common single remedies for various health conditions. Homeopathic remedies can be suggested for at risk groups or those who cannot take other over-the-counter agents because of an existing condition or current medication. There are no known side effects or drug interactions with homeopathy. Homeopathic remedies are easy to administer and cost effective. In addition, homeopathy is safe for the whole family from infants to adults.

Footnotes

1. Frazer, Sir JG, *The Golden Bough*, New York, NY: Macmillan, 1922, 12-42.
2. Note: Other authors have published additional volumes of *Materia Medica* over the years.
3. Fisher P, "The Development of Research Methodology in Homoeopathy," *Complement Ther Nurs Midwifery*, 1995, 1(6):168-74.
4. Coulter H, *Transaction of the American Institute of Homoeopathy*, Vol III, 1901, 304, 460.
5. Kaufman M, *Homeopathy in America*, Baltimore, MD: Johns Hopkins, 1971, 53.
6. Heimlich J, "Homeopathy-New Age, But Not New," *Health & Healing*, 1995, 1-4.
7. Ullman D, *Homeopathy: Medicine for the 21st Century*, Berkeley, CA: North Atlantic Books, 1988, 50.
8. Kleijnen J, Knipschild P, ter Riet G, "Clinical Trials of Homoeopathy," *British Medical Journal*, 1991, 302(6772):316-23; Published erratum appears in *British Medical Journal*, 1991, 302(6780):818.
9. D Reilly, Taylor MA, Beattie NG, et al, "Is Evidence for Homoeopathy Reproducible?" *Lancet*, 1994, 344(8937):1601-6.
10. Jacobs J, Jimenez LM, Gloyd SS, et al, "Homeopathic Treatment of Childhood Diarrhea," *Pediatrics*, 1994, 97(5):778-9.
11. Linde K, Clausius N, Ramirez G, et al, "Are the Clinical Effects of Homeopathy Placebo Effects? A Meta-analysis of Placebo-controlled Trials," *Lancet*, 1997, 350(9081):834-43; Published erratum appears in *Lancet*, 1998, 351(9097):220.
12. No author listed, "Homeopathy Again: A Questionable Meta-analysis," *Prescrire Int*, 1998, 7(35):94-5.
13. Ernst E and Pittler MH, "Efficacy of Homeopathic Arnica: A Systematic Review of Placebo-controlled Clinical Trials," *Arch Surg*, 1998, 133(11):1187-90.
14. Linde K and Melchart D, "Randomized Controlled Trials of Individualized Homeopathy: A State-of-the-Art Review," *J Altern Complement Med*, 1998, 4(4):371-88.
15. Walach H, "Is Homeopathy Accessible to Research?" *Schweia Rundsch Med Prax*, 1994, 83(51-52):1439-7.
16. Walach H and Righetti M, "Homeopathy: Principles, Status of Research, Research Design; Comment," *Wien Klin Wochenschr*, 1996, 108(20):654-64.
17. Popova TD and Simeonova NK, "Homeopathy as a Therapeutic System," *Vestn Akad Med Nauk*, 1991, SSR(5):52-5.
18. No author listed, Homeopathic Medicines in Acute Winter Ailments, Lyons, France: Boiron Institute, 1997, 11, 17.
19. Bellavite P and Signorini A, *Homeopathy: A Frontier in Medical Science*, Berkeley, CA: North Atlantic Books, 1995.

INTRODUCTION TO GLANDULAR EXTRACTS

Glandular Extracts

Extracts derived from bovine, porcine, or sheep have been used for generations by healers from a wide variety of cultures. The ingestion of gland materials was said to strengthen the corresponding organs or glands within the human body. In fact, Egyptian medicine, Ayurvedic medicine, and even Paracelsus in Greece wrote about the utilization of glandular materials as restorative medicines. In the early part of the twentieth century, glandular therapies (termed organotherapy) became a part of the medical mainstream, with clinical reports of beneficial results occurring in the literally thousands of cases.[1,2]

Use and Composition of Glandular Extracts

Glandular extracts are used for health maintenance, rejuvenation, and conditional support to organ-specific conditions. Glandular extracts consist of peptides, proteins, fatty acids, and traces of hormones, as well as signal or messenger substances. These constituents are thought to contribute to the physiologic effects of the substances. Some active peptides have been identified within various glands; however, it will take years to identify all of the various peptides that have beneficial effects. Isolating single fractions contained in these agents may negate the purpose of providing organ-specific nutrition. They can be thought of as concentrated food sources, supplying certain nutrients to support organ-specific function.

Clinical Research

In general, there is a scarcity of clinical evidence supporting the use of glandular extracts in humans. However, thymus extracts are a good example of preparations with sound science behind their use in immune deficiencies and depressed immunity.[3,4] Glandular extracts, such as aortic extracts and pancreatic enzyme extracts, have some supportive science behind them. Others have been studied to varying degrees, but will probably report beneficial use with future studies. From a practical standpoint, professionals involved in natural medicine have utilized glandular extracts as cornerposts of their repertory and the authors have seen the benefits of these agents in clinical settings.

Quality of Glandular Extracts

There are several variables related to the quality of glandular extracts. The first is the selection of glandular materials. Sourcing materials can be difficult. The condition of many bovine sources in the United States is poor. Animals are fed antibiotics and growth hormones. They graze on land that has been sprayed with insecticides and pesticides. Their death experience results in the "mass kill" effect, which modifies the hormone pattern in the glandular material. Concern over contamination from bovine spongiform encephalopathy (BSE) is a current issue. Ascertaining that glandular sources are certified BSE-free becomes essential.

Other relevant considerations about the source of glandular extracts include whether the animal is raised free of pesticides, insecticides, hormones, and other chemicals and is allowed to graze freely. Is the animal killed in a humane way so as not to invoke the hormone rush in mass kill rooms? Does a veterinarian excise the glands? Is the animal inspected both pre- and postmortem to investigate its overall health? Reviewing all of these factors, there is really only one consistent world source that supplies an edible grade, fully inspected gland.

Manufacturing Glandular Extracts

There are several processes used in manufacturing glandular extracts:

- **Desiccation** involves using a heating process to thoroughly change a product, yet prevent damage to intact proteins and peptides.

- **Azeotropic** processing is when a solvent is driven though the material under low temperature. The solvents strip some of the lipid soluble nutrients from the finished product. Complete removal of the chemical solvent is an added concern.

- **Salt precipitation** involves glandular material being mixed with a salt and water solution. The fat-soluble material is filtered off after the mixture is emulsified and separated. There are no solvents involved but therapeutically important lipid portions are lost and the salt content is undesirable.

- **Freeze-drying** and **lyophilization** offer the cleanest, purest methods of product development. Low temperatures allow for proteins, peptides, and enzymes that are typically destroyed under heat to remain intact. By freeze-drying and then removing water, the lipid-soluble fraction remains within the final product, securing the hormone and fatty acid content.

- **Predigestion** is another way of processing glandular material. This consists of using enzymes to begin breaking down glandular material. The theory is that absorption of substances that have been partially digested seems to be more efficient. The extraction process is also able to separate out smaller versus larger peptides, which might be desirable in some instances.

Freeze-drying and predigestion should deliver the best results from a therapeutic perspective.

Absorption and Effectiveness of Glandular Extracts

Historically, there has been concern over whether certain proteins and large molecular polysaccharides could actually be absorbed and then whether the nutrients actually get delivered to the organ. However, recent evidence (animal and human studies) supports the conclusion that large macromolecules do pass intact from the human gut into the bloodstream under normal conditions.[5,6] Examples include human albumin, lactalbumin, bovine albumin, ovalbumin, lactoglobulin, ferritin, chymotrypsinogen, elastase, and other large molecules.

Proteins, polypeptides, and various hormones that are absorbed intact from the gut can exert effects on target tissues. For example, several peptide hormones are biologically active when administered orally, including luteinizing hormone-releasing factor and thyrotropin-releasing hormone.[7] These data suggest that there may be larger molecules in glandular products that are absorbed intact, which may exert therapeutic hormonal or hormone-like effects. Science is still trying to determine the cellular communication network.

Footnotes

1. *Organotherapy in General Practice*, New York, NY: GW Carnick Co, 1924.
2. Harrower HR, *Practical Hormone Therapy – A Manual of Organotherapy for General Practitioners*, New York, NY: American Medical Publishing Co, 1916, 1-17.
3. Tovo PA, "Thymus Extract Therapy in Immunodepressed Patients With Malignancies and Herpes Virus Infections," *Thymus*, 1980, 2:41-8.
4. Schulof RS, Simon GL, Sztein MB, et al, " Phase I/II Trial of Thymosin Fraction 5 and Thymosin Alpha One in HTLV-III Seropositive Subjects," *J Biol Response Mod*, 1986, 5(5):429-43.
5. Gardener ML, "Gastrointestinal Absorption of Intact Proteins," *Annu Rev Nutr*, 1988, 8:329-50.
6. Hemmings WA and Williams EW, "Transport of Large Breakdown Products of Dietary Protein Through the Gut Wall," *Gut*, 1978, 19(8):715-23.
7. Amoss M, Rivier J, and Guillemin R, "Release of Gonadotropins by Oral Administration of Synthetic LRF or a Tripeptide Fragment of LRF," *J Clin Endocrinol Metab*, 1972, 35(1):175-7.

PART II. CONDITIONS
TABLE OF CONTENTS

Introduction to Conditions 41
Acne Vulgaris 44
Allergies / Hay Fever 48
Alzheimer's Disease / Senility 52
Amenorrhea 56
Arthritis (Osteo) 60
Arthritis (Rheumatoid) 64
Asthma 68
Athlete's Foot / Jock Itch 72
Attention Deficit Disorder (ADD) /
    Attention Deficit Hyperactivity Disorder (ADHD) 76
Benign Prostatic Hypertrophy (BPH) 80
Breast-Feeding 84
Candidiasis 88
Cataracts 92
Cervical Dysplasia 96
Chemotherapy and Radiation 100
Chronic Fatigue Syndrome (CFS) 106
Circulation (Peripheral) Problems 110
Cold / Flu 114
Colic 118
Constipation 122
Contact Dermatitis *see Eczema* 162
Contact Dermatitis *see Poison Ivy / Poison Oak* 306
Cough 126
Crohn's Disease 130
Croup 134
Depression 138
Diaper Rash 142
Diarrhea 146
Diverticulitis 150
Dyslipidemia 154
Dysmenorrhea 158
Eczema 162
Endometriosis 166
Epilepsy 170
Fatigue 174
Fever 178
Fibrocystic Breast Disease (FBD) 182
Fibromyalgia 186
Gallbladder / Gallstones 190
Gingivitis 194
Glaucoma 198
Halitosis 202

PART II. CONDITIONS *(Continued)*

Headache / Migraine Headache 206
Hemorrhoids 210
Herpes Simplex 1 214
Herpes Simplex 2 218
Hyperglycemia / Diabetes / Insulin Resistance 222
Hypertension (High Blood Pressure) 226
Hyperthyroidism 230
Hypoglycemia 234
Hypothyroidism 238
Indigestion / Heartburn 242
Insomnia 246
Irritable Bowel Syndrome (IBS) 250
Macular Degeneration 254
Memory Problems 258
Menopause 262
Menorrhagia 266
Minor Injury / Wound Healing 270
Motion Sickness 274
Multiple Sclerosis (MS) 278
Muscle Soreness / Stiffness 282
Nausea / Vomiting 286
Osteoporosis 290
Otitis Media 294
Parkinson's Disease 298
Performance Enhancement 302
Poison Ivy / Poison Oak 306
Premenstrual Syndrome (PMS) 310
Psoriasis 314
Rosacea 318
Scleroderma 322
Sexual Vitality (Females) 326
Sexual Vitality (Males) 330
Sinusitis 334
Sore Throat 338
Stress / Anxiety 342
Sunburn 346
Systemic Lupus Erythematosus (SLE) 350
Teething 354
Ulcer (Aphthous) 358
Ulcer (Duodenal and Peptic) 362
Ulcer (Gastric) *see Ulcer (Duodenal and Peptic)* 362
Ulcerative Colitis 366
Urinary Tract Infection (UTI) 370
Venous Stasis *see Circulation (Peripheral) Problems* 110
Weight Management 374

INTRODUCTION TO CONDITIONS

In the Conditions section of the Pocket Guide, the authors have selected a number of common health conditions for which natural products are likely to play an important role in the support of a specific complaint. For each condition, five distinct areas of material are provided to assist healthcare providers in identifying how natural products might be applied to someone with the particular condition. These five specific areas are as follows:

1. **Condition Overview:** A general overview of the condition, with basic information on its etiology, typical symptoms, who may be affected, associated disorders, common interventions to provide relief, general complications, and the predicted duration of the condition.

2. **Lifestyle Recommendations:** Suggestions are offered for lifestyle changes for each condition. Most of these recommendations revolve around certain behavioral modifications that are likely to provide benefit. General lifestyle recommendations are provided as options that may provide benefit to an individual with the specific condition.

3. **Decision Tree:** A decision tree is provided for each condition to assist healthcare providers in determining when to apply natural products. Each decision tree takes the healthcare provider through a series of questions that aids them in determining situation complexity. Decision points are identified in the trees to assist the healthcare provider in deciding how to proceed based on an individual's particular situation. The components of each decision tree box include:

    Box 1: Identification of a client with a specific condition who is interested in using natural products for the condition

    Box 2: Healthcare provider interacting with the client requests basic background information; general questions to be asked of the client and issues to be reviewed by the healthcare provider prior to considering natural products for the condition are listed

    Box 3: Emphasizes the need for the healthcare provider to review the information obtained in Box 2 before deciding how to proceed with the client

    Box 4A, 4B: Based on the information obtained in Box 2,

    > **Box 4A** – It is determined that the client is a candidate for natural products for the condition
    >
    > **Box 4B** – It is determined that the client is NOT a candidate for natural products for the condition

    Box 5: The client is a candidate for natural products, and several condition-specific questions are offered for review. The responses to these questions offer the healthcare provider a second level of screening of the individual to determine situation complexity, beyond the general information obtained in Box 2. In most situations, the individual's responses to these questions will assist the healthcare provider in directing the client to a specific category or categories of products for the condition. However, there will be times when the responses suggest that the client's situation and/or severity of the disease process is more complex than originally thought, and a referral for additional medical evaluation should be made prior to using natural products (ie, this information sends the healthcare provider back to Box 4B). At this stage, it is important to use effective interview techniques beyond these preliminary questions, and to exercise skilled professional judgement in order to avoid delays in seeking specific treatment or to coordinate natural product support with physician's treatment plan.

INTRODUCTION TO CONDITIONS *(Continued)*

Box 6: Healthcare provider is directed to a listing of natural products to consider for the specific condition

4. **Table of Natural Product Suggestions**: This table lists common natural products used to support each medical condition. Each table has the following three fields of information:

- **Category**: The left column of the table indicates the type of natural product to consider – herb, nutritional/nutraceutical, homeopathic, and other supplements.

- **Natural Products to Consider**: The middle column of the table lists the specific natural product, including condition-specific dosages for nutritional/nutraceutical agents. The authors have limited the list of suggestions to those products that are most commonly used and those that have some degree of scientific support for their usage. The condition-specific dosage represents the **total suggested daily dosage for a specific agent**. If other products containing the same natural agent are being consumed, these dosages must be taken into consideration prior to deciding how much of the agent to use for the specific condition. For example, if the suggested condition-specific dosage for vitamin E is 800 int. units daily, and the individual is already consuming 400 int. units daily as part of a basic wellness program (or for another reason), 400 int. units would be added to the existing amount being taken to reach the target daily dosage of 800 int. units. For further information on suggested daily dosages of specific nutrients, refer to the **Suggested Daily Intake of Nutritional Supplements** *on page 27*.

- **DOC**: The right column of the table represents an abbreviation for Documentation. The authors have developed a classification system for each natural product, based on the type of published information that exists for using that product for the specific condition. Five classifications are utilized:

  HT: Human Trials – published data (structured studies such as double-blind, placebo-controlled, and randomized clinical trials) that support a relationship between the natural product and a specific condition or use

  HD: Human Data – human data (case reports and anecdotal evidence) reported in the literature but not as scientifically sound as human trials

  HE: Historical Evidence – traditional uses of a particular natural product for some conditions have been reported, as well as other reports of clinical experience

  PA: Pharmacological Activity – potential benefit may be observed for a specific condition based on the proposed pharmacological activity of the natural product

  PD: Proving Data – information exists to support the value of using a specific homeopathic remedy for a particular condition

Applying the data in the Natural Products to Consider tables to specific situations requires consideration of the patient's individual needs. It is important for the healthcare provider to consider all symptoms related to the condition, while at the same time reviewing the pharmacology and mechanisms of action for the natural products. There may be considerable differences in how two products within the same classification provide benefit for the same condition.

The selection of products for a specific condition varies due to the scope of the symptoms, patient-specific factors, and the healthcare provider's experience. The use of multiple natural products to support a medical condition must be made on an individual basis. Certain individuals will have complex situations and the healthcare provider might opt to suggest adding one product at a time to their regimen. Other individuals may have a situation of moderate complexity where several products could be added. With experience, the healthcare provider's suggestions will become as familiar as suggestions for traditional drug therapy.

Because of the chemical nature of herbal pharmacology, the authors suggest adding herbs conservatively to a regimen or to support a condition, until experience is obtained regarding the benefits and potential effects of the herbs being used. This is especially true for individuals who have more than one chronic medical condition and/or who are taking chronic prescription medications. There are complex situations where a conservative approach with herbs is warranted and where close supervision by a primary care provider is recommended. There are many combination products, containing two or more herbs, which are designed for specific functional support. Healthcare providers should consider each of the ingredients in a combination product as they relate to the client. In contrast, the profile of many nutritionals, nutraceuticals, and homeopathics would suggest that these could be used in combination very early in a supportive and preventive role.

Natural products with very similar mechanisms of action should not be used together for the same condition so as to avoid duplicate effects. If multiple products are chosen to support a condition, it is recommended that each work differently in order to provide the greatest opportunity for broad support. However, using supplements for prevention and enhancement can be approached differently. In this situation, a variety of natural agents with similar function (for example, mixed antioxidants) could be used for specific goals.

5. **Special Considerations:** The information in this section is extracted from the monographs on individual herbs, nutritionals, and nutraceuticals. It is included in the Conditions section to provide a quick reference to important risk issues for each product. This section provides information that is important to consider when deciding how to apply natural products to a specific condition. It also reduces the need to page back and forth between the Conditions and the Monographs. The information is customized for each medical condition. For more detail, the healthcare provider is referred to the individual product monographs or the appropriate charts.

ACNE VULGARIS

Acne is an inflammatory disease of the sebaceous glands and hair follicles of the skin. The development of acne is influenced by multiple factors, including hormones (particularly androgens), increased sebum production, and proliferation of certain species of bacteria within the clogged follicle. Acne develops in areas where sebaceous glands are most numerous, affecting the face, scalp, neck, chest, back, upper arms, and shoulders. Acne lesions include comedones (blackheads), as well as papules, nodules, and pustules (whiteheads).

Acne usually starts between the ages of 10 and 13 years of age and lasts for 5-10 years. By their midteens, more than 40% of adolescents have acne severe enough to require some physician-directed treatment. While acne normally disappears in the early twenties, it may persist into the late twenties or thirties. Acne affects young men and young women about equally. Young men are more likely to have severe acne and are less likely to consult a dermatologist. In contrast, young women are more likely to have intermittent acne related to their menstrual cycle or acne caused by cosmetics.

Acne is not caused by dirt or surface skin oils. Vigorous washing and scrubbing will actually irritate the skin and may worsen acne. Gentle washing two to three times a day with a mild soap is recommended, along with an appropriate acne treatment. Although scientific studies have not found a clear relationship between diet and acne, some people may note that certain foods affect their acne and these foods may need to be avoided.

Physician referral may be necessary if lesions are large and painful, if results achieved with nonprescription acne products are unsatisfactory, if acne interferes with emotional well-being, if scarring has occurred, or if the acne is causing dark pigmentation patches in individuals with dark skin.

LIFESTYLE RECOMMENDATIONS

- Continuation/initiation of diet and exercise program
- Use an OTC drying lotion/cream
- Wash daily
- Use a water-based make-up
- Avoid prolonged exposure to sunlight
- Do not pick at the lesions!

ACNE VULGARIS DECISION TREE

1. Client with acne vulgaris is interested in using natural products (NP) to support this condition

2. Healthcare provider requests basic background information.
   The following issues are addressed with the client:
   * Allergies?
   * Prescription (Rx)/OTC meds?
   * Natural products?
   * Other medical conditions?
   * Nutrition/diet program?
   * Exercise program?

3. Above data reviewed; if **yes** to Rx/OTC meds, review **Drug-Induced Nutrient Depletion Chart** in Appendix

4A. Client is a candidate for natural products

   * An appropriate homeopathic remedy can be used at any time

4B. Client's case is too complicated at this point; needs additional support from MD before initiating NP program

5. Condition-specific questions:
   * How often do you use antibiotics for this condition?
   * For women: Do you notice any relationship between the onset or worsening of acne and your menstrual cycle?

6. See table on following page

ACNE VULGARIS *(Continued)*

ACNE VULGARIS*

Category	Natural Products to Consider	DOC
Herb	**Chasteberry/Vitex** *on page 408*	HD
	Tea Tree (Topical) *on page 509*	HD
	Olive Leaf *on page 483*	PA
Vitamin/Mineral/ Trace Element/ Nutraceutical	**Vitamin A** *on page 518* Condition-specific dosage: 5000-10,000 int. units/day	HD
	Zinc *on page 534* Condition-specific dosage: 25 mg/day until clear **WITH** **Copper** *on page 416* Condition-specific dosage: 2 mg/day until clear	HT
	Vitamin B₃ (Niacinamide) *on page 521* Condition-specific dosage: 4% topical (if available)	HT
Homeopathic Remedy	Homeopathic combination formulas are available for many conditions. Listed below are some of the most common single homeopathic remedies for acne vulgaris. Also see the **Homeopathic Quick Reference Chart for Common Complaints** *on page 587*	
	Baptisia tinctoria	PD
	Hepar sulphuris calcareum	PD
	Kali bromatum	PD
	Pulsatilla	PD
	Sulphur	PD
Additional supplements to consider	**Fish Oils** *on page 434* Condition-specific dosage: 750 mg 2-3 times/day **OR** **Flaxseed Oil** *on page 435* Condition-specific dosage: 1 Tbsp/day	HD
	Selenium *on page 502* Condition-specific dosage: 200 mcg/day **WITH** **Vitamin E** *on page 529* Condition-specific dosage: 200-400 int. units/day	HD

*Refer to **Introduction to Conditions** *on page 41* for more details on how to apply the information in this table to individuals with this condition.

SPECIAL CONSIDERATIONS

Chasteberry/Vitex
- Contraindicated in pregnancy
- Mainly used in women
- Potential interaction with hormonal replacements or oral contraceptives

Tea Tree
- May cause allergic dermatitis in sensitive individuals
- Not for ingestion

Olive Leaf
- No reported toxicity in humans at normal intakes

Vitamin A
- Contraindicated in pregnancy or in women who may become pregnant

Zinc
- No reported toxicity in humans at normal intakes

Copper
- Contraindicated in Wilson's disease

Vitamin B_3 (Niacinamide)
- For topical use only in the treatment of acne

Fish Oils
- High doses may cause GI upset, loose stools, nausea
- May alter glucose regulation; use with caution in diabetes
- Caution in individuals receiving oral hypoglycemics or insulin; monitor blood glucose closely and coordinate with prescriber
- Potential interaction with anticoagulants (warfarin), aspirin, NSAIDs, anti-platelet agents

Flaxseed Oil
- No reported toxicity in humans at normal intakes

Selenium
- No reported toxicity in humans at normal intakes

Vitamin E
- Use with caution when taking anticoagulants (vitamin E ≥200 int. units increases prothrombin times)
- Interrupt or reduce dosage one week prior to dental or surgical procedures

ALLERGIES / HAY FEVER

Up to 20% of the U.S. population suffers from some form of allergy. Common allergens include animal dander, dust mites, molds, and pharmaceutical agents. One of the most cornmon forms of allergy is hay fever, an allergic reaction to plant pollen produced in large quantities by weeds, grasses, and trees. Symptoms include sneezing, itchy, watery eyes, sinus drainage or congestion, and throat or mouth scratchiness. These may be confused with symptoms of a cold.

The treatment of allergic reactions includes prevention, medication, and immunotherapy. Prevention of hay fever consists of limiting outdoor activities, especially when pollen levels are high. A number of foods have also been associated with allergies and allergy testing by a specialist is frequently helpful in identifying the cause of a person's allergies.

Allergic rhinitis is frequently associated with ear and sinus problems. In particular, children with allergies tend to have reoccurring middle ear infections. Sinus problems are often associated with clear, yellow, or green nasal mucus. A nighttime cough often occurs. Although adults with sinus problems normally complain of headaches, children with allergies do not often complain of this symptom.

Homeopathy in particular, has reported a lot of promise for allergy relief.

LIFESTYLE RECOMMENDATIONS

- Continuation/initiation of diet and exercise programs
- Allergen avoidance program
- Address mattress/pillow covers
- Heating/cooling system filters, air filtration systems, periodic cleaning, maintenance
- If seasonal allergies, watch pollen counts, etc

ALLERGIES DECISION TREE

1. Client with allergies is interested in using natural products (NP) to support this condition

2. Healthcare provider requests basic background information. The following issues are addressed with the client:
   * Allergies? Obtain as much detail as possible
   * Prescription (Rx)/OTC meds?
   * Natural products?
   * Other medical conditions?
   * Nutrition/diet program?
   * Exercise program?

3. Above data reviewed; if **yes** to Rx/OTC meds, review **Drug-Induced Nutrient Depletion Chart** in Appendix

4A. Client is a candidate for natural products

   * An appropriate homeopathic remedy can be used at any time

4B. Client's case is too complicated at this point; needs additional support from MD before initiating NP program

5. Condition-specific questions:
   * Are you seeing a specialist to treat the problem with allergies? If so, what interventions were recommended? Compare to what is listed in the **Lifestyle Recommendations**
   * What triggers cause allergies to worsen?
   * How often does problem with allergies lead to an infection? Is this a situation that is predictable? If so, develop a preventive plan to address.

6. See table on following page

ALLERGIES / HAY FEVER *(Continued)*

ALLERGIES*

Category	Natural Products to Consider	DOC
Herb	**Grape Seed** *on page 451*	PA
	Stinging Nettle (Leaf) *on page 505*	HD
	Coleus *on page 413*	PA
Vitamin/Mineral/ Trace Element/ Nutraceutical	**Vitamin C** *on page 526* Condition-specific dosage: 500-1000 mg twice daily	HT
	Quercetin *on page 494* Condition-specific dosage: 300-400 mg 3 times/day	HD
	Methyl Sulfonyl Methane (MSM) *on page 479* Condition-specific dosage: 2000-5000 mg/day	PA
Homeopathic Remedy	Homeopathic combination formulas are available for many conditions. Listed below are some of the most common single homeopathic remedies for allergies/ hay fever. Also see **Homeopathic Quick Reference Chart for Common Complaints** *on page 587*	
	Allium cepa	PD
	Ambrosia	PD
	Arsenicum album	PD
	Arundo mauritanica	PD
	Drosera rotundifolia	PD
	Histaminum	PD
	Kali bichromicum	PD
	Sabadilla	PD
Additional supplements to consider	**Vitamin B Complex-25** *on page 526* Condition-specific dosage: 25 mg 1-2 times/day	PA

*Refer to **Introduction to Conditions** *on page 41* for more details on how to apply the information in this table to individuals with this condition.

SPECIAL CONSIDERATIONS

Grape Seed
- Contraindicated in active bleeding (eg, peptic ulcer, intracranial bleeding)
- Caution in hemostatic disorders/history of bleeding
- Potential interaction with anticoagulants (warfarin), aspirin, NSAIDs, antiplatelet agents, methotrexate
- Discontinue use prior to dental or surgical procedures (14 days before)

Stinging Nettle
- Contraindicated in pregnancy

Coleus
- Contraindicated in active bleeding (eg, peptic ulcer, intracranial bleeding)
- May cause hypotension; use with caution in cerebrovascular or cardiovascular disease
- Caution in hemostatic disorders/history of bleeding
- Potential interaction with anticoagulants (warfarin), aspirin, NSAIDs, antiplatelet agents
- Potential interaction with antihistamines, decongestants, antihypertensives
- Discontinue use prior to dental or surgical procedures (14 days before)

Vitamin C
- Excess intake in diabetics may give falsely elevated blood glucose readings

Quercetin
- No reported toxicities in humans at normal intakes

Methyl Sulfonyl Methane
- No reported toxicities in humans at normal intakes

Vitamin B Complex-25
- No reported toxicities in humans at normal intakes

ALZHEIMER'S DISEASE / SENILITY

Alzheimer's disease is a progressive, degenerative, neurologic disorder that results in memory impairment and deterioration in cognitive function, reasoning, and behavior. Alzheimer's disease is the most common form of dementia, accounting for >60% of late life disorders of cognitive dysfunction. The loss of intellectual function initially interferes with daily life, and after a course that may last for many years, eventually results in death. Death is not due to the disease itself, but results from the complications of sepsis, nutritional deficiency, pneumonia, aspiration, or trauma.

Neuronal destruction that manifests as cortical atrophy, degeneration of cholinergic neurons, accumulation of neuritic plaques, and neurofibrillary tangles are observed in the brains of individuals afflicted with Alzheimer's. A specific protein, beta amyloid, is found at the center of neuritic plaques. Other factors that may mediate the progression of the disease include concentrations of apolipoprotein E, inflammatory mediators such as prostaglandins, and the degree of cholinergic neuron activity. Hormonal fluctuations may influence the disease process, as demonstrated by a protective effect of estrogen observed in some studies.

A number of illnesses and medications may interfere with memory. To rule out these potentially reversible causes, a complete physical, psychiatric, and neurologic evaluation should be performed by a physician experienced in the diagnosis of Alzheimer's.

Alzheimer's disease begins with almost imperceptible changes. As the disease progresses, gradual memory loss, a decline in performance of routine tasks, increasing disorientation, impaired judgment, personality changes, difficulty in learning, and loss of language skills are observed. Progression of these changes demonstrates a high degree of variability, with courses lasting from 3-20 years. Average survival is between 4 and 8 years following diagnosis.

LIFESTYLE RECOMMENDATIONS

- Continuation/initiation of diet and exercise program

- Eliminate risky situations in the home that may cause injury (burns, falls, etc)

- Follow adherence devices to ensure medications and natural products are taken as ordered or suggested

- Interact as often as possible with caregiver to provide assistance and educational materials

ALZHEIMER'S DISEASE / SENILITY / DEMENTIA
DECISION TREE

1. Client with Alzheimer's disease/senility/dementia is interested in using natural products (NP) to support this condition

2. Healthcare provider requests basic background information. The following issues are addressed with the client:

* Allergies?
* Prescription (Rx)/OTC meds?
* Natural products?

* Other medical conditions?
* Nutrition/diet program?
* Exercise program?

3. Above data reviewed; if **yes** to Rx/OTC meds, review **Drug-Induced Nutrient Depletion Chart** in Appendix

4A. Client is a candidate for natural products

* An appropriate homeopathic remedy can be used at any time

4B. Client's case is too complicated at this point; needs additional support from MD before initiating NP program

5. Condition-specific questions:
* Review meds to ensure they are not contributing to condition:
  Antidepressants, antiparkinson therapy, antipsychotics, anticholinergics, beta-blockers, digoxin, sedative/hypnotics
  If any are identified, refer to MD for review and action
* Determine if caregiver is involved and provide information to this individual

6. See table on following page

ALZHEIMER'S DISEASE / SENILITY *(Continued)*

ALZHEIMER'S DISEASE / SENILITY*

Category	Natural Products to Consider	DOC
Herb	**Ginkgo** *on page 441*	HT
	Vinpocetine *on page 517*	PA
	HuperzineA *on page 460*	PA
	Bacopa *on page 389*	PA
Vitamin/Mineral/ Trace Element/ Nutraceutical	**Phosphatidyl Choline** *on page 488* Condition-specific dosage: 500-1500 mg 2-3 times/day	HT
	Phosphatidyl Serine *on page 489* Condition-specific dosage: 100 mg 3 times/day	HT
	Acetyl-L-Carnitine *on page 380* Condition-specific dosage: 500-2000 mg/day in divided doses	HT
	Vitamin E *on page 529* Condition-specific dosage: 200-800 int. units/day	HT
Homeopathic Remedy	Homeopathic combination formulas are available for many conditions. Listed below are some of the most common single homeopathic remedies for Alzheimer's disease. Also see **Homeopathic Quick Reference Chart for Common Complaints** *on page 587*	
	Alumina	PD
	Hyoscyamus niger	PD
Additional supplements to consider	No recommendations	

*Refer to **Introduction to Conditions** *on page 41* for more details on how to apply the information in this table to individuals with this condition.

SPECIAL CONSIDERATIONS

Ginkgo
- Contraindicated in active bleeding (eg, peptic ulcer, intracranial bleeding)
- Caution in hemostatic disorders/history of bleeding
- Potential interaction with anticoagulants (warfarin), aspirin, NSAIDs, anti-platelet agents
- Theoretical interaction with MAO inhibitors and acetylcholinesterase inhibitors (eg, tacrine, donepezil)
- Discontinue use prior to dental or surgical procedures (14 days before)

Vinpocetine
- No reported toxicity in humans at normal intakes

HuperzineA
- Theoretical interaction with acetylcholinesterase inhibitors (eg, tacrine, donepezil)

Bacopa
- No reported toxicity in humans at normal intakes

Phosphatidyl Choline
- No reported toxicity in humans at normal intakes

Phosphatidyl Serine
- No reported toxicity in humans at normal intakes

Acetyl-L-Carnitine
- Occasionally, mild abdominal discomfort, restlessness, vertigo, and headache have been reported

Vitamin E
- Use with caution when taking anticoagulants (vitamin E ≥200 int. units increases prothrombin times)
- Interrupt or reduce dosage one week prior to dental or surgical procedures

AMENORRHEA

Amenorrhea is the absence of menstrual periods and may be classified as either primary or secondary. In primary amenorrhea, menstruation has never occurred. In the majority of cases, this is merely due to late onset of puberty. If menstruation has not occurred by the age of 17, a physician should perform a full gynecologic examination. Other causes of primary amenorrhea include uterine, ovarian, or pituitary gland disorders.

Secondary amenorrhea is defined by missing three or more periods after establishment of a regular menstrual cycle. The most common cause of secondary amenorrhea is pregnancy. Menstrual patterns may be altered by anemia, emotional stress, illness, certain medications, oral contraceptives, eating disorders, weight loss, and excessive exercise.

LIFESTYLE RECOMMENDATIONS

- Continue with present diet and exercise programs and ensure close monitoring by healthcare provider

- Do not wait too long to seek medical attention if symptoms persist

- Changes in stress levels? If yes, may be contributing to problem, and stress reduction program may be beneficial.

AMENORRHEA DECISION TREE

---

1. Client with amenorrhea is interested in using natural products (NP) to support this condition

---

2. Healthcare provider requests basic background information.
   The following issues are addressed with the client:
   * Allergies?
   * Prescription (Rx)/OTC meds?
     Hormone therapy, OCs,
     NSAIDs - may be contributing to
     problem - see MD to review
   * Natural products?
   * Other medical conditions?
   * Nutrition/diet program?
   * Exercise program?

---

3. Above data reviewed; if **yes** to Rx/OTC meds, review
   Drug-Induced Nutrient Depletion Chart in Appendix

4A. Client is a candidate for natural products

* An appropriate homeopathic remedy can be used at any time

4B. Client's case is too complicated at this point; needs additional support from MD before initiating NP program

---

5. Condition-specific questions:
   * Symptoms for how long? Sought medical attention? If appears to be significant, refer to MD
   * Recent changes in diet, appetite? Anorexia/bulimia can contribute to problem - if this type of behavior is suspected, refer to MD
   * Pregnancy test recently? If pregnancy is possible, refer to have test
   * Associated with pain? Significant: Refer to MD

---

6. See table on following page

AMENORRHEA *(Continued)*

AMENORRHEA*

Category	Natural Products to Consider	DOC
Herb	Chasteberry/Vitex *on page 408*	HD
	Dong Quai *on page 425*	PA
	Evening Primrose *on page 430*	PA
Vitamin/Mineral/ Trace Element/ Nutraceutical	No recommendations	
Homeopathic Remedy	Homeopathic combination formulas are available for many conditions. Listed below are some of the most common single homeopathic remedies for amenorrhea. Also see **Homeopathic Quick Reference Chart for Common Complaints** *on page 587*	
	Ferrum metallicum	PD
	Pulsatilla	PD
Additional supplements to consider	No recommendations	

*Refer to **Introduction to Conditions** *on page 41* for more details on how to apply the information in this table to individuals with this condition.

SPECIAL CONSIDERATIONS

Chasteberry/Vitex
- Contraindicated in pregnancy
- Potential interaction with hormonal replacements or oral contraceptives

Dong Quai
- Caution in pregnancy and breast-feeding
- Contraindicated in active bleeding (eg, peptic ulcer, intracranial bleeding)
- Use caution in those at risk of estrogen-dependent tumors, endometrial cancer, thromboembolic disease, or stroke
- Potential interaction with anticoagulants (warfarin), aspirin, NSAIDs, anti-platelet agents
- Potential interaction with oral contraceptives or hormonal replacement therapy
- Caution in hemostatic disorders/history of bleeding
- Potential interaction with antihypertensives, photosensitizing agents
- Discontinue use prior to dental or surgical procedures (14 days before)

Evening Primrose
- Contraindicated in seizure disorders, schizophrenia, or in persons receiving anticonvulsant or antipsychotic medications
- Contraindicated in active bleeding (eg, peptic ulcer, intracranial bleeding)
- Caution in hemostatic disorders/history of bleeding
- Potential interaction with anticoagulants (warfarin), aspirin, NSAIDs, anti-platelet agents
- Discontinue use prior to dental or surgical procedures (14 days before)

ARTHRITIS (OSTEO)

Up to 66% of individuals older than 60 years of age demonstrate evidence of osteoarthritis. The natural design of moveable (articular) joints allows friction-less movement between the two bony surfaces due to the smooth, lubricated cartilage surface. In addition, this surface facilitates dispersing the force of impact on a joint. In osteoarthritis, joint damage involves injury to this shock-distributing cartilage pad. Trauma to the joint, which is often repetitive (such as in high-impact athletic activities or occupational risks), frays the molecular structure of the cartilage, increasing the friction and damaging its structural integrity. In osteoarthritis, the lining of the joint capsule (synovium) demonstrates minimal inflammation, however, the bone surfaces beneath the cartilage often show signs of bone remodeling and fracture.

In many cases, breakdown of the cartilage may be due to a number of factors besides trauma. For example, genetic abnormalities of cartilage (type II collagen mutation) have been demonstrated which impair smooth, friction-reducing qualities of the cartilage surface. Immune responses, as well as accumulation of some forms of crystals within the joint, have also been implicated.

Factors that increase the risk of osteoarthritis include obesity, advancing age, trauma, and joint instability. Management involves pain reduction and avoidance of exacerbating factors.

Symptoms of osteoarthritis include joint stiffness that often worsens with activity and may be particularly acute on the day after exertion. Pain, which may originate from surrounding structures (tendon, muscle stretching), is generally relieved by resting the joint. Osteoarthritis shows a greater predisposition for specific joints, particularly the hip, knee, cervical spine, and the distal and proximal interphalangeal joints. In the early stages, osteoarthritis is uncomfortable and may limit activity. In advanced stages, or with aggressive disease, the joint damage may be deforming.

LIFESTYLE RECOMMENDATIONS

- Continuation/initiation of diet and exercise program
- Discuss use of heat and cold on affected joints
- Discuss weight loss, where appropriate

ARTHRITIS (OSTEO) DECISION TREE

1. Client with arthritis (osteo) is interested in using natural products
   (NP) to support this condition

2. Healthcare provider requests basic background information.
   The following issues are addressed with the client:

   * Allergies?   * Other medical conditions?
   * Prescription (Rx)/OTC meds?   * Nutrition/diet program?
   * Natural products?   * Exercise program?

3. Above data reviewed; if **yes** to Rx/OTC meds, review
   Drug-Induced Nutrient Depletion Chart in Appendix

4A. Client is a candidate for
    natural products

    * An appropriate homeopathic
      remedy can be used at any time

4B. Client's case is too
    complicated at this point;
    needs additional support
    from MD before initiating
    NP program

5. Condition-specific questions:
   * Any triggers that worsen the symptoms?
   * Describe pain: Intermittent, constant, localized, where, etc
   * How does the condition affect specific joints?
   * Effect on quality of life?

6. See table on following page

ARTHRITIS (OSTEO) *(Continued)*

ARTHRITIS (OSTEO)*

Category	Natural Products to Consider	DOC
Herb	**Boswellia** *on page 397*	HD
	Ginger *on page 440*	HT
	Grape Seed *on page 451*	PA
	Cat's Claw *on page 404*	HT
	Turmeric *on page 512*	PA
Vitamin/Mineral/ Trace Element/ Nutraceutical	**Chondroitin Sulfate** *on page 410* Condition-specific dosage: 300-1500 mg/day **WITH** **Glucosamine Sulfate** *on page 446* Condition-specific dosage: 1500-2000 mg/day **OR** **Glucosamine Hydrochloride** *on page 446* Condition-specific dosage: 1500-2000 mg/day	HT
	Methyl Sulfonyl Methane (MSM) *on page 479* Condition-specific dosage: 2000-5000 mg/day	PA
	SAMe (S-adenosylmethionine) *on page 498* Condition-specific dosage: 400-1600 mg/day	HT
	Collagen *on page 414* Condition-specific dosage: 200 mg 3 times/day	HD
Homeopathic Remedy	Homeopathic combination formulas are available for many conditions. Listed below are some of the most common single homeopathic remedies for osteoarthritis. Also see **Homeopathic Quick Reference Chart for Common Complaints** *on page 587*	
	Arnica montana	PD
	Bryonia alba	PD
	Calcarea phosphorica	PD
	Dulcamara	PD
	Rhus toxicodendron	PD
Additional supplements to consider	**Boron** *on page 397* Condition-specific dosage: 3-6 mg/day	HT

*Refer to **Introduction to Conditions** *on page 41* for more details on how to apply the information in this table to individuals with this condition.

SPECIAL CONSIDERATIONS

Boswellia
- No reported toxicity in humans at normal intakes

Ginger
- Contraindicated in active bleeding (eg, peptic ulcer, intracranial bleeding)
- Caution in hemostatic disorders/history of bleeding
- Potential interaction with anticoagulants (warfarin), aspirin, NSAIDs, anti-platelet agents, cardiac glycosides (digoxin)
- Discontinue use prior to dental or surgical procedures (14 days before)

Grape Seed
- Contraindicated in active bleeding (eg, peptic ulcer, intracranial bleeding)
- Caution in hemostatic disorders/history of bleeding
- Potential interaction with anticoagulants (warfarin), aspirin, NSAIDs, anti-platelet agents, methotrexate
- Discontinue use prior to dental or surgical procedures (14 days before)

Cat's Claw
- Contraindicated in transplant recipients, individuals receiving I.V. immuno-globulins or immunosuppressants
- Contraindicated in active bleeding (eg, peptic ulcer, intracranial bleeding)
- Caution in hemostatic disorders/history of bleeding
- Potential interaction with anticoagulants (warfarin), aspirin, NSAIDs, anti-platelet agents
- Discontinue use prior to dental or surgical procedures (14 days before)

Turmeric
- Caution in biliary obstruction
- Contraindicated in ulcerative gastrointestinal disease (eg, peptic ulcer disease, ulcerative colitis, Crohn's)
- Contraindicated in active bleeding (eg, peptic ulcer, intracranial bleeding)
- Caution in hemostatic disorders/history of bleeding
- Potential interaction with anticoagulants (warfarin), aspirin, NSAIDs, anti-platelet agents
- Discontinue use prior to dental or surgical procedures (14 days before)

Chondroitin Sulfate
- No reported toxicity in humans at normal intakes

Glucosamine Hydrochloride/Sulfate
- Theoretically, may alter glucose control in individuals with diabetes

Methyl Sulfonyl Methane
- No reported toxicity in humans at normal intakes

SAMe (S-adenosylmethionine)
- Use caution when combining SAMe with other antidepressants

Collagen
- No reported toxicity in humans at normal intakes

Boron
- No reported toxicity in humans at normal intakes

ARTHRITIS (RHEUMATOID)

Rheumatoid arthritis is a chronic inflammatory autoimmune disease that is characterized by widespread, chronic synovial inflammation of the joints. It follows a highly variable course with progressive deformity leading to a loss of function. Rheumatoid arthritis includes a variant that has its onset in adolescence (juvenile rheumatoid arthritis).

Autoimmune inflammation may involve many organ systems, including the lungs, heart, nervous system, eyes, hematologic system, and skin. Classically, joint symptoms are characterized by stiffness that increases during periods of rest or immobility, improving with movement. Usually, it affects joints on both sides of the body simultaneously and is often localized to the metacarpophalangeal joint (a joint seldom affected by osteoarthritis). Significant deformity is caused by severe inflammation of the lining of the joint and breakdown of normal tissue structure.

Treatment may involve pain management, reduction of inflammation, protection of the affected joints (splints and assist devices), surgery, and modification of the immune response.

LIFESTYLE RECOMMENDATIONS

- Continuation/initiation of diet and exercise program; exercise program should be supervised by qualified healthcare provider

- Determine if a candidate for splints or prosthesis of any kind

- Understand the use of heat and cold

- Avoid stressing the affected joints

RHEUMATOID ARTHRITIS DECISION TREE

1. Client with rheumatoid arthritis is interested in using natural products (NP) to support this condition

2. Healthcare provider requests basic background information. The following issues are addressed with the client:

* Allergies?
* Prescription (Rx)/OTC meds?
* Natural products?
* Other medical conditions?
* Nutrition/diet program?
* Exercise program?

3. Above data reviewed; if **yes** to Rx/OTC meds, review **Drug-Induced Nutrient Depletion Chart** in Appendix

4A. Client is a candidate for natural products

* An appropriate homeopathic remedy can be used at any time

4B. Client's case is too complicated at this point; needs additional support from MD before initiating NP program

5. Condition-specific questions:
* Any triggers that worsen symptoms?
* Describe specific symptoms with regards to joints involved, for how long, etc
* Describe effectiveness of other interventions

6. See table on following page

ARTHRITIS (RHEUMATOID) *(Continued)*

ARTHRITIS (RHEUMATOID)*

Category	Natural Products to Consider	DOC
Herb	Cat's Claw *on page 404*	HT
	Boswellia *on page 397*	HT
	Devil's Claw *on page 422*	HD
	Evening Primrose *on page 430*	HT
	Turmeric *on page 512*	HT
	Bromelain *on page 399*	PA
Vitamin/Mineral/ Trace Element/ Nutraceutical	Shark Cartilage *on page 503* Condition-specific dosage: 3000 mg 3 times/day	HD
	Methyl Sulfonyl Methane (MSM) *on page 479* Condition-specific dosage: 2000-5000 mg/day	HD
	Collagen *on page 414* Condition-specific dosage: 200 mg 3 times/day	HT
	Chondroitin Sulfate *on page 410* Condition-specific dosage: 300-1500 mg **WITH** Glucosamine Sulfate *on page 446* Condition-specific dosage: 1500-2000 mg/day **OR** Glucosamine Hydrochloride *on page 446* Condition-specific dosage: 1000-2000 mg/day	PA
	Vitamin B$_5$ (Pantothenic Acid) *on page 522* Condition-specific dosage: 500 mg twice daily	
	Vitamin E *on page 529* Condition-specific dosage: Up to 800 int. units/day	
	Copper Salicylate *on page 416* Condition-specific dosage: 64 mg 1-2 times/day	
Homeopathic Remedy	Homeopathic combination formulas are available for many conditions. Listed below are some of the most common single homeopathic remedies for rheumatoid arthritis. Also see **Homeopathic Quick Reference Chart for Common Complaints** *on page 587*	
	Apis mellifica	PD
	Arnica montana	PD
	Causticum	PD
	Colchicum autumnale	PD
	Ledum palustre	PD
	Rhus toxicodendron	PD
Additional supplements to consider	Boron *on page 397* Condition-specific dosage: 3-6 mg/day	PA
	Fish Oils *on page 434* Condition-specific dosage: 750 mg 2-3 times/day **OR** Flaxseed Oil *on page 435* Condition-specific dosage: 1 Tbsp/day	PA

*Refer to **Introduction to Conditions** *on page 41* for more details on how to apply the information in this table to individuals with this condition.

SPECIAL CONSIDERATIONS

Cat's Claw
- Contraindicated in transplant recipients, individuals receiving I.V. immunoglobulins or immunosuppressants; in active bleeding (eg, peptic ulcer, intracranial bleeding)
- Caution in hemostatic disorders/history of bleeding
- Potential interaction with anticoagulants (warfarin), aspirin, NSAIDs, antiplatelet agents
- Discontinue use prior to dental or surgical procedures (14 days before)

Boswellia – No reported toxicity in humans at normal intakes

Devil's Claw
- Contraindicated in pregnancy and breast-feeding
- Caution in individuals with GI disease (eg, peptic ulcer, inflammatory bowel disease); asthma, edema, or CHF

Evening Primrose
- Contraindicated in seizure disorders, schizophrenia, or in persons receiving anticonvulsant or antipsychotic medications; in active bleeding (eg, peptic ulcer, intracranial bleeding)
- Caution in hemostatic disorders/history of bleeding
- Potential interaction with anticoagulants (warfarin), aspirin, NSAIDs, antiplatelet agents
- Discontinue use prior to dental or surgical procedures (14 days before)

Turmeric – See Arthritis (Osteo) *on page 60*

Bromelain
- Contraindicated in active bleeding (eg, peptic ulcer, intracranial bleeding)
- Potential interaction with anticoagulants (warfarin), aspirin, NSAIDs, antiplatelet agents
- Caution in individuals with GI ulceration and/or cardiovascular disorders (hypertension); in hemostatic disorders/history of bleeding
- Discontinue use prior to dental or surgical procedures (14 days before)

Shark Cartilage – May cause gastrointestinal upset (nausea)

Methyl Sulfonyl Methane – No reported toxicity in humans at normal intakes

Collagen – No reported toxicity in humans at normal intakes

Chondroitin Sulfate – No reported toxicity in humans at normal intakes

Glucosamine Hydrochloride/Sulfate – Theoretically, may alter glucose control in individuals with diabetes

Vitamin B$_5$ (Pantothenic Acid) – No reported toxicity in humans at normal intakes

Vitamin E
- Use with caution when taking anticoagulants (vitamin E ≥200 int. units increases prothrombin times)
- Interrupt or reduce dosage one week prior to dental or surgical procedures

Copper Salicylate – Contraindicated in Wilson's disease

Boron – No reported toxicity in humans at normal intakes

Fish Oils
- High doses may cause GI upset, loose stools, nausea
- May alter glucose regulation; use with caution in diabetes
- Caution in individuals receiving oral hypoglycemics or insulin; monitor blood glucose closely and coordinate with prescriber
- Potential interaction with anticoagulants (warfarin), aspirin, NSAIDs, antiplatelet agents

Flaxseed Oil – No reported toxicity in humans at normal intakes

ASTHMA

Asthma is a chronic, inflammatory lung disease in which spasms of the bronchial passages restrict the flow of air in and out of the lungs. Approximately 5% of the United States population is affected (14-15 million people).

A key feature of the disease is a hyper-responsiveness of the airways to various triggering stimuli, which cause the airways to react to irritation with severe bronchospasm and inflammation. Symptoms include wheezing, shortness of breath, and tachycardia. Nighttime awakenings are common.

Triggers of an asthmatic episode include a wide variety of environmental substances, allergens, cold, exercise, nutrient deficiency, food intolerance, digestive incompetence, emotional factors, infection, and drugs (such as NSAIDs). A variety of classification schemes have been based on an ability to identify the trigger or the severity of symptoms. The currently accepted classification of asthma emphasizes only the degree of airflow limitation (mild-moderate-severe) and the persistence of these changes (persistent versus intermittent).

Deterioration in airflow may precede overt symptoms. This has prompted an increased use of self-monitoring, using peak flow (PF) meters to adjust therapy and address inflammation prior to dramatic deterioration in symptoms. This approach has demonstrated an ability to reduce hospitalizations, loss of productivity, cost of care, physician office appointments, and emergency room visits.

Of children with asthma, between 30% to 70% will demonstrate substantial improvement in symptoms as they mature. Only about 30% of individuals will have chronic disease, although a predisposition to airway irritability may persist. Lung tissue is usually normal in appearance during the periods between exacerbations, so deterioration in lung function over time is uncommon.

LIFESTYLE RECOMMENDATIONS

- Continuation/initiation of home peak flow monitoring, diet, and exercise programs

- Follow self-management program established with physician and know target PF readings, when to call the physician, when to go to the emergency department, etc

- Keep a diary of important events leading to improvement/worsening

- Investigate possibility of improving filtering system in home heating/cooling and air system

- Address mattress/pillow covers, pets, carpeting, etc

- Drink plenty of water

- Investigate other potential immune-triggering agents in the home (eg, cleaning products, outgassing of new flooring, etc)

ASTHMA DECISION TREE

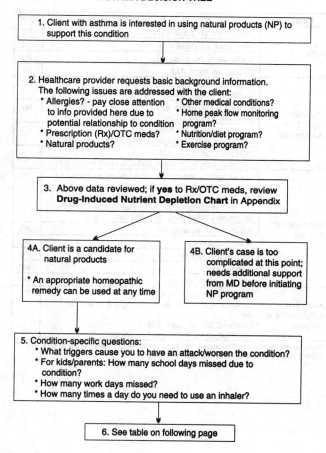

1. Client with asthma is interested in using natural products (NP) to support this condition

2. Healthcare provider requests basic background information. The following issues are addressed with the client:
   * Allergies? - pay close attention to info provided here due to potential relationship to condition
   * Prescription (Rx)/OTC meds?
   * Natural products?
   * Other medical conditions?
   * Home peak flow monitoring program?
   * Nutrition/diet program?
   * Exercise program?

3. Above data reviewed; if **yes** to Rx/OTC meds, review **Drug-Induced Nutrient Depletion Chart** in Appendix

4A. Client is a candidate for natural products
   * An appropriate homeopathic remedy can be used at any time

4B. Client's case is too complicated at this point; needs additional support from MD before initiating NP program

5. Condition-specific questions:
   * What triggers cause you to have an attack/worsen the condition?
   * For kids/parents: How many school days missed due to condition?
   * How many work days missed?
   * How many times a day do you need to use an inhaler?

6. See table on following page

ASTHMA *(Continued)*

ASTHMA*

Category	Natural Products to Consider	DOC
Herb	Cordyceps *on page 417*	PA
	Tylophora *on page 513*	HT
	Grape Seed *on page 451*	PA
	Coleus *on page 413*	HT
Vitamin/Mineral/ Trace Element/ Nutraceutical	Magnesium *on page 473* Condition-specific dosage: 400-600 mg/day	HT
	Vitamin B₆ *on page 523* Condition-specific dosage: 10-20 mg/day	HT
	Vitamin C *on page 526* Condition-specific dosage: 500-1000 mg twice daily	HT
	Quercetin *on page 494* Condition-specific dosage: 300–400 mg 3 times/day	PA
Homeopathic Remedy	Homeopathic combination formulas are available for many conditions. Listed below are some of the most common single homeopathic remedies for asthma. Also see **Homeopathic Quick Reference Chart for Common Complaints** *on page 587*	
	Antimonium tartaricum	PD
	Aralia racemosa	PD
	Arsenicum album	PD
	Ipecacuanha	PD
	Natrum sulphuricum	PD
Additional supplements to consider	Fish Oils *on page 434* Condition-specific dosage: 750 mg 2-3 times/day **OR** Flaxseed Oil *on page 435* Condition-specific dosage: 1 Tbsp/day	PA

*Refer to **Introduction to Conditions** *on page 41* for more details on how to apply the information in this table to individuals with this condition.

SPECIAL CONSIDERATIONS

Cordyceps

- Caution if allergic to molds or fungi, and in hemostatic disorders/history of bleeding
- Theoretical interaction in individuals receiving MAO inhibitors
- Contraindicated in active bleeding (eg, peptic ulcer, intracranial bleeding)
- Potential interaction with anticoagulants (warfarin), aspirin, NSAIDs, antiplatelet agents
- Discontinue use prior to dental or surgical procedures (14 days before)

Tylophora

- Caution in diabetes, fluid retention, edema, or CHF
- Until further studies are conducted, contraindicated in serious infection, organ transplant recipients, major systemic disease, or recent major surgery
- Theoretical interaction with bronchodilator medications, corticosteroids, oral hypoglycemics, beta-blockers, beta-agonists, sympathomimetics, leukotriene modifiers

Grape Seed

- Contraindicated in active bleeding (eg, peptic ulcer, intracranial bleeding)
- Caution in hemostatic disorders/history of bleeding
- Potential interaction with anticoagulants (warfarin), aspirin, NSAIDs, antiplatelet agents, methotrexate
- Discontinue use prior to dental or surgical procedures (14 days before)

Coleus

- Contraindicated in active bleeding (eg, peptic ulcer, intracranial bleeding)
- May cause hypotension; use with caution in cerebrovascular or cardiovascular disease
- Caution in hemostatic disorders/history of bleeding
- Potential interaction with anticoagulants (warfarin), aspirin, NSAIDs, antiplatelet agents, antihistamines, decongestants, antihypertensives
- Discontinue use prior to dental or surgical procedures (14 days before)

Magnesium

- Use caution in renal impairment
- May cause diarrhea

Vitamin B_6

- No reported toxicity in humans at normal intakes

Vitamin C

- Excess intake in diabetics may give falsely elevated blood glucose readings

Quercetin

- No reported toxicity in humans at normal intakes

Fish Oils

- High doses may cause GI upset, loose stools, nausea
- May alter glucose regulation; use with caution in diabetes
- Caution in individuals receiving oral hypoglycemics or insulin; monitor blood glucose closely and coordinate with prescriber
- Potential interaction with anticoagulants (warfarin), aspirin, NSAIDs, antiplatelet agents

Flaxseed Oil

- No reported toxicity in humans at normal intakes

ATHLETE'S FOOT (TINEA PEDIS) / JOCK ITCH (TINEA CRURIS)

Athlete's Foot (Tinea Pedis)

This disease is the most common fungal infection of the skin, affecting >80% of men in their lifetime. The infection is localized between the toes and on the plantar surfaces of the foot, and is characterized by an odorous rash often accompanied by burning, stinging, and itching. Occasionally, the inflammation is severe and blistering may occur.

The fungi that cause athlete's foot thrive in moist, warm environments. For this reason, the occurrence may be associated with hot weather and wearing shoes that do not allow the feet to "breathe." Individuals with a previous fungal infection, adult men, individuals whose feet perspire, and persons with a weakened immune system are at greater risk of infection. Transmission occurs via direct contact, most commonly from walking barefoot over wet floors around swimming pools, locker rooms, and public showers contaminated with the fungus.

Jock Itch (Tinea Cruris)

The symptoms of jock itch are redness, itching, and scaling in the groin and thigh area. The same fungus that causes athlete's foot usually causes jock itch. Jock itch can also result from a bacterial infection, reactions to chemicals in clothing, irritating garments, or exposure to some medications. Despite its name, the affliction is not restricted to males. Under similar conditions, women can also develop this problem.

Self-care recommendations for both conditions include cleansing the affected area repeatedly and drying thoroughly (twice daily if possible), daily change of clothes (socks or underwear), and use of cotton clothing for better absorption of moisture. The use of deodorant soaps is not recommended; the application of talc or other powders may help to keep these areas dry.

LIFESTYLE RECOMMENDATIONS

- Jock itch: Use towels once; wear clean cotton undergarments; wash clothes in hot water; take extra precautions if you have diabetes, asthma, or are overweight

- Athlete's foot: Keep feet clean; wash socks after wearing once; do not walk barefoot in gym, shower, or pool area; do not wear occlusive footwear

- Remove refined sugars and refined carbohydrates from diet

ATHLETE'S FOOT / JOCK ITCH DECISION TREE

1. Client with athlete's foot / jock itch is interested in using natural products (NP) to support this condition

2. Healthcare provider requests basic background information.
   The following issues are addressed with the client:
   * Allergies?
   * Prescription (Rx)/OTC meds?
   * Natural products?
   * Other medical conditions?
   * Nutrition/diet program?
   * Exercise program?

3. Above data reviewed; if **yes** to Rx/OTC meds, review **Drug-Induced Nutrient Depletion Chart** in Appendix

4A. Client is a candidate for natural products

   * An appropriate homeopathic remedy can be used at any time

4B. Client's case is too complicated at this point; needs additional support from MD before initiating NP program

5. Condition-specific questions:
   Present symptoms, situation to be addressed:
   Jock itch:
   * How often do you work out? Do you use a different towel after each shower?
   Athlete's foot:
   * Is there nail involvement? Any odor? Serious inflammation? Oozing vesicles, whitish color between toes? **Yes?** - Refer to MD
   * Any specific climate/environmental conditions that contribute to development? Barefoot in pool/shower area? Wear occlusive footwear?

6. See table on following page

ATHLETE'S FOOT (TINEA PEDIS) / JOCK ITCH (TINEA CRURIS) *(Continued)*

ATHLETE'S FOOT (Tinea pedis) / JOCK ITCH (Tinea cruris)*

Category	Natural Products to Consider	DOC
Herb	Cat's Claw *on page 404*	PA
	Tea Tree (Topical) *on page 509*	PA
	Olive Leaf *on page 483*	PA
	Garlic *on page 438*	PA
Vitamin/Mineral/ Trace Element/ Nutraceutical	*Lactobacillus acidophilus on page 467* and *Bifidobacterium bifidum on page 391* Condition-specific dosage: 10-15 billion CFU twice daily for 2 weeks, then 1-2 billion CFU twice daily with food for 2 months (dairy free)	PA
	Zinc, Undecylenate *on page 534* Condition-specific dosage: Powder: Use topically	PA
Homeopathic Remedy	Homeopathic combination formulas are available for many conditions. Listed below are some of the most common single homeopathic remedies for athlete's foot/jock itch. Also see **Homeopathic Quick Reference Chart for Common Complaints** *on page 587*	
	Agaricus muscarius	PD
	Arsenicum iodatum	PD
	Borax	PD
	Lycopodium clavatum	PD
Additional supplements to consider	No recommendations	

*Refer to **Introduction to Conditions** *on page 41* for more details on how to apply the information in this table to individuals with this condition.

SPECIAL CONSIDERATIONS

Cat's Claw
- Contraindicated in transplant recipients, individuals receiving I.V. immunoglobulins or immunosuppressants
- Contraindicated in active bleeding (eg, peptic ulcer, intracranial bleeding)
- Caution in hemostatic disorders/history of bleeding
- Potential interaction with anticoagulants (warfarin), aspirin, NSAIDs, antiplatelet agents
- Discontinue use prior to dental or surgical procedures (14 days before)

Tea Tree
- May cause allergic dermatitis in sensitive individuals
- Not for ingestion

Olive Leaf
- No reported toxicity in humans at normal intakes

Garlic
- Contraindicated in active bleeding (eg, peptic ulcer, intracranial bleeding)
- Caution in hemostatic disorders/history of bleeding
- Discontinue use prior to dental or surgical procedures (14 days before)
- Caution in individuals at risk due to hypotension or orthostasis (elderly, cerebrovascular or cardiovascular disease)
- Potential interaction with anticoagulants (warfarin), aspirin, NSAIDs, antiplatelet agents, hypolipidemics, antihypertensives
- Caution in diabetes

Lactobacillus acidophilus
- No known toxicity or serious side effects

Bifidobacterium bifidum
- No known toxicity or serious side effects

Zinc, Undecylenate
- No known toxicity or serious side effects

ATTENTION DEFICIT DISORDER (ADD) / ATTENTION DEFICIT HYPERACTIVITY DISORDER (ADHD)

Attention deficit disorder (ADD) is characterized by disorganized, nonproductive, inappropriate behavior, unusual sleeping patterns, and/or over-reaction to stimuli. ADD may or may not be accompanied by hyperactivity. Attention deficit hyperactivity disorder (ADHD) is characterized by a persistent pattern of inattention, hyperactivity, or impulsiveness that may occur in a variety of settings. In the United States, both disorders are diagnosed according to criteria specified in the *Diagnostic and Statistical Manual of Mental Disorders 4th Edition (DSM-IV)*.

Problems with attention include making careless mistakes, failing to complete tasks, problems with organization, and a tendency to be easily distracted. Hyperactivity can include excessive fidgeting, squirming, running, or climbing when it is not appropriate. There is a tendency for excessive talking and the individual may appear to be in constant motion. Impulsivity may be exhibited as impatience, difficulty waiting their turn, blurting out answers, or frequent interruption of others. Although many individuals with ADHD display both inattentive and hyperactive/impulsive symptoms, some individuals show symptoms from one group but not the other.

The exact cause of ADD/ADHD remains uncertain, but some forms may have a hereditary basis, and they appear to affect boys more often than girls. Children with ADD may develop low self-esteem, high levels of frustration, noncompliance, and aggressive behavior. Often, the child has poor peer relationships. The age of onset may be as early as 2 or 3 years, but usually children are not diagnosed until they enter an academic setting. Many adults also have ADD and may have experienced difficulties for many years without diagnosis.

Factors that may be evaluated in ADD and ADHD include: Magnesium status, hyperinsulinemia, heavy metal toxicity, and a history of extensive antibiotic use, dysbiosis, and fatty acid deficiency. Several studies have reported beneficial effects for children with ADD / ADHD when refined sugars, food additives, and dyes were reduced or eliminated and the quality of food selection, including fresh vegetables, was improved.

LIFESTYLE RECOMMENDATIONS

- Continuation/initiation of diet and exercise programs
- Reduce or eliminate refined sugars, food additives, and dyes
- Watch for changes in appetite and sleep patterns
- Monitor for behavior changes
- Keep in touch with teachers
- Keep on a schedule
- Provide positive reinforcement

**ATTENTION DEFICIT DISORDER (ADD) /
ATTENTION DEFICIT HYPERACTIVITY DISORDER (ADHD)
DECISION TREE**

1. Client with ADD/ADHD is interested in using natural products (NP) to support this condition

2. Healthcare provider requests basic background information.
   The following issues are addressed with the client:
   * Allergies?
   * Prescription (Rx)/OTC meds?
   * Natural products?
   * Other medical conditions?
   * Nutrition/diet program?
   * Exercise program?

3. Above data reviewed; if **yes** to Rx/OTC meds, review **Drug-Induced Nutrient Depletion Chart** in Appendix

4A. Client is a candidate for natural products

   * An appropriate homeopathic remedy can be used at any time

4B. Client's case is too complicated at this point; needs additional support from MD before initiating NP program

5. Condition-specific questions:
   * Has the MD established evaluation tools to monitor progress?
     If no, refer (back) to MD
   * If child, how is the teacher involved in monitoring?
   * How does the condition affect quality of life, home life? If appears significant, refer (back) to MD
   * Any triggers that cause worsening of condition? If appear significant and unresponsive to therapy, refer (back) to MD
   * Any meds that may contribute to worsening: Antihistamines, decongestants? If YES, recommend discussing discontinuing with MD
   * If pharmacologic intervention, how is client being monitored for AE (changes in appetite, tics, etc)? Recommend client/parent discuss with MD
   * If pharmacologic intervention for at least a year, any drug holidays? If NO, recommend client/parent discuss with MD

6. See table on following page

ATTENTION DEFICIT DISORDER (ADD) / ATTENTION DEFICIT HYPERACTIVITY DISORDER (ADHD) *(Continued)*

ADD / ADHD*

Category	Natural Products to Consider	DOC
Herb	Grape Seed *on page 451*	PA
	Kava Kava *on page 466*	PA
	Olive Leaf *on page 483*	PA
	Evening Primrose *on page 430*	HD
	Grapefruit Seed Extract *on page 450*	PA
Vitamin/Mineral/ Trace Element/ Nutraceutical	*Lactobacillus acidophilus on page 467* and *Bifidobacterium bifidum on page 391* Condition-specific dosage: 2-5 billion CFU daily for 1 month	HD
	Docosahexaenoic Acid (DHA) *on page 424* Condition-specific dosage: 200-500 mg/day (children <12 years); 500-1000 mg/day (adults)	PA
	Chromium *on page 410* Condition-specific dosage: 200-400 mcg/day	PA
	Magnesium *on page 473* Condition-specific dosage: 400 mg/day (children <12 years); 400-600 mg/day (adults)	HT
Homeopathic Remedy	Homeopathic combination formulas are available for many conditions. Listed below are some of the most common single homeopathic remedies for ADD/ADHD. Also see **Homeopathic Quick Reference Chart for Common Complaints** *on page 587*	
	Agaricus muscarius	PD
	Baryta carbonica	PD
	Hyoscyamus niger	PD
	Stramonium	PD
	Tarentula hispana	PD
Additional supplements to consider	No recommendations	

*Refer to **Introduction to Conditions** *on page 41* for more details on how to apply the information in this table to individuals with this condition.

SPECIAL CONSIDERATIONS

Grape Seed

- Contraindicated in active bleeding (eg, peptic ulcer, intracranial bleeding)
- Caution in hemostatic disorders/history of bleeding
- Potential interaction with anticoagulants (warfarin), aspirin, NSAIDs, anti-platelet agents, methotrexate
- Discontinue use prior to dental or surgical procedures (14 days before)

Kava Kava

- Contraindicated in pregnancy and breast-feeding, or Parkinson's disease
- May cause drowsiness or sedation (higher doses); caution when driving/ performing hazardous tasks
- Potential interactions with ethanol, CNS depressants (benzodiazepines, antidepressants, sedative-hypnotics)

Olive Leaf

- No reported toxicity in humans at normal intakes

Evening Primrose

- Contraindicated in seizure disorders, schizophrenia, or in persons receiving anticonvulsant or antipsychotic medications
- Contraindicated in active bleeding (eg, peptic ulcer, intracranial bleeding)
- Caution in hemostatic disorders/history of bleeding
- Potential interaction with anticoagulants (warfarin), aspirin, NSAIDs, anti-platelet agents
- Discontinue use prior to dental or surgical procedures (14 days before)

Grapefruit Seed Extract

- Grapefruit seed extract is not equivalent to grapefruit juice/pulp. Juice/pulp has been associated with many drug interactions; see Grapefruit Seed *on page 450*
- Until further information is available, it is reasonable to avoid some medications (terfenadine, astemizole, cisapride). Use other medications metabolized by CYP3A4 with caution.

Lactobacillus acidophilus

- No known toxicity or serious side effects

Bifidobacterium bifidum

- No known toxicity or serious side effects

Docosahexaenoic Acid (DHA)

- Contraindicated in active bleeding (eg, peptic ulcer, intracranial bleeding)
- Caution in hemostatic disorders/history of bleeding
- Potential interaction with anticoagulants (warfarin), aspirin, NSAIDs, anti-platelet agents
- Discontinue use prior to dental or surgical procedures (14 days before)

Chromium

- Caution in individuals receiving oral hypoglycemics or insulin; monitor blood glucose closely and coordinate with prescriber

Magnesium

- Use caution in renal impairment
- May cause diarrhea at high intakes

BENIGN PROSTATIC HYPERTROPHY (BPH)

Benign prostatic hypertrophy or hyperplasia (BPH) is a noncancerous increase in the mass of the prostate gland. More than 50% of all men >60 years of age have BPH. By age 80, about 8 out of 10 men have it. Fewer than 50% of all men with BPH exhibit symptoms of the disease.

Common symptoms of BPH involve difficulty in urination, including difficulty initiating or straining at the start of the urine stream, interruption or weakness in the urine stream, dribbling at the end of urination, a sense of incomplete emptying, and increased frequency, urgency, or frequent awakenings at night to urinate. As the prostate enlarges, it impinges upon the urethra, causing narrowing and difficulty in urination.

Although BPH does not cause cancer, some men may have BPH and prostatic carcinoma concurrently. If BPH is left untreated, surgery will ultimately be required. Current evidence suggests that an increase in the conversion of testosterone to dihydrotestosterone (DHT) and a decrease in the testosterone/ estrogen ratio play a major role in stimulating prostate enlargement.

Cancer should be excluded by prostatic exam and laboratory studies (PSA) prior to using natural products for symptoms of BPH. Possible reduction in symptoms involves the use of substances that inhibit the conversion of testosterone to DHT and/or block DHT's activity, as well as the use of phytoestrogens to block endogenous estrogen binding.

LIFESTYLE RECOMMENDATIONS

- Continuation/initiation of diet and exercise program

- Avoid decongestants and other medications with alpha-adrenergic, anticholinergic activity

- Avoid consuming large amounts of water after evening meal

- If antibiotics are needed, recommend *Lactobacillus/Bifidobacterium*

- Eliminate tobacco, alcohol, caffeine, spicy foods

BENIGN PROSTATIC HYPERTROPHY (BPH)
DECISION TREE

1. Client with BPH is interested in using natural products (NP) to support this condition

2. Healthcare provider requests basic background information. The following issues are addressed with the client:
   * Allergies?
   * Prescription (Rx)/OTC meds?
   * Natural products?
   * Other medical conditions?
   * Nutrition/diet program?
   * Exercise program?

3. Above data reviewed; if **yes** to Rx/OTC meds, review **Drug-Induced Nutrient Depletion Chart** in Appendix

4A. Client is a candidate for natural products

   * An appropriate homeopathic remedy can be used at any time

4B. Client's case is too complicated at this point; needs additional support from MD before initiating NP program

5. Condition-specific questions:
   * Has this condition been diagnosed by MD? If no, refer client to MD for specific testing (ie, PSA)
   * If symptoms interfere with normal activity, client should be referred to MD in addition to natural products
   * If client taking prescription meds for BPH, recommend taking at bedtime

6. See table on following page

BENIGN PROSTATIC HYPERTROPHY (BPH) *(Continued)*

BENIGN PROSTATIC HYPERTROPHY (BPH)*

Category	Natural Products to Consider	DOC
Herb	Saw Palmetto *on page 500*	HT
	Pygeum *on page 493*	HT
	Stinging Nettle (Root) *on page 505*	HT
Vitamin/Mineral/ Trace Element/ Nutraceutical	Isoflavones *on page 465* Condition-specific dosage: 100-400 mg/day	PA
	Lycopene *on page 472* Condition-specific dosage: 5 mg twice daily	PA
	Fish Oils *on page 434* Condition-specific dosage: 750 mg twice daily	HT
	Zinc *on page 534* Condition-specific dosage: 15-35 mg/day	HT
Homeopathic Remedy	Homeopathic combination formulas are available for many conditions. Listed below are some of the most common single homeopathic remedies for BPH. Also see **Homeopathic Quick Reference Chart for Common Complaints** *on page 587*	
	Apis mellifica	PD
	Sabal serrulata	PD
	Thuja occidentalis	PD
Additional supplements to consider	Vitamin E *on page 529* Condition-specific dosage: 400 int. units/day	HD

*Refer to **Introduction to Conditions** *on page 41* for more details on how to apply the information in this table to individuals with this condition.

SPECIAL CONSIDERATIONS

Saw Palmetto
- No reported toxicity in humans at normal intakes

Pygeum
- No reported toxicity in humans at normal intakes

Stinging Nettle
- No reported toxicity in humans at normal intakes

Isoflavones
- Caution in estrogen-dependent tumors, endometrial cancer
- Women who are taking estrogen-containing medications (oral contraceptives, hormonal replacement) should consult their physician prior to use

Lycopene
- No reported toxicity in humans at normal intakes

Fish Oils
- High doses may cause GI upset, loose stools, nausea
- May alter glucose regulation; use with caution in diabetes
- Caution in individuals receiving oral hypoglycemics or insulin; monitor blood glucose closely and coordinate with prescriber
- Potential interaction with anticoagulants (warfarin), aspirin, NSAIDs, antiplatelet agents

Zinc
- No known toxicity or serious side effects

Vitamin E
- Use with caution when taking anticoagulants (vitamin E ≥200 int. units increases prothrombin times)
- Interrupt or reduce dosage one week prior to dental or surgical procedures

BREAST-FEEDING

Breast milk contains many nutrients and natural immunity factors that cannot be duplicated in formulas. Breast-fed babies tend to have less gastrointestinal problems, including constipation, diarrhea, and odor. Breast-feeding also provides the baby with antibodies that help fight infection. In addition, it offers a special closeness that strengthens the psychological and emotional bonding between mother and child.

It has been learned that mother's milk also contains substances that promote the growth and proliferation of beneficial bacteria in the baby's gastrointestinal tract. Proper gastrointestinal microflora play an important role in the digestion and absorption of nutrients as well as promoting a healthy immune system.

Breast-feeding may be inconvenient, particularly for mothers who work outside the home. A nursing mother should recognize that her diet may affect the baby. In particular, a healthcare provider should be consulted when taking medication or drinking alcohol.

LIFESTYLE RECOMMENDATIONS

- Continuation/initiation of exercise program; diet should be monitored by healthcare specialist
- Drink plenty of fluids
- Rest whenever possible
- If heat is necessary to express milk, use a heating pad or hot water bottle
- Do not abruptly discontinue breast-feeding; this could cause problems with the ducts. If interested in doing this, physician evaluation is necessary.

BREAST-FEEDING DECISION TREE

1. Client who is breast-feeding is interested in using natural products (NP) to support this condition

2. Healthcare provider requests basic background information. The following issues are addressed with the client:

   * Allergies?   * Other medical conditions?
   * Prescription (Rx)/OTC meds?   * Nutrition/diet program?
   * Natural products?   * Exercise program?

3. Above data reviewed; if **yes** to Rx/OTC meds, review **Drug-Induced Nutrient Depletion Chart** in Appendix

4A. Client is a candidate for natural products

   * An appropriate homeopathic remedy can be used at any time

4B. Client's case is too complicated at this point; needs additional support from MD before initiating NP program

5. Condition-specific questions:
   * Any problems with excessively sore nipples?
     If **yes,** may be sign of infection - refer to MD
   * Any problems with consistent breast-feeding?
     If **yes,** possibly refer to lactation consultant specialist

6. See table on following page

BREAST-FEEDING *(Continued)*

BREAST-FEEDING*

Category	Natural Products to Consider	DOC
Herb	**Chasteberry/Vitex** (Short-term use) *on page 408*	HE
Vitamin/Mineral/ Trace Element/ Nutraceutical	**Fish Oils** *on page 434* Condition-specific dosage: 750 mg capsule 2-3 times/ day	PA
Homeopathic Remedy	Homeopathic combination formulas are available for many conditions. Listed below are some of the most common single homeopathic remedies for breast-feeding. Also see **Homeopathic Quick Reference Chart for Common Complaints** *on page 587*	
	Cinchona officinalis (China)	PD
	Pulsatilla	PD
Additional supplements to consider	No recommendations	

*Refer to **Introduction to Conditions** *on page 41* for more details on how to apply the information in this table to individuals with this condition.

SPECIAL CONSIDERATIONS

Chasteberry/Vitex
- Contraindicated in pregnancy
- Potential interaction with hormonal replacements or oral contraceptives

Fish Oils
- High doses may cause GI upset, loose stools, nausea
- May alter glucose regulation; use with caution in diabetes
- Caution in individuals receiving oral hypoglycemics or insulin; monitor blood glucose closely and coordinate with prescriber
- Potential interaction with anticoagulants (warfarin), aspirin, NSAIDs, anti-platelet agents

CANDIDIASIS

Candidiasis is an infection caused by a fungus of the genus *Candida* (especially *Candida albicans*). It is commonly referred to as a yeast infection. Superficial infections of the vagina or skin are common and generally not severe. However, systemic infection with this organism, particularly in immunocompromised individuals, may be severe and potentially life-threatening.

Vaginal yeast infections may be a major source of discomfort for women. Symptoms include burning and itching, sometimes accompanied by a thick, white discharge, and redness of the vaginal tissues due to localized inflammation. Individuals with diabetes and women who are pregnant or menstruating are at increased risk. In addition, individuals who are receiving an antibiotic, oral contraceptives, or immunosuppressants such as corticosteroids are more susceptible. The risk of yeast infections may be limited by good personal hygiene, wearing cotton undergarments, avoiding snug-fitting clothing, and limiting dietary intake of sugar.

It should be noted that males may be asymptomatic carriers of the fungus. A frequent pattern of reinfection should prompt additional individual evaluation and/or treatment of the sexual partner.

LIFESTYLE RECOMMENDATIONS

- Continuation/initiation of diet and exercise program
- Increase intake of fresh vegetables
- Can increase intake of *Lactobacillus*- fortified yogurt
- Avoid refined sugars and refined carbohydrates
- Avoid wheat
- Avoid fermented foods

CANDIDIASIS DECISION TREE

1. Client with candidiasis is interested in using natural products (NP) to support this condition

2. Healthcare provider requests basic background information.
   The following issues are addressed with the client:

   * Allergies?
   * Prescription (Rx)/OTC meds?
   * Natural products?
   * Other medical conditions?
   * Nutrition/diet program?
   * Exercise program?

3. Above data reviewed; if **yes** to Rx/OTC meds, review **Drug-Induced Nutrient Depletion Chart** in Appendix

4A. Client is a candidate for natural products

   * An appropriate homeopathic remedy can be used at any time

4B. Client's case is too complicated at this point; needs additional support from MD before initiating NP program

5. Condition-specific questions:
   * Do you have a history of antibiotic use, oral contraceptive or corticosteroid use, immunosuppressant agents, chemotherapy or radiation?
   * Have you been exposed to heavy metals, pesticides, or other industrial toxins?
   * Is your diet high in refined sugars, carbs?
   * Was condition diagnosed by MD? If **yes,** what were the recommendations? If **no,** refer to MD.
   * Is this the first episode of this type of infection? If **no,** what was used in the past? Outcome?
   * Any recent course of antibiotics? If **yes,** explore details; may be cause.
   * Recent episode of athlete's foot? Jock itch? Nail fungus? If **yes,** obtain details; possible referral to MD.
   * Has client ever used an antifungal agent? If **yes,** what was the outcome? May need again - possible referral to MD.

6. See table on following page

CANDIDIASIS *(Continued)*

CANDIDIASIS*

Category	Natural Products to Consider	DOC
Herb	Olive Leaf *on page 483*	PA
	Grapefruit Seed Extract *on page 450*	PA
	Cat's Claw *on page 404*	PA
	Garlic *on page 438*	PA
Vitamin/Mineral/ Trace Element/ Nutraceutical	*Lactobacillus acidophilus on page 467* and *Bifidobacterium bifidum on page 391* Condition-specific dosage: 10-15 billion CFU twice daily for 2 weeks, then 1-2 billion CFU twice daily with food for 2 months	HT
	Thymus Extract *on page 510* Condition-specific dosage: 250 mg 3 times/day	HT
	Spleen Extract *on page 505* Condition-specific dosage: 150 mg 3 times/day	HD
	Caprylic Acid *on page 402* Condition-specific dosage: 250 mg 3 times/day	HD
Homeopathic Remedy	Homeopathic combination formulas are available for many conditions. Listed below are some of the most common single homeopathic remedies for candidiasis. Also see **Homeopathic Quick Reference Chart for Common Complaints** *on page 587*	
	Agaricus muscarius	PD
	Arsenicum album	PD
	Borax	PD
	Zincum metallicum	PD
Additional supplements to consider	Magnesium *on page 473* Condition-specific dosage: 400-600 mg/day	PA

*Refer to **Introduction to Conditions** *on page 41* for more details on how to apply the information in this table to individuals with this condition.

SPECIAL CONSIDERATIONS

Olive Leaf
- No reported toxicity in humans at normal intakes

Grapefruit Seed Extract
- Grapefruit seed extract is not equivalent to grapefruit juice/pulp. Juice/pulp has been associated with many drug interactions; see Grapefruit Seed *on page 450*
- Until further information is available, it is reasonable to avoid some medications (terfenadine, astemizole, cisapride). Use other medications metabolized by CYP3A4 with caution.

Cat's Claw
- Contraindicated in transplant recipients, individuals receiving I.V. immunoglobulins or immunosuppressants
- Contraindicated in active bleeding (eg, peptic ulcer, intracranial bleeding)
- Caution in hemostatic disorders/history of bleeding
- Potential interaction with anticoagulants (warfarin), aspirin, NSAIDs, antiplatelet agents
- Discontinue use prior to dental or surgical procedures (14 days before)

Garlic
- May cause GI distress or irritation
- Contraindicated in active bleeding (eg, peptic ulcer, intracranial bleeding)
- Caution in hemostatic disorders/history of bleeding
- Discontinue use prior to dental or surgical procedures (14 days before)
- Caution in individuals at risk due to hypotension or orthostasis (elderly, cerebrovascular or cardiovascular disease)
- Potential interaction with anticoagulants (warfarin), aspirin, NSAIDs, antiplatelet agents
- May potentiate antihypertensives, insulin, oral hypoglycemics
- Caution in diabetes

Lactobacillus acidophilus
- No known toxicity or serious side effects

Bifidobacterium bifidum
- No known toxicity or serious side effects

Thymus Extract
- No known toxicity or serious side effects

Spleen Extract
- No known toxicity or serious side effects

Caprylic Acid
- No known toxicity or serious side effects

Magnesium
- Use caution in renal impairment
- May cause diarrhea at high intakes

CATARACTS

Cataracts occur when the lens of the eye becomes cloudy or distorted. About half of Americans 65-75 years of age have some form of cataract. Symptoms include blurred or dimmed vision, poor night vision, and sensitivity to light or glare. Reduced distance vision may also be noted. Individuals may become aware of vision changes only after noticing a need for brighter lighting for reading or a frequent need to change eyeglass prescriptions.

Age is the single greatest risk factor for cataracts. To some extent, nearly everyone >65 years of age has lens clouding. Factors that increase the risk of developing cataracts include diabetes, a family history of cataracts, previous eye injury, corticosteroid use, excessive alcohol consumption, high amounts of exposure to sunlight, and smoking.

The etiology of cataracts has not been completely defined. Cataracts are known to be associated with a change in the chemical composition of the lens. A variety of factors have been implicated, including exposure to ultraviolet light, low antioxidant levels, and excessive free radical damage.

The degree of visual impairment caused by a cataract is highly variable. However, cataract development tends to be progressive, with a gradual loss of visual acuity. Surgical lens replacement is an option for some individuals. In the presence of other diseases of the eye, such as glaucoma or macular degeneration, surgical lens replacement will not be beneficial.

LIFESTYLE RECOMMENDATIONS

- Continuation/initiation of diet and exercise program

- Avoid dairy products, fats, and anything that might lead to free radical formation

- Avoid OTC antihistamines

- Avoid sugars

- If a smoker, consider enrolling in a smoking cessation program

CATARACTS DECISION TREE

1. Client with cataracts is interested in using natural products (NP) to support this condition

2. Healthcare provider requests basic background information.
   The following issues are addressed with the client:
   * Allergies? * Prescription (Rx)/OTC meds?
   Depending on information obtained above, patient should be questioned about prescription steroid use. If significant, recommend patient discuss this with their MD.
   * Natural products? * Other medical conditions?
   Any other recent change in vision? If yes, refer to MD
   * Nutrition/diet program? * Exercise program?

3. Above data reviewed; if yes to Rx/OTC meds, review **Drug-Induced Nutrient Depletion Chart** in Appendix

4A. Client is a candidate for natural products

   * An appropriate homeopathic remedy can be used at any time

4B. Client's case is too complicated at this point; needs additional support from MD before initiating NP program

5. Condition-specific questions:
   * When was the condition diagnosed?
   * If patient is using eye drops, reinforce proper administration technique and maintain a sterile preparation
   * Any other recent change in vision? If yes, refer to MD

6. See table on following page

CATARACTS *(Continued)*

CATARACTS*

Category	Natural Products to Consider	DOC
Herb	Bilberry *on page 392*	PA
	Ginkgo *on page 441*	PA
	Green Tea *on page 452*	PA
Vitamin/Mineral/ Trace Element/ Nutraceutical	*N*-Acetyl Cysteine *on page 482* Condition-specific dosage: 200-600 mg twice daily	PA
	Lutein *on page 472* Condition-specific dosage: 2-6 mg/day	PA
Homeopathic Remedy	Homeopathic combination formulas are available for many conditions. Listed below are some of the most common single homeopathic remedies for cataracts. Also see **Homeopathic Quick Reference Chart for Common Complaints** *on page 587*	
	Calcarea carbonica	PD
	Cineraria maritima	PD
	Phosphorus	PD
	Silicea	PD
Additional supplements to consider	Selenium *on page 502* Condition-specific dosage: 200 mcg/day	PA
	Vitamin C *on page 526* Condition-specific dosage: 500-1000 mg twice daily	PA
	Vitamin E *on page 529* Condition-specific dosage: 200-400 int. units/day	PA
	Zinc *on page 534* Condition-specific dosage: 15-35 mg/day **WITH** Copper *on page 416* Dosage: 2 mg/day	PA

*Refer to **Introduction to Conditions** *on page 41* for more details on how to apply the information in this table to individuals with this condition.

SPECIAL CONSIDERATIONS

Bilberry (Berry)

- Contraindicated in active bleeding (eg, peptic ulcer, intracranial bleeding)
- Caution in hemostatic disorders/history of bleeding
- Potential interaction with anticoagulants (warfarin), aspirin, NSAIDs, anti-platelet agents
- Discontinue use prior to dental or surgical procedures (14 days before)

Ginkgo

- Contraindicated in active bleeding (eg, peptic ulcer, intracranial bleeding)
- Caution in hemostatic disorders/history of bleeding
- Potential interaction with anticoagulants (warfarin), aspirin, NSAIDs, anti-platelet agents
- Potential interaction with MAO inhibitors, acetylcholinesterase inhibitors (eg, tacrine, donepezil)
- Discontinue use prior to dental or surgical procedures (14 days before)

Green Tea

- Decaffeinated products are recommended
- Caffeine may cause multiple CNS and CV effects; caution in peptic ulcer disease or cardiovascular disease
- Contraindicated in active bleeding (eg, peptic ulcer, intracranial bleeding)
- Caution in hemostatic disorders/history of bleeding
- Discontinue use prior to dental or surgical procedures (14 days before)
- Potential interactions with anticoagulants (warfarin), aspirin, NSAIDs, antiplatelet agents
- See Green Tea *on page 452* for additional potential interactions

N-Acetyl Cysteine

- No known toxicity or serious side effects

Lutein

- No known toxicity or serious side effects

Selenium

- No known toxicity or serious side effects

Vitamin C

- Excess intake in diabetics may give falsely elevated blood glucose readings

Vitamin E

- Use with caution when taking anticoagulants (vitamin E ≥200 int. units increases prothrombin times)
- Interrupt or reduce dosage one week prior to dental or surgical procedures

Zinc

- No known toxicity or serious side effects

Copper

- Contraindicated in Wilson's disease

CERVICAL DYSPLASIA

Cervical dysplasia is an abnormal growth of the epithelial tissue on the surface of the cervix. It may be referred to as cervical intraepithelial neoplasia (CIN), squamous intraepithelial lesion (SIL), or precancerous changes of the cervix. The cause of cervical dysplasia is unknown. Risk factors include multiple sexual partners, early onset of sexual activity (<18 years of age), early childbearing (<16 years of age), past history of diethylstilbestrol (DES) exposure, or a history of sexually transmitted diseases, especially HPV (genital warts), genital herpes, or HIV.

Other factors that have been suggested to play a role in development of the disease include smoking, birth control pills, dysbiosis, and deficiencies of vitamin A, vitamin C, and folic acid. It may occur in women ≥15 years of age, with the peak in women 25-35 years of age. Individuals are normally asymptomatic and diagnosis is usually made based on a routine Pap smear.

Treatment of cervical dysplasia depends on the degree of dysplasia. Treatments range from careful observation with repeat Pap smears at 3- to 6-month intervals to eradication of the abnormal tissue by a variety of methods (cryotherapy, electrocauterization, or a surgical hysterectomy). Clinicians should also evaluate folic acid status. Many studies have reported that nutritional supplements can play an important role in reversing some cases of cervical dysplasia.

If identified early, cervical dysplasia may almost always be cured, provided the individual receives adequate evaluation, treatment, and followup. However, without treatment, up to 50% of cervical dysplasia may progress to invasive cancer. In addition, recurrence of dysplasia may occur after initial eradication.

LIFESTYLE RECOMMENDATIONS

- Continuation/initiation of diet and exercise program
- Discuss birth control options (if interested in this practice) with physician
- Have regular Pap tests done
- Drink 8-10 glasses of water per day
- Increase consumption of fruits, vegetables, grains, and fiber
- Eliminate tobacco, caffeine, and alcohol

CERVICAL DYSPLASIA DECISION TREE

1. Client with cervical dysplasia is interested in using natural products (NP) to support this condition

2. Healthcare provider requests basic background information.
   The following issues are addressed with the client:
   * Allergies?
   * Prescription (Rx)/OTC meds?
   * Natural products?
   * Other medical conditions?
   * Nutrition/diet program?
   * Exercise program?

3. Above data reviewed; if **yes** to Rx/OTC meds, review **Drug-Induced Nutrient Depletion Chart** in Appendix

4A. Client is a candidate for natural products

   * An appropriate homeopathic remedy can be used at any time

4B. Client's case is too complicated at this point; needs additional support from MD before initiating NP program

5. Condition-specific questions:
   * Diagnosed by MD? If **yes**, what was the recommended treatment plan? Effective?
   * Triggers for condition/symptom onset? Worsening?
   * If client is still in her reproductive years and is interested in birth control, need to discuss options with her MD.
   * History of vaginal infection? Treated completely? Make sure it was, and take necessary steps to try to prevent further infections.
   * What is the client's plan for follow-up with MD? Needs to be on a regular basis.

6. See table on following page

CERVICAL DYSPLASIA *(Continued)*

CERVICAL DYSPLASIA*

Category	Natural Products to Consider	DOC
Herb	**Chasteberry/Vitex** *on page 408*	PA, HE
	Cat's Claw *on page 404*	PA, HE
	Bromelain *on page 399*	HE
Vitamin/Mineral/ Trave Element/ Nutraceutical	**Isoflavones** *on page 465* Condition-specific dosage: 100-400 mg/day	PA
	Lactobacillus acidophilus *on page 467* and ***Bifidobacterium bifidum*** *on page 391* Condition-specific dosage: 10 billion CFU twice daily (dairy free)	PA
Homeopathic Remedy	**Note:** This is a complex health issue that should be addressed by someone experienced in homeopathy.	
Additional Supplements to Consider	**Beta-Carotene** *on page 390* Condition-specific dosage: 50,000 int. units/day	HD
	Vitamin A *on page 518* Condition-specific dosage: 10,000-35,000 int. units/ day	HD
	Vitamin C *on page 526* Condition-specific dosage: 250-1000 mg/day	HD
	Vitamin E *on page 529* Condition-specific dosage: 50-400 int. units/day	HD
	Folic Acid *on page 435* Condition-specific dosage: 400-800 mcg/day	PA

*Refer to **Introduction to Conditions** *on page 41* for more details on how to apply the information in this table to individuals with this condition.

SPECIAL CONSIDERATIONS

Chasteberry/Vitex
- Contraindicated in pregnancy
- Potential interaction with hormonal replacements or oral contraceptives

Cat's Claw
- Contraindicated in transplant recipients, individuals receiving I.V. immuno-globulins or immunosuppressants
- Contraindicated in active bleeding (eg, peptic ulcer, intracranial bleeding)
- Caution in hemostatic disorders/history of bleeding
- Potential interaction with anticoagulants (warfarin), aspirin, NSAIDs, anti-platelet agents
- Discontinue use prior to dental or surgical procedures (14 days before)

Bromelain
- Contraindicated in active bleeding (eg, peptic ulcer, intracranial bleeding)
- Potential interaction with anticoagulants (warfarin), aspirin, NSAIDs, anti-platelet agents
- Use with caution in individuals with GI ulceration and/or cardiovascular disorders (hypertension)
- Caution in hemostatic disorders/history of bleeding
- Discontinue use prior to dental or surgical procedures (14 days before)

Isoflavones
- Caution in estrogen-dependent tumors, endometrial cancer
- Women who are taking estrogen-containing medications (oral contraceptives, hormonal replacement) should consult their physician prior to use

Lactobacillus acidophilus
- No known toxicity or serious side effects

Bifidobacterium bifidum
- No known toxicity or serious side effects

Beta-Carotene
- No known toxicity or serious side effects

Vitamin A
- Contraindicated in pregnancy or in women who may become pregnant

Vitamin C
- Excess intake in diabetics may give falsely elevated blood glucose readings

Vitamin E
- Use with caution when taking anticoagulants (vitamin E ≥200 int. units increases prothrombin times)
- Interrupt or reduce dosage one week prior to dental or surgical procedures

Folic Acid
- Does not reverse cervical dysplasia; however, levels are low in many cases and replacement may limit recurrence

CHEMOTHERAPY AND RADIATION

Agents used in cancer chemotherapy may have potent effects on an individual's nutritional status, immune function, and organ function. The impact on general nutritional status may be profound. Nutritional compromise results from two major effects of chemotherapy. Nutrient intake may be decreased by tumor or chemotherapy-induced nausea, and nutrient absorption may be limited due to toxic destruction of cells lining the gastrointestinal tract. There is wide variability between individual chemotherapeutic agents and their relative potential to cause these two effects.

Decreased nutrient intake caused by chemotherapy-induced nausea, vomiting, and anorexia may be mediated through the central nervous system or by local gastrointestinal factors. The emetogenic effects of most agents are limited to the first few hours following administration, but occasionally may be persistent. For example, cisplatin may induce severe nausea and vomiting for up to a week following administration. Widespread general nutritional compromise may be anticipated only in persistent cases.

Both chemotherapy and radiation can cause painful inflammation and/or ulceration in the gastrointestinal tract and/or oral cavity, which makes eating difficult or impossible. Treatment may damage the colon and cause diarrhea. Without the normal absorptive and protective functions of gastrointestinal cells, nutrition may be severely compromised. These forms of injury can result in significant malnutrition because they take a longer time to heal.

Immune suppression often accompanies chemotherapy or radiation. The effects on the production of immune cell populations may be profound, rendering the individual at increased risk of potentially life-threatening infection (especially fungal, see Candidiasis). In an immunosuppressed individual, no symptom of infection, especially fever, should be considered benign or self-limited, and should prompt immediate medical attention and/or physician referral.

Beyond gastrointestinal and immunologic effects, individual chemotherapeutic agents are associated with specific toxicities including neurotoxic reactions, impairment of renal function, anaphylaxis, and depression of myocardial contractility resulting in CHF. An individual's ability to tolerate a given chemotherapeutic regimen is highly variable, and may be difficult to anticipate. The administration of intravenous nutrition several times weekly has proven to be very helpful to cancer patients during the period when they have trouble eating or absorbing nutrients. Nutraceutical agents, herbs, and nutrition intervention may reduce the side effects of chemotherapy and radiation and enhance its effectiveness.

LIFESTYLE RECOMMENDATIONS

- Continuation/initiation of diet and exercise program

- Reduce intake of dairy products, except for yogurt that contains *Lactobacillus acidophilus*

- Reduce refined sugars and refined carbohydrates

- Increase intake of vegetables and fruits, specifically those that contain pectin (consider organic produce only)

- Evaluate fat intake and adjust appropriately

- Offer information on alternative therapies, such as relaxation methods, stress reduction, etc, and discuss these with physician

CHEMOTHERAPY / RADIATION THERAPY DECISION TREE

1. Client who has undergone chemotherapy/radiation therapy is interested in using natural products (NP) to support this condition

↓

2. Healthcare provider requests basic background information. The following issues are addressed with the client:
   * Allergies?
   * Prescription (Rx)/OTC meds?   * Other medical conditions?
     See **Note** below   * Nutrition/diet program?
   * Natural products?   * Exercise program?

Note: Specific attention to meds, other than chemo meds, that could be contributing to nausea/vomiting (narcotics, digoxin, antibiotics)

↓

3. Above data reviewed; if **yes** to Rx/OTC meds, review **Drug-Induced Nutrient Depletion Chart** in Appendix

4A. Client is a candidate for natural products

   * An appropriate homeopathic remedy can be used at any time

4B. Client's case is too complicated at this point; needs additional support from MD before initiating NP program

↓

5. Condition-specific questions:
   * Describe the course of therapy: past, present, future - this should assist in tailoring a regimen to meet client's needs
   * Any relationship between symptoms and other interventions or therapies? Look for a cause and effect relationship
   * Any interventions successful?

↓

6. See table on following page

CHEMOTHERAPY AND RADIATION *(Continued)*

CHEMOTHERAPY & RADIATION*

Category	Natural Products to Consider	DOC
Herb	Arabinoxylane *on page 384*	HT
	Ashwaganda *on page 387*	PA
	Astragalus *on page 388*	PA
	Cat's Claw *on page 404*	PA
	Cordyceps *on page 417*	HD
	Ginger *on page 440*	PA
	Ginseng, Siberian *on page 444*	PA
	Green Tea *on page 452*	HD
	Milk Thistle *on page 479*	PA
	Reishi *on page 497*	
Vitamin/Mineral/ Trace Element/ Nutraceutical	Modified Citrus Pectin (MCP) *on page 480* Condition-specific dosage: 1 g 4 times/day	PA
	Isoflavones *on page 465* Condition-specific dosage: 100-400 mg/day	PA
	Spleen Extract *on page 505* Condition-specific dosage: 300 mg 3 times/day	HD
	Thymus Extract *on page 510* Condition-specific dosage: 500 mg 3 times/day	HT
	Coenzyme Q$_{10}$ *on page 412* Condition-specific dosage: 100-300 mg/day	PA
	Lactobacillus acidophilus *on page 467* and Bifidobacterium bifidum *on page 391* Condition-specific dosage: 10-15 billion CFU twice daily	HD
	Glutamine *on page 446* Condition-specific dosage: 5000 mg 2-3 times/day; swish and swallow	HT
	Selenium *on page 502* Condition-specific dosage: 200-400 mcg/day	HT
	Vitamin C *on page 526* Condition-specific dosage: 500-1000 mg twice daily	HT
	Inositol Hexaphosphate *on page 462* Condition-specific dosage: 600-800 mg 3-4 times/day taken with 200-250 mg inositol	PA
Homeopathic Remedy	Homeopathic combination formulas are available for many conditions. Listed below are some of the most common single homeopathic remedies for chemotherapy/radiation therapy. Also see **Homeopathic Quick Reference Chart for Common Complaints** *on page 587*	
	Cadmium sulphuricum	PD
	Ipecacuanha	PD
	Solanum nigrum	PD
	Conium maculatum	PD
	Phytolacca decandra	PD
Additional supplements to consider	Vitamin A *on page 518* Condition-specific dosage: 10,000-35,000 int. units/day	PA
	Vitamin E *on page 529* Condition-specific dosage: 400 int. units/day	PA
	Alpha-Lipoic Acid *on page 381* Condition-specific dosage: 100-200 mg twice daily	PA
	N-Acetyl Cysteine (NAC) *on page 482* Condition-specific dosage: 500 mg 2-3 times/day	PA

*Refer to **Introduction to Conditions** *on page 41* for more details on how to apply the information in this table to individuals with this condition.

SPECIAL CONSIDERATIONS

Arabinoxylane

* Use with caution in renal failure due to relatively high phosphorus content

Ashwaganda

* Contraindicated in pregnancy and breast-feeding

Astragalus

* May interact with immune stimulants or immunosuppressants

Cat's Claw

* Contraindicated in transplant recipients, individuals receiving I.V. immunoglobulins or immunosuppressants
* Contraindicated in active bleeding (eg, peptic ulcer, intracranial bleeding)
* Caution in hemostatic disorders/history of bleeding
* Potential interaction with anticoagulants (warfarin), aspirin, NSAIDs, antiplatelet agents
* Discontinue use prior to dental or surgical procedures (14 days before)

Cordyceps

* Caution if allergic to molds or fungi
* Theoretical interaction in individuals receiving MAO inhibitors
* Contraindicated in active bleeding (eg, peptic ulcer, intracranial bleeding)
* Caution in hemostatic disorders/history of bleeding
* Potential interaction with anticoagulants (warfarin), aspirin, NSAIDs, antiplatelet agents
* Discontinue use prior to dental or surgical procedures (14 days before)

Ginger

* Contraindicated in active bleeding (eg, peptic ulcer, intracranial bleeding)
* Caution in hemostatic disorders/history of bleeding
* Potential interaction with anticoagulants (warfarin), aspirin, NSAIDs, antiplatelet agents, cardiac glycosides (digoxin)
* Discontinue use prior to dental or surgical procedures (14 days before)

Ginseng, Siberian

* Contraindicated with digoxin, hexobarbital
* Caution with stimulant medications, decongestants, caffeine
* A cycle of 4 weeks on, followed by 2 weeks off is recommended for maximum benefit
* Caution in hypertension or in individuals at risk of hypotension (elderly, cerebrovascular or cardiovascular disease); or those taking antihypertensives
* May alter blood glucose regulation; monitor blood glucose carefully in individuals with diabetes or hypoglycemia
* Contraindicated in active bleeding (eg, peptic ulcer, intracranial bleeding
* Caution in hemostatic disorders/history of bleeding
* Potential interactions with anticoagulants (warfarin), aspirin, NSAIDs, antiplatelet agents, sedative-hypnotics (barbiturates), insulin, oral hypoglycemics, antihypertensives, stimulants, caffeine
* Discontinue use prior to dental or surgical procedures (14 days before)

Green Tea

* Decaffeinated products are recommended
* Caffeine may cause multiple CNS and CV effects; caution in peptic ulcer disease or cardiovascular disease
* Contraindicated in active bleeding (eg, peptic ulcer, intracranial bleeding)
* Caution in hemostatic disorders/history of bleeding
* Discontinue use prior to dental or surgical procedures (14 days before)
* Potential interactions with anticoagulants (warfarin), aspirin, NSAIDs, antiplatelet agents

CHEMOTHERAPY AND RADIATION *(Continued)*

- See Green Tea *on page 452* for other potential interactions

Milk Thistle
- No reported toxicity in humans at normal intakes

Reishi
- Contraindicated in active bleeding (eg, peptic ulcer, intracranial bleeding)
- Caution in hemostatic disorders/history of bleeding
- Potential interactions with anticoagulants, anticonvulsants, antihypertensives, NSAIDs, aspirin, antiplatelet agents
- Discontinue use prior to dental or surgical procedures (14 days before)

Modified Citrus Pectin
- Do not use in individuals who are allergic to citrus.
- Use with caution in renal failure

Isoflavones
- Caution in estrogen-dependent tumors, endometrial cancer, thromboembolic disease, or stroke
- Women who are taking estrogen-containing medications (eg, oral contraceptives, hormonal replacement) should consult their physician prior to use

Spleen Extract
- No known toxicity or serious side effects

Thymus Extract
- No known toxicity or serious side effects

Coenzyme Q_{10}
- No known toxicity or serious side effects
- Caution in individuals receiving anticoagulants

Lactobacillus acidophilus
- No known toxicity or serious side effects

Bifidobacterium bifidum
- No known toxicity or serious side effects

Glutamine
- No known toxicity or serious side effects

Selenium
- Intake should be restricted to no more than 700 mcg/day unless supervised by a physician
- Rarely may cause thrombocytopenia or hepatorenal dysfunction

Vitamin C
- Excess intake in diabetics may give falsely elevated blood glucose readings

Inositol Hexaphosphate
- No known toxicity or serious side effects at normal intakes

Vitamin A
- Contraindicated in pregnancy or in women who may become pregnant

Vitamin E
- Use with caution when taking anticoagulants (vitamin E ≥200 int. units increases prothrombin times)
- Interrupt or reduce dosage one week prior to dental or surgical procedures

Alpha-Lipoic Acid
- No known toxicity or serious side effects at normal intakes
- Caution in individuals receiving oral hypoglycemics or insulin; monitor blood glucose closely and coordinate with prescriber

N-Acetyl Cysteine
- No known toxicity or serious side effects at normal intakes

CHRONIC FATIGUE SYNDROME (CFS)

The diagnostic criteria for chronic fatigue syndrome is 6 months of "debilitating fatigue," in addition to four or more of the following symptoms: Self-reported impairment in short-term memory or concentration (severe enough to cause substantial reduction in previous levels of occupational, educational, social, or personal activities); sore throat; tender cervical or axillary lymph nodes; muscle discomfort or pain; joint pain without joint swelling or redness; headaches of a new type, pattern, or severity; unrefreshing sleep; and postexertional malaise (lasting more than 24 hours).

Individuals may exhibit a range of additional manifestations, such as muscle weakness, swollen underarm (axillary) glands, sleep disturbances, visual disturbances, orthostatic hypotension, cognitive difficulties, syncope, dizziness, depression, irritability, and anxiety. Many individuals report mild to moderate symptoms of anxiety or depression; however 20% to 40% do not have any form of psychiatric illness. Most individuals appear to suffer from a severe metabolic abnormality in which the body shifts rapidly from resting to anaerobic metabolism. As a consequence, normal activities become both difficult and damaging.

The onset of disease is usually abrupt, often following an acute flu-like illness or mononucleosis. The natural history is variable, but tends to stabilize over the first 1-2 years. Regardless of intervention, approximately 45% of individuals return to at least 80% of previous function in 5 years; while 45% remain at <50% of previous function after 10 years. However, some estimates note that >80% of individuals remain chronically debilitated. Relapse has also been noted to occur in some individuals.

A number of agents have been speculated to trigger CFS. Among these are viruses (including herpes virus, enterovirus, Coxsackie virus, or Epstein-Barr virus). In addition, infections with *Mycoplasma* spp, *Chlamydia pneumoniae*, and cytomegalovirus have also been associated with CFS. However, it is difficult to determine whether these infections are causative or simply represent impairment in the immune function of individuals with CFS. Environmental toxins, dysbiosis, altered thyroid function, prolonged stress, and poor nutrient status leading to uncoupling of the Krebs cycle energy system, are also potential cofactors in CFS. Evaluation may be very complicated and referral for complete metabolic and endocrine evaluation should be encouraged. Potential neuropsychiatric causes should be evaluated by an appropriate healthcare professional.

LIFESTYLE RECOMMENDATIONS

- Continued/initiation of diet and exercise program
- Get plenty of rest, but do not rest all day
- Support groups are available
- If relying too heavily on pain/sleep medications, physician evaluation is necessary.
- Drink plenty of water
- Avoid fried foods, caffeinated beverages, sugar
- Increase intake of fiber
- Consider testing for food intolerances
- Evaluate metabolic efficiency through lab assessment

CHRONIC FATIGUE SYNDROME DECISION TREE

1. Client with chronic fatigue syndrome is interested in using natural products (NP) to support this condition

2. Healthcare provider requests basic background information. The following issues are addressed with the client:

* Allergies?
* Prescription (Rx)/OTC meds?
* Natural products?
* Other medical conditions?
* Nutrition/diet program?
* Exercise program?

3. Above data reviewed; if **yes** to Rx/OTC meds, review **Drug-Induced Nutrient Depletion Chart** in Appendix

4A. Client is a candidate for natural products

* An appropriate homeopathic remedy can be used at any time

4B. Client's case is too complicated at this point; needs additional support from MD before initiating NP program

5. Condition-specific questions:
* Was condition diagnosed by MD? If **self-diagnosed**, stress the importance of an accurate diagnosis prior to the development of a natural products plan
* Do the symptoms cycle or are they continuous?
* Any precipitating factors?
* Any recent changes in lifestyle or occupation?
* Any recent changes in the amount of or quality of sleep and rest the client is getting? Evaluate for sleep apnea
* Has the client had their thyroid function checked?
* Evaluate stress level - recommend discussing with healthcare professional
* See section on Candidiasis also.

6. See table on following page

CHRONIC FATIGUE SYNDROME (CFS) *(Continued)*

CHRONIC FATIGUE SYNDROME*

Category	Natural Products to Consider	DOC
Herb	**Cordyceps** on page 417	PA
	Schisandra on page 501	PA
	Ginseng, Siberian on page 444	PA
	Reishi on page 497	PA
	Bupleurum on page 400	PA
Vitamin/Mineral/ Trace Element/ Nutraceutical	**Nicotinamide Adenine Dinucleotide (NADH)** on page 483 Condition-specific dosage: 2.5-5 mg/day	HT
	Coenzyme Q$_{10}$ on page 412 Condition-specific dosage: 30-50 mg 2-3 times/day	HD
	Adrenal Extract on page 380 Condition-specific dosage: 250 mg 2-3 times/day	PA
	Thymus Extract on page 510 Condition-specific dosage: 250 mg 2-3 times/day	PA
	Thyroid Extract on page 510 Condition-specific dosage: 60 mg 1-3 times/day	PA
	Lactobacillus acidophilus on page 467 and ***Bifidobacterium bifidum*** on page 391 Condition-specific dosage: (dairy free)	PA
Homeopathic Remedy	Homeopathic combination formulas are available for many conditions. Listed below are some of the most common single homeopathic remedies for chronic fatigue syndrome. Also see **Homeopathic Quick Reference Chart for Common Complaints** on page 587	
	Arsenicum album	PD
	Gelsemium sempervirens	PD
	Phosphoricum acidum	PD
Additional supplements to consider	**Vitamin B Complex-25** on page 526 Condition-specific dosage: 25 mg twice daily	PA
	Spleen Extract on page 505 Condition-specific dosage: 150-300 mg 2-3 times/day	PA
	***N*-Acetyl Cysteine** on page 482 Condition-specific dosage: 500 mg twice daily	HD

*Refer to **Introduction to Conditions** on page 41 for more details on how to apply the information in this table to individuals with this condition.

SPECIAL CONSIDERATIONS

Cordyceps
- Caution if allergic to molds or fungi; and in hemostatic disorders/history of bleeding
- Theoretical interaction in individuals receiving MAO inhibitors
- Contraindicated in active bleeding (eg, peptic ulcer, intracranial bleeding)
- Potential interaction with anticoagulants (warfarin), aspirin, NSAIDs, antiplatelet agents
- Discontinue use prior to dental or surgical procedures (14 days before)

Schisandra
- Contraindicated in pregnancy (due to uterine stimulation);
- Potential interaction with calcium channel blockers

Ginseng, Siberian
- Contraindicated with digoxin, hexobarbital; and in active bleeding (eg, peptic ulcer, intracranial bleeding)
- Caution with stimulant medications, decongestants, caffeine; and in hemostatic disorders/history of bleeding
- A cycle of 4 weeks on, followed by 2 weeks off is recommended for maximum benefit
- Caution in hypertension or in individuals at risk of hypotension (elderly, cerebrovascular or cardiovascular disease); or those taking antihypertensives
- May alter blood glucose regulation; monitor blood glucose carefully in individuals with diabetes or hypoglycemia
- Potential interactions with anticoagulants (warfarin), aspirin, NSAIDs, antiplatelet agents, sedative-hypnotics (barbiturates), insulin, oral hypoglycemics, antihypertensives, stimulants, caffeine
- Discontinue use prior to dental or surgical procedures (14 days before)

Reishi
- Contraindicated in active bleeding (eg, peptic ulcer, intracranial bleeding)
- Caution in hemostatic disorders/history of bleeding
- Potential interactions with anticoagulants, anticonvulsants, antihypertensives, NSAIDs, aspirin, antiplatelet agents
- Discontinue use prior to dental or surgical procedures (14 days before)

Bupleurum
- Use with caution in diabetes, HTN, edema
- Theoretical interaction with corticosteroids, diuretics, antihypertensives, and antidiabetic agents

NADH – No known toxicity or serious side effects

Coenzyme Q_{10} – No known toxicity or serious side effects; caution in individuals receiving anticoagulants

Adrenal Extract – May cause excitability when taken in large doses

Thymus Extract – No known toxicity or serious side effects

Thyroid Extract
- Use with caution in individuals taking thyroid medication and in individuals with hypertension or cardiovascular disease
- Potential interactions with levothyroxine, propylthiouracil, lithium
- Use with caution in individuals with CNS disorders

Lactobacillus acidophilus – No known toxicity or serious side effects

Bifidobacterium bifidum – No known toxicity or serious side effects

Vitamin B Complex-25 – No reported toxicity in humans at normal intakes

Spleen Extract – No known toxicity or serious side effects

N-Acetyl Cysteine – No known toxicity or serious side effects

CIRCULATION (PERIPHERAL) PROBLEMS
COLD HANDS / FEET

One of the most common symptoms of circulatory insufficiency may be cold extremities (hands and feet). There may be a number of causes of this complaint, including both subclinical and overt hypothyroidism, low cardiac output, diminished blood volume, anemia (inadequate oxygen-carrying capacity), limited ability of the blood cells to pass through capillary networks, and limitations to blood flow (including vessel constriction or obstruction).

Vascular disease, particularly due to atherosclerotic obstruction or diminished cardiac output may be accompanied by easy fatigue, weakness of the extremities, or muscle pain with activity. In chronic vascular insufficiency associated with capillary rupture, pigment deposits (hemosiderin) under the skin may produce a reddish-brown discoloration. Diminished cardiac output, as well as venous or lymphatic insufficiency, is often accompanied by peripheral edema. Spasms of the vasculature, particularly in the terminal arterioles (just before the capillaries), may also limit peripheral circulation. Extreme vasospasm in response to specific environmental or physiologic triggers (such as cold temperature or beta-blocking drugs) is referred to as Raynaud's syndrome. The consequences of insufficiency range from discomfort and inconvenience of cold hands and feet, to necrosis and the potential loss of digits or portions of a limb due to ischemia.

It is important to evaluate causes of peripheral insufficiency as well as to avoid exacerbating factors such as environmental triggers or vasoconstricting medications.

LIFESTYLE RECOMMENDATIONS

- Continuation/initiation of diet and exercise program

- Dress warmly, protecting the extremities

- Avoid cold temperatures, tobacco, extreme emotional swings, standing for prolonged periods of time

- If the feet are involved, have daily foot baths; apply an emollient cream to the feet daily or as needed

CIRCULATION (PERIPHERAL) DECISION TREE

1. Client with circulation (peripheral) problems is interested in using natural products (NP) to support this condition

2. Healthcare provider requests basic background information. The following issues are addressed with the client:

   * Allergies?   * Other medical conditions?
   * Prescription (Rx)/OTC meds?   * Nutrition/diet program?
   * Natural products?   * Exercise program?

3. Above data reviewed; if **yes** to Rx/OTC meds, review **Drug-Induced Nutrient Depletion Chart** in Appendix

4A. Client is a candidate for natural products

   * An appropriate homeopathic remedy can be used at any time

4B. Client's case is too complicated at this point; needs additional support from MD before initiating NP program

5. Condition-specific questions:
   * Specific symptoms: Single vs bilateral, hands vs feet vs both; degree of coldness, color change?
   * Triggers for worsening of symptoms
   * Tobacco use? If **yes,** recommend smoking cessation program
   * Has thyroid function been checked? If **no,** may want to discuss with MD
   * Increase in the number of infections in the extremities?
   * If diabetic, see **Diabetes** Decision Tree
   * Aching in legs and/or calves when walking? If **yes,** refer to MD
   * Discuss hormone replacement therapy with MD if client is taking

6. See table on following page

CIRCULATION (PERIPHERAL) PROBLEMS *(Continued)*

CIRCULATION (PERIPHERAL)*

Category	Natural Products to Consider	DOC
Herb	Ginkgo *on page 441*	PA
	Hawthorn *on page 456*	HD
	Cayenne *on page 405*	PA
	Bilberry *on page 392*	PA
	Horse Chestnut *on page 458*	HT
Vitamin/Mineral/ Trace Element/ Nutraceutical	Arginine *on page 385* Condition-specific dosage: 2-4 g/day in divided doses	PA
	Fish Oils *on page 434* Condition-specific dosage: 1 capsule twice daily	HT
	Magnesium *on page 473* Condition-specific dosage: 600 mg/day	PA
	Vitamin B₃ (Niacin or Inositol Hexaniacinate) *on page 521* Condition-specific dosage: Niacin: 25-50 mg; inositol hexaniacinate: 650 mg 2-3 times/day	HT
	Vitamin E *on page 529* Condition-specific dosage: 400-800 int. units/day	HT
Homeopathic Remedy	Homeopathic combination formulas are available for many conditions. Listed below are some of the most common single homeopathic remedies for circulation (peripheral) problems. Also see **Homeopathic Quick Reference Chart for Common Complaints** *on page 587*	
	Cactus grandiflorus	PD
	Dulcamara	PD
	Lachesis mutus	PD
	Secale cornutum	PD
Additional supplements to consider	Alpha-Lipoic Acid *on page 381* Condition-specific dosage: 100-300 mg/day	PA
	Selenium *on page 502* Condition-specific dosage: 200 mcg/day	PA
	Vitamin A *on page 518* Condition-specific dosage: 10,000-35,000 int. units/day	PA
	Vitamin C *on page 526* Condition-specific dosage: 250-1000 mg/day	PA

*Refer to **Introduction to Conditions** *on page 41* for more details on how to apply the information in this table to individuals with this condition.

SPECIAL CONSIDERATIONS

Gingko
- Contraindicated in active bleeding (eg, peptic ulcer, intracranial bleeding)
- Caution in hemostatic disorders/history of bleeding
- Potential interaction with anticoagulants (warfarin), aspirin, NSAIDs, antiplatelet agents
- Theoretical interaction with MAO inhibitors, acetylcholinesterase inhibitors (tacrine, donepezil)
- Discontinue use prior to dental or surgical procedures (14 days before)

Hawthorn
- Use with caution in pregnancy, in hypertension, or in individuals at risk of hypotension (elderly, cerebrovascular or cardiovascular disease)
- Theoretical interaction with antiarrhythmics, antihypertensives, cardiac glycosides, ACE inhibitors, angiotensin blockers

Cayenne
- Caution in GI ulceration and in hemostatic disorders/history of bleeding
- Contraindicated in active bleeding (eg, peptic ulcer, intracranial bleeding)
- Potential interaction with anticoagulants (warfarin), aspirin, NSAIDs, antiplatelet agents
- Potential interference with MAO inhibitors and antihypertensives
- Discontinue use prior to dental or surgical procedures (14 days before)

Bilberry
- Contraindicated in active bleeding (eg, peptic ulcer, intracranial bleeding)
- Caution in hemostatic disorders/history of bleeding
- Potential interaction with anticoagulants (warfarin), aspirin, NSAIDs, antiplatelet agents
- Discontinue use prior to dental or surgical procedures (14 days before)

Horse Chestnut
- Contraindicated in active bleeding (eg, peptic ulcer, intracranial bleeding)
- Caution in hemostatic disorders/history of bleeding and in hepatic or renal impairment
- Potential interactions with anticoagulants (warfarin), aspirin, NSAIDs, antiplatelet agents
- Discontinue use prior to dental or surgical procedures (14 days before)

Arginine – No known toxicity or serious side effects

Fish Oils
- High doses may cause GI upset, loose stools, nausea
- May alter glucose regulation; use with caution in diabetes
- Caution in individuals receiving oral hypoglycemics or insulin; monitor blood glucose closely and coordinate with prescriber
- Potential interaction with anticoagulants (warfarin), aspirin, NSAIDs, antiplatelet agents

Magnesium
- Use caution in renal impairment
- May cause diarrhea in high intakes

Vitamin B$_3$ (Niacin or Inositol Hexaniacinate))
- Caution in individuals with diabetes, gout
- Potential adverse effects may include headache, nausea, skin flushing and tingling, sweating

Vitamin E
- Use with caution when taking anticoagulants (vitamin E ≥ 200 int. units increases prothrombin times)
- Interrupt or reduce dosage one week prior to dental or surgical procedures

Alpha-Lipoic Acid – No known toxicity or serious side effects at normal intakes; caution in individuals receiving oral hypoglycemics or insulin; monitor blood glucose closely and coordinate with prescriber

Selenium – No reported toxicity in humans at normal intakes

Vitamin A – Contraindicated in pregnancy or in women who may become pregnant

Vitamin C – Excess intake in diabetics may give falsely elevated blood glucose readings

COLD / FLU

The most common acute illness in the United States is the common cold. Colds are infections that can be caused by a number of viruses, which can be transmitted in a variety of ways. Estimates of episodes per year number over 66 million. Preschoolers have the highest rate of infection, experiencing 6-10 episodes per year, while adults average 2-4 colds per year. In addition to age, the person's immune status, smoking status, rate of environmental exposure (ie, presence of school age or preschool children in the home environment), and nutritional status are associated with frequency of infection. Symptoms of nasal congestion, nasal drainage, fatigue, malaise, and muscle aches are common. Fever, if present, is generally low grade.

In common usage, the term "flu" often refers to gastrointestinal complaints of nausea, vomiting, and diarrhea. Gastrointestinal complaints are usually due to bacterial or viral infections, which produce symptoms of weakness, fever, myalgia, and somnolence. The course of most infections is self-limiting, but in high-risk individuals or in those with prolonged symptoms, medical intervention may be required (antibiotics, intravenous rehydration).

The elderly are at particular risk and should consider a proactive immune support program utilizing natural products

Individuals should be encouraged to drink large quantities of pure water to aid in detoxification and rehydration.

LIFESTYLE RECOMMENDATIONS

- Increase rest; reduce physical activity

- Eliminate refined sugars

- Maintain/increase intake of proper foods to support the immune system and one's body

- Increase fluid intake

- Take extra care to wash hands thoroughly

- Gargle with salt water or diluted grapefruit seed extract (4 drops in water) to reduce sore throat

COLD / FLU DECISION TREE

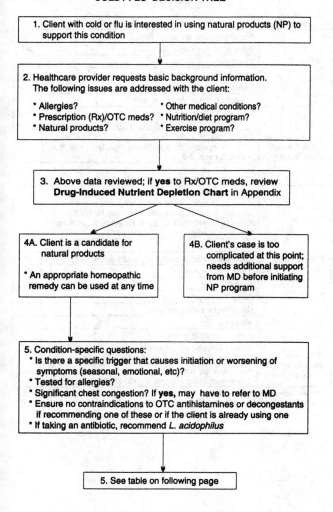

1. Client with cold or flu is interested in using natural products (NP) to support this condition

2. Healthcare provider requests basic background information. The following issues are addressed with the client:

* Allergies?
* Prescription (Rx)/OTC meds?
* Natural products?
* Other medical conditions?
* Nutrition/diet program?
* Exercise program?

3. Above data reviewed; if **yes** to Rx/OTC meds, review **Drug-Induced Nutrient Depletion Chart** in Appendix

4A. Client is a candidate for natural products

* An appropriate homeopathic remedy can be used at any time

4B. Client's case is too complicated at this point; needs additional support from MD before initiating NP program

5. Condition-specific questions:
* Is there a specific trigger that causes initiation or worsening of symptoms (seasonal, emotional, etc)?
* Tested for allergies?
* Significant chest congestion? If **yes,** may have to refer to MD
* Ensure no contraindications to OTC antihistamines or decongestants if recommending one of these or if the client is already using one
* If taking an antibiotic, recommend *L. acidophilus*

5. See table on following page

COLD / FLU *(Continued)*

COLD / FLU*

Category	Natural Products to Consider	DOC
Herb	Arabinoxylane *on page 384*	PA
	Echinacea *on page 426*	HT
	Elderberry *on page 428*	HD
	Astragalus *on page 388*	PA
	Golden Seal *on page 448*	PA
	Grapefruit Seed *on page 450*	PA
Vitamin/Mineral/ Trace Element/ Nutraceutical	Thymus Extract *on page 510* Condition-specific dosage: 250 mg 4 times/day	PA
	Zinc (Lozenges) *on page 534* Condition-specific dosage: Slowly dissolve 1 lozenge in mouth every 2-3 hours	HT
	Vitamin C *on page 526* Condition-specific dosage: 250-1000 mg/day	HT
Homeopathic Remedy	Homeopathic combination formulas are available for many conditions. Listed below are some of the most common single homeopathic remedies for cold/flu. Also see **Homeopathic Quick Reference Chart for Common Complaints** *on page 587*	
	Aconitum napellus	PD
	Anas barbariae (hepatis et cordis extractum)	PD
	Atropa belladonna	PD
	Bryonia alba	PD
	Ferrum phosphoricum	PD
	Gelsemium sempervirens	PD
	Mercuris vivus	PD
	Natrum muriaticum	PD
Additional supplements to consider	Spleen Extract *on page 505* Condition-specific dosage: 150 mg 3 times/day	PA
	Vitamin A *on page 518* Condition-specific dosage: 10,000-35,000 int. units/day	PA

*Refer to **Introduction to Conditions** *on page 41* for more details on how to apply the information in this table to individuals with this condition.

SPECIAL CONSIDERATIONS

Arabinoxylane
* Use with caution in renal failure due to relatively high phosphorus content

Echinacea
* Not recommended for use longer than 10 days (acute treatment) or in immunosuppressed individuals
* If used as prophylaxis, cycle 3 weeks on/1 week off
* Potential interaction with therapeutic immunosuppressants and corticosteroids
* Caution in renal impairment (may cause electrolyte imbalance)
* Use with caution in individuals with allergies to *Asteraceae/Compositae* family (ragweed, daisy, aster, chrysanthemum) and other pollens

Elderberry
* No reported toxicity in humans at normal intakes

Astragalus
* May interact with immune stimulants or immunosuppressants

Golden Seal
* Contraindicated during pregnancy

Grapefruit Seed Extract
* Grapefruit seed extract is not equivalent to grapefruit juice/pulp. Juice/pulp has been associated with many drug interactions; see Grapefruit Seed *on page 450*
* Until further information is available, it is reasonable to avoid some medications (terfenadine, astemizole, cisapride). Use other medications metabolized by CYP3A4 with caution.

Thymus Extract
* No known toxicity or serious side effects

Zinc
* No known toxicity or serious side effects at normal intakes

Vitamin C
* Excess intake in diabetics may give falsely elevated blood glucose readings

Spleen Extract
* No known toxicity or serious side effects

Vitamin A
* Contraindicated in pregnancy or in women who may become pregnant

COLIC

Colic is a condition that begins within the first few weeks of life, in which a baby cries for prolonged periods of time, often lifting his head or legs and appearing to be in pain. The condition affects up to 33% of all babies. Crying may be worse in the late afternoon, often lasting for hours at a time. Babies with colic may refuse to eat or may begin crying after feeding for only a brief time. In addition, the baby may have sleeping difficulties. Parents may become stressed and frustrated due to inability to comfort the child.

Infants with colic maintain normal growth and weight gain despite crying and feeding difficulties. There is no clear cause for colic. In general, it appears to be due to an immature gastrointestinal tract, with cramping and slow development of normal motility. For this reason, the only real cure is to be patient while waiting for the baby to grow through the first few months of life. Children who do not grow normally or gain weight should be evaluated, regardless of the presence of colic.

A number of suggestions have been proposed to comfort babies with colic, including the following:

1. Use a different formula or feed the baby with a different kind of bottle (curved bottle or bottle with a collapsible bag). Protein hydrolysate formulas are available specifically for infants with colic.
2. Use special techniques to feed, carry and/or burp the baby.
3. Keep the baby wrapped snugly in a blanket (swaddling).
4. Give the baby gentle belly massages.
5. Place the child in an infant swing.
6. If the mother is breast-feeding, a change in the mother's diet, such as limiting or avoiding milk products, gas-forming vegetables (eg, beans/legumes, cauliflower, broccoli, cabbage), eggs, and avoiding caffeine may be helpful

LIFESTYLE RECOMMENDATIONS

- Continuation/initiation of normal feeding/diet unless otherwise prescribed

- Try motion-related activities (stroller, swing)

- Change to hypoallergenic formula for allergy-sensitive child

- Have parents/caregivers work together and work in shifts to reduce parental stress

- Massage the abdomen

- Place the child on a warm heating pad, warm blanket, or warm towel to try and relax

COLIC DECISION TREE

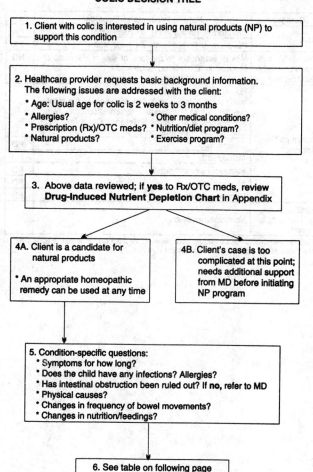

1. Client with colic is interested in using natural products (NP) to support this condition

2. Healthcare provider requests basic background information. The following issues are addressed with the client:
   * Age: Usual age for colic is 2 weeks to 3 months
   * Allergies?   * Other medical conditions?
   * Prescription (Rx)/OTC meds?   * Nutrition/diet program?
   * Natural products?   * Exercise program?

3. Above data reviewed; if **yes** to Rx/OTC meds, review **Drug-Induced Nutrient Depletion Chart** in Appendix

4A. Client is a candidate for natural products
   * An appropriate homeopathic remedy can be used at any time

4B. Client's case is too complicated at this point; needs additional support from MD before initiating NP program

5. Condition-specific questions:
   * Symptoms for how long?
   * Does the child have any infections? Allergies?
   * Has intestinal obstruction been ruled out? If **no**, refer to MD
   * Physical causes?
   * Changes in frequency of bowel movements?
   * Changes in nutrition/feedings?

6. See table on following page

COLIC *(Continued)*

COLIC*

Category	Natural Products to Consider	DOC
Herb	**Chamomile** (In tea form) *on page 407*	PA
	Peppermint (In tea form) *on page 486*	PA
Vitamin/Mineral/ Trace Element/ Nutraceutical	**Milk of Magnesia** (in the form of Milk of Magnesia or Magnesium Citrate) *on page 473* Condition-specific dosage: ½ tsp/day	HD
Homeopathic Remedy	Homeopathic combination formulas are available for many conditions. Listed below are some of the most common single homeopathic remedies for colic. Also see **Homeopathic Quick Reference Chart for Common Complaints** *on page 587*	
	Chamomilla	PD
	Colocynthis	PD
	Magnesia phosphorica	PD
	Nux vomica	PD
	Veratrum album	PD
Additional supplements to consider	No recommendations	

*Refer to **Introduction to Conditions** *on page 41* for more details on how to apply the information in this table to individuals with this condition.

SPECIAL CONSIDERATIONS

Chamomile

- May cause drowsiness; caution in driving/performing hazardous tasks
- Use with caution in individuals with allergies to *Asteraceae/Compositae* family (chrysanthemum, daisy) or ragweed pollens

Peppermint

- Contraindicated in biliary tract obstruction, cholecystitis, severe liver damage, gallstones, hiatal hernia

Milk of Magnesia

- Use caution in renal impairment
- May cause diarrhea at high intakes

CONSTIPATION

Constipation is estimated to occur in as many as 4 million people in the United States with a frequency sufficient to prompt treatment. Discomfort, distention, bloating, and/or lower back pain may accompany constipation. Other symptoms may include headache, fatigue, and loss of appetite. Constipation is a symptom and not a disease in and of itself. It is often associated with hard, dry feces resulting in difficult or painful passage that may be subjectively incomplete. It represents an imbalance in motility due to impaired muscular contractions or changes in stool composition.

Contributing factors include ingestion of constipating foods, inadequate fluid intake, lack of fiber, and inactivity. A number of medications, particularly those with high anticholinergic activity may also decrease bowel motility. In addition, a number of conditions may alter gastrointestinal motility such as diabetes, hypercalcemia, hypothyroidism, pregnancy, multiple sclerosis, dysbiosis, and Parkinson's disease.

Abuse of stimulant laxatives may worsen the responsiveness of normal gastrointestinal factors. Physical abnormalities of the bowel such as stricture, adhesions, or masses (tumor) will also disrupt movement of stool, often with serious consequences. Constipation may contribute to straining during defecation, leading to the development of hemorrhoids or resulting in dizziness from vagal responses. In severe forms, impaction or obstruction of the bowel may occur.

Individuals should be evaluated for potential causes or complications. Dietary habits and medications should be reviewed for the potential to cause constipation. Often, ingestion of high-fiber foods, elimination of low-fiber processed foods, and drinking large quantities of water will relieve the condition.

LIFESTYLE RECOMMENDATIONS

- Continuation/initiation of diet and exercise program
- Increased intake of fluids
- Increase intake of fiber: fruits, vegetables, prunes, grains, fiber supplements
- Minimize laxative use

CONSTIPATION DECISION TREE

1. Client with constipation is interested in using natural products (NP) to support this condition

2. Healthcare provider requests basic background information. The following issues are addressed with the client:
   * Allergies?
   * Prescription (Rx)/OTC meds?
   * Natural products
   * Other medical conditions?
   * Nutrition/diet program?
   * Exercise program?

3. Above data reviewed; if **yes** to Rx/OTC meds, review **Drug-Induced Nutrient Depletion Chart** in Appendix

4A. Client is a candidate for natural products

   * An appropriate homeopathic remedy can be used at any time

4B. Client's case is too complicated at this point; needs additional support from MD before initiating NP program

5. Condition-specific questions:
   * Recent lifestyle changes? Diet, fluid intake, etc?
   * Recent changes in meds? Specific focus here should be on those that can cause constipation, eg, pain meds, calcium supplements, iron products, vitamins, aluminum-containing antacids, diuretics, antidepressants
   * Other symptoms: Fever, nausea, vomiting, weight gain/loss, abdominal pain? If significant, refer to MD
   * Laxative use? If chronic, stress importance of limited PRN use, potential for abuse
   * Blood/mucus in stool? If **yes**, refer to MD

6. See table on following page

CONSTIPATION *(Continued)*

CONSTIPATION*

Category	Natural Products to Consider	DOC
Herb	Cascara *on page 404*	HD
	Milk Thistle *on page 479*	HE
	Psyllium *on page 492*	HT
	Senna *on page 503*	HT
Vitamin/Mineral/ Trace Element/ Nutraceutical	Flaxseed Oil *on page 435* Condition-specific dosage: 1 Tbsp/day	HD
	Lactobacillus acidophilus *on page 467* and *Bifidobacterium bifidum* *on page 391* Condition-specific dosage: 10-15 billion CFU twice daily for 2 weeks (dairy free)	HD
Homeopathic Remedy	Homeopathic combination formulas are available for many conditions. Listed below are some of the most common single homeopathic remedies for constipation. Also see **Homeopathic Quick Reference Chart for Common Complaints** *on page 587*	
	Graphites	PD
	Hydrastis canadensis	PD
	Nux vomica	PD
	Plumbum metallicum	PD
	Veratrum album	PD
Additional Supplements to Consider	Vitamin C *on page 526* Condition-specific dosage: Dose to bowel tolerance	HD

*Refer to **Introduction to Conditions** *on page 41* for more details on how to apply the information in this table to individuals with this condition.

SPECIAL CONSIDERATIONS

Cascara
- Use with caution in bowel disorders, inflammatory bowel disease (ulcerative colitis, Crohn's disease), and appendicitis
- Avoid use in children <12 years of age
- May decrease absorption of some oral medications
- Excessive use may lead to electrolyte disturbances
- Avoid use in bowel obstruction
- Potential interaction with antiarrhythmics, digoxin, phenytoin, laxatives, lithium, theophylline

Milk Thistle
- No reported toxicity in humans at normal intakes

Psyllium
- Avoid use in bowel obstruction

Senna
- Use with caution in bowel disorders, inflammatory bowel disease (ulcerative colitis, Crohn's disease), and appendicitis
- Avoid use in children <12 years of age
- May decrease absorption of some oral medications
- Excessive use may lead to electrolyte disturbances
- Avoid use in bowel obstruction
- Potential interaction with antiarrhythmics, digoxin, phenytoin, laxatives, lithium, theophylline

Flaxseed Oil
- No known toxicity or serious side effects

Lactobacillus acidophilus
- No known toxicity or serious side effects

Bifidobacterium bifidum
- No known toxicity or serious side effects

Vitamin C
- Excess intake in diabetics may give falsely elevated blood glucose readings

COUGH

The cough reflex is a natural defense against irritations and infections. Layers of mucus (phlegm) lining the nose and airways trap particles such as pollen or dust, chemicals, and infectious organisms that may enter from the environment. In response to the irritation or infection, mucous production is increased.

Coughing is a protective reflex that occurs when an irritant stimulates one of several cough receptors in the airways. Coughing helps clear the airways of mucus, along with the irritants trapped in the sticky secretion.

A harsh or forceful cough can cause additional irritation to the airways. Repeated coughing can lead to inflamed membranes, helping to perpetuate cough. For this reason, individuals should be instructed to try to limit coughing. Some measures which may be of assistance include increasing fluid intake (unless on a fluid-restricted diet), increasing the humidity of inhaled air (with a vaporizer or by taking a shower), sucking on hard candy or lozenges, as well as drinking tea sweetened with honey to soothe irritated passageways. Interventions should always include a vigorous review and potential elimination of the cause. For symptomatic relief, an expectorant or a suppressant, or a combination may be used.

Expectorants work to loosen mucus in the airways. Suppressants, or antitussives, act on the CNS cough center. In general, suppressants should not be encouraged with a productive cough. However, if a cough is frequent and produces small amounts of mucus, particularly if the cough is interrupting sleep, temporary use of an expectorant in combination with a suppressant may be considered. If a cough lasts longer than 2-3 weeks, the individual should see a physician.

LIFESTYLE RECOMMENDATIONS

- Avoid refined sugars, refined carbohydrates, fried foods, dairy products, any mucous-producing foods

- Increase consumption of water

- Avoid triggers, such as cold weather, dust, tobacco smoke, others

- If a smoker, consider enrolling in a smoking cessation program

- Use of a vaporizer may be beneficial

- If cough is persistent or recurs often, may want to consider installing a more sophisticated air-filtering system inside the home

PART II. CONDITIONS / DECISION TREES / CONSIDERATIONS

COUGH DECISION TREE

1. Client with cough is interested in using natural products (NP) to support this condition

2. Healthcare provider requests basic background information. The following issues are addressed with the client:
   * Allergies? Obtain as much detail as possible re: environmental allergens
   * Prescription (Rx)/OTC meds?
   * Natural products?
   * Other medical conditions? Focus on recent viral conditions, asthma
   * Nutrition, diet program?
   * Exercise program?

3. Above data reviewed; if **yes** to Rx/OTC meds, review **Drug-Induced Nutrient Depletion Chart** in Appendix

4A. Client is a candidate for natural products
   * An appropriate homeopathic remedy can be used at any time

4B. Client's case is too complicated at this point; needs additional support is needed before initiating NP program

5. Condition-specific questions:
   * Evaluated by MD? If **yes**, what was the recommended treatment plan? Effective?
   * Triggers for condition/symptom onset? Worsening?
   * Accompanying symptoms such as fever, headache, runny nose, watery eyes; anything that might reflect a viral condition, cold, flu?
   * Any problems with heartburn, digestion? If **yes**, may be related to cough and should be discussed with MD
   * Any problems with breathing, painful breathing? If **yes**, may be related to cough and should be discussed with MD
   * Any new medications? If patient is taking angiotensin-converting enzyme inhibitor (ACEI), this class of antihypertensive agents has been shown to cause cough; if **yes**, discuss with pharmacist or MD

6. See table on following page

127

COUGH (Continued)

COUGH*

Category	Natural Products to Consider	DOC
Herb	Ground Ivy *on page 454*	PA
	Thyme *on page 509*	PA, HE
	Licorice *on page 470*	PA, HE
	Marshmallow *on page 476*	PA
Vitamin/Mineral/ Trace Element/ Nutraceutical	No recommendations	
Homeopathic Remedy	Homeopathic combination formulas are available for many conditions. Listed below are some of the most common single homeopathic remedies for croup. Also see **Homeopathic Quick Reference Chart for Common Complaints** *on page 587*	PD
	Aconitum napellus	PD
	Bryonia alba	PD
	Grindelia	PD
	Phosphorus	PD
	Spongia tosta	PD
Additional Supplements to Consider	No recommendations	

*Refer to **Introduction to Conditions** *on page 41* for more details on how to apply the information in this table to individuals with this condition.

SPECIAL CONSIDERATIONS

Ground Ivy

- Contraindicated in individuals with epilepsy

Thyme

- Use with caution in individuals with allergy to oregano or *Labitae* spp
- Use with caution in individuals with urinary tract or gastrointestinal inflammation

Licorice

- Contraindicated in pregnancy and breast-feeding
- Contraindicated in hepatic impairment, renal impairment, hypertension, arrhythmias, congestive heart failure, or edematous states
- May cause sodium and water retention
- Caution in estrogen-dependent tumors, endometrial cancer, thromboembolic disease, or stroke
- Potential interactions with laxatives, corticosteroids, cardiac glycosides, antihypertensives, diuretics
- Avoid use in hypokalemic states
- High doses may cause pseudoaldosteronism

Marshmallow

- May alter blood glucose; monitor blood sugar closely in diabetics or those predisposed to hypoglycemia
- Potential interactions with insulin, oral hypoglycemic agents

CROHN'S DISEASE

Crohn's disease is an inflammatory condition that affects the last section of the small intestine and the beginning section of the colon. It often causes bloody stools and malabsorption. Abdominal cramping, fever, malaise, and general fatigue are also frequent symptoms. Crohn's disease is also referred to as ileitis or regional enteritis. It is a relatively rare condition, but its frequency appears to be increasing. Diagnosis often requires visualization and biopsy of tissue.

The inflammatory process in Crohn's disease affects the entire thickness of the bowel wall, with areas of disease often separated by normal appearing bowel. The cause of Crohn's disease is unknown. A genetic predisposition has been defined and exposure to environmental or infectious agents may contribute. Food allergies have also been found to be contributing factors for some individuals. Crohn's may represent a form of autoimmune reaction stemming from localized immune reactions. Dysbiosis may contribute to this condition.

The disease tends to be chronic with periods of alternating remission and progression. It is not associated with an increased risk of colon cancer. Crohn's is associated with fistula formation (communications formed by fusion between loops of bowel, bladder, or the skin). Nutritional compromise due to decreased nutrient absorption is common, and systemic inflammatory changes such as arthritis and ocular inflammation may occur. Toxic megacolon, perforation of the bowel, and septic shock may rarely occur. Immunosuppressive therapy and surgical removal of diseased tissue are often required. However, many people improve by eliminating allergic foods and high sugar foods, decreasing consumption of animal protein foods, and instituting a good nutritional supplement program with special emphasis on essential fatty acids (DHA and EPA).

LIFESTYLE RECOMMENDATIONS

- Continuation/initiation of diet and exercise program - ensure proper nutritional intake
- Option for pain control may be biofeedback
- If a smoker, consider enrolling in a smoking cessation program
- Avoid dairy products, refined sugars, refined carbohydrates, and raw vegetables
- Reduce stress

CROHN'S DISEASE DECISION TREE

1. Client with Crohn's disease is interested in using natural products (NP) to support this condition

2. Healthcare provider requests basic background information. The following issues are addressed with the client:
   * Allergies?   * Other medical conditions?
   * Prescription (Rx)/OTC meds?   * Nutrition/diet program?
   * Natural products?   * Exercise program?

3. Above data reviewed; if **yes** to Rx/OTC meds, review **Drug-Induced Nutrient Depletion Chart** in Appendix

4A. Client is a candidate for natural products

   * An appropriate homeopathic remedy can be used at any time

4B. Client's case is too complicated at this point; needs additional support from MD before initiating NP program

5. Condition-specific questions:
   * Treatment plan assembled by MD?
   * History of parasitic or fungal diagnosis?
   * What has been the effectiveness of pharmacologic therapy?
   * Depending on specifics of condition, has medication absorption been addressed?
   * See the section on Candidiasis also.

6. See table on following page

CROHN'S DISEASE *(Continued)*

CROHN'S DISEASE*

Category	Natural Products to Consider	DOC
Herb	Cat's Claw *on page 404*	PA
	Olive Leaf *on page 483*	PA
	Licorice (DGL) *on page 470*	PA
Vitamin/Mineral/ Trace Element/ Nutraceutical	Caprylic Acid *on page 402* Condition-specific dosage: 250 mg 3 times/day	PA
	Fish Oils *on page 434* Condition-specific dosage: 1 capsule twice daily	HT
	Glutamine (Buffered) *on page 446* Condition-specific dosage: 5 g 2-3 times/day for 2 months, then maintenance dose of 500 mg 3 times/ day	HD
	Lactobacillus acidophilus *on page 467* and *Bifidobacterium bifidum* *on page 391* Condition-specific dosage: 10-15 billion CFU twice daily for 4 months, then 1-2 billion CFU twice daily with food for 2 months (dairy free)	PA
	Zinc *on page 534* Condition-specific dosage: 15-35 mg/day	HD
	Vitamin A *on page 518* Condition-specific dosage: 10,000-35,000 int. units daily (reduce amount after improvement)	HD
	Vitamin C *on page 526* Condition-specific dosage: 500-1000 mg twice daily	HD
Homeopathic Remedy	Homeopathic combination formulas are available for many conditions. Listed below are some of the most common single homeopathic remedies for Crohn's disease. Also see **Homeopathic Quick Reference Chart for Common Complaints** *on page 587*	
	Aloe socotrina	PD
	Cinchona officinalis (China)	PD
Additional Supplements to Consider	Folic Acid *on page 435* Condition-specific dosage: 400-800 mcg/day	HD

*Refer to **Introduction to Conditions** *on page 41* for more details on how to apply the information in this table to individuals with this condition.

SPECIAL CONSIDERATIONS

Cat's Claw

- Contraindicated in transplant recipients, individuals receiving I.V. immunoglobulins or immunosuppressants
- Contraindicated in active bleeding (eg, peptic ulcer, intracranial bleeding)
- Caution in hemostatic disorders/history of bleeding
- Potential interaction with anticoagulants (warfarin), aspirin, NSAIDs, antiplatelet agents
- Discontinue use prior to dental or surgical procedures (14 days before)

Olive Leaf

- No reported toxicity in humans at normal intakes

Licorice (DGL)

- Contraindicated in pregnancy and breast-feeding
- Potential interactions with nitrofurantoin

Caprylic Acid

- No known toxicity or serious side effects

Fish Oils

- High doses may cause GI upset, loose stools, nausea
- May alter glucose regulation; use with caution in diabetes
- Caution in individuals receiving oral hypoglycemics or insulin; monitor blood glucose closely and coordinate with prescriber
- Potential interaction with anticoagulants (warfarin), aspirin, NSAIDs, antiplatelet agents

Glutamine

- No known toxicity or serious side effects

Lactobacillus acidophilus

- No known toxicity or serious side effects

Bifidobacterium bifidum

- No known toxicity or serious side effects

Zinc

- Prolonged intake at levels >150 mg/day may be associated with toxicity

Vitamin A

- Contraindicated in pregnancy and in women who may become pregnant

Vitamin C

- Excess intake in diabetics may give falsely elevated blood glucose readings

Folic Acid

- No known toxicity or serious side effects

CROUP

Croup is a respiratory symptom characterized by hoarseness, coughing, and wheezing. It is a common manifestation of respiratory infection in childhood. The disease primarily affects children <3 years of age, and attacks typically occur during the night. Breathing becomes strained and difficult, and the child may become frightened. It is important to comfort the child, since anxiety may increase breathing difficulties.

Croup is caused by inflammation and swelling of the nasal passages, larynx, and trachea. Swelling occurs as a result of viral or other infection. Common home treatments include the use of a cool mist vaporizer or steam from a shower to relieve swelling and congestion. In some cases, exposure to cold air may be beneficial. Symptom reversal may be dramatic. In general, if the child starts breathing normally, he or she should be able to fall back to sleep. Urgent treatment should be sought if there is no sign of improvement after 20 minutes or immediately if the child's lips become cyanotic (begin turning blue). Obstruction of the airway may be life threatening and delay in treatment should be avoided.

LIFESTYLE RECOMMENDATIONS

- Remain calm, try to keep child calm, comfortable
- Use warm mist (shower steam) - avoid direct close exposure to steam to avoid burn potential
- If using warm mist is ineffective, use cool air - a cool mist vaporizer, outside cool air
- Increase intake of fluids
- Use acetaminophen to reduce fever
- Avoid dairy products and mucous-producing foods
- Avoid fruit juices
- Avoid refined sugars

Breathing problems can be very serious; if little or no response to interventions or parenteral concern, physician or emergency department evaluation is necessary.

CROUP DECISION TREE

1. Client with croup is interested in using natural products (NP) to support this condition

2. Healthcare provider requests basic background information. The following issues are addressed with the client:
   * Allergies? Obtain as much detail as possible re: environmental allergens
   * Other medical conditions? Focus on recent viral conditions, asthma
   * Prescription (Rx)/OTC meds?
   * Natural products?
   * Nutrition, diet program?
   * Exercise program?

3. Above data reviewed; if **yes** to Rx/OTC meds, review **Drug-Induced Nutrient Depletion Chart** in Appendix

4A. Client is a candidate for natural products
   * An appropriate homeopathic remedy can be used at any time

4B. Client's case is too complicated at this point; needs additional support is needed before initiating NP program

5. Condition-specific questions:
   * Recent viral illness? What was the treatment program prescribed by the physician?
   * Accompanying symptoms - fever, GI, etc?
   * If symptoms worsen or do not improve within 20 minutes, refer to MD
   * Breathing problems can be very serious, if little or no response to interventions or parenteral concern, refer to MD/ED

6. See table on following page

CROUP *(Continued)*

CROUP*

Category	Natural Products to Consider	DOC
Herb	Ground Ivy *on page 454*	PA
	Thyme *on page 509*	PA
	Licorice *on page 470*	PA
	Marshmallow *on page 476*	PA
Vitamin/Mineral/ Trace Element/ Nutraceutical	No recommendations	
Homeopathic Remedy	Homeopathic combination formulas are available for many conditions. Listed below are some of the most common single homeopathic remedies for croup. Also see the Also see **Homeopathic Quick Reference Chart for Common Complaints** *on page 587*	
	Cuprum metallicum	PD
	Drosera rotundifolia	PD
	Rumex crispus	PD
	Spongia tosta	PD
	Sticta pulmonaria	PD
Additional Supplements to Consider	No recommendations	

*Refer to **Introduction to Conditions** *on page 41* for more details on how to apply the information in this table to individuals with this condition.

SPECIAL CONSIDERATIONS

Ground Ivy

* Contraindicated in individuals with epilepsy

Thyme

* Use with caution in individuals with allergy to oregano or *Labitae* spp
* Use with caution in individuals with urinary tract or gastrointestinal inflammation

Licorice

* Contraindicated in hepatic impairment, renal impairment, hypertension, arrhythmias, congestive heart failure, or edematous states
* May cause sodium and water retention
* Potential interactions with laxatives, corticosteroids, cardiac glycosides, antihypertensives, diuretics
* Avoid use in hypokalemic states
* High doses may cause pseudoaldosteronism

Marshmallow

* May alter blood glucose; monitor blood sugar closely in diabetics or those predisposed to hypoglycemia
* Potential interactions with insulin, oral hypoglycemic agents

DEPRESSION

Depression can be caused by stressful events, drug-induced nutrient depletions, hypoglycemia, hypothyroidism, food and environmental reactions, hormonal imbalances, biochemical abnormalities, environmental toxin exposure, or other causes. Occasional mild depression that passes quickly may not require treatment. However, if depression is prolonged, recurrent, or severe, a licensed counselor, psychologist, or psychiatrist should diagnose it.

Major depressive disorder, or unipolar mood disorder, is characterized by persistently depressed mood or anhedonia, and presence of a variety of other symptoms including significant weight change, sleep disturbance, psychomotor agitation or retardation, decreased energy, feelings of worthlessness or inappropriate guilt, diminished concentration, and thoughts of death. Symptom severity may fluctuate and may present in some individuals with a diurnal pattern, usually of greatest severity in the morning.

Major depression is a common disorder with a lifetime prevalence of 15%. Women are nearly twice as likely as men to develop major depression. Mean age of onset for major depression is approximately 40 years. Depression in the elderly is more common than in younger populations, with prevalence rates up to 40% in some older adult populations. Major depression may be chronic or have a tendency for relapse.

The etiology of mood disorders is not clear. Biological causes have been the focus of investigation, however, situational/relational factors certainly contribute. The neurotransmitters, norepinephrine and serotonin, have been the most frequently implicated and well-studied,

Depression is perceived by the individual as distressing and is associated with impairments in work or social functioning. Severely depressed individuals may have psychotic features in addition to depressive symptoms. Another subgroup of depressed individuals present atypically with increased sleep, increased appetite, and weight gain. Depressed individuals have a greater risk for suicide, with 10% to 15% eventually committing suicide. Those with psychotic depression may be at greater risk for suicide. Careful monitoring of suicide risk is essential in all phases of treatment of the depressed individual.

Concurrent use of natural products with antidepressant activity and other antidepressants should be considered only under the supervision of a physician. Mild to moderate depression is commonly treated with prescription drugs. However, supplementation with amino acids, which are metabolic precursors to various neurotransmitters, and various herbs are gaining in popularity because they are generally effective and without side effects.

LIFESTYLE RECOMMENDATIONS

- Continuation/initiation of diet and exercise program

- Adhere to medication regimens as prescribed

- When adding any product, discuss with healthcare provider first to ensure no interactions

- Recognize what causes worsening of symptoms and focus attention and interventions here

- Recognize what makes the client feel better and capitalize on opportunities for more of these situations/experiences

- If seasonal, light therapy (SAD light) may provide improvement.

- Establish a support network

DEPRESSION DECISION TREE

1. Client with depression is interested in using natural products (NP) to support this condition

2. Healthcare provider requests basic background information. The following issues are addressed with the client:

* Allergies?
* Prescription (Rx)/OTC meds?
* Natural products?
* Other medical conditions?
* Nutrition/diet program?
* Exercise program?

3. Above data reviewed; if **yes** to Rx/OTC meds, review **Drug-Induced Nutrient Depletion Chart** in Appendix

4A. Client is a candidate for natural products

* An appropriate homeopathic remedy can be used at any time

4B. Client's case is too complicated at this point; Needs additional support from MD before initiating NP program

5. Condition-specific questions:
* Diagnosed by MD/mental health professional? If **yes**, what was recommended treatment plan? Effective?
* Seasonal? Might recommend light therapy
* Recent changes in lifestyle/home situation?
* Any specific precipitating factors that can be eliminated, reduce exposure?
* Ensure client shares all pertinent information regarding therapies so possible interactions, adverse effects, can be reviewed
* Any suggestions or evidence of suicidal thoughts or plan, as well as potentially violent behavior, should prompt immediate referral to a mental health professional

6. See table on following page

DEPRESSION *(Continued)*

DEPRESSION*

Category	Natural Products to Consider	DOC
Herb	St John's Wort *on page 506*	HT
	Ginkgo *on page 441*	HT
Vitamin/Mineral/ Trace Element/ Nutraceutical	**Adrenal Extract** *on page 380* Condition-specific dosage: 150-200 mg 2-3 times/day	HD
	Dehydroepiandrosterone (DHEA) *on page 421* Condition-specific dosage: Determined by clinician	HD
	5-Hydroxytryptophan (5-HTP) *on page 461* Condition-specific dosage: 50-100 mg 1-3 times/day	HD
	SAMe (S-adenosylmethionine) *on page 498* Condition-specific dosage: 400-1600 mg/day	HT
	Tyrosine *on page 514* Condition-specific dosage: 1000-5000 mg/day **OR** **DL Phenylalanine (DLPA)** *on page 487* Condition-specific dosage: 1200 mg/day	HT
	Vitamin B₆ *on page 523* Condition-specific dosage: 10-20 mg/day	HT
Homeopathic Remedy	Homeopathic combination formulas are available for many conditions. Listed below are some of the most common single homeopathic remedies for depression. Also see **Homeopathic Quick Reference Chart for Common Complaints** *on page 587*	
	Aurum metcallicum	PD
	Kali bromatum	PD
	Sepia	PD
Additional supplements to consider	**Borage Oil, see Evening Primrose Oil** *on page 430* Condition-specific dosage: 500 mg twice daily	HD

*Refer to **Introduction to Conditions** *on page 41* for more details on how to apply the information in this table to individuals with this condition.

SPECIAL CONSIDERATIONS

St John's Wort
- Contraindicated in pregnancy
- Not for use in severe depression
- May cause drowsiness (mild); caution in driving/performing hazardous tasks
- May cause photosensitivity (rare) at high doses
- Potential interactions with antidepressants (including SSRIs, tricyclics, MAO inhibitors), narcotics, other CNS depressants, reserpine, digoxin

Ginkgo
- Contraindicated in active bleeding (eg, peptic ulcer, intracranial bleeding)
- Caution in hemostatic disorders/history of bleeding
- Potential interaction with anticoagulants (warfarin), aspirin, NSAIDs, anti-platelet agents
- Potential interaction with MAO inhibitors, acetylcholinesterase inhibitors (tacrine, donepezil)
- Discontinue use prior to dental or surgical procedures (14 days before)

Adrenal Extract
- May cause excitability when taken in large doses

Dehydroepiandrosterone (DHEA)
- Caution in individuals with congestive heart failure
- Contraindicated in hypertension
- Contraindicated in individuals with a history of prostate or breast cancer
- Potential interaction with hormonal agents, hypoglycemics, insulin

5-Hydroxytryptophan (5-HTP)
- May have additive effects with antidepressants (including SSRIs, MAO inhibitors, and tricyclic antidepressants)
- 5-HTP, St John's wort, tryptophan, and/or SAMe may have additive effects
- May cause mild-moderate gastrointestinal distress

SAMe (S-adenosylmethionine)
- Use caution when combining SAMe with other antidepressants

Tyrosine
- No known toxicity or serious side effects at normal intakes

DL Phenylalanine (DLPA)
- Caution in hyperactive children and individuals that suffer from migraine headaches
- Phenylketonuria (PKU), a genetic abnormality causing toxicity from elevated phenylalanine, results in severe mental retardation
- Ingestion of the artificial sweetener aspartame causes a rapid increase in brain levels of phenylalanine

Vitamin B$_6$
- No known toxicity or serious side effects at normal intakes

Evening Primrose Oil
- Contraindicated in seizure disorders, schizophrenia, or in persons receiving anticonvulsant or antipsychotic medications
- Contraindicated in active bleeding (eg, peptic ulcer, intracranial bleeding)
- Caution in hemostatic disorders/history of bleeding
- Potential interaction with anticoagulants (warfarin), aspirin, NSAIDs, anti-platelet agents
- Discontinue use prior to dental or surgical procedures (14 days before)

DIAPER RASH

Diaper rash is a generally benign dermatologic condition that affects most babies at some time. Diaper rash can be any rash that develops inside the diaper area. Risk factors for development of rash include frequent stools, transition to eating solid foods, and antibiotic exposure (including nursing babies when the mother is taking antibiotics). The risk of diaper rash is generally related to the ability to keep the baby clean and dry. Mild cases clear up within 3-4 days without any intervention. A pediatrician should be consulted if the rash has blisters or pustules, fails to resolve in 48-72 hours, or worsens. In addition, persistent rash or redeveloping rash after any interventions should prompt additional consultation and evaluation.

Causes of rash may include excessive moisture, chafing, prolonged contact with urine or feces, yeast infection, allergic reactions, teething, diet, and ammonia in the urine. In particular, moisture on the skin may render it more susceptible to irritation and breakdown. Infants taking antibiotics are at increased risk of yeast infections, which are characterized by a bright red rash with reddish spots at the edges.

Prevention tips: Promptly change diaper after soiling or wetting; avoid creation of an airtight area when fastening the diaper, particularly when worn overnight; gently cleanse the diaper area with water during changing, use soap only when the stool does not come off easily. Avoid over-cleansing with commercial wipes that may contain alcohol or perfume; these may dry the skin or sensitize the baby's skin.

If diaper rash develops, change wet or soiled diapers often. Use clear water to cleanse the diaper area with each diaper change. Blot dry without rubbing and allow to air dry completely. The application of a thick layer of protective ointment or cream (zinc oxide or petrolatum) is often helpful. These do not have to be completely removed at the next diaper change, since heavy scrubbing or rubbing may damage the skin.

LIFESTYLE RECOMMENDATIONS

- Continue with the same feedings, foods, etc, for the child unless they might be contributing to the condition - then change ASAP

- Change diapers frequently

- Use water to rinse, wash the bottom, and allow to dry

- Do not treat with an OTC antifungal without the recommendation of the physician

- If using an ointment, zinc oxide and petroleum jelly appear to work the best. Do not use either of these if there are severe cracks in the skin.

DIAPER RASH DECISION TREE

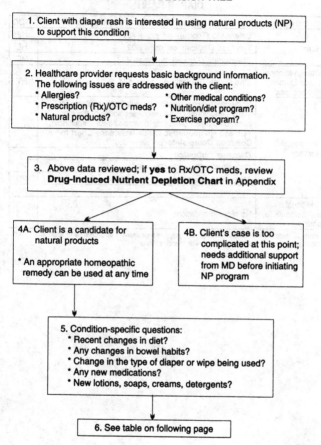

1. Client with diaper rash is interested in using natural products (NP) to support this condition

2. Healthcare provider requests basic background information. The following issues are addressed with the client:
   * Allergies?
   * Prescription (Rx)/OTC meds?
   * Natural products?
   * Other medical conditions?
   * Nutrition/diet program?
   * Exercise program?

3. Above data reviewed; if **yes** to Rx/OTC meds, review **Drug-Induced Nutrient Depletion Chart** in Appendix

4A. Client is a candidate for natural products

   * An appropriate homeopathic remedy can be used at any time

4B. Client's case is too complicated at this point; needs additional support from MD before initiating NP program

5. Condition-specific questions:
   * Recent changes in diet?
   * Any changes in bowel habits?
   * Change in the type of diaper or wipe being used?
   * Any new medications?
   * New lotions, soaps, creams, detergents?

6. See table on following page

DIAPER RASH *(Continued)*

DIAPER RASH*

Category	Natural Products to Consider	DOC
Herb	**Calendula** (Topical) *on page 401*	HE
	Tea Tree (Topical) *on page 509*	HE
	Chamomile (Topical) *on page 407*	HE
Vitamin/Mineral/ Trace Element/ Nutraceutical	**Zinc Oxide** (Topical) *on page 534*	HT
Homeopathic Remedy	Homeopathic combination formulas are available for many conditions. Listed below are some of the most common single homeopathic remedies for diaper rash. Also see **Homeopathic Quick Reference Chart for Common Complaints** *on page 587*	
	Calcarea carbonica	PD
	Calendula officinalis (Topical)	PD
	Mercurius corrosivus	PD
	Sulphur	PD
Additional supplements to consider	No recommendations	

*Refer to **Introduction to Conditions** *on page 41* for more details on how to apply the information in this table to individuals with this condition.

SPECIAL CONSIDERATIONS

Calendula
- No reported toxicity in humans at normal intakes

Tea Tree
- May cause allergic dermatitis in sensitive individuals
- Not for ingestion

Chamomile (Topical)
- Avoid use in individuals with allergies to *Asteraceae/Compositae* family (chrysanthemum, daisy)

Zinc Oxide
- No known toxicity or serious side effects with topical product

DIARRHEA

An abnormal frequency of unformed, semisolid or liquid stools is characterized as diarrhea. Excessive fluidity of stool may be caused by hypersecretion, hypermotility, inflammation, ingestion of high amounts of nonabsorbable solutes, or disruption of the microflora of the gastrointestinal tract. It may be accompanied by high amounts of mucous or blood in the stool. Systemic symptoms may include fever, weakness, malaise, myalgias, vomiting, abdominal cramping, and anorexia. Diarrhea is usually due to infectious agents or drugs. Occasionally, it may be caused by inadequate absorptive surface, tumors that secrete vasoactive compounds, secretion of excessive amounts of fluid by the gastrointestinal cells, or impaired absorptive function.

It is usually acute in nature but some forms may be chronic (lasting longer than 2-4 weeks). It is important to consider the causes of diarrhea. Viral, bacterial, and/or parasitic infections, drugs, toxin ingestion from contaminated food or water, changes in diet, or stress may contribute. Blood in the stool is particularly important and may signify hemorrhage, infection, inflammation, or neoplastic disease. Diseases of the small bowel tend to produce nonbloody, highly fluid stools. Neurologic disorders may also cause diarrhea. A notorious secondary invader, often following exposure to broad-spectrum antibiotics, *Clostridium difficile* produces a toxin that causes desquamation (shedding) of villi. Individuals with diarrhea >5 days; or diarrhea associated with bloody stools, high fever (>101°F), symptoms of dehydration (such as orthostatic hypotension, dizziness, or tachycardia), or severe cramping should be referred for evaluation. Extra fluids should be consumed to prevent dehydration.

Chronic or prolonged diarrhea may result in malabsorption and increase the excretion of all vitamins and minerals.

LIFESTYLE RECOMMENDATIONS

- Drink plenty of fluids to avoid dehydration

- Avoid beverages with alcohol, caffeine, dairy products, and artificial sweeteners

- If food poisoning, usually let it run its course; if after a few days condition is no better, or worse, seek medical attention

- Consider BRAT diet - **B** ananas, **R** ice, **A** pplesauce, and **T** oast

- Avoid consistent use of antidiarrheal medications - PRN use over a couple days is reasonable; any longer and medical attention should be sought

DIARRHEA DECISION TREE

1. Client with diarrhea is interested in using natural products (NP) to support this condition

2. Healthcare provider requests basic background information. The following issues are addressed with the client:
   * Allergies?
   * Prescription (Rx)/OTC meds?
   * Natural products?
   * Other medical conditions?
   * Nutrition/diet program?
   * Exercise program?

ADULTS

INFANTS

Duration <2 days

Duration ≥2 days

Additional symptoms: Fever, nausea, vomiting, blood/mucus in stool? — **YES** → Refer to MD

NO ↓   **YES**

Review profile for possible drug-induced condition — **NO** → Refer to Considerations and Lifestyle Recommendations

ADULTS

3. Above data reviewed; if **yes** to Rx/OTC meds, review **Drug-Induced Nutrient Depletion Chart** in Appendix

4A. Client is a candidate for natural products

* An appropriate homeopathic remedy can be used at any time

4B. Client's case is too complicated at this point; needs additional support from MD before initiating NP program

5. Condition-specific questions:
   * Stools contain blood/mucus? Refer to MD
   * How often having bowel movements?
   * Other symptoms: Nausea, fever, stomach ache, vomiting, weakness? If severe, refer to MD
   * Recent foreign travel?
   * Any chance it is food poisoning?
   * Swimming in pond, lake, river?
   * Changes in diet that coincide?
   * New medications, specifically antibiotics?

6. See table on following page

DIARRHEA *(Continued)*

DIARRHEA*

Category	Natural Products to Consider	DOC
Herb	**Grapefruit Seed Extract** *on page 450*	PA
	Olive Leaf *on page 483*	PA
	Green Tea *on page 452*	PA
	Bilberry *on page 392*	PA
Vitamin/Mineral/ Trace Element/ Nutraceutical	*Lactobacillus acidophilus on page 467* and *Bifidobacterium bifidum on page 391* Condition-specific dosage: 15 billion CFU twice daily for 2 weeks, then 1-2 billion CFU twice daily with food for 2 months (dairy free)	HT
Homeopathic Remedy	Homeopathic combination formulas are available for many conditions. Listed below are some of the most common single homeopathic remedies for diarrhea. Also see **Homeopathic Quick Reference Chart for Common Complaints** *on page 587*	
	Arsenicum album	PD
	Colocynthis	PD
	Natrum sulphuricum	PD
	Podophyllum peltatum	PD
	Veratrum album	PD
Additional supplements to consider	No recommendations	

*Refer to **Introduction to Conditions** *on page 41* for more details on how to apply the information in this table to individuals with this condition.

SPECIAL CONSIDERATIONS

Grapefruit Seed Extract

- Grapefruit seed extract is not equivalent to grapefruit juice/pulp. Juice/pulp has been associated with many drug interactions; see Grapefruit Seed *on page 450*
- Until further information is available, it is reasonable to avoid some medications (terfenadine, astemizole, cisapride). Use other medications metabolized by CYP3A4 with caution.

Olive Leaf

- No reported toxicity in humans at normal intakes

Green Tea

- Decaffeinated products are recommended
- Caffeine may cause multiple CNS and CV effects; caution in peptic ulcer disease or cardiovascular disease
- Contraindicated in active bleeding (eg, peptic ulcer, intracranial bleeding)
- Caution in hemostatic disorders/history of bleeding
- Potential interaction with anticoagulants (warfarin), aspirin, NSAIDs, antiplatelet agents
- See Green Tea *on page 452* for additional potential interactions

Bilberry (Berry)

- Contraindicated in active bleeding (eg, peptic ulcer, intracranial bleeding)
- Caution in hemostatic disorders/history of bleeding
- Potential interaction with anticoagulants (warfarin), aspirin, NSAIDs, antiplatelet agents
- Discontinue use prior to dental or surgical procedures (14 days before)

Lactobacillus acidophilus

- No known toxicity or serious side effects

Bifidobacterium bifidum

- No known toxicity or serious side effects

DIVERTICULITIS

Diverticulitis is a condition in which small pouches form in the walls of the intestine (known as diverticula) and become inflamed. This inflammation may affect single or multiple diverticula. It is most common in the sixth through eighth decade of life and may affect up to 60% to 80% of the elderly population. Symptoms are usually mild and may consist of abdominal pain, constipation, and diarrhea. Sometimes severe attacks occur, consisting of intense abdominal pain and fever. A palpable abdominal mass may be present. Fistulae may form between the inflamed bowel and the skin, adjacent bowel loop, or bladder. Attacks are usually sudden in onset and may be recurrent.

There is no known cause of diverticular disease, although defects in colonic wall strength and diminished fecal volume have been proposed as contributors. Diverticulitis is associated with a low fiber diet; therefore, a high fiber diet may help to prevent this condition. Depending on the severity of the attacks, a change in diet, antibiotics, and bedrest may be used to ease the symptoms.

Diverticulitis should be differentiated from a variety of other gastrointestinal diseases, including irritable bowel disease, infections, and inflammatory bowel disease. Qualified medical personnel should immediately evaluate severe or persistent symptoms.

LIFESTYLE RECOMMENDATIONS

- Continuation/initiation of diet and exercise program

- Increase fluid intake

- Increase fiber intake - fruits, vegetables, grains, prunes, fiber products

- If client is taking antibiotics, suggest *Lactobacillus acidophilus/Bifidobacterium bifidum*

DIVERTICULITIS DECISION TREE

1. Client with diverticulitis is interested in using natural products (NP) to support this condition

2. Healthcare provider requests basic background information. The following issues are addressed with the client:
   * Allergies?   * Other medical conditions?
   * Prescription (Rx)/OTC meds?   * Nutrition/diet program?
   * Natural products?   * Exercise program?

3. Above data reviewed; if **yes** to Rx/OTC meds, review **Drug-Induced Nutrient Depletion Chart** in Appendix

4A. Client is a candidate for natural products

   * An appropriate homeopathic remedy can be used at any time

4B. Client's case is too complicated at this point; needs additional support from MD before initiating NP program

5. Condition-specific questions:
   * Frequency of symptoms? How often do flare-ups require antibiotics?
   * Any rectal bleeding, fever, or abdominal distention? Sought medical attention for this? If **no**, refer to MD

6. See table on following page

DIVERTICULITIS *(Continued)*

DIVERTICULITIS*

Category	Natural Products to Consider	DOC
Herb	Cat's Claw *on page 404*	PA
	Ginger *on page 440*	PA
	Grapefruit Seed Extract *on page 450*	PA
	Olive Leaf *on page 483*	PA
Vitamin/Mineral/ Trace Element/ Nutraceutical	***Lactobacillus acidophilus*** *on page 467* and ***Bifidobacterium bifidum*** *on page 391* Condition-specific dosage: 2-5 billion CFU twice daily (dairy free)	PA
Homeopathic Remedy	Homeopathic combination formulas are available for many conditions. Listed below are some of the most common single homeopathic remedies for diverticulitis. Also see **Homeopathic Quick Reference Chart for Common Complaints** *on page 587*	
	Argentum nitricum	PD
	Arsenicum album	PD
	Colycynthis	PD
Additional supplements to consider	**Vitamin A** *on page 518* Condition-specific dosage: 10,000-35,000 int. units daily for 1 month	PA
	Vitamin C (buffered) *on page 526* Condition-specific dosage: 250-1000 mg twice daily	PA
	Zinc *on page 534* Condition-specific dosage: 15-35 mg/day	PA

*Refer to **Introduction to Conditions** *on page 41* for more details on how to apply the information in this table to individuals with this condition.

SPECIAL CONSIDERATIONS

Cat's Claw

- Contraindicated in transplant recipients, individuals receiving I.V. immuno-globulins or immunosuppressants
- Contraindicated in active bleeding (eg, peptic ulcer, intracranial bleeding)
- Caution in hemostatic disorders/history of bleeding
- Potential interaction with anticoagulants (warfarin), aspirin, NSAIDs, anti-platelet agents
- Discontinue use prior to dental or surgical procedures (14 days before)

Ginger

- Contraindicated in active bleeding (eg, peptic ulcer, intracranial bleeding)
- Caution in hemostatic disorders/history of bleeding
- Potential interaction with anticoagulants (warfarin), aspirin, NSAIDs, anti-platelet agents, cardiac glycosides (digoxin)
- Discontinue use prior to dental or surgical procedures (14 days before)

Grapefruit Seed Extract

- Grapefruit seed extract is not equivalent to grapefruit juice/pulp. Juice/pulp has been associated with many drug interactions; see Grapefruit Seed *on page 450*
- Until further information is available, it is reasonable to avoid some medications (terfenadine, astemizole, cisapride). Use other medications metabolized by CYP3A4 with caution.

Olive Leaf

- No reported toxicity in humans at normal intakes

Lactobacillus acidophilus

- No known toxicity or serious side effects

Bifidobacterium bifidum

- No known toxicity or serious side effects

Vitamin A

- Contraindicated in pregnancy and in women who may become pregnant

Vitamin C

- Excess intake in diabetics may give falsely elevated blood glucose readings

Zinc

- No known toxicity or serious side effects

DYSLIPIDEMIA

Cholesterol is an important component of cell membranes and a precursor in the synthesis of the sex and steroid hormones. Most of our cholesterol is manufactured in the liver, but we also ingest it from saturated fats in our diets.

HDL (high-density lipoprotein) is considered to be the "good" cholesterol, while LDL (low-density lipoprotein) is known as the "bad" cholesterol. Cholesterol itself is not "bad," but the oxidation of LDL cholesterol is associated with the build-up of atherosclerotic plaque, which is one of the most serious risk factors in cardiovascular disease. Therefore, an elevated level of LDL cholesterol, and a lack of appropriate antioxidant nutrients are two factors that create a major risk for developing atherosclerotic heart disease.

A total cholesterol level <200 mg/dL is generally considered appropriate. Levels of 200-240 mg/dL warrant caution, and levels >240 mg/dL signal danger. However, knowing the HDL and LDL levels is more important than knowing total cholesterol.

The American Heart Association (AHA) recommends limiting daily caloric intake from saturated fat to <10% of all calories and reducing total dietary fat to <30% of all daily calories. Others promote total fat consumption at 20%. Saturated fats, which are oils from animal products and some plants, raise blood cholesterol levels. Examples of saturated fats are meat fat, butter, cream, coconut oil, palm oil, and shortening.

People should be advised to avoid **ALL** foods containing partially hydrogenated fats and oils. Partially hydrogenated fats and oils contain substances known as trans-fatty acids, which are fats that have been altered structurally. Trans-fatty acids block the body's ability to metabolize and eliminate cholesterol, thus elevating cholesterol levels and increasing the risk of cardiovascular disease.

Recommendations include periodic cholesterol screening, limiting ingestion of high cholesterol foods, substituting monounsaturated fats (such as olive and canola oil) in cooking, and exercising regularly (which increases the body's levels of high-density lipoprotein).

LIFESTYLE RECOMMENDATIONS

- Continuation/initiation of diet and exercise program. Specific focus for diet should be on the Step I and Step II diets, with increasing fiber, more fish, less red meat, substituting monounsaturated and polyunsaturated fats (safflower, corn, and olive oils), decreasing fats

- Maintaining nonpharmacologic interventions even with drug therapy is important

- If a smoker, consider enrolling in a smoking cessation program

- If on a medication requiring monitoring (ie, HMG-CoA reductase inhibitor), discuss monitoring plan with physician

- Have lipid panel checked on a regular basis (every 3-6 months) to evaluate success of intervention program

DYSLIPIDEMIA DECISION TREE

1. Client with dyslipidemia (cholesterol problems) is interested in using natural products (NP) to support this condition

↓

2. Healthcare provider requests basic background information. The following issues are addressed with the client:
   * Allergies?
   * Prescription (Rx)/OTC meds?
   * Natural products?
   * Lipid monitoring program with healthcare provider?
   * Other medical conditions?
   * Nutrition/diet program?
   * Exercise program?

↓

3. Above data reviewed; if **yes** to Rx/OTC meds, review **Drug-Induced Nutrient Depletion Chart** in Appendix

↓

4A. Client is a candidate for natural products

   * An appropriate homeopathic remedy can be used at any time

4B. Client's case is too complicated at this point; needs additional support from MD before initiating NP program

↓

5. Condition-specific questions:
Review NCEP II Guidelines to determine number of risk factors and target LDL value
   * **Positive risk factors:**
      Male: ≥45 years of age; Female: ≥55 years of age, or premature menopause and no estrogen replacement therapy
      Family history of premature coronary heart disease
      Hypertension
      Diabetes
      HDL ≤35 mg/dL

   * **Negative risk factor:** HDL ≥60 mg/dL
   * Is a treatment plan being overseen by MD? If **yes**, have client describe plan. If **no**, recommend a plan be put together.
   * If using an HMG-CoA reductase inhibitor, recommend coenzyme Q10

↓

6. See table on following page

DYSLIPIDEMIA *(Continued)*

DYSLIPIDEMIA*

Category	Natural Products to Consider	DOC
Herb	Red Yeast Rice *on page 496*	HT
	Garlic *on page 438*	HT
	Guggul *on page 454*	HT
Vitamin/Mineral/ Trace Element/ Nutraceutical	Borage Oil, see Evening Primrose Oil *on page 430* Condition-specific dosage:	PA
	Chromium *on page 410* Condition-specific dosage: 200–400 mg/day	HT
	Vitamin B₃ (Inositol Hexaniacinate) *on page 521* Condition-specific dosage: 650 mg 2-3 times/day	PA
	Carnitine *on page 403* Condition-specific dosage: 500-2000 mg/day in divided doses	PA
	Coenzyme Q₁₀ *on page 412* Condition-specific dosage: 50-100 mg/day	PA
	Vitamin E *on page 529* Condition-specific dosage: 200-400 int. units/day	HD
	Tocotrienols *on page 511* Condition-specific dosage: 50 mg/day	HT
Homeopathic Remedy	Homeopathic combination formulas are available for many conditions. Listed below are some of the most common single homeopathic remedies for dyslipidemia. Also see **Homeopathic Quick Reference Chart for Common Complaints** *on page 587*	
	Carduus marianus	PD
	Chelidonium majus	PD
	Cholesterinum	PD
	Petroleum	PD
Additional supplements to consider	No recommendations	

*Refer to **Introduction to Conditions** *on page 41* for more details on how to apply the information in this table to individuals with this condition.

SPECIAL CONSIDERATIONS

Red Yeast Rice
- Contraindicated in pregnancy or breast-feeding, known hypersensitivity to rice or yeast
- Do not use in individuals with hepatic disease, serious infection, recent surgery, serious systemic disease, transplant recipients, persons consuming more than two alcohol-containing drinks per day
- Keep out of reach of children; do not use in individuals <20 years of age
- Adverse effects include gastrointestinal upset
- HMG-CoA reductase inhibitors have been associated with rare but serious adverse hepatic and skeletal muscle effects; risk may be increased by concomitant drug therapy (not specifically reported for red yeast rice)
- Discontinue at the first sign of hepatic dysfunction
- Potential interactions with HMG-CoA reductase inhibitors, other cholesterol-lowering agents, anticoagulants, gemfibrozil, erythromycin, itraconazole, cyclosporin, niacin

Garlic
- Contraindicated in active bleeding (eg, peptic ulcer, intracranial bleeding)
- Caution in hemostatic disorders/history of bleeding; in individuals at risk due to hypotension or orthostasis (elderly, cerebrovascular or cardiovascular disease); in diabetes
- Discontinue use prior to dental or surgical procedures (14 days before)
- Potential interaction with anticoagulants (warfarin), aspirin, NSAIDs, antiplatelet agents, antihypertensives, hypolipidemics

Guggul
- Contraindicated during pregnancy and breast-feeding
- Contraindicated in active bleeding (eg, peptic ulcer, intracranial bleeding)
- Caution in thyroid disease and in hemostatic disorders/history of bleeding
- Potential interaction with anticoagulants (warfarin), aspirin, NSAIDs, antiplatelet agents
- Discontinue use prior to dental or surgical procedures (14 days before)
- Potential interactions with antihypertensives (serum levels of propranolol and diltiazem may be increased)

Evening Primrose Oil
- Contraindicated in seizure disorders, schizophrenia, or in persons receiving anticonvulsant or antipsychotic medications
- Contraindicated in active bleeding (eg, peptic ulcer, intracranial bleeding)
- Caution in hemostatic disorders/history of bleeding
- Potential interaction with anticoagulants (warfarin), aspirin, NSAIDs, antiplatelet agents
- Discontinue use prior to dental or surgical procedures (14 days before)

Chromium
- Caution in individuals receiving oral hypoglycemics or insulin; monitor blood glucose closely and coordinate with prescriber

Vitamin B_3 (Inositol Hexaniacinate) – No known toxicity or serious side effects

Carnitine – No known toxicity or serious side effects

Coenzyme Q_{10}
- No known toxicity or serious side effects; caution in individuals receiving anticoagulants

Vitamin E
- Use with caution when taking anticoagulants (vitamin E ≥200 int. units increases prothrombin times)
- Interrupt or reduce dosage one week prior to dental or surgical procedures

Tocotrienols – No known toxicity or serious side effects

DYSMENORRHEA

Dysmenorrhea usually begins 2-3 years following the onset of menses, but may occur much later. It consists of abdominal pain which is usually described as crampy, which starts 1-2 days prior to the beginning of a menstrual period. Generally, the pain lasts 1-2 additional days into the period and then subsides. Pain may be mild to severe and may be associated with nausea, vomiting, constipation, or diarrhea.

Dysmenorrhea is a common gynecological complaint, particularly in adolescents. Most cases are not associated with underlying disease. These cases are termed "functional" dysmenorrhea. However, some cases are associated with diseases such as endometriosis or pelvic inflammatory disease. In particular, in adolescents, the increasing frequency of sexually-transmitted disease has increased the frequency of dysmenorrhea which may be associated with underlying disease.

A complete history and physical exam by a qualified healthcare provider is required to differentiate between functional dysmenorrhea and cases caused by a more severe medical condition. Functional dysmenorrhea is not associated with complications; however, disease-induced dysmenorrhea may be associated with significant complications.

In general, efforts are focused on pain relief with mild analgesics and/or anti-inflammatory agents. In some cases, hormonal regulation is incorporated. If an underlying disease state is responsible for the complaints, improvement accompanies definitive treatment of the disease.

LIFESTYLE RECOMMENDATIONS

- If a smoker, consider enrolling in a smoking cessation program

- Avoid refined sugars, refined carbohydrates, fried foods, caffeine, excess dietary fat

- Increase intake of fiber, fresh fruits, and vegetables

- Increase consumption of water

- Applying heat to the lower abdomen (in the form of a heating pad, hot water bottle, or a warm bath) may provide some relief of the symptoms

DYSMENORRHEA DECISION TREE

1. Client with dysmenorrhea is interested in using natural products (NP) to support this condition

2. Healthcare provider requests basic background information. The following issues are addressed with the client:
   * Allergies?
   * Prescription (Rx)/OTC meds?
   * Other medical conditions?
   * Nutrition/diet program?
   * Exercise program?

3. Above data reviewed; if **yes** to Rx/OTC meds, review **Drug-Induced Nutrient Depletion Chart** in Appendix

4A. Client is a candidate for natural products

   * An appropriate homeopathic remedy can be used at any time

4B. Client's case is too complicated at this point; needs additional support from MD before initiating NP program

5. Condition-specific questions:
   * Diagnosed by MD? If **yes**, what was the recommended treatment plan? Effective?
   * Triggers for condition/symptom onset? Worsening?
   * How does the onset of symptoms relate to the menstrual cycle? How long do the symptoms last? If extend beyond the traditional 48- to 72-hour maximum time, seek medical attention
   * Are menstrual cycles regular? If **no**, seek medical attention
   * Using an intrauterine device (IUD)? If **yes**, this may be the primary cause of the symptoms, or at the very least, is contributing to symptoms.

6. See table on following page

DYSMENORRHEA *(Continued)*

DYSMENORRHEA*

Category	Natural Products to Consider	DOC
Herb	Dong Quai *on page 425*	PA
	Turmeric *on page 512*	PA
Vitamin/Mineral/ Trace Element/ Nutraceutical	**Magnesium** *on page 473* Condition-specific dosage: 400-600 mg/day	HT
	Progesterone *on page 491* Condition-specific dosage: On days 7-28 of cycle, 1/8 to 1/4 tsp applied topically daily	PA
	Fish Oils *on page 434* Condition-specific dosage: 750 mg 2-3 times/day	HT
Homeopathic Remedy	Homeopathic combination formulas are available for many conditions. Listed below are some of the most common single homeopathic remedies for dysmenorrhea. Also see **Homeopathic Quick Reference Chart for Common Complaints** *on page 587*	
	Chamomilla	PD
	Cimicifuga racemosa	PD
	Magnesia phosphorica	PD
Additional supplements to consider	No recommendations	

*Refer to **Introduction to Conditions** *on page 41* for more details on how to apply the information in this table to individuals with this condition.

SPECIAL CONSIDERATIONS

Dong Quai

- Caution in pregnancy and breast-feeding
- Contraindicated in active bleeding (eg, peptic ulcer, intracranial bleeding)
- Use caution in those at risk of estrogen-dependent tumors, endometrial cancer, thromboembolic disease, or stroke
- Potential interaction with anticoagulants (warfarin), aspirin, NSAIDs, anti-platelet agents
- Potential interaction with oral contraceptives or hormonal replacement therapy
- Caution in hemostatic disorders/history of bleeding
- Potential interaction with antihypertensives, photosensitizing agents
- Discontinue use prior to dental or surgical procedures (14 days before)

Turmeric

- Caution in biliary obstruction
- Caution in ulcerative gastrointestinal disease (eg, peptic ulcer disease, ulcerative colitis, Crohn's)
- Contraindicated in active bleeding (eg, peptic ulcer, intracranial bleeding)
- Caution in hemostatic disorders/history of bleeding
- Potential interaction with anticoagulants (warfarin), aspirin, NSAIDs, anti-platelet agents
- Discontinue use prior to dental or surgical procedures (14 days before)

Magnesium

- Use caution in renal impairment
- May cause diarrhea in high intakes

Progesterone

- May alter hormonal regulation
- Not to be used with oral contraceptives without medical supervision

Fish Oils

- High doses may cause GI upset, loose stools, nausea
- May alter glucose regulation; use with caution in diabetes
- Caution in individuals receiving oral hypoglycemics or insulin; monitor blood glucose closely and coordinate with prescriber
- Potential interaction with anticoagulants (warfarin), aspirin, NSAIDs, anti-platelet agents

ECZEMA

Eczema is a general term used to describe a variety of acute or chronic inflammatory conditions of the skin. These conditions are characterized by an itchy, red rash, edema, papules, vesicles, and crusting. Numerous skin conditions can cause similar rashes, so it is important to have a proper diagnosis.

Two forms of eczema are atopic dermatitis or contact dermatitis. Atopic dermatitis is usually genetically inherited and develops in infancy. Contact dermatitis is more common and develops from exposure to an allergic or irritant substance. Both forms of eczema are frequently due to allergic reactions and these individuals frequently have allergies to other things such as foods, inhalants, etc.

Dry eczema is associated with low humidity and winter. This condition may be related to diminished intradermal lipids. This condition is particularly common in elderly individuals, beginning with dry, scaly skin followed by cracks and fissures. Erythema may be noted in these cracks. Individuals often complain of stinging and tight skin.

In children, a typical progression towards eczema includes repeated rounds of antibiotics (ie, otitis media) leading to eczema, then leading to asthma. Dysbiosis and reduced immune competence may be implicated.

LIFESTYLE RECOMMENDATIONS

- Continuation/initiation of diet and exercise program
- Avoid wheat, refined sugar, dairy
- Only use creams and ointments on **dry** skin
- Use liquids and lotions on areas with "oozing"
- Use hypoallergenic soap, detergents, cosmetics, and cleansing products
- Use moisturizing lotion after shower and bath to prevent dryness
- If condition is related to stress, seek stress management program, look for relaxation techniques
- Check for food intolerances

ECZEMA / DERMATITIS DECISION TREE

1. Client with eczema or dermatitis is interested in using natural products (NP) to support this condition

2. Healthcare provider requests basic background information. The following issues are addressed with the client:

* Allergies?
* Prescription (Rx)/OTC meds?
* Natural products?
* Other medical conditions?
* Nutrition/diet program?
* Exercise program?

3. Above data reviewed; if **yes** to Rx/OTC meds, review **Drug-Induced Nutrient Depletion Chart** in Appendix

4A. Client is a candidate for natural products

* An appropriate homeopathic remedy can be used at any time

4B. Client's case is too complicated at this point; needs additional support from MD before initiating NP program

5. Condition-specific questions:
* Triggers that cause worsening of symptoms (such as certain foods, clothing, lotions, shampoos, soaps, cosmetics, stress, seasonal issues)
* Itching? What relieves this? Make sure client does not scratch until it bleeds
* Is the skin broken or look infected?
If **yes**, refer to MD for further evaluation

6. See table on following page

ECZEMA *(Continued)*

ECZEMA*

Category	Natural Products to Consider	DOC
Herb	Milk Thistle *on page 479*	PA, HE
	Evening Primrose *on page 430*	PA
	Grapefruit Seed Extract *on page 450*	PA
	Olive Leaf *on page 483*	PA
	Artichoke *on page 386*	PA
Vitamin/Mineral/ Trace Element/ Nutraceutical	*Lactobacillus acidophilus on page 467* and *Bifidobacterium bifidum on page 391* Condition-specific dosage: 10-15 billion CFU twice daily for 2 weeks, then 1-2 billion CFU twice daily (dairy free)	HD
	Fish Oils *on page 434* Condition-specific dosage: 750 mg 2-3 times/day	HT
	Vitamin A *on page 518* Condition-specific dosage: 10,000-35,000 int. units/ day	PA
	Vitamin C *on page 526* Condition-specific dosage: 250-1000 mg/day	HT
Homeopathic Remedy	Homeopathic combination formulas are available for many conditions. Listed below are some of the most common single homeopathic remedies for eczema. Also see **Homeopathic Quick Reference Chart for Common Complaints** *on page 587*	
	Calcarea carbonica	PD
	Cantharis	PD
	Croton tiglium	PD
	Graphites	PD
	Mezereum	PD
	Sulphur	PD
Additional supplements to consider	Selenium *on page 502* Condition-specific dosage: 200 mcg/day	HD
	Vitamin E *on page 529* Condition-specific dosage: 200-400 int. units/day	PA
	Zinc *on page 534* Condition-specific dosage: 15-35 mg/day	HD

*Refer to **Introduction to Conditions** *on page 41* for more details on how to apply the information in this table to individuals with this condition.

SPECIAL CONSIDERATIONS

Milk Thistle
- No known toxicity or serious side effects

Evening Primrose
- Contraindicated in active bleeding (eg, peptic ulcer, intracranial bleeding), in seizure disorders, schizophrenia, or in persons receiving anticonvulsant or antipsychotic medications
- Caution in hemostatic disorders/history of bleeding
- Potential interaction with anticoagulants (warfarin), aspirin, NSAIDs, antiplatelet agents
- Discontinue use prior to dental or surgical procedures (14 days before)

Grapefruit Seed Extract
- Grapefruit seed extract is not equivalent to grapefruit juice/pulp. Juice/pulp has been associated with many drug interactions; see Grapefruit Seed *on page 450*
- Until further information is available, it is reasonable to avoid some medications (terfenadine, astemizole, cisapride). Use other medications metabolized by CYP3A4 with caution.

Olive Leaf
- No reported toxicity in humans at normal intakes

Artichoke
- Contraindicated in bile duct obstruction
- Avoid use in individuals with allergies to *Asteraceae/Compositae* family (chrysanthemum, daisy)

Lactobacillus acidophilus
- No known toxicity or serious side effects

Bifidobacterium bifidum
- No known toxicity or serious side effects

Fish Oils
- High doses may cause GI upset, loose stools, nausea
- May alter glucose regulation; use with caution in diabetes
- Caution in individuals receiving oral hypoglycemics or insulin; monitor blood glucose closely and coordinate with prescriber
- Potential interaction with anticoagulants (warfarin), aspirin, NSAIDs, antiplatelet agents

Vitamin A
- Contraindicated in pregnancy and in women who may become pregnant

Vitamin C
- Excess intake in diabetics may give falsely elevated blood glucose readings

Selenium
- No known toxicity or serious side effects at normal intakes

Vitamin E
- Use with caution when taking anticoagulants (vitamin E ≥200 int. units increases prothrombin times)
- Interrupt or reduce dosage one week prior to dental or surgical procedures

Zinc
- No known toxicity or serious side effects at normal intakes

ENDOMETRIOSIS

The endometrium is the membrane lining the uterine surface. Endometriosis involves the development of endometrial tissue outside the uterus, usually on the ovaries, but potentially on other sites within the abdominal cavity. Endometriosis is usually diagnosed in women during their thirties; however, it is likely that the problem begins much earlier, possibly at the beginning of regular menstruation. Endometriosis occurs in roughly 10% to 20% of women during their reproductive years. The incidence approaches 15% to 40% in women with infertility.

A higher risk has been noted in first degree relatives of women with endometriosis, a menstrual cycle length of 27 days or less, early onset of menstrual periods, and periods lasting 7 or more days. The cause of endometriosis is unknown, although several theories have been proposed. What is known is that fragments of endometrial tissue are found growing in other parts of the pelvic cavity, which respond to hormonal changes of the menstrual cycle similar to normal intrauterine endometrial tissue. The tissue fills with blood, creating blood-filled sacs, or cysts. An ongoing process of scar formation and healing of tissue may lead to adhesions in the fallopian tubes and ovaries. Elevated estrogen/progesterone levels may be implicated.

Common symptoms of endometriosis include lower abdominal pain which is most pronounced during menstruation, irregular menstrual cycles, and pain during sexual intercourse. Less common symptoms include pain with bowel movements or low back pain. In some women, endometriosis may be asymptomatic. The degree of discomfort does not bear an absolute relationship to the extent of tissue involved. In some women, pregnancy diminishes symptoms during subsequent periods.

LIFESTYLE RECOMMENDATIONS

- Increase consumption of fiber, fruits, vegetables, easy-to-digest foods
- Avoid sugars, alcohol, caffeine, tobacco, dairy products
- Avoid use of tampons; use sanitary pads
- Seek assistance from a support group
- Stress management may be important

ENDOMETRIOSIS DECISION TREE

1. Client with endometriosis is interested in using natural products (NP) to support this condition

2. Healthcare provider requests basic background information. The following issues are addressed with the client:
   * Allergies?
   * Prescription (Rx)/OTC meds?
   * Natural products?
   * Other medical conditions?
   * Nutrition/diet program?
   * Exercise program?

3. Above data reviewed; if **yes** to Rx/OTC meds, review **Drug-Induced Nutrient Depletion Chart** in Appendix

4A. Client is a candidate for natural products

   * An appropriate homeopathic remedy can be used at any time

4B. Client's case is too complicated at this point; needs additional support from MD before initiating NP program

5. Condition-specific questions:
   * Diagnosed by MD? If **yes**, what was the recommended treatment plan? Effective?
   * Triggers for condition/symptom onset? Worsening?
   * Is the client pre-/peri-/postmenopausal? Discuss with MD how the condition may relate to client's status
   * Any relationship between symptoms and changes in menstruation?

6. See table on following page

II. CONDITIONS / DECISION TREES / CONSIDERATIONS

ENDOMETRIOSIS *(Continued)*

ENDOMETRIOSIS*

Category	Natural Products to Consider	DOC
Herb	Cat's Claw *on page 404*	PA
	Chasteberry/Vitex *on page 408*	PA, HE
	Evening Primrose *on page 430*	HT
	Grapefruit Seed Extract *on page 450*	PA
	Olive Leaf *on page 483*	PA
	Red Clover *on page 495*	PA, HE
Vitamin/Mineral/ Trace Element/ Nutraceutical	**Progesterone** *on page 491* Condition-specific dosage: On days 7-28 of cycle, topically apply 1/8 to 1/4 tsp twice daily	HD
	Isoflavones *on page 465* Condition-specific dosage: 500-1000 mg of soy extract/day	PA
	Lactobacillus acidophilus *on page 467* and **Bifidobacterium bifidum** *on page 391* Condition-specific dosage: 10 billion CFU twice daily (dairy free)	PA
Homeopathic Remedy	Homeopathic combination formulas are available for many conditions. Listed below are some of the most common single homeopathic remedies for endometriosis. Also see **Homeopathic Quick Reference Chart for Common Complaints** *on page 587*	
	Apis mellifica	PD
	Atropa belladonna	PD
	Kali iodatum	PD
	Lachesis mutus	PD
	Vitamin C *on page 526* Condition-specific dosage: 500-1000 mg/day	PA
	Vitamin E *on page 529* Condition-specific dosage: 400 int. units/day	PA

*Refer to **Introduction to Conditions** *on page 41* for more details on how to apply the information in this table to individuals with this condition.

168

SPECIAL CONSIDERATIONS

Cat's Claw

- Contraindicated in transplant recipients, individuals receiving I.V. immuno-globulins or immunosuppressants; in active bleeding (eg, peptic ulcer, intra-cranial bleeding)
- Caution in hemostatic disorders/history of bleeding
- Potential interaction with anticoagulants (warfarin), aspirin, NSAIDs, anti-platelet agents
- Discontinue use prior to dental or surgical procedures (14 days before)

Chasteberry/Vitex

- Contraindicated in pregnancy
- Potential interaction with hormonal replacements or oral contraceptives

Evening Primrose

- Contraindicated in seizure disorders, schizophrenia, or in persons receiving anticonvulsant or antipsychotic medications; in active bleeding (eg, peptic ulcer, intracranial bleeding)
- Caution in hemostatic disorders/history of bleeding
- Potential interaction with anticoagulants (warfarin), aspirin, NSAIDs, anti-platelet agents
- Discontinue use prior to dental or surgical procedures (14 days before)

Grapefruit Seed Extract

- Grapefruit seed extract is not equivalent to grapefruit juice/pulp. Juice/pulp has been associated with many drug interactions; see Grapefruit Seed *on page 450*
- Until further information is available, it is reasonable to avoid some medica-tions (terfenadine, astemizole, cisapride). Use other medications metabo-lized by CYP3A4 with caution.

Olive Leaf

- No reported toxicity in humans at normal intakes

Red Clover

- Contraindicated in active bleeding (eg, peptic ulcer, intracranial bleeding)
- Caution in individuals at risk of estrogen-dependent tumors, endometrial cancer, thromboembolic disease, or stroke; in hemostatic disorders/history of bleeding
- Potential interactions with hormonal replacement therapy, oral contracep-tives, anticoagulants, aspirin, NSAIDs, antiplatelet agents
- Discontinue use prior to surgical or dental procedures (14 days before)

Progesterone

- Hormonal regulation may be disrupted
- Not to be used with oral contraceptives without medical supervision

Isoflavones

- Caution in estrogen-dependent tumors, endometrial cancer
- Women who are taking estrogen-containing medications (oral contracep-tives, hormonal replacement) should consult their physician prior to use

Lactobacillus acidophilus – No known toxicity or serious side effects

Bifidobacterium bifidum – No known toxicity or serious side effects

Vitamin C

- Excess intake in diabetics may give falsely elevated blood glucose readings

Vitamin E

- Use with caution when taking anticoagulants (vitamin E ≥200 int. units increases prothrombin times)
- Interrupt or reduce dosage one week prior to dental or surgical procedures

EPILEPSY

Epilepsy is a chronic, recurrent medical condition characterized by sudden, abnormal electrical discharges in the brain. Approximately 125,000 cases of epilepsy are diagnosed annually. Of these, 30% occur in individuals <18 years of age. Seizure type tends to vary with the age of diagnosis. These discharges may be manifested as abnormal motor, behavioral, or sensory activity. The most common perception of seizures are the tonic-clonic form, which involve wide-scale intermittent contractions and relaxation of muscle groups, associated with a loss consciousness and possibly bladder control. However, other forms of seizure activity may be demonstrated by subtle symptoms such as a prolonged, blank stare or abnormal, occasionally bizarre behaviors. Epilepsy represents a chronic, recurrent condition and should be differentiated from seizures caused by electrolyte disorders, hypoglycemia, central nervous system infection, fever, drug overdose, or withdrawal syndromes.

Causes of epilepsy include genetic disorders, head injury, nutritional disorders, environmental toxins, blood sugar disturbances, brain tumor, and stroke. In addition, there are idiopathic causes. Epilepsy is classified by the initial involvement of specific regions of the brain and the degree of generalization to other areas. Seizures do not generally cause additional brain injury unless they occur in rapid succession (status epilepticus), which may result in significant metabolic derangements, cardiovascular strain, and respiratory compromise. Complications of seizures may include aspiration pneumonia or trauma.

LIFESTYLE RECOMMENDATIONS

- Reduce or eliminate refined sugars
- Ensure there is a plan in place to address emergency situations
- Discuss medication regimen and reinforce importance of adherence
- Make sure all interventions are approved and overseen by a physician

EPILEPSY / SEIZURE DISORDER DECISION TREE

---

1. Client with epilepsy/seizure disorder is interested in using natural products (NP) to support this condition

---

2. Healthcare provider requests basic background information. The following issues are addressed with the client:

* Allergies?
* Prescription (Rx)/OTC meds?
* Natural products?
* Other medical conditions?
* Nutrition/diet program?
* Exercise program?

---

3. Above data reviewed; if **yes** to Rx/OTC meds, review **Drug-Induced Nutrient Depletion Chart** in Appendix

---

4A. Client is a candidate for natural products

* An appropriate homeopathic remedy can be used at any time

4B. Client's case is too complicated at this point; needs additional support from MD before initiating NP program

---

5. Condition-specific questions:
* MD treatment plan in place? Is there a plan to support client during emergency situation? Ensure this is in place; review meds and other interventions
* Precipitating factors? Work to minimize exposure to them
* Any contributing factors: Environment, meds (antidepressants, benzodiazepines), and discuss with client and work to minimize

---

6. See table on following page

171

EPILEPSY *(Continued)*

EPILEPSY / SEIZURE DISORDER*

Category	Natural Products to Consider	DOC
Herb	Ginkgo *on page 441*	PA
	Gymnema (if related to blood sugar) *on page 455*	PA
	Bitter Melon (if related to blood sugar) *on page 394*	PA
Vitamin/Mineral/ Trace Element/ Nutraceutical	Taurine *on page 508* Condition-specific dosage: 1.5-3 g/day	HT
	Chromium (if not related to blood sugar) *on page 410* Condition-specific dosage: 200-600 mcg/day	PA
	Magnesium *on page 473* Condition-specific dosage: 400-600 mg/day	HD
	Manganese *on page 475* Condition-specific dosage: 5-10 mg/day	HD
Homeopathic Remedy	Homeopathic combination formulas are available for many conditions. Listed below are some of the most common single homeopathic remedies for epilepsy. Also see **Homeopathic Quick Reference Chart for Common Complaints** *on page 587*	
	Bufo rana	PD
	Calcarea carbonica	PD
	Causticum	PD
	Cicuta virosa	PD
	Cuprum metallicum	PD
	Hyoscyamus niger	PD
Additional supplements to consider	Selenium *on page 502* Condition-specific dosage: 200 mcg/day	PA
	Vitamin E *on page 529* Condition-specific dosage: 200-400 int. units/day	PA

*Refer to **Introduction to Conditions** *on page 41* for more details on how to apply the information in this table to individuals with this condition.

SPECIAL CONSIDERATIONS

Ginkgo
- Contraindicated in active bleeding (eg, peptic ulcer, intracranial bleeding)
- Caution in hemostatic disorders/history of bleeding
- Potential interaction with anticoagulants (warfarin), aspirin, NSAIDs, anti-platelet agents
- Theoretical interaction with MAO inhibitors, acetylcholinesterase inhibitors (tacrine, donepezil)
- Discontinue use prior to dental or surgical procedures (14 days before)

Gymnema
- May alter blood glucose; use caution in individuals with diabetes or predisposition to hypoglycemia
- Monitor blood sugar closely in individuals with diabetes
- Potential interactions with insulin, oral hypoglycemics

Bitter Melon
- Contraindicated in pregnancy
- May alter blood glucose; use caution in individuals with diabetes or predisposition to hypoglycemia
- Monitor blood sugar closely in individuals with diabetes
- Potential interactions with insulin, oral hypoglycemics

Taurine
- No known toxicity or serious side effects

Chromium
- Caution in individuals receiving oral hypoglycemics or insulin; monitor blood glucose closely and coordinate with prescriber

Magnesium
- Use caution in renal impairment
- May cause diarrhea at high intakes

Manganese
- Use caution in individuals with liver disease

Selenium
- No known toxicity at normal intakes

Vitamin E
- Use with caution when taking anticoagulants (vitamin E $\geq$200 int. units increases prothrombin times)
- Interrupt or reduce dosage one week prior to dental or surgical procedures

FATIGUE

Fatigue is a nonspecific subjective symptom often described as a lack of energy or strength. It is often a symptom of general systemic disease. It is normal to experience fatigue following a period of mental or physical activity. This fatigue is characterized by a lessened capacity for work, usually accompanied by a feeling of weariness, sleepiness, or irritability. Technically, fatigue may occur at any time when energy expenditure outstrips the ability to supply oxygen and/or nutrients to the metabolizing organ or body system. The resistance to fatigue is dependent upon multiple factors, including individual conditioning, nutrition, psychological factors, and functional status of key organ systems. A complete medical history and physical exam may be required to determine any potential cause of fatigue. For this reason, persistent fatigue, or any acute degeneration in resistance to fatigue, should be evaluated to determine any potential systemic causes.

LIFESTYLE RECOMMENDATIONS

- Continuation/initiation of diet and exercise program

- Avoid refined sugars, refined carbohydrates, fried foods, caffeine, excess dietary fat

- Increase intake of fiber, fresh fruits, and vegetables

- Increase consumption of quality water

- Do not rely on medications to help with sleep. If using medications consistently for longer than 2 weeks, seek medical attention.

- Get plenty of rest, but do not rest all day

- If fatigue is persistent and testing for thyroid problems or allergies has not been done, seek medical attention

FATIGUE DECISION TREE

1. Client with fatigue is interested in using natural products (NP) to support this condition

2. Healthcare provider requests basic background information. The following issues are addressed with the client:

   * Allergies?
   * Prescription (Rx)/OTC meds?
   * Natural products?
   * Other medical conditions?
   * Nutrition/diet program?
   * Exercise program?

3. Above data reviewed; if **yes** to Rx/OTC meds, review **Drug-Induced Nutrient Depletion Chart** in Appendix

4A. Client is a candidate for natural products

   * An appropriate homeopathic remedy can be used at any time

4B. Client's case is too Complicated at this point; needs additional support from MD before initiating NP program

5. Condition-specific questions:
   * Individual evaluated by a physician? If **yes**, what was recommended treatment plan?
   * Triggers for condition/symptom onset? Worsening?
   * Precipitating factor(s), such as changes in lifestyle or occupation?
   * Review list of medical conditions to see if any might be contributing, such as anemia, blood sugar fluctuations, allergies, circulatory problems, hypothyroidism
   * Does the individual spend considerable time in high heat, high humidity environment? If **yes**, this is probably contributing to the condition
   * Accompanying symptoms, such as fever, headache, congestion, sore throat? If **yes**, may need to be evaluated by MD
   * Any noticeable changes in sleep patterns?
   * Any new medication/medication change that may be contributing

6. See table on following page

FATIGUE *(Continued)*

FATIGUE *

Category	Natural Products to Consider	DOC
Herb	Cordyceps *on page 417*	HT
	Ginseng, Siberian *on page 444*	HT
	Schisandra *on page 501*	PA, HE
	Evening Primrose *on page 430*	HT
Vitamin/Mineral/ Trace Element/ Nutraceutical	Coenzyme Q$_{10}$ *on page 412* Condition-specific dosage: 30-50 mg twice daily	HD
	Magnesium *on page 473* Condition-specific dosage: 400 mg/day	HT
	Adrenal Extract *on page 380* Condition-specific dosage: 200 mg 3 times/day	HD
	Nicotinamide Adenine Dinucleotide (NADH) *on page 483* Condition-specific dosage: 2.5-5 mg/day	HT
	Fish Oils *on page 434* Condition-specific dosage: 750 mg, 1-2 times/day	HT
Homeopathic Remedy	Homeopathic combination formulas are available for many conditions. Listed below are some of the most common single homeopathic remedies for fatigue. Also see **Homeopathic Quick Reference Chart for Common Complaints** *on page 587*	
	Arsenicum album	PD
	Carbo vegetabilis	PD
	Natrum muriaticum	PD
Additional supplements to consider	Vitamin B Complex-25 *on page 526* Condition-specific dosage: 25-50 mg twice daily	PA
	Vitamin C *on page 526* Condition-specific dosage: 250-1000 mg daily	PA

*Refer to **Introduction to Conditions** *on page 41* for more details on how to apply the information in this table to individuals with this condition.

SPECIAL CONSIDERATIONS

Cordyceps

- Caution if allergic to molds or fungi; and in hemostatic disorders/history of bleeding
- Theoretical interaction in individuals receiving MAO inhibitors
- Contraindicated in active bleeding (eg, peptic ulcer, intracranial bleeding)
- Potential interaction with anticoagulants (warfarin), aspirin, NSAIDs, anti-platelet agents
- Discontinue use prior to dental or surgical procedures (14 days before)

Ginseng, Siberian

- Contraindicated with digoxin, hexobarbital; and in active bleeding (eg, peptic ulcer, intracranial bleeding)
- Caution with stimulant medications, decongestants, caffeine
- A cycle of 4 weeks on, followed by 2 weeks off is recommended for maximum benefit
- Caution in hypertension or in individuals at risk of hypotension (elderly, cerebrovascular or cardiovascular disease); or those taking antihypertensives
- May alter blood glucose regulation; monitor blood glucose carefully in individuals with diabetes or hypoglycemia
- Caution in hemostatic disorders/history of bleeding
- Potential interactions with anticoagulants (warfarin), aspirin, NSAIDs, anti-platelet agents, sedative-hypnotics (barbiturates), insulin, oral hypoglycemics, antihypertensives, stimulants, caffeine
- Discontinue use prior to dental or surgical procedures (14 days before)

Schisandra

- Contraindicated in pregnancy (due to uterine stimulation)
- Potential interaction with calcium channel blockers

Evening Primrose

- Contraindicated in seizure disorders, schizophrenia, or in persons receiving anticonvulsant or antipsychotic medications
- Contraindicated in active bleeding (eg, peptic ulcer, intracranial bleeding)
- Caution in hemostatic disorders/history of bleeding
- Potential interaction with anticoagulants (warfarin), aspirin, NSAIDs, anti-platelet agents
- Discontinue use prior to dental or surgical procedures (14 days before)

Coenzyme Q$_{10}$ – No known toxicity or serious side effects; caution in individuals receiving anticoagulants

Magnesium

- Use caution in renal impairment
- May cause diarrhea at high intakes

Adrenal Extract – May cause excitability when taken in large doses

NADH – No known toxicity or serious side effects

Fish Oils

- High doses may cause GI upset, loose stools, nausea
- May alter glucose regulation; use with caution in diabetes
- Caution in individuals receiving oral hypoglycemics or insulin; monitor blood glucose closely and coordinate with prescriber
- Potential interaction with anticoagulants (warfarin), aspirin, NSAIDs, anti-platelet agents

Vitamin B Complex-25 – No side effects at the RDI or ODA doses

Vitamin C – Excess intake in diabetics may give falsely elevated blood glucose readings

FEVER

Fever refers to an elevation in the body's temperature above normal. The normal oral temperature is 98.6°F and an individual's temperature may be considered normal if it is 1° above or 2° below this value. Fever is a nonspecific response that can be triggered by a number of insults, such as infection, immune reactions (autoimmune disorders), drugs, metabolic disorders, or dehydration.

An increase in body temperature is a natural response that assists the normal immune response to infection. Children tend to have pronounced fever with little stimulation. At the other extreme, the ability to develop a fever may be limited in some individuals. The elderly, in particular, may actually have a decrease in body temperature as a result of infection.

Fever may have value in promoting activation of immune responses and/or limiting growth/replication of invading organisms. However, extreme elevations may increase metabolic demands, resulting in cardiovascular strain, or may cause neurologic changes, including seizures. An individual's sensitivity to the adverse effects of fever varies widely. In particular, the elderly or medically-compromised individuals tend to tolerate the increased demand poorly, and individuals with neurologic disease, including those receiving drugs that lower the seizure threshold, may be much more prone to febrile seizures.

Evaluation is essential to identify causes of fever and address potential complications of the underlying disease that results in a fever.

LIFESTYLE RECOMMENDATIONS

- Do not use aspirin or willow bark in children

- If adult with GI problems, use acetaminophen; avoid aspirin, NSAIDs, and willow bark

- If taking anticoagulants or undergoing antiplatelet therapy, use acetaminophen (with supervision of physician if longer than 7 days)

- Do not use willow bark, if allergic to aspirin

- For adults, may not have to use interventions unless uncomfortable or temperature is >102°

- Sponge baths may be beneficial, but not with cold water; use lukewarm water

- Avoid prolonged exposure to excessive heat; avoid clothing that might be too warm

- Increase fluid consumption

- Use antipyretics sparingly

FEVER DECISION TREE

---

1. Client with fever is interested in using natural products (NP) to support this condition

---

2. Healthcare provider requests basic background information. The following issues are addressed with the client:

  * Allergies?
  * Prescription (Rx)/OTC meds?
  * Natural products?

  * Other medical conditions?
  * Nutrition/diet program?
  * Exercise program?

---

3. Above data reviewed; if **yes** to Rx/OTC meds, review **Drug-Induced Nutrient Depletion Chart** in Appendix

---

4A. Client is a candidate for natural products

  * An appropriate homeopathic remedy can be used at any time

4B. Client's case is too complicated at this point; needs additional support from MD before initiating NP program

---

5. Condition-specific questions:
   * History of seizure disorder? If **yes and peds patient**, refer to MD.
   * How long has temperature been elevated? If >102° for longer than 24 hours with treatment, refer.
   * Any new medications where the timing of initiation coincides with temperature increase (tricyclics, meds with anticholinergic properties)?
   * What has been used so far to try to normalize temperature? Effectiveness?
   * Accompanying symptoms: Cough, nausea, vomiting, headache, sore throat, sinus pain, lethargy, malaise - if appears serious, refer to MD.
   * Med conditions that might be contributing: Some autoimmune conditions, hyperthyroidism
   * How is temperature being measured? Normals are:
     - Per rectum: 101° to 102°; oral: 100°; axillary and via ear: 99°
     - Preferred methods of measuring: Per rectum for child >3 months of age; axillary for child 3 months to 5 years
   * Seek medical attention in the following pediatric situations:
     - Age ≤1 month: Temperature ≥2° above normal (per rectum)
     - 1-3 months: Temperature ≥2.5° above normal (per rectum)
     - 3 months to 2 years: Temperature ≥4° above normal (axillary)
     - >2 years: Temperature ≥5° above normal (axillary)

---

6. See table on following page

FEVER *(Continued)*

FEVER*

Category	Natural Products to Consider	DOC
Herb	White Willow *on page 532*	PA, HE
	Golden Seal *on page 448*	PA, HE
	Elderberry *on page 428*	PA, HE
Vitamin/Mineral/ Trace Element/ Nutraceutical	**Vitamin C** *on page 526* Condition-specific dosage: 500-1000 mg 2-3 times/day	PA
Homeopathic Remedy	Homeopathic combination formulas are available for many conditions. Listed below are some of the most common single homeopathic remedies for fever. Also see **Homeopathic Quick Reference Chart for Common Complaints** *on page 587*	
	Aconitum napellus	PD
	Atropa belladonna	PD
	Bryonia alba	PD
	Ferrum phosphoricum	PD
	Gelsemium sempervirens	PD
	Phosphorus	PD
Additional supplements to consider	No recommendations	

*Refer to **Introduction to Conditions** *on page 41* for more details on how to apply the information in this table to individuals with this condition.

SPECIAL CONSIDERATIONS

White Willow
- Contraindicated in aspirin allergy or hypersensitivity
- Do not use in children (potential for Reye's syndrome)
- Potential interactions with aspirin, anticoagulants, methotrexate, metoclopramide, phenytoin, probenecid, spironolactone, valproic acid, antiplatelet agents, NSAIDs

Golden Seal
- Contraindicated in pregnancy

Elderberry
- No reported toxicity in humans at normal intakes

Vitamin C
- Excess intake in diabetics may give falsely elevated blood glucose readings

FIBROCYSTIC BREAST DISEASE (FBD)

Fibrocystic breast disease represents a common, benign syndrome of breast changes. It has also been called mammary dysplasia, chronic cystic mastitis, benign breast disease, and diffuse cystic mastopathy. It has been estimated to occur in as many as 60% of all women, and is most common between the ages of 30 and 50. Women taking oral contraceptives have a lower incidence. Risk factors may include genetic predisposition, excessive dietary fat, and consumption of caffeine-containing foods or beverages. The cause of fibrocystic breast changes is not completely understood, but appears to be related to hormonal changes, since the disease usually subsides after menopause.

Symptoms may include a dull heavy pain and tenderness of the breast, breast discomfort, a sensation of breast fullness, nipple sensation changes, and itching. A dense, irregular, and bumpy consistency of the breast is usually noted, in addition to mobile breast "masses" which are usually rounded, with smooth borders. Tenderness and swelling is pronounced during the premenstrual phase. A number of diagnostic tests and procedures are recommended to rule out the possibility of breast cancer. Oral contraceptives are occasionally prescribed, and other medications may be used in rare situations. A reduction in dietary fat and caffeine intake is recommended.

Apart from general discomfort, the major complication of fibrocystic changes involves the masking of breast cancer symptoms. These changes may make breast examination and mammography more difficult to interpret, which may in turn make the recognition of early cancerous lesions more difficult.

LIFESTYLE RECOMMENDATIONS

- Eliminate caffeine from the diet, including drinks and chocolate
- Reduce/eliminate sugar, dairy products, alcohol, tobacco, commercially-raised meat (may have been given hormones), saturated fat, salt
- Reduce stress
- Increase fiber, fruits, vegetables, and fish (salmon, mackerel, trout)
- Wear a support bra and loose-fitting clothing

FIBROCYSTIC BREAST DISEASE DECISION TREE

1. Client with fibrocystic breast disease is interested in using natural products (NP) to support this condition

2. Healthcare provider requests basic background information. The following issues are addressed with the client:
   * Allergies?
   * Prescription (Rx)/OTC meds?
   * Natural products?
   * Other medical conditions?
   * Nutrition/diet program?
   * Exercise program?

3. Above data reviewed; if **yes** to Rx/OTC meds, review **Drug-Induced Nutrient Depletion Chart** in Appendix

4A. Client is a candidate for natural products

   * An appropriate homeopathic remedy can be used at any time

4B. Client's case is too complicated at this point; needs additional support from MD before initiating NP program

5. Condition-specific questions:
   * Diagnosed by MD? If **yes**, what was the recommended treatment plan? Effective?
   * Triggers for condition/symptom onset? Worsening?
   * Is the client taking any form of estrogen, such as birth control pills? If **yes**, refer to MD to explore the option of discontinuing and using another form of birth control.
   * How often does client perform breast self-examinations? Should be done monthly during the week after her period.
   * Do symptoms change during the menstrual cycle, such as increasing just prior to her period starting, and improving at the end of the cycle?
   * Clients definitely need to be evaluated by MD to share the following information: When was/were lump(s) detected? Has there been a change in size? How does/do it/they feel? Is there history of breast disease, breast cancer in the family? When was her last period? Any discharge from the nipple area?

6. See table on following page

183

FIBROCYSTIC BREAST DISEASE (FBD) *(Continued)*

FIBROCYSTIC BREAST DISEASE (FBD)*

Category	Natural Products to Consider	DOC
Herb	Evening Primrose *on page 430*	PA
	Bladderwrack *(Fucus vesiculosus) on page 396*	PA
Vitamin/Mineral/ Trace Element/ Nutraceutical	**Vitamin E** *on page 529* Condition-specific dosage: 200-400 int. units/day	PA
Homeopathic Remedy	Homeopathic combination formulas are available for many conditions. Listed below are some of the most common single homeopathic remedies for fibrocystic breast disease. Also see **Homeopathic Quick Reference Chart for Common Complaints** *on page 587*	
	Graphites	PD
	Phytolacca decandra	PD
Additional supplements to consider	**Iodine** *on page 463* Condition-specific dosage: 150-250 mcg/day	HD
	Vitamin A *on page 518* Condition-specific dosage: 10,000-35,000 int. units/day	HD
	Vitamin B₆ *on page 523* Condition-specific dosage: 50-100 mg/day	PA
	Vitamin C *on page 526* Condition-specific dosage: 250-1000 mg/day	PA

*Refer to **Introduction to Conditions** *on page 41* for more details on how to apply the information in this table to individuals with this condition.

184

SPECIAL CONSIDERATIONS

Evening Primrose
- Contraindicated in seizure disorders, schizophrenia, or in persons receiving anticonvulsant or antipsychotic medications
- Contraindicated in active bleeding (eg, peptic ulcer, intracranial bleeding)
- Caution in hemostatic disorders/history of bleeding
- Potential interaction with anticoagulants (warfarin), aspirin, NSAIDs, anti-platelet agents
- Discontinue use prior to dental or surgical procedures (14 days before)

Bladderwrack
- Caution in hyperthyroidism
- May increase serum potassium; caution in renal failure
- Potential interaction with thyroid agents or antithyroid drugs
- Avoid use in individuals with iodine sensitivity

Vitamin E
- Use with caution when taking anticoagulants (vitamin E ≥200 int. units increases prothrombin times)
- Interrupt or reduce dosage one week prior to dental or surgical procedures

Iodine
- In cases of existing hyperthyroidism, doses as small as 1 mg can result in cessation of thyroid hormone production and thyrotoxicosis
- Extensive long-term intake can result in thyroid goiter

Vitamin A
- Contraindicated in pregnancy or in women who may become pregnant

Vitamin B₆
- Prolonged excesses can cause reversible nerve damage

Vitamin C
- Excess intake in diabetics may give falsely elevated blood glucose readings

FIBROMYALGIA

Fibromyalgia is a syndrome of prolonged fatigue with widespread muscle aches and pains. Recurrent sore throat, headache, low fever, and depression are also common symptoms. Characteristically, fibromyalgia is diagnosed by the existence of at least 10 distinct sites of deep muscle tenderness that are painful when pressure is applied. Sites include the side of the neck, the top of the shoulder blade, the outside of the upper buttock and hip joint, and the inside of the knee.

Fibromyalgia (sometimes referred to as fibrositis) affects 3-6 million Americans. The syndrome appears to have considerable overlap with symptoms of depression, and some experts believe it represents a variant of chronic fatigue syndrome (CFS).

The cause of fibromyalgia has not been defined. Some researchers believe chemical or hormonal influences contribute to the syndrome. Environmental, viral, and emotional factors have been suggested. Sleep disturbance as well as physical or emotional stress may trigger fibromyalgia. One theory is that localized accumulation of lactic acid in muscle tissue, caused by the incomplete burning of fuel in the Krebs cycle, may result in muscle pain. A genetic susceptibility has also been suggested. Other factors that may predispose to fibromyalgia include physical deconditioning, depression, low self-esteem, or obsessive personalities. However, fibromyalgia is not generally regarded as a psychiatric disorder.

LIFESTYLE RECOMMENDATIONS

- Increase consumption of canola, flaxseed, and walnut oils; dark leafy greens; fish; fruits (except citrus); legumes; oats; vegetables

- Decrease consumption of alcohol, artificial sweeteners, butter, caffeine, carbonated beverages, citrus, dairy products, meat, monosodium glutamate (MSG), nuts, sugars, white flour

- Consider other therapies: Acupuncture, massage therapy, aerobic exercise, physical therapy, muscle relaxation, stress management

- Work to improve sleep patterns (preferably without medication)

- Look to join a support group

FIBROMYALGIA DECISION TREE

1. Client with fibromyalgia is interested in using natural products (NP) to support this condition

2. Healthcare provider requests basic background information. The following issues are addressed with the client:

   * Allergies? Work up as it relates specifically to this condition
   * Prescription (Rx)/OTC meds?
   * Natural products?
   * Other medical conditions?
   * Nutrition/diet program? Details on successes, benefits, challenges
   * Exercise program? Details on successes, benefits

3. Above data reviewed; if **yes** to Rx/OTC meds, review **Drug-Induced Nutrient Depletion Chart** in Appendix

4A. Client is a candidate for natural products

   * An appropriate homeopathic remedy can be used at any time

4B. Client's case is too complicated at this point; needs additional support from MD before initiating NP program

5. Condition-specific questions:
   * Individual evaluated by a physician? If **yes**, what was was recommended treatment plan?
   * Trigger points?
   * Sleep disturbances?
   * Depressive symptoms?
   * Recent viral illness?
   * Precipitating factors?
   * If using Rx meds, monitor for adverse events that might worsen condition

6. See table on following page

FIBROMYALGIA *(Continued)*

FIBROMYALGIA*

Category	Natural Products to Consider	DOC
Herb	Turmeric *on page 512*	PA
	Cat's Claw *on page 404*	PA
	Cordyceps *on page 417*	PA
	Kava Kava *on page 466*	PA
Vitamin/Mineral/ Trace Element/ Nutraceutical	Adrenal Extract *on page 380* Condition-specific dosage: 200 mg 2-3 times/day	HD
	Lactobacillus acidophilus on page 467 and *Bifidobacterium bifidum on page 391* Condition-specific dosage: 10 billion CFU twice daily (dairy free)	PA
	Magnesium malate *on page 473* Condition-specific dosage: 400-800 mg 3 times/day	
	Vitamin C *on page 526* Condition-specific dosage: 250-1000 mg/day	PA
	Glutamine *on page 446* Condition-specific dosage: 10 g daily for 2 months, then maintenance dose of 500 mg 3 times/day	PA
Homeopathic Remedy	Homeopathic combination formulas are available for many conditions. Listed below are some of the most common single homeopathic remedies for fibromyalgia. Also see **Homeopathic Quick Reference Chart for Common Complaints** *on page 587*	
	Lacticum acidum	PD
	Magnesia phosphorica	PD
	Rhus toxicodendron	PD
Additional supplements to consider	Coenzyme Q₁₀ *on page 412* Condition-specific dosage: 30-50 mg twice daily	PA
	Thyroid Extract *on page 510* Condition-specific dosage: 60 mg 2-3 times/day	HD
	Vitamin B₁ *on page 519* Condition-specific dosage: 25-50 mg twice daily	PA

*Refer to **Introduction to Conditions** *on page 41* for more details on how to apply the information in this table to individuals with this condition.

SPECIAL CONSIDERATIONS

Turmeric

- Caution in biliary obstruction; in ulcerative gastrointestinal disease (eg, peptic ulcer disease, ulcerative colitis, Crohn's); hemostatic disorders/history of bleeding
- Contraindicated in active bleeding (eg, peptic ulcer, intracranial bleeding)
- Potential interaction with anticoagulants (warfarin), aspirin, NSAIDs, anti-platelet agents
- Discontinue use prior to dental or surgical procedures (14 days before)

Cat's Claw

- Contraindicated in transplant recipients, individuals receiving I.V. immunoglobulins or immunosuppressants; and in active bleeding (eg, peptic ulcer, intracranial bleeding)
- Caution in hemostatic disorders/history of bleeding
- Potential interaction with anticoagulants (warfarin), aspirin, NSAIDs, anti-platelet agents
- Discontinue use prior to dental or surgical procedures (14 days before)

Cordyceps

- Caution if allergic to molds or fungi, and in hemostatic disorders/history of bleeding
- Theoretical interactions in individuals receiving MAO inhibitors
- Contraindicated in active bleeding (eg, peptic ulcer, intracranial bleeding)
- Potential interactions with anticoagulants (warfarin), aspirin, NSAIDs, anti-platelet agents
- Discontinue use prior to dental or surgical procedures (14 days before)

Kava Kava

- Contraindicated in pregnancy and breast-feeding, or Parkinson's disease
- May cause drowsiness or sedation (higher doses); caution when driving/performing hazardous tasks
- Potential interactions with ethanol, CNS depressants (benzodiazepines, antidepressants, sedative-hypnotics)

Adrenal Extract – May cause excitability when taken in large doses

Lactobacillus acidophilus – No known toxicity or serious side effects

Bifidobacterium bifidum – No known toxicity or serious side effects

Magnesium Malate

- Use caution in renal impairment
- May cause diarrhea at high intakes

Vitamin C – Excess intake in diabetics may give falsely elevated blood glucose readings

Glutamine – No known toxicity or serious side effects

Coenzyme Q_{10} – No known toxicity or serious side effects; caution in individuals receiving anticoagulants

Thyroid Extract

- Use with caution in individuals taking thyroid medication, and in individuals with hypertension or cardiovascular disease, and in those with CNS disorders
- Potential interactions with levothyroxine, propylthiouracil, lithium

Vitamin B_1 – No known toxicity or serious side effects

GALLBLADDER / GALLSTONES

Gallstones form when the chemical composition of the bile becomes imbalanced. An excess of cholesterol or deficiency of bile salts may allow some of the cholesterol to precipitate out of solution and form crystals. Other contributing factors may include incomplete or infrequent emptying of the gallbladder which allows the bile to overconcentrate, as well as an imbalance of secreted proteins in the bile which may facilitate cholesterol crystallization.

The chance of having gallstones increases with age. Ten to 15% of men and 25% to 30% of women will eventually develop gallstones. Women are more prone to gallbladder disease. Additional risk factors include a genetic predisposition (particularly in certain ethnic groups), advancing age, pregnancy, and obesity (even being moderately overweight will increase cholesterol in the bile). Medications, such as oral contraceptives and hormone replacement therapy, increase the risk of gallstones. Although controversial, diets high in fat and sugar may also increase risk. In addition, rapid weight loss diets may precipitate gallstone formation. There is no diet that has been clearly demonstrated to have an effect on the disappearance of gallstones.

Gallstones usually consist of a mixture of cholesterol, bilirubin, and protein. They occasionally enter the ducts to the liver, pancreas, and small intestine, which can cause serious complications such as pancreatitis and systemic inflammatory responses mimicking septic shock that may be fatal if untreated. Immediate medical attention should be sought if the following signs or symptoms occur: Severe, steady pain in the right to mid to upper abdomen, urine discoloration (tea- or coffee-colored), fever, disorientation, rigors, or jaundice.

Symptomatic gallstone disease is often treated by removing the gallbladder (cholecystectomy). For years, herbalists and naturopaths have suggested gallbladder flushes. Though generally thought to be safe, there is a potential for a stone to lodge during the flushing process. Nonsurgical methods of gallstone removal are used very rarely. The disadvantage of nonsurgical alternatives is that stones usually redevelop.

LIFESTYLE RECOMMENDATIONS

- Continuation/initiation of diet and exercise program

- Use moisturizing lotion for dry skin

- Use OTC antihistamines for itching; counsel on drowsiness with OTC products

- Increase calcium intake provided it is not contraindicated based on condition (ie, history of calcium oxalate stones)

- Restrict intake of fat

- Increase fiber intake

GALLBLADDER / GALL STONES DISORDER DECISION TREE

1. Client with gallbladder disorder or gall stones is interested in using natural products (NP) to support this condition

2. Healthcare provider requests basic background information. The following issues are addressed with the client:

   * Allergies?
   * Prescription (Rx)/OTC meds?
   * Natural products?
   * Other medical conditions?
   * Nutrition/diet program?
   * Exercise program?

3. Above data reviewed; if **yes** to Rx/OTC meds, review **Drug-Induced Nutrient Depletion Chart** in Appendix

4A. Client is a candidate for natural products

   * An appropriate homeopathic remedy can be used at any time

4B. Client's case is too complicated at this point; needs additional support from MD before initiating NP program

5. Condition-specific questions:

   * Fever? If **yes,** evaluate severity of situation and refer when necessary
   * Fatigue? If **yes,** how is this being managed?
   * Excessive itching? If **yes,** how is this being managed?
   * What is MD plan for overall management?

6. See table on following page

GALLBLADDER / GALLSTONES *(Continued)*

GALLBLADDER / GALLSTONES*

Category	Natural Products to Consider	DOC
Herb	**Milk Thistle** *on page 479*	PA, HE
	Artichoke *on page 386*	PA, HE
	Golden Seal *on page 448*	PA, HE
Vitamin/Mineral/ Trace Element/ Nutraceutical	**Phosphatidyl Choline** *on page 488* Condition-specific dosage: 500-1500 mg 2-3 times/day	HD
	Taurine *on page 508* Condition-specific dosage: 1.5-3 g/day	PA
	Magnesium *on page 473* Condition-specific dosage: 400-600 mg/day	PA
Homeopathic Remedy	Homeopathic combination formulas are available for many conditions. Listed below are some of the most common single homeopathic remedies for gallbladder/gallstones. Also see **Homeopathic Quick Reference Chart for Common Complaints** *on page 587*	
	Berberis vulgaris	PD
	Cinchona officinalis(China)	PD
	Lycopodium clavatum	PD
Additional supplements to consider	**Vitamin C** *on page 526* Condition-specific dosage: 250-1000 mg/day	PA
	Vitamin E *on page 529* Condition-specific dosage: 200-400 int. units/day	PA

*Refer to **Introduction to Conditions** *on page 41* for more details on how to apply the information in this table to individuals with this condition.

SPECIAL CONSIDERATIONS

Milk Thistle
- No reported toxicity in humans at normal intakes

Artichoke
- Use with caution in individuals with allergies to *Asteraceae/Compositae* family (chrysanthemum, daisy)

Golden Seal
- Contraindicated in pregnancy

Phosphatidyl Choline
- No known toxicity or serious side effects

Taurine
- No known toxicity or serious side effects

Magnesium
- Use caution in renal impairment
- May cause diarrhea at high intakes

Vitamin C
- Excess intake in diabetics may give falsely elevated blood glucose readings

Vitamin E
- Use with caution when taking anticoagulants (vitamin E ≥200 int. units increases prothrombin times)
- Interrupt or reduce dosage one week prior to dental or surgical procedures

GINGIVITIS

The soft tissue supporting the teeth is known as the gingiva. Inflammation of this tissue is called gingivitis. Bacterial organisms and toxins have been implicated in this condition, particularly anaerobic organisms. Initial gum sensitivity, which inhibits removal of debris and organisms, may lead to further inflammation, bleeding, and deterioration of gum tissue. This cycle results in toothaches and halitosis, as well as a receding gum line, episodic swelling, or abscesses. Gingivitis may also extend to the bone and ligaments that support the tissue, resulting in periodontitis. If this process is left to progress without interruption, severe pain and tooth loss may result.

A number of factors contribute to the development of gingivitis, including genetics, diet, lifestyle, and hygiene. In addition, the activity of an individual's collagenase and local prostaglandins, which break down supporting structures, help to determine the rate and extent of progression. This disorder has a relationship to uncontrolled diabetes, cardiovascular disease, myocardial infarction, and stroke. In addition, possible relationships to respiratory diseases, HIV, and cancer have been noted.

Appropriate dental cleaning may prevent gingivitis. Proper nutrition also plays an important role in prevention.

LIFESTYLE RECOMMENDATIONS

- Use soft-bristled toothbrush
- Use tartar-control toothpaste
- Brush teeth, tongue, and gums regularly
- Avoid using dental floss in area aggravated by condition
- Avoid sugar
- Avoid tobacco

GINGIVITIS DECISION TREE

1. Client with gingivitis is interested in using natural products (NP) to support this condition

2. Healthcare provider requests basic background information. The following issues are addressed with the client:

   * Allergies?
   * Prescription (Rx)/OTC meds?
   * Natural products?
   * Other medical conditions?
   * Nutrition/diet program?
   * Exercise program?

3. Above data reviewed; if **yes** to Rx/OTC meds, review **Drug-Induced Nutrient Depletion Chart** in Appendix

4A. Client is a candidate for natural products

   * An appropriate homeopathic remedy can be used at any time

4B. Client's case is too complicated at this point; needs additional support from MD before initiating NP program

5. Condition-specific questions:
   * How do you brush your teeth?
   * Swelling, bleeding severity when brushing?
   * Associated sinus infection, ear infection, cold, fever?
   * How often do you see your dentist?
   * Any loose teeth?
   * Increased pain, pressure, other changes with any teeth recently?
   * History of heart disease?
   * Use oral contraceptives or anticholinergic meds? May increase risk

6. See table on following page

GINGIVITIS *(Continued)*

GINGIVITIS*

Category	Natural Products to Consider	DOC
Herb	Grapefruit Seed Extract (Oral rinse) *on page 450*	
	White Oak Bark (Oral rinse) *on page 531*	PA
	Tea Tree *on page 509*	HD
	Green Tea *on page 452*	PA
	Chamomile (Oral rinse) *on page 407*	PA
	Aloe (Oral rinse) *on page 381*	PA
	Grape Seed *on page 451*	PA
Vitamin/Mineral/ Trace Element/ Nutraceutical	Coenzyme Q$_{10}$ *on page 412* Condition-specific dosage: 30 mg twice daily	HD
	Vitamin C *on page 526* Condition-specific dosage: 500-1000 mg twice daily	PA
	Folic Acid *on page 435* Condition-specific dosage: Rinse mouth with 5 mL of a 0.1% folic acid mouthwash twice daily for 1 minute	HT
Homeopathic Remedy	Homeopathic combination formulas are available for many conditions. Listed below are some of the most common single homeopathic remedies for gingivitis. Also see **Homeopathic Quick Reference Chart for Common Complaints** *on page 587*	
	Kreosotum	PD
	Phosphorus	PD
Additional supplements to consider	No recommendations	

*Refer to **Introduction to Conditions** *on page 41* for more details on how to apply the information in this table to individuals with this condition.

SPECIAL CONSIDERATIONS

Grapefruit Seed Extract

- Grapefruit seed extract is not equivalent to grapefruit juice/pulp. Juice/pulp has been associated with many drug interactions; see Grapefruit Seed *on page 450*

- Until further information is available, it is reasonable to avoid some medications (terfenadine, astemizole, cisapride). Use other medications metabolized by CYP3A4 with caution.

White Oak Bark

- No reported toxicity in humans at normal intakes

Tea Tree

- May cause allergic dermatitis in sensitive individuals
- Not for ingestion

Green Tea

- Decaffeinated products recommended
- Caffeine may cause multiple CNS and CV effects (caution in peptic ulcer disease or cardiovascular disease)
- Contraindicated in active bleeding (eg, peptic ulcer, intracranial bleeding)
- Caution in hemostatic disorders/history of bleeding
- Discontinue use prior to dental or surgical procedures (14 days before)
- Potential interaction with anticoagulants (warfarin), aspirin, NSAIDs, anti-platelet agents
- See Green Tea monograph *on page 452* for additional potential interactions

Chamomile

- Avoid use in individuals with allergies to *Asteraceae/Compositae* family (chrysanthemum, daisy) or ragweed pollens
- May cause drowsiness; caution in driving/performing hazardous tasks

Aloe

- May delay wound healing (topical)

Grape Seed

- Contraindicated in active bleeding (eg, peptic ulcer, intracranial bleeding)
- Caution in hemostatic disorders/history of bleeding
- Potential interaction with anticoagulants (warfarin), aspirin, NSAIDs, anti-platelet agents, methotrexate
- Discontinue use prior to dental or surgical procedures (14 days before)

Coenzyme Q$_{10}$

- No known toxicity or serious side effects
- Caution in individuals receiving anticoagulants

Vitamin C

- Excess intake in diabetics may give falsely elevated blood glucose reading

Folic Acid

- No known toxicity or serious side effects

GLAUCOMA

Glaucoma is a group of conditions involving increased pressure within the eye, which can damage the optic nerve. Elevated intraocular pressure develops when fluid in the eye fails to drain properly. It is estimated that 1% to 2% of individuals >40 years of age have chronic glaucoma with about 25% of the cases undetected.

There are two types of glaucoma: Primary, which has no known cause, and secondary, in which the increase in intraocular pressure is due to another eye disease. The most common form of glaucoma is open-angle glaucoma, in which fluid that normally flows through the pupil into the anterior chamber cannot pass through the trabecular meshwork to drain normally. In most individuals, open-angle glaucoma has no symptoms until visual impairment occurs.

In angle-closure glaucoma, the area between the iris and the cornea is closed. This condition can be chronic or acute. Acute angle-closure glaucoma is considered an emergency because optic nerve damage can occur within hours of the onset. Symptoms of acute angle closure glaucoma may include nausea and vomiting, visual halos around light, and ocular pain. Chronic angle-closure glaucoma, like open-angle glaucoma, is usually asymptomatic until visual loss occurs.

Congenital glaucoma, present at birth, is the result of defective development of the structures of the eye, and surgery is required for correction.

The major complication of glaucoma is loss of vision. Untreated acute glaucoma results in severe and permanent vision loss after the onset of symptoms. Vision can be preserved with prompt treatment. Untreated chronic glaucoma can progress to blindness within 20-25 years. Early diagnosis and treatment have excellent success with preserving vision. The outcome for congenital glaucoma varies depending on the age when symptoms begin.

LIFESTYLE RECOMMENDATIONS

- Reinforce proper technique for administering eye drops
- Reinforce need to see eye specialist for management (regular exams and evaluation)
- If sudden change in pain or vision, or GI symptoms, seek medical attention immediately

GLAUCOMA DECISION TREE

1. Client with glaucoma is interested in using natural products (NP) to support this condition

2. Healthcare provider requests basic background information. The following issues are addressed with the client:

* Allergies?
* Prescription (Rx)/OTC meds?
* Natural products?
* Other medical conditions?
* Nutrition/diet program?
* Exercise program?

3. Above data reviewed; if **yes** to Rx/OTC meds, review **Drug-Induced Nutrient Depletion Chart** in Appendix

4A. Client is a candidate for natural products

* An appropriate homeopathic remedy can be used at any time

4B. Client's case is too complicated at this point; needs additional support from MD before initiating NP program

5. Condition-specific questions:
* Describe treatment program; Meds, surgery, etc
* Eye pain? If **yes**, significance?
* Avoid meds that might worsen the condition: Corticosteroids, antihistamines, decongestants, antidepressants - if taking any of these, discuss with MD
* Associated GI symptoms? If **yes,** may be closed-angle glaucoma; a serious situation that could result in permanent eye damage, refer to MD

6. See table on following page

GLAUCOMA *(Continued)*

GLAUCOMA*

Category	Natural Products to Consider	DOC
Herb	**Bilberry** *on page 392* OR **Grape Seed** *on page 451*	PA
Vitamin/Mineral/ Trace Element/ Nutraceutical	**Alpha-Lipoic Acid** *on page 381* Condition-specific dosage: 100-300 mg/day	HT
Homeopathic Remedy	Homeopathic combination formulas are available for many conditions. Listed below are some of the most common single homeopathic remedies for glaucoma. Also see **Homeopathic Quick Reference Chart for Common Complaints** *on page 587*	
	Aconitum napellus	PD
	Atropa belladonna	PD
	Cineraria maritima	PD
Additional supplements to consider	**Vitamin A** *on page 518* Condition-specific dosage: 10,000-35,000 int. units/day	HD
	Vitamin C *on page 526* Condition-specific dosage: 500-1000 mg twice daily	HD

*Refer to **Introduction to Conditions** *on page 41* for more details on how to apply the information in this table to individuals with this condition.

SPECIAL CONSIDERATIONS

Bilberry (Berry)
- Consult with physician if pregnant or breast-feeding
- Contraindicated in active bleeding (eg, peptic ulcer, intracranial bleeding)
- Caution in hemostatic disorders/history of bleeding
- Potential interaction with anticoagulants (warfarin), aspirin, NSAIDs, anti-platelet agents
- Discontinue use prior to dental or surgical procedures (14 days before)

Grape Seed
- Contraindicated in active bleeding (eg, peptic ulcer, intracranial bleeding)
- Caution in hemostatic disorders/history of bleeding
- Potential interaction with anticoagulants (warfarin), aspirin, NSAIDs, anti-platelet agents, methotrexate
- Discontinue use prior to dental or surgical procedures (14 days before)

Alpha-Lipoic Acid
- No known toxicity or serious side effects
- Caution in individuals receiving oral hypoglycemics or insulin; monitor blood glucose closely and coordinate with prescriber

Vitamin A
- Contraindicated in pregnancy or in women who may become pregnant

Vitamin C
- Excess intake in diabetics may give falsely elevated blood glucose readings

HALITOSIS

Halitosis is a foul or disagreeable odor that is often referred to as "bad breath." This condition may chronically affect as many as 25 million people in the United States. It is frequently related to either poor oral hygiene and/or poor digestion. In approximately 85% of cases, the odor is usually caused by bacterial overgrowth in the oral cavity. Some specific strong-smelling foods and smoking are also contributors. Bacterial metabolism, which produces volatile sulfur-containing compounds, appears to be a common issue. For this reason, chronic halitosis is often associated with plaque, gingivitis, periodontitis, and dental caries. Salivary dysfunction and oral carcinoma are rare factors. In some situations, sinusitis, tonsillitis, lung abscess, hepatic failure, hepatic stress, renal failure, or gastrointestinal disorders may contribute.

Decreased nocturnal salivation may contribute to odor on awakening for many individuals with good oral hygiene. The mouth, tongue, and teeth are the most common sources of the odor, although the nose, sinuses, and pharynx may also be the source.

Consideration should be given to the possibility of systemic causes that require referral. As a rare consideration, some individuals may harbor an irrational fear in regard to their oral hygiene. Obsession with this issue may be a presentation of obsessive compulsive disorder.

LIFESTYLE RECOMMENDATIONS

- Continuation/initiation of diet and exercise program
- Use mouthwashes, mints, and breath fresheners sparingly - they will not cure the problem
- Avoid mouthwashes that have a high alcohol content
- If a smoker, consider enrolling in a smoking cessation program
- Avoid alcohol, garlic, and onions
- Brush teeth and tongue, and floss regularly
- Get regular dental check-ups
- Increase consumption of quality water

HALITOSIS DECISION TREE

1. Client with halitosis is interested in using natural products (NP) to support this condition

↓

2. Healthcare provider requests basic background information. The following issues are addressed with the client:

* Allergies?
* Prescription (Rx)/OTC meds?
* Natural products?
* Other medical conditions?
* Nutrition/diet program?
* Exercise program?

↓

3. Above data reviewed; if **yes** to Rx/OTC meds, review **Drug-Induced Nutrient Depletion Chart** in Appendix

4A. Client is a candidate for natural products

* An appropriate homeopathic remedy can be used at any time

4B. Client's case is too complicated at this point; needs additional support from MD before initiating NP program

↓

5. Condition-specific questions:
* Any dental diseases that have not been treated?
* Regular dental check-ups?
* Changes in diet? New foods?
* Possible contributing factors: Diabetes, GI problems, sinusitis, bronchitis

↓

6. See table on following page

HALITOSIS *(Continued)*

HALITOSIS*

Category	Natural Products to Consider	DOC
Herb	Milk Thistle *on page 479*	PA
	Parsley *on page 485*	PA, HE
	Psyllium *on page 492*	PA
	Tea Tree *on page 509*	PA
Vitamin/Mineral/ Trace Element/ Nutraceutical	*Lactobacillus acidophilus on page 467* and *Bifidobacterium bifidum on page 391* Condition-specific dosage: 2-5 billion CFU twice daily for 1 month (dairy free)	HD
	Chlorophyll *on page 409* Condition-specific dosage: 1 tsp or 3-4 tablets 1-2 times/day	HD
Homeopathic Remedy	Homeopathic combination formulas are available for many conditions. Listed below are some of the most common single homeopathic remedies for halitosis. Also see **Homeopathic Quick Reference Chart for Common Complaints** *on page 587*	
	Mercurius solubilis	PD
	Nux vomica	PD
Additional supplements to consider	No recommendations	

*Refer to **Introduction to Conditions** *on page 41* for more details on how to apply the information in this table to individuals with this condition.

SPECIAL CONSIDERATIONS

Milk Thistle
- No reported toxicity in humans at normal intakes

Parsley
- Contraindicated in individuals with renal disease or acute inflammation

Psyllium
- Avoid use in bowel obstruction

Tea Tree
- May cause allergic dermatitis in sensitive individuals
- Not for ingestion

Lactobacillus acidophilus
- No known toxicity or serious side effects

Bifidobacterium bifidum
- No known toxicity or serious side effects

Chlorophyll
- No known toxicity or serious side effects

HEADACHE / MIGRAINE HEADACHE

Headache is a diffuse sensation of pain with an incidence that is difficult to define. Headaches account for at least 18 million outpatient visits annually. They can be caused by muscle tension, increases in pressure within the cerebral blood vessels, underlying illness, environmental toxin exposure, hormonal disturbances, structural alignment problems, altered blood sugar, magnesium status, food intolerances, allergies, or temporomandibular joint dysfunction (TMJ).

The most common causes of simple headache are stress and musculoskeletal tension, which result from prolonged contraction of the neck/shoulder muscles. This may cause constriction of the cranial artery. These tension headaches consist of a dull ache, are bilateral, and involve the back of the neck, temples, and forehead. Tender localized spots in the neck and jaw may be located. They do not have nausea and vomiting associated and physical activity does not aggravate the symptoms.

Migraine headaches are most common in females 12-40 years of age, although both sexes may be affected. These headaches consist of distinct episodes that are often preceded by neurologic symptoms such as numbness, or distinct visual sensations often referred to as an "aura." Nausea and vomiting are common accompanying features. Symptoms appear to be caused by a cascade of events that may include vascular spasm or dilatation, followed by neuronal ischemia with release of excitatory neurotransmitters. Migraines may begin or cease at menopause, and physical activity may trigger or aggravate attacks. Other causes such as stress, food reactivity, and blood sugar disturbances have also been implicated.

Cluster headaches, which occur more commonly in males, tend to be unilateral and localized to the eye or temple. The attacks may last for minutes to hours. Associated symptoms may include nasal congestion and drooping or edematous eyelids. Facial sweating may occur as well. Attacks may occur daily for several days, followed by remissions that may last for months to years. The attacks are not usually accompanied by nausea and/or vomiting, and physical activity does not exacerbate the attacks.

Secondary headaches should be differentiated from the above primary causes. These headaches are associated with a systemic disease, such as infection or central nervous system lesion (such as hemorrhage or tumor). Differentiating these causes may require advanced diagnostic techniques.

LIFESTYLE RECOMMENDATIONS

- Avoid triggers or possible triggers: Aged cheese, artificial sweeteners, monosodium glutamate, chocolate, processed meats, alcohol, caffeine, sugar

- Avoid long-term use of OTC analgesics without seeking medical attention

- Consider massage therapy, stress management

- Review sleep habits and try to improve

- Avoid environmental or chemical triggers

- Drink plenty of quality water

- Improve posture

HEADACHE / MIGRAINE HEADACHE DECISION TREE

1. Client with headache or migraine headache is interested in using natural products (NP) to support this condition

2. Healthcare provider requests basic background information. The following issues are addressed with the client:
   * Allergies?
   * Prescription (Rx)/OTC meds?
   * Natural products?
   * Other medical conditions?
   * Nutrition/diet program?
   * Exercise program?

3. Above data reviewed; if **yes** to Rx/OTC meds, review **Drug-Induced Nutrient Depletion Chart** in Appendix

4A. Client is a candidate for natural products

   * An appropriate homeopathic remedy can be used at any time

4B. Client's case is too complicated at this point; needs additional support from MD before initiating NP program

5. Condition-specific questions:
   * Family history of headaches?
   * Taking specific meds that may contribute (hormone, nitrates)?
   * Specific conditions: Hypertension?
   * If female, related to hormonal changes?
   * Triggers? Sleep, work, stress, etc
   * Specific response to certain interventions?
   * Recent sinus problems or infections?
   * Any associated symptoms? Visual changes, GI, stiff neck, others?
   * How frequent?
   * Unilateral versus bilateral

6. See table on following page

HEADACHE / MIGRAINE HEADACHE *(Continued)*

HEADACHE/MIGRAINE HEADACHE*

Category	Natural Products to Consider	Rank
Herb	**Feverfew** *on page 432*	HT
	White Willow *on page 532*	PA, HE
	Ginkgo *on page 441*	PA
Vitamin/Mineral/ Trace Element/ Nutraceutical	**Magnesium** *on page 473* Condition-specific dosage: 400-600 mg/day	HT
	Vitamin B₂ *on page 520* Condition-specific dosage: 400 mg/day	HT
	Vitamin B₆ *on page 523* Condition-specific dosage: 50 mg twice daily	PA
	SAMe (S-adenosylmethionine) *on page 498* Condition-specific dosage: 200-400 mg twice daily	HT
	Fish Oils *on page 434* Condition-specific dosage: 1000 mg twice daily	HT
Homeopathic Remedy - **Headache**	Homeopathic combination formulas are available for many conditions. Listed below are some of the most common single homeopathic remedies for headaches. Also see **Homeopathic Quick Reference Chart for Common Complaints** *on page 587*	
	Apis mellifica	PD
	Atropa belladonna	PD
	Bryonia alba	PD
	Gelsemium sempervirens	PD
	Glonoinum	PD
	Ignatia amara	PD
	Nux vomica	PD
	Theridion	PD
Homeopathic Remedy - **Migraine**	Homeopathic combination formulas are available for many conditions. Listed below are some of the most common single homeopathic remedies for migraine headaches. Also see **Homeopathic Quick Reference Chart for Common Complaints** *on page 587*	
	Iris versicolor	PD
	Lachesis mutus	PD
	Natrum muriaticum	PD
	Spigelia anthelmia	PD
	Thuja occidentalis	PD
Additional supplements to consider	No recommendations	

*Refer to **Introduction to Conditions** *on page 41* for more details on how to apply the information in this table to individuals with this condition.

208

SPECIAL CONSIDERATIONS

Feverfew

- Contraindicated in pregnancy
- Contraindicated in allergy to *Asteraceae/Compositae* family (chrysanthemum, daisy)
- Contraindicated in active bleeding (eg, peptic ulcer, intracranial bleeding)
- Onset may be delayed for several weeks
- Abrupt discontinuation may increase migraine frequency
- Caution in hemostatic disorders/history of bleeding
- Potential interaction with anticoagulants (warfarin), aspirin, NSAIDs, antiplatelet agents
- Discontinue use prior to dental or surgical procedures (14 days before)

White Willow

- Contraindicated in aspirin allergy or hypersensitivity
- Do not use in children (potential for Reye's syndrome)
- Potential interactions with aspirin, anticoagulants, methotrexate, metoclopramide, phenytoin, probenecid, spironolactone, valproic acid, NSAIDs, antiplatelet agents

Ginkgo

- Contraindicated in active bleeding (eg, peptic ulcer, intracranial bleeding)
- Caution in hemostatic disorders/history of bleeding
- Potential interaction with anticoagulants (warfarin), aspirin, NSAIDs, antiplatelet agents
- Theoretical interaction with MAO inhibitors, acetylcholinesterase inhibitors (tacrine, donepezil)
- Discontinue use prior to dental or surgical procedures (14 days before)

Magnesium

- Use caution in renal impairment
- May cause diarrhea at high intakes

Vitamin B$_2$

- No known toxicity or serious side effects

Vitamin B$_6$

- No reported toxicity in humans at normal intakes

SAMe (S-adenosylmethionine)

- Use caution when combining SAMe with other antidepressants

Fish Oils

- High doses may cause GI upset, loose stools, nausea
- May alter glucose regulation; use with caution in diabetes
- Caution in individuals receiving oral hypoglycemics or insulin; monitor blood glucose closely and coordinate with prescriber
- Potential interaction with anticoagulants (warfarin), aspirin, NSAIDs, antiplatelet agents

HEMORRHOIDS

Hemorrhoid symptoms include perianal itching, burning, pain, or bleeding. Fissure, ulceration, or prolapse may occur in severe cases. Chronic blood loss may be associated with anemia. Other than in pregnancy, hemorrhoids are uncommon in individuals <30 years of age, but increase in frequency to affect 5% of the population by age 50.

Blood vessels that line the lower sphincter area become engorged and dilated. Prolonged sitting or standing, pregnancy, or infection may exacerbate the condition. They become symptomatic as a result of strain or physical disturbances, such as passage of hardened stool or diarrhea. The presence of hemorrhoids may be confirmed by proctoscopic visualization. Additional evaluation of the lower gastrointestinal tract is generally recommended to rule out the possibility of other gastrointestinal disease such as polyps, colitis, or carcinoma.

LIFESTYLE RECOMMENDATIONS

- Avoid nuts, alcohol, caffeine, and heavy lifting
- Clean anorectal area regularly with mild soap
- Use unscented, soft toilet tissue
- Local anesthetics may cause allergic reactions with symptoms resembling the condition (burning, itching)
- Use OTC products for the symptoms **after** a bowel movement
- Increase intake of fiber and water
- Avoid sitting for prolonged periods of time

HEMORRHOIDS DECISION TREE

1. Client with hemorrhoids is interested in using natural products (NP) to support this condition

2. Healthcare provider requests basic background information. The following issues are addressed with the client:

   * Allergies?
   * Prescription (Rx)/OTC meds?
   * Natural products?
   * Other medical conditions?
   * Nutrition/diet program?
   * Exercise program?

3. Above data reviewed; if **yes** to Rx/OTC meds, review **Drug-Induced Nutrient Depletion Chart** in Appendix

4A. Client is a candidate for natural products

   * An appropriate homeopathic remedy can be used at any time

4B. Client's case is too complicated at this point; needs additional support from MD before initiating NP program

5. Condition-specific questions:
   * Constipated? Use laxatives regularly?
   * Use any meds that may contribute to the problem: Narcotics, anticholinergics, antidepressants, calcium channel blockers, aluminum- or calcium-containing antacids, potassium-wasting diuretics?
   * Hypothyroidism? May contribute to condition
   * Diabetes? May contribute to condition
   * Blood from rectum not associated with bowel movement? If **yes**, refer to MD.

6. See table on following page

HEMORRHOIDS *(Continued)*

HEMORRHOIDS*

Category	Natural Products to Consider	Rank
Herb	**Horse Chestnut** (topical) *on page 458*	PA, HE
	Milk Thistle *on page 479*	PA
	Gotu Kola (topical) *on page 449*	PA
	Bilberry *on page 392*	PA
Vitamin/Mineral/ Trace Element/ Nutraceutical	**Flaxseed Oil** *on page 435* Condition-specific dosage: 1 Tbsp/day	PA
Homeopathic Remedy	Homeopathic combination formulas are available for many conditions. Listed below are some of the most common single homeopathic remedies for hemorrhoids. Also see **Homeopathic Quick Reference Chart for Common Complaints** *on page 587*	
	Aesculus hippocastanum	PD
	Carduus marianus	PD
	Hamamelis virginica	PD
	Podophyllum peltatum	PD
	Sulphur	PD
Additional supplements to consider	**Vitamin A** *on page 518* Condition-specific dosage: 10,000-35,000 int. units/ day	PA
	Vitamin C *on page 526* Condition-specific dosage: 250-1000 mg/day	PA
	Vitamin E *on page 529* Condition-specific dosage: 200-400 int. units/day	PA
	Selenium *on page 502* Condition-specific dosage: 200 mcg	PA

*Refer to **Introduction to Conditions** *on page 41* for more details on how to apply the information in this table to individuals with this condition.

SPECIAL CONSIDERATIONS

Horse Chestnut
- Contraindicated in active bleeding (eg, peptic ulcer, intracranial bleeding)
- Caution in hemostatic disorders/history of bleeding
- Potential interactions with anticoagulants (warfarin), aspirin, NSAIDs, antiplatelet agents
- Caution in hepatic or renal impairment
- Discontinue use prior to dental or surgical procedures (14 days before)

Milk Thistle
- No reported toxicity in humans at normal intakes

Gotu Kola
- Contraindicated during pregnancy
- High doses may be sedating; caution when driving/performing hazardous tasks
- May be additive with other CNS sedatives

Bilberry
- Contraindicated in active bleeding, including peptic ulcer
- Caution in hemostatic disorders/history of bleeding
- Potential interaction with anticoagulants (warfarin), aspirin, NSAIDs, antiplatelet agents
- Discontinue use prior to dental or surgical procedures (14 days before)

Flaxseed Oil
- No known toxicity or serious side effects

Vitamin A
- Contraindicated in pregnancy or in women who become pregnant

Vitamin C
- Excess intake in diabetics may give falsely elevated blood glucose readings

Vitamin E
- Use with caution when taking anticoagulants (vitamin E ≥200 int. units increases prothrombin times)
- Interrupt or reduce dosage one week prior to dental or surgical procedures

Selenium
- No reported toxicity in humans at normal intakes

HERPES SIMPLEX 1

Herpes simplex 1 is a virus that usually causes cold sores, also known as fever blisters, and/or herpes labialis. As many as 15% of the population have a primary infection, of which 20% to 45% will have recurrent lesions. Approximately 7% of individuals have two or more occurrences per year. Infections, fever, stress, trauma, hormonal changes, and exposure to sunlight may trigger an eruption.

Eruptions often involve an initial stage of tingling, burning, or numbness, followed by localized erythema and edema. A cluster of small vesicles appears at the top of the lesion that rupture and crust over. An adherent clot will form and the lesion will heal in 10-14 days. These painful lesions, which generally occur along the lip or its borders, are believed to be transmitted by direct contact with the virus. It should be noted that excretion of viral particles might persist for as long as 6 weeks following the initial infection. Shedding of virus after secondary eruptions is considerably shorter.

LIFESTYLE RECOMMENDATIONS

- Avoid triggers: Spicy foods, stress, overexposure to the sun, fatigue, extreme temperature changes

- If symptoms are related to hormonal cycle, may discuss preventive program to reduce frequency/severity of recurrences with healthcare provider.

- OTC anesthetic ointment might relieve pain

- Keep area clean

- Avoid contact of affected area with others until lesions are completely healed

- Rinse mouth regularly with salt water

HERPES SIMPLEX 1 DECISION TREE

---

1. Client with herpes simplex 1 is interested in using natural products (NP) to support this condition

---

2. Healthcare provider requests basic background information. The following issues are addressed with the client:

* Allergies?
* Prescription (Rx)/OTC meds?
* Natural products?
* Other medical conditions?
* Nutrition/diet program?
* Exercise program?

---

3. Above data reviewed; if **yes** to Rx/OTC meds, review **Drug-Induced Nutrient Depletion Chart** in Appendix

---

4A. Client is a candidate for natural products

* An appropriate homeopathic remedy can be used at any time

4B. Client's case is too complicated at this point; needs additional support from MD before initiating NP program

---

5. Condition-specific questions:
* Diagnosed by MD? Treatment plan?
* Triggers: How often exposed to these?
* Using any antivirals?
* Any other infections during the time of the outbreak?
* Any other conditions that might compromise immune function?
* If pregnant or possiblility of pregnancy, refer to MD

---

6. See table on following page

215

HERPES SIMPLEX 1 *(Continued)*

HERPES SIMPLEX 1*

Category	Natural Products to Consider	DOC
Herb	**Lemon Balm/Melissa** *on page 469*	HT
	Grapefruit Seed Extract *on page 450*	PA
	Olive Leaf *on page 483*	PA
	Echinacea purpura *on page 426*	PA
Vitamin/Mineral/ Trace Element/ Nutraceutical	**Lysine** *on page 473* Condition-specific dosage: 500-1000 mg 3 times/day	HT
	Vitamin C *on page 526* Condition-specific dosage: 500-1000 mg twice daily	HT
Homeopathic Remedy	Homeopathic combination formulas are available for many conditions. Listed below are some of the most common single homeopathic remedies for herpes simplex 1. Also see **Homeopathic Quick Reference Chart for Common Complaints** *on page 587*	
	Baptista tinctoria	PD
	Croton tiglium	PD
	Muriaticum acidum	PD
	Rhus toxicodendron	PD
Additional supplements to consider	**Selenium** *on page 502* Condition-specific dosage: 200 mcg/day	PA

*Refer to **Introduction to Conditions** *on page 41* for more details on how to apply the information in this table to individuals with this condition.

SPECIAL CONSIDERATIONS

Lemon Balm/Melissa
- No reported toxicity in humans at normal intakes

Grapefruit Seed Extract
- Grapefruit seed extract is not equivalent to grapefruit juice/pulp. Juice/pulp has been associated with many drug interactions; see Grapefruit Seed *on page 450*
- Until further information is available, it is reasonable to avoid some medications (terfenadine, astemizole, cisapride). Use other medications metabolized by CYP3A4 with caution.

Olive Leaf
- No reported toxicity in humans at normal intakes

Echinacea purpura
- Not recommended for use longer than 10 days (acute treatment) or in immunosuppressed individuals
- If used as prophylaxis, cycle 3 weeks on/1 week off
- Caution in renal impairment (may cause electrolyte imbalance)
- Caution if allergic to *Asteraceae/Compositae* family (ragweed, daisy, aster, chrysanthemum) and other pollens

Lysine
- No known toxicity or serious side effects

Vitamin C
- Excess intake in diabetics may give falsely elevated blood glucose readings

Selenium
- No reported toxicity in humans at normal intakes

HERPES SIMPLEX 2

Genital herpes is a sexually transmitted disease (STD) caused by a strain of the herpes simplex virus (HSV). The virus usually enters the body through small cuts in the skin or mucous membranes, and may be passed to neonates by contact during delivery. Both men and women can be infected.

Signs or symptoms of genital herpes include lesions (sores) on the genitals, buttocks, anus, or thighs; pain, itching, or tenderness around the genitals; painful urination; swollen groin lymph nodes; headache, fever, and other flu-like symptoms.

Lesions begin as small red bumps that form vesicles that coalesce into blisters. The blisters rupture, ooze, or bleed. This is followed by crusting of the lesion. Gradually, the sores scab and heal as the infection resolves. In rare cases, the infection can be active when lesions are not present.

Genital herpes has a unique cycle that may recur for many years. Individuals may experience an episode every month. However, outbreaks are less frequent for most individuals. Some individuals experience only a single outbreak. In others, the symptoms may decrease with time.

Currently, there is no cure for genital herpes. Treatment involves efforts to prevent transmission, limit eruptions, increase the rate of healing, and limit relapses. Genital herpes is highly contagious while lesions are present. Abstinence is the most certain method to prevent transmission. Other efforts to limit transmission include limiting sexual intercourse to periods when no signs or symptoms are present, and using condoms. Good nutrition, careful hygiene, and stress management may help limit eruptions.

The first episode should prompt physician evaluation immediately, since there is a chance of infection with another sexually transmitted disease in addition to HSV. Genital herpes can lead to discomfort or embarrassment, however, it is not generally associated with other serious medical problems.

LIFESTYLE RECOMMENDATIONS

- Avoid triggers

- If symptoms are related to hormonal cycle, may discuss preventive program to reduce frequency/severity of recurrences with healthcare provider

- Avoid risky behaviors that increase chances for outbreak, exposing partners

- Avoid tight-fitting clothes during outbreaks

- Use condoms

- If any partners are at risk, make sure they seek medical attention

- Avoid sexual relations during outbreaks

- Keep area clean

- Avoid contact of affected area with others until lesions are completely healed

HERPES SIMPLEX 2 (GENITAL) DECISION TREE

1. Client with herpes simplex 2 (genital) is interested in using natural products to support their treatment regimen

2. HCP requests basic background information in order to formulate recommendations. The following questions are asked of the client:

* Allergies?
* Rx meds?
* Other meds?
* Natural products?

* Other medical conditions?
* Nutrition/diet program?
* Exercise program?

3. Above data reviewed

4A. Client is a candidate for natural products

4B. Client case too complicated at this point - needs additional support from MD before initiating NP program

5. Condition-specific questions:
* Has condition been diagnosed by MD? Treatment plan?
* Triggers: How often exposed to these?
* Using any antivirals?
* Any other infections during the time of the outbreak?
* Any other conditions that might compromise immune function?
* If pregnant or possibility of pregnancy, refer to MD

6. See recommendations on following pages

HERPES SIMPLEX 2 *(Continued)*

HERPES SIMPLEX 2*

Category	Natural Products to Consider	DOC
Herb	**Arabinoxylane** *on page 384*	PA
	Cat's Claw *on page 404*	PA
	Lemon Balm/Melissa (topical) *on page 469*	HT
	Tea Tree (topical) *on page 509*	PA
	Olive Leaf *on page 483*	PA
	Grapefruit Seed Extract *on page 450*	PA
Vitamin/Mineral/ Trace Element/ Nutraceutical	**Lysine** *on page 473* Condition-specific dosage: 500-1000 mg 3 times/day	HT
	Vitamin C *on page 526* Condition-specific dosage: 500-1000 mg twice daily	HT
	Selenium *on page 502* Condition-specific dosage: 200 mcg/day	PA
	Fish Oils *on page 434* Condition-specific dosage: 1000 mg twice daily	PA
Homeopathic Remedy	Homeopathic combination formulas are available for many conditions. Listed below are some of the most common single homeopathic remedies for herpes simplex 2. Also see **Homeopathic Quick Reference Chart for Common Complaints** *on page 587*	
	Capsicum annuum	PD
	Natrum muriaticum	PD
	Rhus toxicodendron	PD
Additional Supplements to Consider	*Lactobacillus acidophilus* *on page 467* and *Bifidobacterium bifidum* *on page 391* Condition-specific dosage: 2-5 billion CFU twice daily	PA

*Refer to **Introduction to Conditions** *on page 41* for more details on how to apply the information in this table to individuals with this condition.

SPECIAL CONSIDERATIONS

Arabinoxylane

- Do not use in renal failure due to relatively high phosphorus content

Cat's Claw

- Contraindicated in transplant recipients, individuals receiving I.V. immunoglobulins or immunosuppressants
- Contraindicated in active bleeding (eg, peptic ulcer, intracranial bleeding)
- Caution in hemostatic disorders/history of bleeding
- Potential interaction with anticoagulants (warfarin), aspirin, NSAIDs, antiplatelet agents
- Discontinue use prior to dental or surgical procedures (14 days before)

Lemon Balm/Melissa

- No reported toxicity in humans at normal intakes

Tea Tree

- May cause allergic dermatitis in sensitive individuals
- Topical use only; **not for ingestion**

Olive Leaf

- No reported toxicity in humans at normal intakes

Grapefruit Seed Extract

- Grapefruit seed extract is not equivalent to grapefruit juice/pulp. Juice/pulp has been associated with many drug interactions; see Grapefruit Seed *on page 450*
- Until further information is available, it is reasonable to avoid some medications (terfenadine, astemizole, cisapride). Use other medications metabolized by CYP3A4 with caution.

Lysine

- No known toxicity or serious side effects

Vitamin C

- Excess intake in diabetics may give falsely elevated blood glucose readings

Selenium

- No reported toxicity in humans at normal intakes

Fish Oils

- High doses may cause GI upset, loose stools, nausea
- May alter glucose regulation; use with caution in diabetes
- Caution in individuals receiving oral hypoglycemics or insulin; monitor blood glucose closely and coordinate with prescriber
- Potential interaction with anticoagulants (warfarin), aspirin, NSAIDs, antiplatelet agents

Lactobacillus acidophilus

- No known toxicity or serious side effects

Bifidobacterium bifidum

- No known toxicity or serious side effects

HYPERGLYCEMIA / DIABETES / INSULIN RESISTANCE

Diabetes is a chronic disease characterized by hyperglycemia. There are two types of diabetes. Type 1 diabetes is usually diagnosed before age 25 and affects 10% of persons, while type 2 diabetes is much more prevalent and historically has occurred in older adults. However, the mass use of refined sugars is resulting in younger and younger type 2 diabetics. While type 1 diabetes is associated with an absence of insulin production, type 2 diabetes may be related to abnormalities in insulin sensitivity, decreased insulin production, or abnormalities of other hormones that regulate blood glucose.

Type 1 diabetes is evident when >80% of the cells that secrete insulin have been destroyed. This destruction appears to be caused by an autoimmune process, triggered by virus, vaccinations, or endotoxins or xenotoxins. In the absence of insulin, cells cannot use glucose as fuel. Hunger (polyphagia), thirst (polydipsia), and excessive urine production (polyuria) are classic symptoms of type 1 diabetes. Type 2 diabetes may be caused by a number of potential defects in glucose regulation. It represents a spectrum of disorders that share in common the manifestation of hyperglycemia.

Regardless of cause, acute hyperglycemia may cause dehydration, blurred vision, weight loss, and impaired healing. Chronic hyperglycemia may lead to organ dysfunction including retinopathy, neuropathy, and nephropathy. In addition, individuals with diabetes are known to have an increased incidence of MI, stroke, and peripheral vascular disease. Control of diabetes may require dietary adaptation, weight management, insulin replacement, or other pharmacological therapy. It is not uncommon for individuals with diabetes to also receive additional medications to prevent or treat complications of the disease.

LIFESTYLE RECOMMENDATIONS

- Continuation/initiation of diet and exercise program - THIS IS VERY IMPORTANT! MANAGEMENT MAY INVOLVE JUST THESE INTERVENTIONS AND NO MEDICATIONS

- Education must be routine, focused, and reinforced

- Stress adherence to all interventions and timing of medications

- Limit alcohol consumption to two drinks per day

- Inspect feet and skin daily - use lotions to keep skin from getting cracked, dry

- Massage feet to maintain proper circulation

- Make sure client has ID bracelet/ID card to show they have diabetes in case of an emergency

- If prone to hypoglycemia, keep glucose tabs/rescue preparation with client at all times

- Work with dietician to customize nutrition program; learn how to monitor carbohydrate intake; keep log

- Read labels on food and medications, looking for sugar content

- Make sure client knows symptoms of HYPER-, HYPOglycemia:

Signs and symptoms of HYPERglycemia: Increased thirst, hunger, and urination; weight loss, increase in rate of infection, time for wound healing, visual disturbances

Signs and symptoms of HYPOglycemia: Increased heart rate or respiratory rate, pale moist skin, headache, blurred vision, lethargy, weakness, irritability, confusion, hunger, nausea

HYPERGLYCEMIA / DIABETES DECISION TREE

1. Client hyperglycemia/diabetes is interested in using natural products (NP) to support this condition

2. Healthcare provider requests basic background information.
   The following issues are addressed with the client:
   * Allergies?
   * Prescription (Rx)/OTC meds?
   * Natural products?
   * Other medical conditions?
   * Home blood glucose monitoring program?
     What are the numbers? Get the data!
   * Nutrition/diet program? Specific
   * Exercise program? Specifics

3. Above data reviewed; if **yes** to Rx/OTC meds, review
   Drug-Induced Nutrient Depletion Chart in Appendix

4A. Client is a candidate for natural products

   * An appropriate homeopathic remedy can be used at any time

4B. Client's case is too complicated at this point; needs additional support from MD before initiating NP program

5. Condition-specific questions:
   * When diagnosed?
   * Family history? Stress importance of screening of family members
   * Type 1 or 2? Treatment plan?
   * Specialists involved in care? MD, RPh, CDE, RD, etc ?
     Stress importance of team approach to treatment
   * HB A1c blood sugar monitoring? Numbers
   * If using insulin, review technique
   * How often is client symptomatic (both hyper- and hypoglycemic)?
   * Stress adherence to all therapies, timing of medications in relation to meals
   * If taking meds, review to ensure that the meds are not contributing to problem with blood sugar

6. See table on following page

HYPERGLYCEMIA / DIABETES /
INSULIN RESISTANCE *(Continued)*

HYPERGLYCEMIA / DIABETES / INSULIN RESISTANCE*

Category	Natural Products to Consider	DOC
Herb	Gymnema *on page 455*	HT
	Bitter Melon *on page 394*	HT
	Evening Primrose *on page 430*	HT
Vitamin/Mineral/ Trace Element/ Nutraceutical	Chromium *on page 410* Condition-specific dosage: 400-1000 mcg/day	HT
	Cyclo-Hispro *on page 420* Condition-specific dosage: 200-300 mg 4 times/day	HD
	Vanadium (Vanadyl Sulfate) *on page 516* Condition-specific dosage: 250 mcg 3 times/day	HT
	Alpha-Lipoic Acid *on page 381* Condition-specific dosage: 100-200 mg 3 times/day	HT
	Magnesium *on page 473* Condition-specific dosage: 400-600 mg/day	HD
Homeopathic Remedy	Homeopathic combination formulas are available for many conditions. Listed below are some of the most common single homeopathic remedies for hyperglycemia. Also see **Homeopathic Quick Reference Chart for Common Complaints** *on page 587*	
	Lycopodium clavatum	PD
	Phaseolus	PD
	Phosphoricum acidum	PD
	Syzygium jambolanum	PD
	Uranium nitricum	PD
Additional supplements to consider	Vitamin B Complex-25 *on page 526* Condition-specific dosage: 25-50 mg twice daily	HD
	Zinc *on page 534* Condition-specific dosage: 15-35 mg/day	HD

*Refer to **Introduction to Conditions** *on page 41* for more details on how to apply the information in this table to individuals with this condition.

SPECIAL CONSIDERATIONS

Gymnema
- May alter blood glucose; use with caution in individuals with diabetes or predisposition to hypoglycemia
- Monitor blood sugar closely in individuals with diabetes
- Potential interactions with insulin, oral hypoglycemics

Bitter Melon
- Contraindicated in pregnancy
- May alter blood glucose; use with caution in individuals with diabetes or predisposition to hypoglycemia
- Monitor blood sugar closely in individuals with diabetes
- Potential interactions with insulin, oral hypoglycemics

Evening Primrose
- Contraindicated in seizure disorders, schizophrenia, or in persons receiving anticonvulsant or antipsychotic medications
- Contraindicated in active bleeding (eg, peptic ulcer, intracranial bleeding)
- Caution in hemostatic disorders/history of bleeding
- Potential interaction with anticoagulants (warfarin), aspirin, NSAIDs, anti-platelet agents
- Discontinue use prior to dental or surgical procedures (14 days before)

Chromium
- Caution in individuals receiving oral hypoglycemics or insulin; monitor blood glucose closely and coordinate with prescriber

Cyclo-Hispro
- Caution in individuals receiving oral hypoglycemics or insulin; monitor blood glucose closely and coordinate with prescriber

Vanadium (Vanadyl Sulfate)
- Caution in individuals receiving oral hypoglycemics or insulin; monitor blood glucose closely and coordinate with prescriber

Alpha-Lipoic Acid
- Caution in individuals receiving oral hypoglycemics or insulin; monitor blood glucose closely and coordinate with prescriber

Magnesium
- Use caution in renal impairment
- May cause diarrhea at high intakes

Vitamin B Complex-25
- No side effects at the RDI or ODA doses

Zinc
- No known toxicity or serious side effects at normal intakes

HYPERTENSION
(HIGH BLOOD PRESSURE)

More than 60 million Americans may have high blood pressure and about 50% are not aware of their condition. Hypertension can damage vessels in the heart, kidneys, and brain without obvious symptoms. Symptoms of high blood pressure include headache, dizziness, and palpitations. Long-term consequences may involve stroke, kidney failure, impairment of heart function, and coronary heart disease.

High blood pressure or hypertension occurs due to constriction of the arterioles. This increases the work of the heart as it attempts to distribute the blood to the body. In >90% of cases, the specific causal factor is unknown. Systolic blood pressure >140 mm Hg or a diastolic blood pressure >90 mm Hg is considered to represent hypertension. A diagnosis of hypertension should rarely be made on the basis of a single measurement, unless the initial readings are dangerously elevated, and must be made by a physician.

Important approaches to the reducing of high blood pressure are weight reduction, salt and alcohol restriction, avoidance of tobacco, regular exercise, determination of insulin resistance, and relaxation techniques. In addition, prescribed medications may be taken to control blood pressure.

LIFESTYLE RECOMMENDATIONS

- Continuation/initiation of diet and exercise program

- Continuation/initiation of home blood pressure monitoring program

- If a smoker, this behavior will worsen condition; consider enrolling in a smoking cessation program

- Diet: Sodium restriction, weight reduction, alcohol (maximum: 2 drinks/day)

- Avoid stressful situations

HYPERTENSION DECISION TREE

---

1. Client with hypertension is interested in using natural products (NP) to support this condition

↓

2. Healthcare provider requests basic background information. The following issues are addressed with the client:

* Allergies?
* Prescription (Rx)/OTC meds?
* Natural products?
* Other medical conditions?

* Home blood pressure monitoring program? What are the readings? Compare to those of MD's office.
* Nutrition/diet program? Additional fiber? Sodium-restricted?
* Exercise program?

↓

3. Above data reviewed; if **yes** to Rx/OTC meds, review **Drug-Induced Nutrient Depletion Chart** in Appendix

↓

4A. Client is a candidate for natural products

* An appropriate homeopathic remedy can be used at any time

4B. Client's case is too complicated at this point; needs additional support from MD before initiating NP program

↓

5. Condition-specific questions:
* If client is taking drug therapy for hypertension, review effectiveness: Positive and negative outcomes, adherence; have client also share this with MD.
* Client's lipids checked recently? If **yes**, what were the results? Candidate for natural products, see **Dyslipidemia** Decision Tree.

↓

6. See table on following page

HYPERTENSION
(HIGH BLOOD PRESSURE) *(Continued)*

HYPERTENSION*

Category	Natural Products to Consider	DOC
Herb	**Hawthorn** *on page 456*	HD
	Coleus *on page 413*	PA
	Garlic *on page 438*	HT
Vitamin/Mineral/ Trace Element/ Nutraceutical	**Magnesium** *on page 473* Condition-specific dosage: 400-600 mg/day	HT
	Calcium *on page 400* Condition-specific dosage: 1000 mg/day	HT
	Coenzyme Q$_{10}$ *on page 412* Condition-specific dosage: 30-50 mg twice daily	HT
	Fish Oils *on page 434* Condition-specific dosage: 750 mg 2-3 times/day OR **Flaxseed Oil** *on page 435* Condition-specific dosage: 1 Tbsp/day	HT
Homeopathic Remedy	Homeopathic combination formulas are available for many conditions. Listed below are some of the most common single homeopathic remedies for hypertension. Also see **Homeopathic Quick Reference Chart for Common Complaints** *on page 587*	
	Cactus grandiflorus	PD
	Glonoinum	PD
	Natrum muriacticum	PD
Additional supplements to consider	**Alpha-Lipoic Acid** *on page 381* Condition-specific dosage: 200-600 mg/day	HE

*Refer to **Introduction to Conditions** *on page 41* for more details on how to apply the information in this table to individuals with this condition.

SPECIAL CONSIDERATIONS

Hawthorn

- Use with caution in pregnancy
- Use with caution in hypertension or in individuals at risk of hypotension (elderly, cerebrovascular or cardiovascular disease)
- Theoretical interactions with antiarrhythmics, antihypertensives, cardiac glycosides, ACE inhibitors, angiotensin blockers

Coleus

- Contraindicated in active bleeding
- May cause hypotension; use with caution in cerebrovascular or cardiovascular disease
- Caution in hemostatic disorders/history of bleeding
- Potential interactions with anticoagulants (warfarin), aspirin, NSAIDs, antiplatelet agents
- Potential interactions with antihistamines, decongestants, antihypertensives
- Discontinue use prior to dental or surgical procedures (14 days before)

Garlic

- May cause GI distress or irritation
- Contraindicated in active bleeding (eg, peptic ulcer, intracranial bleeding)
- Caution in hemostatic disorders/history of bleeding
- Discontinue use prior to dental or surgical procedures (14 days before)
- Caution in individuals at risk due to hypotension or orthostasis (elderly, cerebrovascular or cardiovascular disease)
- Potential interaction with anticoagulants (warfarin), aspirin, NSAIDs, antiplatelet agents
- May potentiate antihypertensives, antihyperlipidemics
- Caution in diabetes

Magnesium

- Use caution in renal impairment
- May cause diarrhea at high intakes

Calcium

- Calcium supplements may contain lead (check for manufacturers who certify low lead levels)
- Potential interactions with tetracyclines, fluoroquinolones

Coenzyme Q_{10}

- No known toxicity or serious side effects
- Caution in individuals receiving anticoagulants

Fish Oils

- High doses may cause GI upset, loose stools, nausea
- May alter glucose regulation; use with caution in diabetes
- Caution in individuals receiving oral hypoglycemics or insulin; monitor blood glucose closely and coordinate with prescriber
- Potential interaction with anticoagulants (warfarin), aspirin, NSAIDs, antiplatelet agents

Flaxseed Oil

- No known toxicity or serious side effects

Alpha-Lipoic Acid

- No known toxicity or serious side effects
- Caution in individuals receiving oral hypoglycemics or insulin; monitor blood glucose closely and coordinate with prescriber

HYPERTHYROIDISM

Hyperthyroidism is a condition that is due to an overactive thyroid gland secreting excessive amounts of the thyroid hormone, thyroxine. The disease is most prevalent in women; however, males may also be affected.

Signs and symptoms of hyperthyroidism include heat intolerance, nervousness, emotional instability, weight loss, increased bowel activity, palpitation, and proximal muscle weakness. The hair of hyperthyroid individuals is particularly fine and the skin is smooth. Eyelid retraction and lagging of the eyelid are common. Individuals may have hyperdynamic circulation, including hypertension, tachycardia, widened pulse pressure, and a systolic ejection murmur indicative of high flow.

Hyperthyroidism is most commonly attributed to Graves' disease, an autoimmune disorder in which autoantibodies stimulate the thyroid gland to produce excessive amounts of hormone. Another type of hyperthyroidism is known as toxic multinodular goiter, or Plummer's disease. In this condition, some of the thyroid nodules fail to respond to the body's normal chemical messages, which results in the overproduction of thyroid hormone. In some cases, hyperthyroidism results from excessive supplementation (iatrogenic) or a specific medication (such as amiodarone).

Hyperthyroidism may result in thyroid storm, which is a medical emergency characterized by severe hyperthermia, tachycardia, delirium, diarrhea, and coma. Thyroid storm may be precipitated by an acute stress such as surgery, infection, or trauma. Mortality of this disorder is approximately 20%.

LIFESTYLE RECOMMENDATIONS

- Follow physician's recommendations to treat

- Treatment may lead to development of hypothyroidism, which most likely will result in the need for thyroid supplementation

- Avoid other medications that may mimic or exacerbate symptoms (ie, anticholinergic agents)

HYPERTHYROIDISM DECISION TREE

1. Client with hyperthyroidism is interested in using natural products (NP) to support this condition

2. Healthcare provider requests basic background information. The following issues are addressed with the client:

   * Allergies?   * Other medical conditions?
   * Prescription (Rx)/OTC meds?   * Nutrition/diet program?
   * Natural products?   * Exercise program?

3. Above data reviewed; if **yes** to Rx/OTC meds, review **Drug-Induced Nutrient Depletion Chart** in Appendix

4A. Client is a candidate for natural products

   * An appropriate homeopathic remedy can be used at any time

4B. Client's case is too complicated at this point; needs additional support from MD before initiating NP program

5. Condition-specific questions:
   * Diagnosed by MD?
   * Treatment program, plan, effectiveness of interventions to date
   * Sleep problems? May be related to condition
   * Weight problems? May be related to condition

6. See table on following page

231

HYPERTHYROIDISM *(Continued)*

HYPERTHYROIDISM*

Category	Natural Products to Consider	DOC
Herb	**Milk Thistle** *on page 479*	PA
	Passion Flower *on page 486*	PA, HE
	Valerian *on page 515*	PA, HE
Vitamin/Mineral/ Trace Element/ Nutraceutical	**N-Acetyl Cysteine** *on page 482* Condition-specific dosage: 600-1200 mg/day	PA
Homeopathic Remedy	Homeopathic combination formulas are available for many conditions. Listed below are some of the most common single homeopathic remedies for hyperthyroidism. Also see **Homeopathic Quick Reference Chart for Common Complaints** *on page 587*	
	Iodium	PD
	Lycopus virginicus	PD
	Natrum muriaticum	PD
Additional Supplements to Consider	No recommendations	

*Refer to **Introduction to Conditions** *on page 41* for more details on how to apply the information in this table to individuals with this condition.

SPECIAL CONSIDERATIONS

Milk Thistle
- No reported toxicity in humans at normal intakes

Passion Flower
- May cause sedation; may cause drowsiness; caution when driving/performing hazardous tasks
- Potential interactions with antianxiety agent, antidepressants, hexobarbital, hypnotics, sedatives

Valerian
- May cause drowsiness; caution when driving/performing hazardous tasks
- Effects do not appear to be potentiated by ethanol
- Do not use in children <3 years of age; use only valepotriate and baldrinal-free in children <12 years of age due to potential mutagenic properties
- Potential interactions: CNS depressants, sedative-hypnotics (barbiturates), antidepressants, anxiolytics, antihistamines

N-Acetyl Cysteine
- No known toxicity or serious side effects

HYPOGLYCEMIA

Due to dysfunction in the regulation of glucose metabolism, a person's blood sugar may decrease to a level where they become symptomatic due to hypoglycemia. Symptoms may include headache, lightheadedness, confusion, somnolence, tachycardia, sweaty palms, and diaphoresis.

Hypoglycemia may be caused by a number of endocrine disorders, including those that result in increased insulin activity or decreased activity of counter-regulatory compounds such as epinephrine, glucagon, and cortisol. Hypoglycemia may occur in sensitive individuals during fasting or during long intervals between meals. Alcohol ingestion tends to contribute to hypoglycemia. Individuals with diabetes are at risk of this problem as a complication of treatment (excessive dosages of insulin or hypoglycemic agents). Hypoglycemia, if prolonged, may progress to coma and/or result in damage to the central nervous system.

LIFESTYLE RECOMMENDATIONS

- Continuation/initiation of diet and exercise program - make sure that this is not contributing

- Education must be routine, focused, and reinforced

- Stress adherence to all interventions, timing of meds

- Limit alcohol consumption

- Make sure to have ID bracelet/ID card to show that you have low blood sugar in case of an emergency

- If prone to regular, symptomatic hypoglycemia, keep glucose tabs/rescue preparation with you at all times

- Work with dietician to customize nutrition program, learn how to monitor carbohydrate intake, keep log

- Make sure you know the symptoms of hyper-, hypoglycemia:

Signs/symptoms of HYPOglycemia: Increase in heart rate, respiratory rate, pale moist skin, headache, blurred vision, lethargy, weakness, irritability, confusion, hunger, nausea

Signs/symptoms of HYPERglycemia: Increased thirst, hunger, urination; weight loss, increase in rate of infection, time for wound healing, visual disturbances

HYPOGLYCEMIA DECISION TREE

1. Client with hypoglycemia is interested in using natural products (NP) to support this condition

↓

2. Healthcare provider requests basic background information. The following issues are addressed with the client:

* Allergies?
* Prescription (Rx)/OTC meds?
* Natural products?
* Other medical conditions?
* Home blood glucose monitoring program? What are the numbers? Get the data
* Nutrition/diet program? Specifics
* Exercise program? Specifics

↓

3. Above data reviewed; if **yes** to Rx/OTC meds, review **Drug-Induced Nutrient Depletion Chart** in Appendix

↓

4A. Client is a candidate for natural products

* An appropriate homeopathic remedy can be used at any time

4B. Client's case is too complicated at this point; needs additional support from MD before initiating NP program

↓

5. Condition-specific questions:
 * When diagnosed?
 * Treatment plan/effective treatments
 * Specialists involved in care? MD, RPh, CDE, RD, etc: Stress importance of team approach to treatment, education
 * Any recent changes in diet, exercise program that might be contributing?
 * How often is client symptomatic, both hyper- and hypoglycemia?
 * Stress adherence to all therapies, timing of medication in relation to meals
 * If taking any medications, review to ensure they are not contributing to problem with blood sugar

↓

6. See table on following page

HYPOGLYCEMIA *(Continued)*

HYPOGLYCEMIA*

Category	Natural Products to Consider	DOC
Herb	**Bitter Melon** *on page 394*	PA
	Garcinia *on page 437*	PA
Vitamin/Mineral/ Trace Element/ Nutraceutical	**Chromium** *on page 410* Condition-specific dosage: 200-600 mcg/day	HT
	Cyclo-Hispro *on page 420* Condition-specific dosage: 200-300 mg 3-4 times/day	PA
	Vanadium (Vanadyl Sulfate) *on page 516* Condition-specific dosage: 250 mcg 3 times/day	PA
Homeopathic Remedy	Homeopathic combination formulas are available for many conditions. Listed below are some of the most common single homeopathic remedies for hypoglycemia. Also see **Homeopathic Quick Reference Chart for Common Complaints** *on page 587*	
	Lycopodium clavatum	PD
	Phosphorus	PD
	Sulphur	PD
Additional supplements to consider	**Vitamin B Complex-25** *on page 526* Condition-specific dosage: 25-50 mg twice daily	PA
	Magnesium *on page 473* Condition-specific dosage: 400-600 mg/day	PA

*Refer to **Introduction to Conditions** *on page 41* for more details on how to apply the information in this table to individuals with this condition.

SPECIAL CONSIDERATIONS

Bitter Melon
- Contraindicated in pregnancy
- Monitor blood sugar; caution in individuals who may be predisposed to hypoglycemia
- Potential interactions with insulin, oral hypoglycemics

Garcinia
- Monitor blood sugar; caution in individuals who may be predisposed to hypoglycemia
- Potential interaction with insulin, oral hypoglycemics

Chromium
- Caution in individuals receiving oral hypoglycemics or insulin; monitor blood glucose closely and coordinate with prescriber

Cyclo-Hispro
- No known toxicity or serious side effects
- Caution in individuals receiving oral hypoglycemics or insulin; monitor blood glucose closely and coordinate with prescriber

Vanadium (Vanadyl Sulfate)
- No known toxicity or serious side effects
- Caution in individuals receiving oral hypoglycemics or insulin; monitor blood glucose closely and coordinate with prescriber

Vitamin B Complex-25 – No side effects at the RDI or ODA doses

Magnesium
- Use caution in renal impairment
- May cause diarrhea at high intakes

HYPOTHYROIDISM

Hypothyroidism refers to the clinical and biochemical changes related to diminished activity of thyroid hormone. Primary hypothyroidism is related to glandular failure, while secondary hypothyroidism results from pituitary failure. It is more prevalent with advancing age. Hypothyroidism occurs in 1.5% to 2% of women as compared to 0.5% of men.

Symptoms include dry skin, intolerance to cold, weight gain, elevated cholesterol, adrenal insufficiency, weakness, and constipation. Individuals with hypothyroidism experience a generalized slowing of mental and physical capabilities. Depression is a common manifestation. Hoarse slow speech is often a sign, as are coarsening of the skin and hair. The individual may have periorbital puffiness, muscle complaints, and neuropathies. The heart rate is slowed and the contractility is poor. The largest number of cases of hypothyroidism are caused by autoimmune thyroiditis (Hashimoto's disease). Evidence now suggests that dysbiosis and food antigen response may contribute to this condition, along with environmental toxins such as halogens, heavy metals, or endocrine disruptors. Many individuals become hypothyroid as a result of surgical or chemical treatment of hyperthyroidism. Subclinical hypothyroidism is gaining a lot of attention. Individuals exhibit the signs of hypothyroidism, yet blood values for triiodothyronine (T_3) and thyroxine (T_4) are normal. It is important to understand that the functioning of T_3 or T_4 may be different from adequate blood levels.

Iodine deficiency and peripheral resistance to thyroid hormone are two uncommon causes of hypothyroidism. If untreated, hypothyroidism may progress to myxedema with severe hypothermia and coma. The mortality of this complication has been estimated to be as high as 60% to 70%.

LIFESTYLE RECOMMENDATIONS

- Continuation/initiation of diet and exercise program
- Take medications/supplements at the same time each day
- If symptoms do not resolve with selected interventions, seek medical attention - should not be treated without the supervision of physician.

HYPOTHYROIDISM DECISION TREE

1. Client with hypothyroidism is interested in using natural products (NP) to support this condition

2. Healthcare provider requests basic background information. The following issues are addressed with the client:

   * Allergies?
   * Prescription (Rx)/OTC meds?
   * Natural products?
   * Other medical conditions?
   * Nutrition/diet program?
   * Exercise program?

3. Above data reviewed; if **yes** to Rx/OTC meds, review **Drug-Induced Nutrient Depletion Chart** in Appendix

4A. Client is a candidate for natural products

   * An appropriate homeopathic remedy can be used at any time

4B. Client's case is too complicated at this point; needs additional support from MD before initiating NP program

5. Condition-specific questions:
   * Diagnosed by MD?
   * If taking meds to treat, avoid administering with bile acid sequestrant, antacids, sucralfate, iron preparations
   * Had lipids checked? If **no**, recommend having lipids checked
   * Taking any meds that might contribute; Phenytoin, amiodarone, lithium, carbamazepine
   * Pregnant or postpartum? May be related to condition
   * Check for symptoms of disease being treated symptomatically with other drugs, and not being considered as complications of underlying condition (ie, constipation, depression, menstrual irregularities)
   Note: Make sure these issues are discussed with MD, and try to eliminate unnecessary meds
   * If being treated for depression, check for thyroid issues

6. See table on following page

HYPOTHYROIDISM *(Continued)*

HYPOTHYROIDISM*

Category	Natural Products to Consider	DOC
Herb	Bladderwrack *on page 396*	PA
	Guggul *on page 454*	PA
Vitamin/Mineral/ Trace Element/ Nutraceutical	Thyroid Extract *on page 510* Condition-specific dosage: 60 mg 1-3 times/day	HD
	Tyrosine *on page 514* Condition-specific dosage: 3000-5000 mg/day	PA
	Iodine *on page 463* Condition-specific dosage: 250 mcg/day	HT
Homeopathic Remedy	Homeopathic combination formulas are available for many conditions. Listed below are some of the most common single homeopathic remedies for hypothyroidism. Also see **Homeopathic Quick Reference Chart for Common Complaints** *on page 587*	
	Arsenicum album	PD
	Fucus vesiculosus	PD
	Thyroidinum	PD
Additional supplements to consider	Chromium *on page 410* Condition-specific dosage: 200-400 mcg/day	PA
	Selenium *on page 502* Condition-specific dosage: 200 mcg/day	PA
	N-Acetyl Cysteine (NAC) *on page 482* Condition-specific dosage: 500 mg 2-3 times/day	PA

*Refer to **Introduction to Conditions** *on page 41* for more details on how to apply the information in this table to individuals with this condition.

SPECIAL CONSIDERATIONS

Bladderwrack
- Caution in hyperthyroidism
- May increase serum potassium; caution in renal failure
- Potential interaction with thyroid agents or antithyroid drugs
- Avoid use in individuals with iodine sensitivity

Guggul
- Contraindicated during pregnancy and breast-feeding
- Contraindicated in active bleeding (eg, peptic ulcer, intracranial bleeding)
- Caution in individuals with thyroid disease
- Caution in hemostatic disorders/history of bleeding
- Potential interaction with anticoagulants (warfarin), aspirin, NSAIDs, anti-platelet agents
- Discontinue use prior to dental or surgical procedures (14 days before)
- Potential interactions with antihypertensives (serum levels of propranolol and diltiazem may be increased), thyroid medications

Thyroid Extract
- Use with caution in individuals taking thyroid medication
- Caution in individuals with hypertension or cardiovascular disease
- Potential interactions with levothyroxine, propylthiouracil, lithium
- Use with caution in individuals with CNS disorders

Tyrosine
- Contraindicated in individuals on MAO inhibitors

Iodine
- In cases of existing hyperthyroidism, doses as small as 1 mg can result in cessation of thyroid hormone production and thyrotoxicosis
- Extensive long-term intake can result in thyroid goiter

Chromium
- Caution in individuals receiving oral hypoglycemics or insulin; monitor blood glucose closely and coordinate with prescriber

Selenium
- No reported toxicity in humans at normal intakes

N-Acetyl Cysteine
- No known toxicity or serious side effects

INDIGESTION / HEARTBURN

Indigestion or dyspepsia is a broad term used to describe a variety of gastrointestinal complaints. It may refer to epigastric pain, upset stomach, excessive gas production, bloating, nausea, or pain related to the stomach. Often, this may be related to ingestion of foods that are irritating to the stomach, prone to produce large amounts of gas during digestion, or overindulgence. Dyspepsia may be associated with esophageal, gastric, or duodenal erosions, and therefore, may be a symptom of peptic ulcer disease or esophageal reflux.

An evaluation of possible causes should explore changes in diet, new medications, or potential systemic diseases. Prolonged or repeated episodes, particularly if associated with symptoms of fever, pain, diarrhea, or severe distention should prompt referral for additional evaluation.

As many as 7% of adults may experience heartburn on a daily basis. In pregnant women, this may reach 25%. As many as 50% of the individuals who self-medicate for indigestion or heartburn may have esophagitis. Heartburn may be described as a sensation of warmth or burning in the chest which may radiate upward to the neck. Additional symptoms may include difficulty or pain in swallowing, hypersalivation, bronchospasm, morning hoarseness, hiccups, or chest pain.

A reflux of acid from the stomach into the esophagus may cause irritation and inflammation. The esophagus lacks the normal protective mechanisms of the stomach, and is prone to damage from exposure to its acidic secretions and digestive enzymes. Excessive acid production, a deficiency of digestive enzymes, physical/anatomic abnormalities (hiatal hernia), weakness of the lower esophageal sphincter (often exacerbated by drugs or posture), abnormally high intra-abdominal pressure, or decreased mucosal defenses may cause heartburn. The risk of heartburn is increased by obesity, smoking, caffeinated beverages, and/or pregnancy.

The potential for confusion between heartburn and chest pain related to myocardial ischemia should be recognized. It is imperative to allow a qualified diagnostician to make this distinction.

LIFESTYLE RECOMMENDATIONS

- Chew food thoroughly
- Eat last meal of the day at least 3 hours prior to bedtime
- Consider weight loss program if weight is an issue
- Avoid foods that trigger worsening of symptoms, which may include spicy foods, tomatoes, foods with high fat content, large meals, chocolate, dairy products
- Reduce/eliminate tobacco, alcohol, caffeine
- Do not lie down after meals
- Avoid tight-fitting clothing

INDIGESTION / HEARTBURN DECISION TREE

1. Client with indigestion/hearburn is interested in using natural products (NP) to support this condition

↓

2. Healthcare provider requests basic background information. The following issues are addressed with the client:

* Allergies?
* Prescription (Rx)/OTC meds? OTC, H2s, antacids?
* Natural products?
* Other medical conditions? Specific attention to diabetes if diagnosis for client
* Nutrition/diet program?
* Exercise program?

↓

3. Above data reviewed; if **yes** to Rx/OTC meds, review **Drug-Induced Nutrient Depletion Chart** in Appendix

4A. Client is a candidate for natural products

* An appropriate homeopathic remedy can be used at any time

4B. Client's case is too complicated at this point; needs additional support from MD before initiating NP program

↓

5. Condition-specific questions:
  * Diagnosis by MD? Treatment plan?
  * Any meds to treat? (See above)
  * Any foods, behaviors alleviate symptoms? Describe
  * Triggers for worsening of symptoms? Food, stress, meals, pregnancy, meds (theophylline, HRT, narcotics, tricyclic antidepressants, calcium channel blockers, anticholinergic meds, NSAIDs, beta-blockers)?
  * Associated with chest pain? If **yes**, have client describe. If any questions as to whether there is cardiac involvement, refer to MD. Stress the difference to the client (MI = radiating pain, increased sweating, dizziness, shortness of breath, arm pain)
  * Any additional symptoms? Vomiting blood, significant abdominal pain, blood in stool, black tarry stools? Refer to MD

↓

6. See table on following page

INDIGESTION / HEARTBURN (Continued)

INDIGESTION / HEARTBURN*

Category	Natural Products to Consider	DOC
Herb	Bromelain *on page 399*	PA
	Ginger *on page 440*	PA, HE
	Peppermint *on page 486*	HE
	Chamomile *on page 407*	HE
	Cayenne *on page 405*	PA
	Artichoke *on page 386*	PA
Vitamin/Mineral/ Trace Element/ Nutraceutical	***Lactobacillus acidophilus** on page 467* and ***Bifidobacterium bifidum** on page 391* Condition-specific dosage: 2-5 billion CFU twice daily	HD
Homeopathic Remedy	Homeopathic combination formulas are available for many conditions. Listed below are some of the most common single homeopathic remedies for indigestion/heartburn. Also see **Homeopathic Quick Reference Chart for Common Complaints** *on page 587*	
	Argentum nitricum	PD
	Carbo vegetabilis	PD
	Lycopodium clavatum	PD
	Nux vomica (China)	PD
Additional Supplements to Consider	No recommendations	

*Refer to **Introduction to Conditions** *on page 41* for more details on how to apply the information in this table to individuals with this condition.

SPECIAL CONSIDERATIONS

Bromelain

- Contraindicated in active bleeding (eg, peptic ulcer, intracranial bleeding)
- Potential interaction with anticoagulants (warfarin), aspirin, NSAIDs, antiplatelet agents
- Use with caution in individuals with GI ulceration and/or cardiovascular disorders (hypertension)
- Caution in hemostatic disorders/history of bleeding
- Discontinue use prior to dental or surgical procedures (14 days before)

Ginger

- Contraindicated in active bleeding (eg, peptic ulcer, intracranial bleeding)
- Caution in hemostatic disorders/history of bleeding
- Potential interaction with anticoagulants (warfarin), aspirin, NSAIDs, antiplatelet agents, cardiac glycosides (digoxin)
- Discontinue use prior to dental or surgical procedures (14 days before)

Peppermint

- Contraindicated in biliary tract obstruction, cholecystitis, severe liver damage, gallstones, hiatal hernia

Chamomile

- Avoid use in individuals with allergies to *Asteraceae/Compositae* family (chrysanthemum, daisy) or ragweed pollens
- May cause drowsiness; caution in driving/performing hazardous tasks

Cayenne

- Caution in GI ulceration
- Contraindicated in active bleeding (eg, peptic ulcer, intracranial bleeding)
- Caution in hemostatic disorders/history of bleeding
- Potential interaction with anticoagulants (warfarin), aspirin, NSAIDs, antiplatelet agents
- Potential interference with MAO inhibitors, antihypertensives
- Discontinue use prior to dental or surgical procedures (14 days before)

Artichoke

- Avoid use in individuals with allergies to *Asteraceae/Compositae* family (chrysanthemum, daisy)

Lactobacillus acidophilus

- No known toxicity or serious side effects

Bifidobacterium bifidum

- No known toxicity or serious side effects

INSOMNIA

Difficulty sleeping has been estimated to occur in >50% of the population at some point in their lifetime. Usually, insomnia is caused by situational factors such as depression, transient stress, or anxiety. In addition, changes in work shifts and travel across time zones (jet lag) may disturb normal sleep-wake cycles, resulting in a type of situational insomnia.

Transient insomnia lasts only 2-3 days, while insomnia lasting 2-3 weeks is characterized as short-term. Insomnia may occur at the onset of sleep or may manifest as restless sleeping or premature awakening. In addition to medical or psychological conditions, insomnia may be caused by a number of drugs, including stimulants, antidepressants, and steroids. Withdrawal from sedative-hypnotics may also be associated with insomnia. Insomnia which persists longer than a few days should prompt referral for medical evaluation. In addition, daytime fatigue and difficulty concentrating are symptoms which indicate the presence of a serious sleep disorder, and individuals will need referral for treatment of the underlying condition.

Numerous drugs have been found to inhibit the synthesis of melatonin, which is the body's sleep trigger. Therefore, an individual who is suffering from insomnia should have their medications examined to see if that could be causing the problem.

LIFESTYLE RECOMMENDATIONS

- Avoid large meals late at night; make sure not to eat too late at night or consume a chemical (ie, caffeine) too late (ie, within 3 hours of expected bedtime), unless insomnia is induced by hypoglycemia

- Use comfortable mattress/bed

- Participate in relaxing activities at least 1 hour prior to bedtime

- May want to consider relaxation techniques

- Reduce stress - may need to discuss with healthcare provider

- Keep bedroom as dark as possible

- Maintain a regular sleep schedule

- Use the bedroom for sleep and intimacy; not watching TV, eating

- Regular exercise is important, but not close to bedtime (within 3 hours)

- Avoid naps during the day unless absolutely necessary

- Avoid chronic use of OTC sleep aids

INSOMNIA DECISION TREE

1. Client with insomnia is interested in using natural products (NP) to support this condition

2. Healthcare provider requests basic background information. The following issues are addressed with the client:
   * Allergies?
   * Prescription (Rx)/OTC meds?
   * Natural products?
   * Other medical conditions?
   * Nutrition/diet program?
   * Exercise program?

3. Above data reviewed; if **yes** to Rx/OTC meds, review **Drug-Induced Nutrient Depletion Chart** in Appendix

4A. Client is a candidate for natural products

   * An appropriate homeopathic remedy can be used at any time

4B. Client's case is too complicated at this point; needs additional support from MD before initiating NP program

5. Condition-specific questions:
   * Evaluated by MD? Treatment plan?
   * Drugs that may contribute to the problem: Beta agonists (oral, inhaled), SSRIs, some antihypertensives, decongestants, theophylline, medications for ADD/ADHD, caffeine, tobacco
   * If possible, speak with spouse to obtain more information on sleep patterns, habits, behaviors
   * Review eating habits to see if they may be contributing
   * Usually associated with other primary conditions - make sure depression, pain ruled out
   * If using sedative/hypnotic, have client discuss with MD duration of therapy - should be 2 weeks or less

6. See table on following page

INSOMNIA *(Continued)*

INSOMNIA*

Category	Natural Products to Consider	DOC
Herb	Valerian *on page 515*	HT
	Kava Kava *on page 466*	PA
	Passion Flower *on page 486*	PA
	Chamomile *on page 407*	HD
Vitamin/Mineral/ Trace Element/ Nutraceutical	Melatonin *on page 477* Condition-specific dosage: 0.5-3 mg at bedtime	HT
	Vitamin B₆ *on page 523* Condition-specific dosage: 25 mg twice daily	PA
	Magnesium *on page 473* Condition-specific dosage: 400-600 mg/day	HD
Homeopathic Remedy	Homeopathic combination formulas are available for many conditions. Listed below are some of the most common single homeopathic remedies for insomnia. Also see **Homeopathic Quick Reference Chart for Common Complaints** *on page 587*	
	Coffea cruda	PD
	Ignatia amara	PD
	Lycopodium clavatum	PD
	Nux vomica	PD
Additional Supplements to Consider	No recommendations	

*Refer to **Introduction to Conditions** *on page 41* for more details on how to apply the information in this table to individuals with this condition.

SPECIAL CONSIDERATIONS

Valerian

- May cause drowsiness; caution when driving/performing hazardous tasks
- Effects do not appear to be potentiated by ethanol
- Do not use in children <3 years of age; use only valepotriate and baldrinal-free in children <12 years of age due to potential mutagenic properties
- Increased effect/toxicity: CNS depressants, sedative-hypnotics (barbiturates), antidepressants, anxiolytics, antihistamines

Kava Kava

- Contraindicated in pregnancy and breast-feeding, or Parkinson's disease
- May cause drowsiness or sedation (higher doses); caution when driving/performing hazardous tasks
- Potential interactions with ethanol, CNS depressants (benzodiazepines, antidepressants, sedative-hypnotics)

Passion Flower

- May cause sedation; may cause drowsiness; caution when driving/performing hazardous tasks
- Potential interactions with antianxiety agent, antidepressants, hexobarbital, hypnotics, sedatives

Chamomile

- Avoid use in individuals with allergies to *Asteraceae/Compositae* family (chrysanthemum, daisy) family or ragweed pollens
- May cause drowsiness; caution in driving/performing hazardous tasks
- Effects may be additive with CNS depressants

Melatonin

- Long-term human studies have not been conducted
- Excessive dosages may cause morning sedation or drowsiness

Vitamin B$_6$

- No reported toxicity in humans at normal intakes

Magnesium

- Use caution in renal impairment
- May cause diarrhea at high intakes

IRRITABLE BOWEL SYNDROME (IBS)

Irritable bowel syndrome (IBS) is characterized by abdominal pain and altered bowel function. It is an extremely common ailment, and is second only to the common cold as a cause of lost work and school time. It has been estimated that 35 million Americans have IBS, and it accounts for about 3 million physician visits annually. IBS affects nearly 20% of the people in the United States, and women are affected three times as often as men are. IBS has also been called "spastic colon."

Symptoms demonstrate a high degree of intrapatient and interpatient variability. Dramatic changes from diarrhea to constipation are common in individuals with IBS. Symptoms are nonspecific. A key feature is abdominal pain or discomfort relieved with defecation or associated with a change in frequency or consistency of stool. Symptoms include two or more of the following (on at least 25% of occasions or days): Altered stool frequency and form, altered stool passage (straining, urgency, or feeling of incomplete evacuation), passage of mucus, bloating, or a feeling of abdominal distention.

The diagnosis of IBS is one of exclusion. Other gastrointestinal conditions such as Crohn's disease and ulcerative colitis must be ruled out, often by xray or colonoscopy. Abrupt changes in diet, certain gluten-containing foods, fruit, dairy products, refined sugars, allergies, medications, and gastrointestinal infection may trigger symptoms which mimic IBS.

Proposed causes of IBS include changes in the neuronal control in the bowel, including sensation or muscle contractility. Fluctuation in hormonal levels may also contribute, as evidenced by a worsening of symptoms during menstruation. In addition, central nervous system factors may also contribute, as well as changes in bowel flora and slow reactive immune responses.

IBS is not associated with cancer. Complications are rare, but may occur due to loss of electrolytes, dehydration, or nutritional compromise.

Metabolic assessment should include organic acid urinalysis and comprehensive stool analysis. Foods to avoid include gluten and sugar, including fruit sources and dairy products.

LIFESTYLE RECOMMENDATIONS

- Continuation/initiation of diet and exercise program

- Reduce exposure to triggers: Investigate stress reduction programs, avoid foods that precipitate or worsen symptoms

- Increase intake of fiber

- Eat smaller meals more frequently instead of 2-3 large meals daily

- Do not delay bowel movements; go when the need arises

- Avoid products that cause diarrhea, such as dairy (milk), laxatives, sorbitol, refined sugars

- Eliminate from the diet foods that may cause gas production: Broccoli, beans, leafy vegetables, cucumbers, onions, high-fat foods

IRRITABLE BOWEL SYNDROME (IBS) DECISION TREE

1. Client with irritable bowel syndrome (IBS) sincerely interested in using natural products (NP) to support this condition

2. Healthcare provider requests basic background information. The following issues are addressed with the client:

   * Allergies?
   * Prescription (Rx)/OTC meds?
   * Natural products?
   * Other medical conditions?
   * Nutrition/diet program?
   * Exercise program?

3. Above data reviewed; if **yes** to Rx/OTC meds, review **Drug-Induced Nutrient Depletion Chart** in Appendix

4A. Client is a candidate for natural products

   * An appropriate homeopathic remedy can be used at any time

4B. Client's case is too complicated at this point; needs additional support from MD before initiating NP program

5. Condition-specific questions:
   * Diagnosed by MD? A treatment plan outlined?
   * Triggers: Food, stress, anxiety, depression
   * How long has client had condition? Response to intervention?
   * Assess affect on quality of life and ability to perform daily activities

6. See table on following page

IRRITABLE BOWEL SYNDROME (IBS) *(Continued)*

IRRITABLE BOWEL SYNDROME (IBS)*

Category	Natural Products to Consider	DOC
Herb	Cat's Claw *on page 404*	PA
	Grapefruit Seed Extract *on page 450*	PA
	Peppermint (oil) *on page 486*	HT
	Evening Primrose *on page 430*	HT
Vitamin/Mineral/ Trace Element/ Nutraceutical	*Lactobacillus acidophilus on page 467* and *Bifidobacterium bifidum on page 391* Condition-specific dosage: 10-15 billion CFU twice daily for 2 weeks, then 1-2 billion CFU twice daily with food for 2 months (dairy free)	PA
	Glutamine *on page 446* Condition-specific dosage: 3000 mg twice daily	HD
	Vitamin C (Buffered) *on page 526* Condition-specific dosage: 500-1000 mg twice daily	PA
Homeopathic Remedy	Homeopathic combination formulas are available for many conditions. Listed below are some of the most common single homeopathic remedies for IBS. Also see **Homeopathic Quick Reference Chart for Common Complaints** *on page 587*	
	Argentum nitricum	PD
	Colchicum autumnale	PD
	Colocynthis	PD
Additional supplements to consider	No recommendations	

*Refer to **Introduction to Conditions** *on page 41* for more details on how to apply the information in this table to individuals with this condition.

SPECIAL CONSIDERATIONS

Cat's Claw

- Contraindicated in transplant recipients, individuals receiving I.V. immunoglobulins or immunosuppressants
- Contraindicated in active bleeding (eg, peptic ulcer, intracranial bleeding)
- Caution in hemostatic disorders/history of bleeding
- Potential interaction with anticoagulants (warfarin), aspirin, NSAIDs, antiplatelet agents
- Discontinue use prior to dental or surgical procedures (14 days before)

Grapefruit Seed Extract

- Grapefruit seed extract is not equivalent to grapefruit juice/pulp. Juice/pulp has been associated with many drug interactions; see Grapefruit Seed *on page 450*
- Until further information is available, it is reasonable to avoid some medications (terfenadine, astemizole, cisapride). Use other medications metabolized by CYP3A4 with caution.

Peppermint

- Contraindicated in biliary tract obstruction, cholecystitis, severe liver damage, gallstones, hiatal hernia

Evening Primrose

- Contraindicated in seizure disorders, schizophrenia, or in persons receiving anticonvulsant or antipsychotic medications
- Contraindicated in active bleeding (eg, peptic ulcer, intracranial bleeding)
- Caution in hemostatic disorders/history of bleeding
- Potential interaction with anticoagulants (warfarin), aspirin, NSAIDs, antiplatelet agents
- Discontinue use prior to dental or surgical procedures (14 days before)

Lactobacillus acidophilus

- No known toxicity or serious side effects

Bifidobacterium bifidum

- No known toxicity or serious side effects

Glutamine

- No known toxicity or serious side effects

Vitamin C

- Excess intake in diabetics may give falsely elevated blood glucose readings

MACULAR DEGENERATION

The macula is the central portion of the retina that is responsible for transforming light entering the eye into electrical neural impulses. The macula mediates central vision as well as the ability to see color and fine detail. Macular degeneration results in improper processing of images.

Macular degeneration is the leading cause of blindness in elderly Americans. Heredity and aging appear to represent the primary risk factors; however, long-term exposure to blue and ultraviolet light may also contribute. Women and individuals with lighter colored eyes may be at increased risk. Low circulating levels of antioxidants such as vitamins A, C, and E may be associated with a higher risk. Hyperlipidemia and cigarette smoking have also been implicated.

The disease generally takes one of two forms. In both forms, central vision is primarily affected while peripheral vision is preserved. The "dry" form results from thinning of the macula tissue. Symptoms include grayness, haziness, or a blind spot in the center of the visual field. Blurring of words and dimming of colors are often reported. The "wet" form results from abnormal blood vessel growth beneath the retina, resulting in distortion of the macula. Vascular leakage may also result in retinal damage. Visual distortions, such as a wavering of straight lines and a central blind spot are characteristic symptoms. The "dry" form is generally less severe, developing more slowly than its counterpart. It accounts for up to 90% of cases.

Treatment does not appear to reverse damage; however, vision loss may be slowed. The wet form may respond to laser treatment in about 50% of the treated individuals; however, the effects may be temporary. The dry form does not respond to surgical correction. Appropriate nutrition, smoking cessation, and protective measures, such as wearing sunglasses that block out ultraviolet light, are important adjunctive measures. Nutrients associated with improving the integrity of collagen tissues may also be beneficial.

LIFESTYLE RECOMMENDATIONS

- Increase consumption of fruits and vegetables

- Avoid alcohol, tobacco, high fat content foods, sugars, processed foods

- Any significant, abrupt changes in vision? Refer for physician evaluation ASAP.

- Avoid medications that might cause drying of eyes - those with anticholinergic activity

MACULAR DEGENERATION DECISION TREE

1. Client with macular degeneration is interested in using natural products (NP) to support this condition

2. Healthcare provider requests basic background information. The following issues are addressed with the client:
   * Allergies?
   * Prescription (Rx)/OTC meds?
   * Other medical conditions?
   * Nutrition/diet program?
   * Exercise program?

3. Above data reviewed; if **yes** to Rx/OTC meds, review **Drug-Induced Nutrient Depletion Chart** in Appendix

4A. Client is a candidate for natural products

   * An appropriate homeopathic remedy can be used at any time

4B. Client's case is too complicated at this point; needs additional support from MD before initiating NP program

5. Condition-specific questions:
   * Physician treatment plan?
   * Triggers that cause worsening of symptoms?
   * Any interventions that provide relief?
   * If using eye drops, review proper technique

6. See table on following page

MACULAR DEGENERATION *(Continued)*

MACULAR DEGENERATION*

Category	Natural Products to Consider	DOC
Herb	Ginkgo *on page 441*	HT
	Bilberry *on page 392* **OR** Grape Seed *on page 451*	HT
	Gotu Kola *on page 449*	PA
	Green Tea *on page 452*	PA
Vitamin/Mineral/ Trace Element/ Nutraceutical	**N-Acetyl Cysteine** *on page 482* Condition-specific dosage: 200-1200 mg/day	PA
	Lutein *on page 472* Condition-specific dosage: 2-6 mg/day	HT
Homeopathic Remedy	Homeopathic combination formulas are available for many conditions. Listed below are some of the most common single homeopathic remedies for macular degeneration. Also see **Homeopathic Quick Reference Chart for Common Complaints** *on page 587*	
	Carbo vegetabilis	PD
	Secale cornutum	PD
Additional supplements to consider	**Selenium** *on page 502* Condition-specific dosage: 200 mcg/day	PA
	Vitamin E *on page 529* Condition-specific dosage: 50-400 int. units/day	PA

*Refer to **Introduction to Conditions** *on page 41* for more details on how to apply the information in this table to individuals with this condition.

SPECIAL CONSIDERATIONS

Ginkgo

- Contraindicated in active bleeding (eg, peptic ulcer, intracranial bleeding)
- Caution in hemostatic disorders/history of bleeding
- Potential interaction with anticoagulants (warfarin), aspirin, NSAIDs, anti-platelet agents
- Theoretical interaction with MAO inhibitors, acetylcholinesterase inhibitors (tacrine, donezepil)
- Discontinue use prior to dental or surgical procedures (14 days before)

Bilberry

- Contraindicated in active bleeding, including peptic ulcer
- Caution in hemostatic disorders/history of bleeding
- Potential interaction with anticoagulants (warfarin), aspirin, NSAIDs, anti-platelet agents
- Discontinue use prior to dental or surgical procedures (14 days before)

Grape Seed

- Contraindicated in active bleeding (eg, peptic ulcer, intracranial bleeding)
- Caution in hemostatic disorders/history of bleeding
- Potential interaction with anticoagulants (warfarin), aspirin, NSAIDs, anti-platelet agents, methotrexate
- Discontinue use prior to dental or surgical procedures (14 days before)

Gotu Kola

- Contraindicated during pregnancy
- High doses my be sedating; may cause drowsiness; caution when driving/performing hazardous tasks
- Potential interaction with CNS depressants or ethanol

Green Tea

- Decaffeinated products are recommended
- Caffeine may cause multiple CNS and CV effects; caution in peptic ulcer disease or cardiovascular disease
- Contraindicated in active bleeding (eg, peptic ulcer, intracranial bleeding)
- Caution in hemostatic disorders/history of bleeding
- Discontinue use prior to dental or surgical procedures (14 days before)
- Potential interactions with anticoagulants (warfarin), aspirin, NSAIDs, antiplatelet agents
- See Green Tea *on page 452* for additional potential interactions

N-Acetyl Cysteine

- No known toxicity or serious side effects

Lutein

- No known toxicity or serious side effects

Selenium

- No known toxicity or serious side effects at normal intakes

Vitamin E

- Use with caution when taking anticoagulants (vitamin E ≥200 int. units increases prothrombin times)
- Interrupt or reduce dosage one week prior to dental or surgical procedures

MEMORY PROBLEMS

Alzheimer's disease is the most common cause of a loss of intellectual function among older individuals. However, a number of other conditions or exposures may cause development of memory loss as a symptom. These include endocrine disorders (such as thyroid disease), alcoholism, vascular disease, brain tumor, and infections (including HIV or prions).

Depression and nutritional deficiencies may also contribute to memory problems. A number of medications may have an impact on cognitive function and memory. Individuals presenting with memory impairment, particularly of recent onset, should receive a complete medical examination to rule out these causes and evaluate their potential for reversal.

It is now known that certain memory enhancing nutrients, herbs, and drugs may help slow down the process of memory loss and cognitive decline. In some cases, variable amounts of improvement in memory and cognition are achieved.

LIFESTYLE RECOMMENDATIONS

- Eliminate risky situations in the home that may cause injury (burns, falls, etc)

- Adhere to devices that ensure meds and natural products are taken as ordered/recommended

- Interact as often as possible with caregiver to provide assistance, educational materials

- Increase intake of fruits, vegetables, whole grains, fish, soy beans

- Decrease consumption of saturated fats, alcohol, sugars, dairy products, wheat

- If problems remembering daily activities, make lists, write things down, create reminders to help

MEMORY PROBLEMS DECISION TREE

1. Client with memory problems is interested in using natural products (NP) to support this condition

2. Healthcare provider requests basic background information. The following issues are addressed with the client:
   * Allergies?
   * Prescription (Rx)/OTC meds?
   * Natural products?
   * Other medical conditions?
   * Home blood glucose monitoring program?
   * Nutrition/diet program?
   * Exercise program?

3. Above data reviewed; if **yes** to Rx/OTC meds, review **Drug-Induced Nutrient Depletion Chart** in Appendix

4A. Client is a candidate for natural products

   * An appropriate homeopathic remedy can be used at any time

4B. Client's case is too complicated at this point; needs additional support from MD before initiating NP program

5. Condition-specific questions:
   * Evaluated by MD? Treatment plan?
   * Review medications to ensure they are not contributing to condition:
     Antidepressants   Antiparkinson therapy
     Antipsychotics   Anticholinergics
     Beta-blockers   Digoxin
     Sedative/hypnotics
   *** If any identified, refer to MD for review, action ***
   * Determine if caregiver is involved and provide info to this individual
   * Blood sugar checked recently? Low value could be contributing. If a possibility, refer to MD for more complete work-up.

6. See table on following page

MEMORY PROBLEMS *(Continued)*

MEMORY PROBLEMS*

Category	Natural Products to Consider	DOC
Herb	Ginkgo *on page 441*	HT
	Vinpocetine *on page 517*	HT
	HuperzineA *on page 460*	PA
Vitamin/Mineral/ Trace Element/ Nutraceutical	Fish Oils *on page 434* Condition-specific dosage: 750 mg 2-3 times/day	PA
	Phosphatidyl Choline *on page 488* Condition-specific dosage: 500-1500 mg 2-3 times/day	HT
	Phosphatidyl Serine *on page 489* Condition-specific dosage: 100 mg twice daily	HT
	Vitamin B₁₂ *on page 524* Condition-specific dosage: 500-1000 mcg/day	HD
Homeopathic Remedy	Homeopathic combination formulas are available for many conditions. Listed below are some of the most common single homeopathic remedies for memory problems. Also see **Homeopathic Quick Reference Chart for Common Complaints** *on page 587*	
	Anacardium orientale	PD
	Baryta carbonica	PD
	Cocculus indicus	PD
Additional supplements to consider	No recommendations	

*Refer to **Introduction to Conditions** *on page 41* for more details on how to apply the information in this table to individuals with this condition.

SPECIAL CONSIDERATIONS

Ginkgo

- Contraindicated in active bleeding (eg, peptic ulcer, intracranial bleeding)
- Caution in hemostatic disorders/history of bleeding
- Potential interaction with anticoagulants (warfarin), aspirin, NSAIDs, anti-platelet products
- Theoretical interaction with MAO inhibitors, acetylcholinesterase inhibitors (tacrine, donepezil)
- Discontinue use prior to dental or surgical procedures (14 days before)

Vinpocetine

- No reported toxicity in humans at normal intakes

HuperzineA

- Potential interaction with acetylcholinesterase inhibitors (eg, tacrine, donepezil)

Phosphatidyl Choline

- No known toxicity or serious side effects

Phosphatidyl Serine

- No known toxicity or serious side effects

Vitamin B$_{12}$

- No known toxicity or serious side effects

Fish Oils

- High doses may cause GI upset, loose stools, nausea
- May alter glucose regulation; use with caution in diabetes
- Caution in individuals receiving oral hypoglycemics or insulin; monitor blood glucose closely and coordinate with prescriber
- Potential interaction with anticoagulants (warfarin), aspirin, NSAIDs, anti-platelet agents

MENOPAUSE

Menopause is a natural event in a woman's life when ovulation ceases. Menstruation becomes less frequent, less consistent, and eventually stops altogether. Menopause usually occurs between 40-55 years of age. Some women may not experience menopause until their sixties. Menopause may also be referred to as the "change of life" or climacteric phase.

The symptoms of menopause are related to changes in the level of estrogen produced by the ovaries. A high degree of variability may be noted in the symptoms a woman experiences, which may relate to the rapidity of estrogen decline. Hot flashes (vasodilation of the face, neck, chest, and back), vaginal dryness, palpitations, joint pain, headaches, mood changes, and lack of sex drive may occur. Long-term complications include osteoporosis and an increased risk of cardiovascular disease.

For many women, compliance with hormone replacement therapy (HRT) is poor. Natural support for menopause provides new options and hope for increased compliance.

LIFESTYLE RECOMMENDATIONS

- Limit dairy products, meat, alcohol, sugar, caffeine, spicy foods, tobacco
- Increase intake of quality water
- Use caution if mixing natural products with hormone-like activity and prescription HRT; discuss with physician prior to doing so
- If at risk for osteoporosis, use appropriate supplements
- Soy products may be beneficial
- Vaginal dryness may be a concern; use water-soluble lubricants (not Vaseline®)

MENOPAUSE DECISION TREE

1. Client with menopause is interested in using natural products (NP) to support this condition

2. Healthcare provider requests basic background information. The following issues are addressed with the client:
   * Allergies
   * Prescription (Rx)/OTC meds? Hormone replacement therapy?
   * Natural products? Anything with estrogenic, hormone-like properties? Soy-based products?
   * Other medical conditions?
   * Nutrition/diet program?
   * Exercise program?

3. Above data reviewed; if **yes** to Rx/OTC meds, review **Drug-Induced Nutrient Depletion Chart** in Appendix

4A. Client is a candidate for natural products

   * An appropriate homeopathic remedy can be used at any time

4B. Client's case is too complicated at this point; needs additional support from MD before initiating NP program

5. Condition-specific questions:
   * How was menopause initiated? Naturally or surgically-induced?
   * Evaluated by MD? Prescribed HRT/ERT? Obtain details
   * Frequency of symptoms
   * Triggers for worsening, relieving symptoms
   * Any of the following completed/worked up: Thyroid, lipids, blood sugar?
   * Regarding lipids: If panel completed, evaluate risk factors and make appropriate suggestions (see **Dyslipidemia** Decision Tree)
   * History of breast cancer? If **yes**, refer to MD
   * Patients have increased risk for urinary incontinence, UTIs - educate on these issues

6. See table on following page

MENOPAUSE *(Continued)*

MENOPAUSE*

Category	Natural Products to Consider	DOC
Herb	**Black Cohosh** *on page 395*	HT
	Chasteberry/Vitex *on page 408*	PA
	Red Clover *on page 495*	HT
Vitamin/Mineral/ Trace Element/ Nutraceutical	**Progesterone** (natural) *on page 491* Condition-specific dosage: 1/8 to 1/4 tsp applied topically daily on days 7-28 of cycle	HT
	Isoflavones *on page 465* Condition-specific dosage: 500-1000 mg soy isoflavones daily	HT
Homeopathic Remedy	Homeopathic combination formulas are available for many conditions. Listed below are some of the most common single homeopathic remedies for menopause. Also see **Homeopathic Quick Reference Chart for Common Complaints** *on page 587*	
	Kali carbonica	PD
	Lachesis mutus	PD
	Sepia	PD
Additional supplements to consider	No recommendations	

*Refer to **Introduction to Conditions** *on page 41* for more details on how to apply the information in this table to individuals with this condition.

SPECIAL CONSIDERATIONS

Black Cohosh
- Contraindicated in pregnancy and breast-feeding
- Use caution in individuals with allergies to salicylates
- May cause nausea, vomiting, headache and hypotension (at higher dosages)
- Monitoring of serum hormone levels is recommended after 6 months of treatment
- Use with caution in individuals with a history of estrogen-dependent tumors, endometrial cancer, thromboembolic disease, or stroke
- Potential interaction with oral contraceptives, hormonal replacement therapy

Chasteberry/Vitex
- Contraindicated in pregnancy
- Potential interaction with hormonal replacements or oral contraceptives

Red Clover
- Contraindicated in active bleeding (eg, peptic ulcer, intracranial bleeding)
- Caution in individuals at risk of estrogen-dependent tumors, thromboembolic disease, or stroke
- Caution in hemostatic disorders/history of bleeding
- Potential interactions with anticoagulants, aspirin, NSAIDs, antiplatelet agents
- Discontinue use prior to dental or surgical procedures (14 days before)

Progesterone
- May alter hormonal regulation
- Not to be used with oral contraceptives without medical supervision

Isoflavones
- Caution in estrogen-dependent tumors, endometrial cancer
- Women who are taking estrogen-containing medications (oral contraceptives, hormonal replacement) should consult their physician prior to use

MENORRHAGIA

Menorrhagia refers to excessive blood loss during menstruation. Irregular vaginal bleeding is a possible symptom of general menstrual dysfunction, fluctuating hormone levels, vaginitis, and/or ruptured vaginal varicosities. Tumors, polyps, or fibroids of the vagina, cervix, uterus, or fallopian tubes may also cause excessive bleeding.

Any unusual vaginal bleeding should be evaluated by a physician. Physicians generally recommend that all sexually active women, as well as women >18 years of age, should have a yearly pelvic exam and Pap smear (some exceptions apply to this general rule). Most irregular vaginal bleeding has a benign cause. If a woman is experiencing heavy vaginal bleeding (defined as one pad per hour for more than a couple of hours), immediate medical assistance should be sought. Likewise, pregnant women who experience vaginal bleeding should contact their physician immediately.

LIFESTYLE RECOMMENDATIONS

- Continuation/initiation of diet and exercise program

- Increase water intake

- If using iron supplement, keep in childproof container: Iron consumption is the #1 cause of pediatric poisoning!

MENORRHAGIA DECISION TREE

1. Client with menorrhagia is interested in using natural products (NP) to support this condition

2. Healthcare provider requests basic background information. The following issues are addressed with the client:

   * Allergies?
   * Prescription (Rx)/OTC meds?
   * Natural products?
   * Other medical conditions?
   * Nutrition/diet program?
   * Exercise program?

3. Above data reviewed; if **yes** to Rx/OTC meds, review **Drug-Induced Nutrient Depletion Chart** in Appendix

4A. Client is a candidate for natural products

   * An appropriate homeopathic remedy can be used at any time

4B. Client's case is too complicated at this point; needs additional support from MD before initiating NP program

5. Condition-specific questions:
   * Discussed situation with MD/GYN? What were recommendations?
   * Screened for diabetes? Thyroid function?
   * Use IUD? Noticed any changes related to this device?
   * Taking any meds which may contribute: Oral contraceptives, anticoagulants, antiplatelet agents, hormone replacement therapy, chemotherapy
   * Bleeding anywhere else? If **yes,** determine location and refer to MD for evaluation

6. See table on following page

MENORRHAGIA (Continued)

MENORRHAGIA*

Category	Natural Products to Consider	DOC
Herb	Chasteberry/Vitex on page 408	PA
	Red Clover on page 495	PA
	Evening Primrose on page 430	PA
	Dong Quai on page 425	PA
Vitamin/Mineral/ Trace Element/ Nutraceutical	Iron on page 464 Condition-specific dosage: Determined by clinician	HD
Homeopathic Remedy	Homeopathic combination formulas are available for many conditions. Listed below are some of the most common single homeopathic remedies for menorrhagia. Also see **Homeopathic Quick Reference Chart for Common Complaints** on page 587	
	Calcarea carbonica	PD
	Sabina	PD
	Sanguinaria canadensis	PD
	Secale cornutum	PD
Additional supplements to consider	No recommendations	

*Refer to **Introduction to Conditions** on page 41 for more details on how to apply the information in this table to individuals with this condition.

SPECIAL CONSIDERATIONS

Chasteberry/Vitex
- Contraindicated in pregnancy
- Potential interaction with hormonal replacements or oral contraceptives

Red Clover
- Contraindicated in active bleeding (eg, peptic ulcer, intracranial bleeding)
- Caution in individuals at risk of estrogen-dependent tumors, thromboembolic disease, or stroke
- Caution in hemostatic disorders/history of bleeding
- Potential interactions with anticoagulants, aspirin, NSAIDs, antiplatelet agents
- Discontinue use prior to surgical or dental procedures (14 days before)

Evening Primrose
- Contraindicated in seizure disorders, schizophrenia, or in persons receiving anticonvulsant or antipsychotic medications
- Contraindicated in active bleeding (eg, peptic ulcer, intracranial bleeding)
- Caution in hemostatic disorders/history of bleeding
- Potential interaction with anticoagulants (warfarin), aspirin, NSAIDs, antiplatelet agents
- Discontinue use prior to dental or surgical procedures (14 days before)

Dong Quai
- Caution in pregnancy and breast-feeding
- Contraindicated in active bleeding (eg, peptic ulcer, intracranial bleeding)
- Use caution in those at risk of estrogen-dependent tumors, endometrial cancer, thromboembolic disease, or stroke
- Potential interaction with anticoagulants (warfarin), aspirin, NSAIDs, antiplatelet agents
- Potential interaction with oral contraceptives or hormonal replacement therapy
- Caution in hemostatic disorders/history of bleeding
- Potential interaction with antihypertensives, photosensitizing agents
- Discontinue use prior to dental or surgical procedures (14 days before)

Iron
- May interfere with absorption of fluoroquinolones, tetracycline antibiotics

MINOR INJURY / WOUND HEALING

The body is designed to respond to injury or trauma in a consistent, efficient manner. It maintains a "surveillance" network of circulating proteins, platelets, and immune cells to react swiftly to breaks in the integrity of the skin, which serves as the principle protective barrier to the environment. Minor wounds, abrasions, or contusions elicit an initial activation of this response network, which is designed to simultaneously limit loss of blood and recruit appropriate molecules and cells to seal off potential invading organisms.

Many factors influence the rate of healing, including the depth of the injury, involvement of underlying tissues or organs, and type of wound (blunt trauma, incision, or tear). The nutritional and immune status of the individual may greatly influence the rate and success of wound healing.

Wounds should be evaluated for potential to heal without suturing, potential damage to underlying tissues, and possibility for infection. Appropriate cleansing and dressing of the wound is also essential. Nutrient and immune support that could contribute to wound healing should also be evaluated.

LIFESTYLE RECOMMENDATIONS

- Bleeding wound: Keep above level of the heart and apply pressure until the bleeding stops
- Keep wound clean with soap and water
- If wound is in an area that might get dirty, use protective covering
- Keep wound moist; use the proper antiseptic/dressing (alcohol-based are the best)

MINOR INJURY / WOUND HEALING DECISION TREE

1. Client with minor injury/wound healing is interested in using natural products (NP) to support this condition

2. Healthcare provider requests basic background information.
   The following issues are addressed with the client:
   * Allergies?
   * Prescription (Rx)/OTC meds?
   * Natural products?
   * Other medical conditions (specifically diabetes)?
   * If diabetic: Home blood glucose monitoring program?
     Blood sugar values?
   * Nutrition/diet program?
   * Exercise program?

3. Above data reviewed; if **yes** to Rx/OTC meds, review **Drug-Induced Nutrient Depletion Chart** in Appendix

4A. Client is a candidate for natural products

   * An appropriate homeopathic remedy can be used at any time

4B. Client's case is too complicated at this point; needs additional support from MD before initiating NP program

5. Condition-specific questions:
   * Sought medical attention for this problem?
   * What type of wound? Acute versus chronic?
   * Last tetanus immunization?
   * Associated symptoms: Fever, inflammation, pus, erythema?
   If **yes,** to more than one of these, refer to MD
   * Deep wound? Refer to MD

6. See table on following page

MINOR INJURY / WOUND HEALING *(Continued)*

MINOR INJURY / WOUND HEALING*

Category	Natural Products to Consider	DOC
Herb	**Calendula** (Topical) *on page 401*	PA
	Tea Tree (Topical) *on page 509*	PA
	Chamomile (Topical) *on page 407*	HT
	St John's Wort *on page 506*	PA
	Echinacea *on page 426*	HT
Vitamin/Mineral/ Trace Element/ Nutraceutical	**Zinc** (Topical) *on page 534* Condition-specific dosage: Use topically as needed	HT
	Collagen (Topical) *on page 414* Condition-specific dosage: Use topically as needed	HT
Homeopathic Remedy	Homeopathic combination formulas are available for many conditions. Listed below are some of the most common single homeopathic remedies for minor injury/ wound healing. Also see **Homeopathic Quick Reference Chart for Common Complaints** *on page 587*	
Bruises	*Arnica montana*	PD
	Hypericum perforatum	PD
	Ruta graveolens	PD
Burns (Minor)	*Apis mellifica*	PD
	Atropa belladonna	PD
	Calendula officinalis	PD
	Cantharis	PD
	Hypericum perforatum	PD
	Rhus toxicodendron	PD
	Urtica urens	PD
Insect Bites or Stings	*Apis mellifica*	PD
	Calendula officinalis	PD
	Ledum palustre	PD
	Tarentula hispana	PD
Sprains or Strains	*Arnica montana*	PD
	Bellis perennis	PD
	Bryonia alba	PD
	Rhus toxicodendron	PD
	Ruta graveolens	PD
Wounds (Minor) or Cuts/Scrapes	*Apis mellifica*	PD
	Calendula officinalis	PD
	Hepar sulphuris calcareum	PD
	Hypericum perforatum	PD
	Ledum palustre	PD
Additional supplements to consider	No recommendations	

*Refer to **Introduction to Conditions** *on page 41* for more details on how to apply the information in this table to individuals with this condition.

SPECIAL CONSIDERATIONS

Calendula
- No reported toxicity in humans at normal intakes

Tea Tree
- May cause allergic dermatitis in sensitive individuals
- Not for ingestion

Chamomile
- Avoid use in individuals with allergies to *Asteraceae/Compositae* family (chrysanthemum, daisy) or ragweed pollens
- May cause drowsiness; caution in driving/performing hazardous tasks

St John's Wort
- Topical use
- Contraindicated in pregnancy
- May cause photosensitivity (rare)

Echinacea
- Not recommended for use longer than 10 days (acute treatment) or in immunosuppressed individuals
- Potential interaction with therapeutic immunosuppressants and cortico-steroids
- Caution in renal impairment (may cause electrolyte imbalance)
- Caution if allergic to *Asteraceae/Compositae* family (ragweed, daisy, aster, chrysanthemum) and other pollens

Zinc
- No known toxicity or serious side effects

Collagen
- No known toxicity or serious side effects

MOTION SICKNESS

Motion sickness represents a normal physiologic response to excessive stimulation of the vestibular system, which is located in the inner ear, and is responsible for maintaining our sense of balance and equilibrium. Individual susceptibility is highly variable, and individuals often adapt after prolonged stimulation. Motion sickness appears to be related to difficulty interpreting conflicting neural signals from the eyes and positional receptors in the body. Nausea and potentially vomiting are the predominant consequences. Dehydration may become a complicating feature.

Individuals who complain of motion sickness without exposure to situations that would be expected to cause this complaint, should be referred for evaluation.

LIFESTYLE RECOMMENDATIONS

- Continuation/initiation of diet and exercise program
- Stay hydrated
- Eat a small meal/snack prior to the trip
- Sit in the front seat of the vehicle and near an open window
- Avoid alcohol and heavy meals prior to traveling
- Avoid reading or trying to focus on small print/objects
- If taking medications to treat this condition, take them 30-60 minutes prior to the trip

MOTION SICKNESS DECISION TREE

1. Client with motion sickness is interested in using natural products (NP) to support this condition

2. Healthcare provider requests basic background information. The following issues are addressed wtih the client:

   * Allergies?
   * Prescription (Rx)/OTC meds?
   * Natural products?
   * Other medical conditions?
   * Nutrition/diet program?
   * Exercise program?

3. Above data reviewed; if **yes** to Rx/OTC meds, review **Drug-Induced Nutrient Depletion Chart** in Appendix

4A. Client is a candidate for natural products

   * An appropriate homeopathic remedy can be used at any time

4B. Client's case is too complicated at this point; needs additional support from MD before initiating NP program

5. Condition-specific questions:
   * How soon into the trip do symptoms start?
   * What, if any, interventions relieve the symptoms?
   * Is the client taking any meds that might contribute to the stomach upset, dizziness, or other symptoms? If **yes,** avoid taking prior to the trip.

6. See table on following page

MOTION SICKNESS *(Continued)*

MOTION SICKNESS*

Category	Natural Products to Consider	DOC
Herb	**Ginger** *on page 440*	HT
	Peppermint *on page 486*	HE
Vitamin/Mineral/ Trace Element/ Nutraceutical	No recommendations	
Homeopathic Remedy	Homeopathic combination formulas are available for many conditions. Listed below are some of the most common single homeopathic remedies for motion sickness. Also see **Homeopathic Quick Reference Chart for Common Complaints** *on page 587*	
	Ambra grisea	PD
	Cocculus indicus	PD
	Ipecacuanha	PD
	Nux vomica	PD
	Petroleum	PD
	Tabacum	PD
Additional supplements to consider	No recommendations	

*Refer to **Introduction to Conditions** *on page 41* for more details on how to apply the information in this table to individuals with this condition.

SPECIAL CONSIDERATIONS

Ginger
- Contraindicated in active bleeding (eg, peptic ulcer, intracranial bleeding)
- Caution in hemostatic disorders/history of bleeding
- Potential interaction with anticoagulants (warfarin), aspirin, NSAIDs, anti-platelet agents, cardiac glycosides (digoxin)
- Discontinue use prior to dental or surgical procedures (14 days before)

Peppermint
- Contraindicated in biliary tract obstruction, cholecystitis, severe liver damage, gallstones, hiatal hernia

MULTIPLE SCLEROSIS (MS)

Multiple sclerosis (MS) is a potentially debilitating autoimmune disease affecting the brain and spinal cord. In the United States, an estimated 250,000-350,000 individuals have MS. It usually affects individuals between 20-45 years of age. Women are affected at a rate of 2:1 over men. Genetic predisposition, age, environmental, and geographic factors have been associated with a risk of developing the disease.

Up to 20% of people with MS have at least one affected relative. Multiple genes likely contribute to MS susceptibility. It has been proposed that an exposure to common viruses, such as the human herpes virus 6 (HHV-6), or specific bacteria, may trigger the disease in individuals with a genetic tendency. Hormonal factors have also been suggested to predispose women to develop MS. Immune disruption from environmental toxins may also play a role.

The disease appears to represent an autoimmune reaction to myelin surrounding the nerves. The trigger for this reaction has not been identified, but dysbiosis may be partially responsible for the autoimmune response. The myelin sheath of neurons becomes inflamed, swollen, and detached from the nerve fibers. Eventually, the myelin is destroyed. Sclerosed or hardened patches of scar tissue form over the fibers, disrupting normal impulse transmission. Symptoms vary depending on the location of lesions in the central nervous system.

Initially, the symptoms of MS may be subtle. Visual symptoms, including blurred or double vision, are often the first indication of the disease. Other early symptoms include paresthesia, numbness, extremity weakness (particularly in the hands or legs), fatigue, dizziness, and a loss of balance. As the disease progresses, muscle spasms, slurred speech, vision loss, and problems with bladder, bowel, or sexual function occur. Paralysis may develop in some individuals. Mental status changes, including increased forgetfulness or confusion, may occur.

Diagnosis of MS is generally based on a complete medical history and neurological examination. Other causes of symptoms must be excluded. There are several types of MS. The most common form is the relapsing-remitting type, which affects approximately 85% of people with MS. It is characterized by one or two flare-ups every 1-3 years, followed by periods of remission.

Complications of MS include pneumonia, sepsis, and a suicide rate up to seven times that of the general population. Much of the current treatment is geared to the management of specific symptoms. Medications may be used for muscle stiffness, fatigue, depression, pain, and bladder control problems. Because of the autoimmune nature of the disease, immune modulators and immunosuppressant medications may slow MS in some cases.

LIFESTYLE RECOMMENDATIONS

- Specific foods to avoid: Saturated fats, chocolate, alcohol, caffeine, sugars, gluten-containing products
- Increase consumption of seafood, vegetables, seeds, fiber
- Manage stress - classes, massage therapy
- Avoid exposure to excessive temperatures
- Investigate joining a support group
- Avoid exposure to pesticides, insecticides, heavy metals, and other immune irritants

MULTIPLE SCLEROSIS DECISION TREE

1. Client with multiple sclerosis is interested in using natural products (NP) to support this condition

2. Healthcare provider requests basic background information. The following issues are addressed with the client:

* Allergies? Tested for gluten, dairy?
* Prescription (Rx)/OTC meds?
* Natural products?
* Other medical conditions?
* Nutrition/diet program?
* Exercise program?

3. Above data reviewed; if **yes** to Rx/OTC meds, review **Drug-Induced Nutrient Depletion Chart** in Appendix

4A. Client is a candidate for natural products

* An appropriate homeopathic remedy can be used at any time

4B. Client's case is too complicated at this point; needs additional support from MD before initiating NP program

5. Condition-specific questions:
* Diagnosis by MD? Treatment plan outlined?
* How often does client experience exacerbations/flare-ups. How are these managed?
* Does client have a significant amount of mercury fillings in teeth? If **yes,** may wish to discuss with client the option of seeing dentist to discuss replacing these
* Has client been evaluated for candidal infection? Lyme disease? Discuss these options with MD

6. See table on following page

MULTIPLE SCLEROSIS (MS) *(Continued)*

MULTIPLE SCLEROSIS*

Category	Natural Products to Consider	DOC
Herb	**Astragalus** *on page 388*	PA
	Cat's Claw *on page 404*	PA
	Evening Primrose *on page 430*	HT
	Grape Seed *on page 451*	PA
	Olive Leaf *on page 483*	PA
Vitamin/Mineral/ Trace Element/ Nutraceutical	**Coenzyme Q₁₀** *on page 412* Condition-specific dosage: 60 mg twice daily	PA
	N-Acetyl Cysteine *on page 482* Condition-specific dosage: 600-1200 mg/day	PA
	Lactobacillus acidophilus *on page 467* and **Bifidobacterium bifidum** *on page 391* Condition-specific dosage: 2-5 billion CFU twice daily	PA
	Alpha-Lipoic Acid *on page 381* Condition-specific dosage: 100 mg 1-3 times/day	PA
	Magnesium *on page 473* Condition-specific dosage: 400-600 mg/day	PA
Homeopathic Remedy	Homeopathic combination formulas are available for many conditions. Listed below are some of the most common single homeopathic remedies for multiple sclerosis. Also see **Homeopathic Quick Reference Chart for Common Complaints** *on page 587*	
	Carboneum sulphuratum	PD
	Causticum	PD
	Lathyrus sativus	PD
	Phosphorus	PD
Additional supplements to consider	**Fish Oils** *on page 434* Condition-specific dosage: 1 capsule twice daily **OR** **Flaxseed Oil** *on page 435* Condition-specific dosage: 1 Tbsp daily	HD
	Vitamin B₁₂ *on page 524* Condition-specific dosage: 100 mcg/day	HD
	Vitamin C *on page 526* Condition-specific dosage: 250-1000 mg/day	PA
	Vitamin E *on page 529* Condition-specific dosage: 50-400 int. units/day	PA

*Refer to **Introduction to Conditions** *on page 41* for more details on how to apply the information in this table to individuals with this condition.

SPECIAL CONSIDERATIONS

Astragalus – May interact with immune stimulants or immunosuppressants

Cat's Claw
- Contraindicated in transplant recipients, individuals receiving I.V. immuno-globulins or immunosuppressants; and in active bleeding (eg, peptic ulcer, intracranial bleeding)
- Caution in hemostatic disorders/history of bleeding
- Potential interaction with anticoagulants (warfarin), aspirin, NSAIDs, anti-platelet agents
- Discontinue use prior to dental or surgical procedures (14 days before)

Evening Primrose
- Contraindicated in active bleeding (eg, peptic ulcer, intracranial bleeding), and in seizure disorders, schizophrenia, or in persons receiving anticonvulsant or antipsychotic medications
- Caution in hemostatic disorders/history of bleeding
- Potential interaction with anticoagulants (warfarin), aspirin, NSAIDs, anti-platelet agents
- Discontinue use prior to dental or surgical procedures (14 days before)

Grape Seed
- Contraindicated in active bleeding (eg, peptic ulcer, intracranial bleeding)
- Caution in hemostatic disorders/history of bleeding
- Potential interaction with anticoagulants (warfarin), aspirin, NSAIDs, anti-platelet agents, methotrexate
- Discontinue use prior to dental or surgical procedures (14 days before)

Olive Leaf – No reported toxicity in humans at normal intakes

Coenzyme Q$_{10}$ – No known toxicity or serious side effects; caution in individuals receiving anticoagulants

N-Acetyl Cysteine – No known toxicity or serious side effects

Lactobacillus acidophilus – No known toxicity or serious side effects

Bifidobacterium bifidum – No known toxicity or serious side effects

Alpha-Lipoic Acid – Caution in individuals receiving oral hypoglycemics or insulin; monitor blood glucose closely and coordinate with prescriber

Magnesium
- Use caution in renal impairment
- May cause diarrhea at high intakes

Fish Oils
- High doses may cause GI upset, loose stools, nausea
- May alter glucose regulation; use with caution in diabetes
- Caution in individuals receiving oral hypoglycemics or insulin; monitor blood glucose closely and coordinate with prescriber
- Potential interaction with anticoagulants (warfarin), aspirin, NSAIDs, anti-platelet agents

Flaxseed Oil – No known toxicity or serious side effects

Vitamin B$_{12}$ – No known toxicity or serious side effects

Vitamin C – Excess intake in diabetics may give falsely elevated blood glucose readings

Vitamin E
- Use with caution when taking anticoagulants (vitamin E ≥200 int. units increases prothrombin times)
- Interrupt or reduce dosage one week prior to dental or surgical procedures

MUSCLE SORENESS / STIFFNESS

Up to 7 million people in the United States report limitation of activities due to musculoskeletal complaints. Muscle pain is normally referred to as myalgia. Muscle pain may be associated with infection, metabolic disease, endocrine disorders, or toxic effects of drugs or environmental exposures. This type of pain is often gradual in onset and diffuse. Pain related to strain of a particular muscle group may often be attributed to athletic exertion.

Muscle pain may be associated with fatigue, weakness, stiffness, or swelling. The individual often describes a sensation of tightness and may report muscle spasms. Vigorous or strenuous activity is the most common cause of muscle soreness due to damage to individual muscle fibers and inflammatory responses. Muscle that has been depleted of glycogen, fatigued, or unaccustomed to a load may be more easily damaged.

Conditioning makes muscle more difficult to damage and less susceptible to fatigue. Muscle requires approximately 48 hours to repair. Light to moderate stretching prior to exercise will reduce the potential for damage to the muscle or supporting structures.

Individuals complaining of unusual muscle soreness that is unrelated to exertion should be evaluated for potential adverse reactions to specific medications, such as myalgia from HMG-CoA reductase inhibitors or tendonitis from quinolone antibiotics. It should also be noted that fibromyalgia includes pain and tenderness in both muscle and connective tissue. Individuals with consistent complaints of muscle soreness, not associated with exertion, may require referral for medical evaluation.

LIFESTYLE RECOMMENDATIONS

- Avoid sudden intense movements that might exacerbate symptoms

- Increase consumption of fruits and vegetables

- Use cold therapy to treat, primarily for swelling (maximum of 20 minutes, then remove for 10-20 minutes)

- Stretch adequately prior to exercise

- May have to wrap or tape affected area until completely healed, and possibly for awhile thereafter

MUSCLE SORENESS / STIFFNESS DECISION TREE

1. Client with muscle soreness/stiffness is interested in using natural products (NP) to support this condition

2. Healthcare provider requests basic background information.
   The following issues are addressed with the client:

   * Allergies?
   * Prescription (Rx)/OTC meds?
   * Natural products?
   * Other medical conditions?
     Specific attention to fibromyalgia, arthritis, chronic fatigue

   * Nutrition/diet program?
   * Exercise program? **Specifically, what does this involve?**

3. Above data reviewed; if **yes** to Rx/OTC meds, review **Drug-Induced Nutrient Depletion Chart** in Appendix

4A. Client is a candidate for natural products

   * An appropriate homeopathic remedy can be used at any time

4B. Client's case is too complicated at this point; needs additional support from MD before initiating NP program

5. Condition-specific questions:
   * Was there a specific incident/event that caused the problem?
   * Evaluated by MD? If **yes**, treatment plan outlined?
   * Happened previously? What interventions were done/what worked?
   * Triggers for worsening symptoms?
   * Pain near a joint? Other symptoms of problem that may be related to a joint, such as erythema, inflammation, warmth, tenderness? If **yes**, refer to MD

6. See table on following page

MUSCLE SORENESS / STIFFNESS (Continued)

MUSCLE SORENESS*

Category	Natural Products to Consider	DOC
Herb	Feverfew *on page 432*	PA
	Kava Kava *on page 466*	PA
	Turmeric *on page 512*	PA
Vitamin/Mineral/ Trace Element/ Nutraceutical	**Magnesium Malate** *on page 473* Condition-specific dosage: 600-800 mg 3 times/day	HD
Homeopathic Remedy	Homeopathic combination formulas are available for many conditions. Listed below are some of the most common single homeopathic remedies for muscle soreness/stiffness. Also see **Homeopathic Quick Reference Chart for Common Complaints** *on page 587*	
	Arnica montana (Topical and Internal)	PD
	Rhododendron chrysanthum	PD
	Rhus toxicodendron	PD
	Ruta graveolens	PD
Additional supplements to consider	No recommendations	

*Refer to **Introduction to Conditions** *on page 41* for more details on how to apply the information in this table to individuals with this condition.

SPECIAL CONSIDERATIONS

Feverfew

- Contraindicated in pregnancy
- Contraindicated in allergy to *Asteraceae/Compositae* family (chrysanthemum, daisy)
- Contraindicated in active bleeding (eg, peptic ulcer, intracranial bleeding)
- Onset may be delayed for several weeks
- Abrupt discontinuation may increase migraine frequency
- Caution in hemostatic disorders/history of bleeding
- Potential interaction with anticoagulants (warfarin), aspirin, NSAIDs, antiplatelet agents
- Discontinue use prior to dental or surgical procedures (14 days before)

Kava Kava

- Contraindicated in pregnancy and breast-feeding, or Parkinson's disease
- May cause drowsiness or sedation (higher doses); caution when driving/performing hazardous tasks
- Potential interactions with ethanol, CNS depressants (benzodiazepines, antidepressants, sedative-hypnotics)

Turmeric

- Caution in biliary obstruction
- Caution in ulcerative gastrointestinal disease (eg, peptic ulcer disease, ulcerative colitis, Crohn's)
- Contraindicated in active bleeding (eg, peptic ulcer, intracranial bleeding)
- Caution in hemostatic disorders/history of bleeding
- Potential interaction with anticoagulants (warfarin), aspirin, NSAIDs, antiplatelet agents
- Discontinue use prior to dental or surgical procedures (14 days before)

Magnesium Malate

- Caution in renal impairment
- May cause diarrhea at high intakes

NAUSEA / VOMITING

Nausea is an uncomfortable sensation or queasiness that often precedes the urge to vomit. It may be accompanied by hypersalivation, sweating, pallor, and tachycardia. Depending on the cause, nausea may also be associated with a constellation of symptoms including fever, confusion, obtundation, and chest pain. It is a nonspecific response to a number of precipitating causes.

Causes of nausea include local factors that irritate the gastric mucosa as well as agents that directly stimulate chemoreceptors in the vomiting center of the brain. A number of psychological factors, local gastrointestinal irritation, endocrine abnormalities, and metabolic derangements may precipitate an episode. Additional causes include infection, drugs, and intestinal obstruction or inflammation (such as in pancreatitis or gallstones).

The act of vomiting is initiated by a site within the central nervous system, and represents a coordinated effort of several muscle groups, including the diaphragm and abdominal muscles, to expel the contents of the stomach. In effect, it is a defense against the ingestion of noxious compounds.

Complications of vomiting include dehydration, electrolyte disturbances, and aspiration of vomitus into the lungs, resulting in a chemical pneumonitis or mixed aerobic-anaerobic infection. Children are at particular risk for dehydration and electrolyte shifts.

LIFESTYLE RECOMMENDATIONS

- Continuation/initiation of diet and exercise program

- Keep hydrated; drink as much water/clear fluid as possible

- Eat small amounts of bland food

- May need to start consumption of solid foods with ice chips

- Avoid treating symptoms for >48 hours without addressing the underlying cause

- If considering inducing vomiting, use ipecac only under the supervision of a physician

NAUSEA / VOMITING DECISION TREE

1. Client with nausea/vomiting is interested in using natural products (NP) to support this condition

2. Healthcare provider requests basic background information. The following issues are addressed with the client:
   * Allergies?
   * Prescription (Rx)/OTC meds?
   * Natural products?
   * Other medical conditions?
   * Nutrition/diet program?
   * Exercise program?

3. Above data reviewed; if **yes** to Rx/OTC meds, review **Drug-Induced Nutrient Depletion Chart** in Appendix

4A. Client is a candidate for natural products

   * An appropriate homeopathic remedy can be used at any time

4B. Client's case is too complicated at this point; needs additional support From MD before initiating NP program

5. Condition-specific questions:
   * Symptoms addressed by MD? If YES, what was the recommended treatment plan? Effective?
   * Triggers for condition/symptom onset? Worsening?
   * Taking any meds that may precipitate these symptoms, such as antibiotics, digoxin, narcotics, chemotherapy?
   * Has the client eaten anything recently that may have caused food poisoning?
   * Any recent changes in medications, diet, eating habits?
   * Does the client have diabetes?
   * Any blood in the vomitus?
   * Possible pregnancy?
   * Other symptoms, such as fever, headache, dizziness, diarrhea, abdominal pain?
   * Are the symptoms positional, related to any activity?

6. See table on following page

NAUSEA / VOMITING *(Continued)*

NAUSEA / VOMITING*

Category	Natural Products to Consider	DOC
Herb	**Ginger** *on page 440*	HT
	Chamomile *on page 407*	PA, HE
Vitamin/Mineral/ Trace Element/ Nutraceutical	No recommendations	
Homeopathic Remedy	Homeopathic combination formulas are available for many conditions. Listed below are some of the most common single homeopathic remedies for nausea/ vomiting. Also see **Homeopathic Quick Reference Chart for Common Complaints** *on page 587*	
	Ipecacuanha	PD
	Nux vomica	PD
	Pulsatilla	PD
	Tabacum	PD
Additional supplements to consider	No recommendations	

*Refer to **Introduction to Conditions** *on page 41* for more details on how to apply the information in this table to individuals with this condition.

SPECIAL CONSIDERATIONS

Ginger

- Contraindicated in active bleeding (eg, peptic ulcer, intracranial bleeding)
- Caution in hemostatic disorders/history of bleeding
- Potential interaction with anticoagulants (warfarin), aspirin, NSAIDs, anti-platelet agents, cardiac glycosides (digoxin)
- Discontinue use prior to dental or surgical procedures (14 days before)

Chamomile

- Avoid use in individuals with allergies to *Asteraceae/Compositae* family (chrysanthemum, daisy) or ragweed pollens
- May cause drowsiness; caution in driving/performing hazardous tasks

OSTEOPOROSIS

Osteoporosis is a condition in which the bones become porous, brittle, and weak. It results from either a failure to form new bone and/or as a result of excessive bone resorption. The resulting reduction in bone density increases the likelihood of fracture. Usually, loss of bone density occurs over a period of many years. A fracture is often the first indication of the disease. Unfortunately, by the time a fracture occurs, bone loss has usually progressed to severe levels.

Researchers estimate that about 23% of American women >50 years of age have osteoporosis. An additional 40% to 50% of women have an abnormally low bone density, or osteopenia, which may deteriorate to osteoporosis if untreated. Risk factors, in addition to menopause, include genetic and ethnic background. White or Asian women, particularly with a positive family history of osteoporosis, are at increased risk. Additional risk factors include a low intake of several nutrients including calcium, magnesium, vitamin D, vitamin K, boron, copper, manganese, and zinc. Other risk factors include smoking, alcohol use, eating disorders, and use of certain medications such as steroids.

Osteoporosis usually has no obvious symptoms. It may cause pain in the back, ribs, or limbs. As the disease progresses, a loss of height may be noted. This is caused by compression of the vertebrae, as well as an increased spinal curvature.

There are a number of causes of osteoporosis. Hormone deficiency is the greatest factor. Women >60 years of age are most frequently affected due to the loss of estrogenic activity at menopause, with subsequent loss of bone mineralization. Other causes include Cushing's disease (corticosteroid excess), hyperthyroidism, hyperparathyroidism, immobilization, bone malignancies, and genetic disorders.

The major consequence of osteoporosis is fracture. Approximately 50% of women >50 years of age will suffer a fracture, while only 13% of men will experience this type of event. The hip, wrist, or vertebra are common fracture locations. Regular exercise can reduce the likelihood of fractures in osteoporosis. However, exercise that carries a risk of falling should be avoided.

LIFESTYLE RECOMMENDATIONS

- Continuation/initiation of diet and exercise program

- Ensure optimal consumption of calcium, magnesium, trace minerals, and vitamin D

- Pursue options for weight-bearing exercises, provided there are no physical barriers

- Reduce opportunities for falls

- If postmenopausal female is not on HRT, recommend discussing with physician as soon as possible

- Avoid antacid products that propose to provide calcium; these do not allow for calcium to be absorbed adequately

- Recommend screening of children, if applicable, and starting a prevention program as early as in their twenties

OSTEOPOROSIS DECISION TREE

1. Client with osteoporosis is interested in using natural products (NP) to support this condition

2. Healthcare provider requests basic background information. The following issues are addressed with the client:

* Allergies?
* Prescription (Rx)/OTC meds? Any hormone replacement therapy?
* Natural products?
* Other medical conditions?
* Nutrition/diet program?
* Exercise program? Weight-bearing?

3. Above data reviewed; if **yes** to Rx/OTC meds, review **Drug-Nutrient Depletion Chart** in Appendix

4A. Client is a candidate for natural products

* An appropriate homeopathic remedy can be used at any time

4B. Client's case is too complicated at this point; needs additional support from MD before initiating NP program

5. Condition-specific questions:
* Diagnosed by MD? If **yes,** what was the recommended treatment plan? Effective?
* Triggers for condition/symptom onset? Worsening?
* Any PPT factors: Smoker, excess use of alcohol, caffeine, steroid use? If **yes** to any, recommend stopping ASAP, except discuss steroid options with MD
* If postmenopausal female not on HRT, recommend discussing with MD ASAP
* Taking antacids or acid-reducing medications may affect calcium absorption; do not take within 2 hours of calcium supplement
* Medications that may decrease calcium: Furosemide, estrogen, corticosteroids, cholestyramine, phosphates, some anticonvulsants - discuss with healthcare provider

6. See table on following page

OSTEOPOROSIS *(Continued)*

OSTEOPOROSIS*

Category	Natural Products to Consider	DOC
Herb	**Horsetail** *on page 459*	PA
Vitamin/Mineral/ Trace Element/ Nutraceutical	**Boron** *on page 397* Condition-specific dosage: 1 mg/day	HT
	Calcium *on page 400* Condition-specific dosage: 1000-1500 mg/day	HT
	Isoflavones *on page 465* Condition-specific dosage: 500-1000 mg of soy isoflavones daily	HT
	Magnesium *on page 473* Condition-specific dosage: 600-800 mg/day	HT
	Vitamin D *on page 528* Condition-specific dosage: 200-400 int. units/day	HD
	Vitamin K *on page 531* Condition-specific dosage: Food source or by prescription only	HT
Homeopathic Remedy	Homeopathic combination formulas are available for many conditions. Listed below are some of the most common single homeopathic remedies for osteoporosis. Also see **Homeopathic Quick Reference Chart for Common Complaints** *on page 587*	
	Calcarea carbonica	PD
	Calcarea fluorica	PD
	Calcarea phosphorica	PD
	Hekla lava	PD
Additional supplements to consider	**Copper** *on page 416* Condition-specific dosage: 2-3 mg/day	PA
	Manganese *on page 475* Condition-specific dosage: 2 mg/day	PA
	Vitamin C *on page 526* Condition-specific dosage: 250-1000 mg/day	PA

*Refer to **Introduction to Conditions** *on page 41* for more details on how to apply the information in this table to individuals with this condition.

SPECIAL CONSIDERATIONS

Horsetail
- May cause electrolyte disturbances
- Potential interactions: antiarrhythmics, digoxin, phenytoin, diuretics, lithium, theophylline, vitamin B_1 (depletion)

Boron
- No known toxicity or serious side effects

Calcium
- Calcium supplements may contain lead (check for manufacturers who certify low lead levels)
- Potential interactions with tetracyclines, fluoroquinolones

Isoflavones
- Caution in estrogen-dependent tumors, endometrial cancer
- Women who are taking estrogen-containing medications (oral contraceptives, hormonal replacement) should consult their physician prior to use

Magnesium
- Use caution in renal impairment
- May cause diarrhea at high intakes

Vitamin D
- Toxicity symptoms: Excessive thirst, dehydration, anorexia, nausea, vomiting, headache, constipation, weakness, weight loss, hypercalcemia, kidney stones, arterial calcium deposits

Vitamin K
- Large doses of Vitamin K_3(synthetic form) can cause hemolytic anemia in animals and jaundice in infants

Copper
- Contraindicated in Wilson's disease

Manganese
- Use caution in individuals with liver disease

Vitamin C
- Excess intake in diabetics may give falsely elevated blood glucose readings

OTITIS MEDIA

Otitis media, or infection of the middle ear, occurs most frequently in children. A significant number of children experience multiple episodes. The incidence of allergy among children with recurrent ear infections is much higher than among the general public. Studies have reported that as many as 50% of all children with recurrent ear infections suffer from food allergies. Removal of offending foods from the diet led to significant improvement in >80% of allergic children. Milk and dairy products seem to be the class of foods that most frequently cause this condition.

A large percentage of recurrent otitis media infections can be explained as follows: The eustachian tube normally allows drainage from the middle ear into the back of the throat. Food allergies create an inflammatory response and the resulting swelling causes the tiny eustachian canal to become blocked. Blockage prevents drainage, causing painful pressure and stagnation of fluid in the inner ear. This allows bacteria to grow and create an infection.

Symptoms of middle ear infection include a feeling of fullness in the ear, earache, fever, chills, nausea, diarrhea, irritability, and temporary hearing loss. Infants may pull or rub their ears and cry in pain for long periods of time.

Analgesics and antibiotics are commonly prescribed in the United States, but are rarely used by physicians in Europe, and some researchers claim these efforts are not effective. Many children with recurrent infections undergo myringotomy, which is the surgical insertion of tubes in the ears to facilitate drainage. This procedure has not been consistently successful. In children who have food allergies, antibiotics and surgery only treat the symptoms, not the cause.

Children with repeated infections may eventually suffer from perforation or scarring of the tympanic membrane (eardrum), or damage to the structures of the middle ear, which may lead to loss of hearing acuity. Recent research has also reported that a high percentage of children with attention deficit disorder (ADD) and attention deficit hyperactivity disorder (ADHD), had recurrent inner ear infections and repeated rounds of antibiotics as younger children. Thus, parents should be encouraged to have their children tested for food allergies. Although this is not a panacea, many parents have been grateful to learn that removal of offending foods from the child's diet abruptly breaks the cycle of recurrent inner ear infections.

LIFESTYLE RECOMMENDATIONS

- May apply warm compresses to affected ear to decrease pain

- Do not instill anything in the ear (such as drops) unless specifically instructed to do so by physician

- If a swimmer, customized ear plugs may be of benefit; discuss with physician

- If any changes in hearing or possible hearing loss, see a specialist

- Check for food intolerances

- Eliminate dairy products and refined sugars, wheat

- If more than one episode and not yet tested for allergies, recommend being checked as soon as possible

- Check for environmental exposure or link

OTITIS MEDIA DECISION TREE

1. Client with otitis media is interested in using natural products (NP) to support this condition

2. Healthcare provider requests basic background information. The following issues are addressed with the client:
   * Allergies?
   * Other medical conditions?
   * Prescription (Rx)/OTC meds?
   * Nutrition/diet program?
   * Natural products?
   * Exercise program?

3. Above data reviewed; if **yes** to Rx/OTC meds, review **Drug-Induced Nutrient Depletion Chart** in Appendix

4A. Client is a candidate for natural products

   * An appropriate homeopathic remedy can be used at any time

4B. Client's case is too complicated at this point; needs additional support from MD before initiating NP program

5. Condition-specific questions:
   * Diagnosed by MD? If **yes**, what was the recommended treatment plan? Effective?
   * Triggers for condition/symptom onset? Worsening? Cold, flu, travel (flying), swimming?
   * First episode? If **no**, what happened in the past? Response to therapy, interventions?
   * Does client have myringotomy tubes? If **yes**, do not use anything locally in the ears unless specifically instructed to do so by the physician.
   * Accompanying symptoms: Fever, drainage from the ear, pain, malaise, sore throat, pulling at the affected ear, irritability, changes in eating patterns? If patient is experiencing some of these changes, refer to MD.

6. See table on following page

OTITIS MEDIA *(Continued)*

OTITIS MEDIA*

Category	Natural Products to Consider	DOC
Herb	**Echinacea** *on page 426*	PA, HE
	Astragalus *on page 388*	PA
	Olive Leaf *on page 483*	PA
Vitamin/Mineral/ Trace Element/ Nutraceutical	***Lactobacillus acidophilus*** *on page 467* and ***Bifidobacterium bifidum*** *on page 391* Condition-specific dosage: 2-5 billion CFU twice daily	PA
	Thymus Extract *on page 510* Condition-specific dosage: 250 mg twice daily	PA
Homeopathic Remedy	Homeopathic combination formulas are available for many conditions. Listed below are some of the most common single homeopathic remedies for otitis media. Also see **Homeopathic Quick Reference Chart for Common Complaints** *on page 587*	
	Atropa belladonna	PD
	Chamomilla	PD
	Mercuris solubilis	PD
Additional supplements to consider	**Vitamin A** *on page 518* Condition-specific dosage: 5,000 int. units/day	PA
	Vitamin C *on page 526* Condition-specific dosage: 100-500 mg/day	PA
	Zinc *on page 534* Condition-specific dosage: Children (<12 years): 5 mg/day; Adults: 25 mg/day	PA

*Refer to **Introduction to Conditions** *on page 41* for more details on how to apply the information in this table to individuals with this condition.

SPECIAL CONSIDERATIONS

Echinacea

- Not recommended for use longer than 10 days (acute treatment) or in immunosuppressed individuals
- Potential interaction with therapeutic immunosuppressants and cortico-steroids
- Caution in renal impairment (may cause electrolyte imbalance)
- Caution if allergic to *Asteraceae/Compositae* family (ragweed, daisy, aster, chrysanthemum) and other pollens

Astragalus

- May interact with immune stimulants or immunosuppressants

Olive Leaf

- No reported toxicity in humans at normal intakes

Lactobacillus acidophilus

- No known toxicity or serious side effects

Bifidobacterium bifidum

- No known toxicity or serious side effects

Thymus Extract

- No known toxicity or serious side effects

Vitamin A

- Contraindicated in pregnancy or in women who may become pregnant

Vitamin C

- Excess intake in diabetics may give falsely elevated blood glucose readings

Zinc

- No reported toxicity in humans at normal intakes

PARKINSON'S DISEASE

Parkinson's disease is a chronic, progressive neurologic disorder that results from the loss of dopamine-producing neurons. In North America, the annual incidence is approximately 20 per 100,000 population. It is generally a disease of older individuals, with a mean onset at 65 years of age; however, the range of onset is extremely broad, from 31-83 years of age.

The etiology of Parkinson's disease is unknown. A genetic association may be present in some forms. Many researchers believe it may be the result of some cumulative process, due to its tendency to appear late in life. Current theories include environmental toxicity. A breakdown in antioxidant defense mechanisms within and outside neurons has also been suggested to play a role. Damage is localized primarily to the substantia nigra, an area of the brain that governs smooth, controlled motor activity. By the time symptoms appear, a large percentage of dopamine-producing cells have already been destroyed.

The classic symptoms of Parkinson's include tremor, rigidity, impaired balance, and slow movement (bradykinesia). Occasionally, symptoms are more prevalent on one side of the body and may be confused with stroke. In up to 33% of individuals, progression may lead to dementia, including loss or impairment of memory, judgment, and abstract thinking, as well as personality changes.

The diagnosis of Parkinson's disease is primarily based upon neurological examination. It is not contagious. Although no cure exists, treatment may provide dramatic relief of symptoms. New approaches to slow progression and potentially restore function are being investigated.

LIFESTYLE RECOMMENDATIONS

- Structured stress management may provide assistance

- Understand how condition affects daily living, ability to be independent

- Rehab may be indicated

- Support groups are available and are of value

PARKINSON'S DISEASE DECISION TREE

1. Client with Parkinson's disease is interested in using natural products (NP) to support this condition

2. Healthcare provider requests basic background information.
   The following issues are addressed with the client:
   * Allergies?   * Other medical conditions?
   * Prescription (Rx)/OTC meds?   * Nutrition/diet program?
   * Natural products?   * Exercise program?

3. Above data reviewed; if **yes** to Rx/OTC meds, review **Drug-Induced Nutrient Depletion Chart** in Appendix

4A. Client is a candidate for natural products

* An appropriate homeopathic remedy can be used at any time

4B. Client's case is too complicated at this point; needs additional support from MD before initiating NP program

5. Condition-specific questions:
   * Diagnosed by MD? If **yes**, what was the recommended treatment plan? Effective?
   * Is the client taking any meds that may contribute to worsening of condition, such as metoclopramide, neuroleptics?

6. See table on following page

PARKINSON'S DISEASE *(Continued)*

PARKINSON'S DISEASE*

Category	Natural Products to Consider	DOC
Herb	Ginkgo *on page 441*	PA
	Grape Seed *on page 451*	PA
Vitamin/Mineral/ Trace Element/ Nutraceutical	Nicotinamide Adenine Dinucleotide (NADH) *on page 483* Condition-specific dosage: 3-4 times/day	HD
	Acetyl-L-Carnitine *on page 380* Condition-specific dosage: 500-2000 mg/day in divided doses	PA
	N-Acetyl Cysteine (NAC) *on page 482* Condition-specific dosage: 500 mg 2-3 times/day	PA
	Magnesium *on page 473* Condition-specific dosage: 400-600 mg/day	PA
Homeopathic Remedy	Homeopathic combination formulas are available for many conditions. Listed below are some of the most common single homeopathic remedies for Parkinson's disease. Also see **Homeopathic Quick Reference Chart for Common Complaints** *on page 587*	
	Cuprum metallicum	PD
	Mercurius solubilis	PD
	Thuja occidentalis	PD
	Zincum metallicum	PD
Additional supplements to consider	Vitamin C *on page 526* Condition-specific dosage: 250-1000 mg/day	HD

*Refer to **Introduction to Conditions** *on page 41* for more details on how to apply the information in this table to individuals with this condition.

SPECIAL CONSIDERATIONS

Ginkgo
- Contraindicated in active bleeding (eg, peptic ulcer, intracranial bleeding)
- Caution in hemostatic disorders/history of bleeding
- Potential interaction with anticoagulants (warfarin), aspirin, NSAIDs, anti-platelet agents
- Theoretical interaction with MAO inhibitors, acetylcholinesterase inhibitors (tacrine, donepezil)
- Discontinue use prior to dental or surgical procedures (14 days before)

Grape Seed
- Contraindicated in active bleeding (eg, peptic ulcer, intracranial bleeding)
- Caution in hemostatic disorders/history of bleeding
- Potential interaction with anticoagulants (warfarin), aspirin, NSAIDs, anti-platelet agents, methotrexate
- Discontinue use prior to dental or surgical procedures (14 days before)

NADH
- No known toxicity or serious side effects

Acetyl-L-Carnitine
- Occasionally, mild abdominal discomfort, restlessness, vertigo, and headache have been reported

N-Acetyl Cysteine
- No known toxicity or serious side effects

Magnesium
- Use caution in renal impairment
- May cause diarrhea at high intakes

Vitamin C
- Excess intake in diabetics may give falsely elevated blood glucose readings

PERFORMANCE ENHANCEMENT

There are a number of products and programs available for athletes who want to enhance their performance. Areas of emphasis include bodybuilding, muscle enhancement and development, fat loss, improvement of lean body mass, increasing strength, speed and stamina, reducing risk of injury, and supporting immune function.

Although much has appeared in the media about illegal performance enhancement aids such as steroids and blood doping, it is important for athletes to know that there are healthy, legal methods to achieve performance enhancement. Nutritional science and sports medicine have paved the way for the development of newer, more effective ergogenic aids, substances used to improve athletic performance.

Highly specialized combinations of protein and amino acid supplements have been formulated to maximize building muscle and strength. Pyruvate products help with fat burning and energy production; glutamine supplements reduce catabolism of muscle, while enhancing glycogen replenishment and growth hormone release; creatine monohydrate increases cell volume in muscles and improves recovery after exercise. Products are also available that help improve the performer's supply and utilization of oxygen.

Other areas of specialty for performance enhancement include mental and psychological training aids, psychological energizers, psychological relaxants, and a wide range of specialized sports training equipment.

In short, performance enhancement has gone "high tech." There are products and programs that can be individually designed to enhance the performance of any type of athlete in any type of sport or competition.

LIFESTYLE RECOMMENDATIONS

- Avoid alcohol, caffeine, and tobacco
- Stress management may provide some assistance
- Decrease consumption of red meat, sugar, fats, processed foods
- Increase consumption of fresh fruits, vegetables, protein
- Drink plenty of quality water

PERFORMANCE ENHANCEMENT DECISION TREE

1. Client with a desire for performance enhancement is interested in using natural products (NP) to support this condition

2. Healthcare provider requests basic background information.
   The following issues are addressed with the client:
   * Allergies?
   * Other medical conditions?
   * Prescription (Rx)/OTC meds?
   * Nutrition/diet program?
   * Natural products?
   * Exercise program?

3. Above data reviewed; if **yes** to Rx/OTC meds, review **Drug-Induced Nutrient Depletion Chart** in Appendix

4A. Client is a candidate for natural products

   * An appropriate homeopathic remedy can be used at any time

4B. Client's case is too complicated at this point; needs additional support from MD before initiating NP program

5. Condition-specific questions:
   * Why is the client looking for performance enhancement?
   * Any specific interests (ie, sports)?
   * Recent change in lifestyle, behaviors resulting in this decision?
   * Thyroid, allergy testing? If **no**, recommend discussing with MD?

6. See table on following page

303

PERFORMANCE ENHANCEMENT *(Continued)*

PERFORMANCE ENHANCEMENT*

Category	Natural Products to Consider	DOC
Herb	**Ginseng, Siberian** *on page 444*	HT
	Tribulis *on page 511*	PA
	Cordyceps *on page 417*	HD
Vitamin/Mineral/ Trace Element/ Nutraceutical	**Colostrum** *on page 415* Condition-specific dosage: 500 mg 3 times/day	HD
	Glutamine *on page 446* Condition-specific dosage: 1000-2000 mg 3 times/day	HT
	Creatine *on page 419* Condition-specific dosage: 10 g/day in divided doses for 5 days, then 5 g/day in divided doses for 6 weeks; take 4 weeks off, then repeat cycle	HT
	Pyruvate *on page 494* Condition-specific dosage: 500-1000 mg 3 times/day	HD
Homeopathic Remedy	Homeopathic combination formulas are available for many conditions. Listed below are some of the most common single homeopathic remedies for performance enhancement. Also see **Homeopathic Quick Reference Chart for Common Complaints** *on page 587*	
	Arnica montana	PD
	Lacticum acidum	PD
Additional supplements to consider	No recommendations	

*Refer to **Introduction to Conditions** *on page 41* for more details on how to apply the information in this table to individuals with this condition.

SPECIAL CONSIDERATIONS

Ginseng, Siberian
- Contraindicated with digoxin, hexobarbital
- Caution with stimulant medications, decongestants, caffeine
- A cycle of 4 weeks on, followed by 2 weeks off is recommended for maximum benefit
- Caution in hypertension or in individuals at risk of hypotension (elderly, cerebrovascular or cardiovascular disease); or those taking antihypertensives
- May alter blood glucose regulation; monitor blood glucose carefully in individuals with diabetes or hypoglycemia
- Contraindicated in active bleeding (eg, peptic ulcer, intracranial bleeding)
- Caution in hemostatic disorders/history of bleeding
- Potential interactions with anticoagulants (warfarin), aspirin, NSAIDs, antiplatelet agents, sedative-hypnotics (barbiturates), insulin, oral hypoglycemics, antihypertensives, stimulants, caffeine
- Discontinue use prior to dental or surgical procedures (14 days before)

Tribulis
- Caution in individuals taking steroidal medications

Cordyceps
- Caution if allergic to molds or fungi
- Theoretical interaction in individuals receiving MAO inhibitors
- Contraindicated in active bleeding (eg, peptic ulcer, intracranial bleeding)
- Caution in hemostatic disorders/history of bleeding
- Potential interaction with anticoagulants (warfarin), aspirin, NSAIDs, antiplatelet agents
- Discontinue use prior to dental or surgical procedures (14 days before)

Colostrum
- No known toxicity or serious side effects

Glutamine
- No known toxicity or serious side effects

Creatine
- Use with caution in renal or hepatic disease

Pyruvate
- Large doses may cause gas, bloating, and diarrhea

POISON IVY / POISON OAK

Poison ivy and poison oak are specific types of contact dermatitis that develop from contact with these plants. The ensuing allergic rash is a reaction to a substance contained in leaves, stems, and roots of these poisonous plants. These plants thrive and are most abundant in the springtime, which is when the majority of cases are reported.

In addition to direct contact with the plant, rash can also occur by touching things that have come into contact with the plants, such as clothing or garden tools. Inhalation of smoke from burning plants can provide a serious exposure.

The allergic response can develop within hours, or a day or two after contact. The rash usually produces a very annoying itch and reddish skin that sometimes progresses to tiny fluid-filled blisters. Care should be taken to not rub one's eyes with the hands during the time of contact or while cleaning and scrubbing after contact.

Careful washing of the exposed areas is advised. Calamine lotion and/or over-the-counter antihistamines are usually sufficient for most cases.

LIFESTYLE RECOMMENDATIONS

- Client should treat itching so as to avoid scratching, which increases risk for developing infection
- Wash area thoroughly; keep clean to avoid secondary infection
- Clean clothes, other items that may have been exposed to the plant (such as garden tools, pets, gloves)
- Try to avoid 3-leaf plants
- When in an area where the plant may grow, wear protective clothing

POISON IVY DECISION TREE

1. Client with poison ivy is interested in using natural products (NP) to support this condition

2. Healthcare provider requests basic background information. The following issues are addressed with the client:
   * Allergies?
   * Prescription (Rx)/OTC meds?
   * Natural products?
   * Other medical conditions?
   * Nutrition/diet program?
   * Exercise program?

3. Above data reviewed; if **yes** to Rx/OTC meds, review **Drug-Induced Nutrient Depletion Chart** in Appendix

4A. Client is a candidate for natural products

   * An appropriate homeopathic remedy can be used at any time

4B. Client's case is too complicated at this point; needs additional support from MD before initiating NP program

5. Condition-specific questions:
   * Sought medical attention? If **yes**, what was the recommended treatment plan? Effective?
   * Triggers for condition/symptom onset? Worsening?
   * How long since exposure to the plant?
   * First time exposure? If **no**, what has/has not worked in the past?
   * What have you tried? Effective?
   * Symptoms may develop/worsen 7-10 days after exposure

6. See table on following page

POISON IVY / POISON OAK (Continued)

POISON IVY / POISON OAK*

Category	Natural Products to Consider	DOC
Herb	Aloe (Topical) on page 381	PA, HE
	Calendula (Topical) on page 401	PA
	Echinacea (Topical) on page 426	PA, HE
Vitamin/Mineral/ Trace Element/ Nutraceutical	Calcium Lactate on page 400 Condition-specific dosage: 2000-5000 mg/day for 3-5 days	HE
Homeopathic Remedy	Homeopathic combination formulas are available for many conditions. Listed below are some of the most common single homeopathic remedies for poison ivy/ poison oak. Also see Homeopathic Quick Reference Chart for Common Complaints on page 587	
	Apis mellifica	PD
	Cantharis	PD
	Croton tiglium	PD
	Mezereum	PD
	Rhus toxicodendron	PD
	Sulphur	PD
Additional supplements to consider	No recommendations	

*Refer to Introduction to Conditions on page 41 for more details on how to apply the information in this table to individuals with this condition.

SPECIAL CONSIDERATIONS

Aloe
- No reported toxicity in humans at normal intakes
- External use only

Calendula
- No reported toxicity in humans at normal intakes
- External use only

Echinacea
- No reported toxicity in humans at normal intakes
- External use only

Calcium Lactate
- Potential interactions with tetracyclines, fluoroquinolones

PREMENSTRUAL SYNDROME (PMS)

PMS is estimated to affect 70% to 90% of women during their childbearing years. PMS may be disabling, and as many as 30% to 40% of women have symptoms severe enough to interfere with daily activities. PMS is most common between 20-40 years of age. Other correlations have been made between PMS and women with at least one child, or a family history of depression or other mood disorder. Symptoms must occur during the second half of the menstrual cycle (14 days or more after the first day of the menstrual period) and be absent for 7 days after the end of the menstrual period, to meet the definition of PMS. Some women have symptoms that last for 2 weeks or longer, while others only feel effects for a few hours. Most women fall somewhere in between.

PMS has been divided into four distinct types depending on which symptoms predominate. Many women have symptoms that overlap into more than one category. The four types include: PMS-A (anxiety) occurs in 65% to 75% of cases with primary symptoms of anxiety, irritability, mood swings, and increased appetite. PMS-C (cravings) occurs in 24% to 35% of cases with primary symptoms of increased appetite, headache, fatigue, dizziness/fainting, and palpitations. PMS-H (hyperhydration) occurs in 65% to 72% of cases with primary symptoms of fluid retention, swollen extremities, breast tenderness, and abdominal bloating. PMS-D (depression) is the least common form of PMS with primary symptoms of depression, crying, forgetfulness, confusion, and insomnia.

The cause of PMS is probably multifactorial. Adequate rest is important to minimize symptoms. Regular exercise and good dietary habits (whole grains, vegetables, fruit, as well as decreased salt, sugar, alcohol, and caffeine) are often helpful. A variety of nutritional and herbal products may also prove helpful for many women.

LIFESTYLE RECOMMENDATIONS

- Continuation/initiation of diet and exercise program
- Decrease consumption of caffeine, sodium, red meat, dairy products, sugar, alcohol
- Reduce stress
- Increase consumption of fruits, vegetables, protein (whole foods)

PMS DECISION TREE

1. Client with premenstrual syndrome is interested in using natural products (NP) to support this condition

2. Healthcare provider requests basic background information.
   The following issues are addressed with the client:
   * Allergies?   * Other medical conditions?
   * Prescription (Rx)/OTC meds?   * Nutrition/diet program?
   * Natural products?   * Exercise program?

3. Above data reviewed; if **yes** to Rx/OTC meds, review **Drug-Induced Nutrient Depletion Chart** in Appendix

4A. Client is a candidate for natural products

* An appropriate homeopathic remedy can be used at any time

4B. Client's case is too complicated at this point; needs additional support from MD before initiating NP program

5. Condition-specific questions:
   * Diagnosed by MD? If **yes**, what was the recommended treatment plan? Effective?
   * Triggers for condition/symptom onset? Worsening?
   * Does the client have a regular cycle? If **no**, does the PMS occur with each period, change month to month?
   * How does this condition affect the client's quality of life? Ability to perform routine daily functions?

6. See table on following page

PREMENSTRUAL SYNDROME (PMS) *(Continued)*

PREMENSTRUAL SYNDROME (PMS)*

Category	Natural Products to Consider	DOC
Herb	Chasteberry/Vitex *on page 408*	HT
	Dong Quai *on page 425*	HT
	Evening Primrose *on page 430*	HT
	Black Cohosh *on page 395*	HT
Vitamin/Mineral/ Trace Element/ Nutraceutical	Chromium *on page 410* Condition-specific dosage: 200-600 mcg/day	PA
	Progesterone *on page 491* Condition-specific dosage: 1/8 to 1/4 tsp applied topically daily on days 7-28 of cycle	HT
	Isoflavones *on page 465* Condition-specific dosage: 500-1000 mg soy isoflavones daily	PA
	Fish Oils *on page 434* Condition-specific dosage: 750 mg 2-3 times/day OR Flaxseed Oil *on page 435* Condition-specific dosage: 1 Tbsp/day	HD
Homeopathic Remedy	Homeopathic combination formulas are available for many conditions. Listed below are some of the most common single homeopathic remedies for premenstrual syndrome (PMS). Also see **Homeopathic Quick Reference Chart for Common Complaints** *on page 587*	
	Apis mellifica	PD
	Lachesis mutus	PD
	Lycopodium clavatum	PD
	Natrum muriaticum	PD
	Pulsatilla	PD
	Sepia	PD
Additional supplements to consider	Magnesium *on page 473* Condition-specific dosage: 400-600 mg/day	HT
	Vitamin B$_6$ *on page 523* Condition-specific dosage: 25 mg twice daily	HT
	Vitamin E *on page 529* Condition-specific dosage: 200-400 int. units/day	HT

*Refer to **Introduction to Conditions** *on page 41* for more details on how to apply the information in this table to individuals with this condition.

SPECIAL CONSIDERATIONS

Chasteberry/Vitex

- Contraindicated in pregnancy
- Potential interaction with hormonal replacements or oral contraceptives

Dong Quai

- Caution in pregnancy and breast-feeding
- Contraindicated in active bleeding (eg, peptic ulcer, intracranial bleeding), and in those at risk of estrogen-dependent tumors, endometrial cancer, thromboembolic disease, or stroke
- Potential interaction with anticoagulants (warfarin), aspirin, NSAIDs, antiplatelet agents, and with oral contraceptives or hormonal replacement therapy
- Caution in hemostatic disorders/history of bleeding
- Potential interaction with antihypertensives, photosensitizing agents
- Discontinue use prior to dental or surgical procedures (14 days before)

Evening Primrose

- Contraindicated in seizure disorders, schizophrenia, or in persons receiving anticonvulsant or antipsychotic medications, and in active bleeding (eg, peptic ulcer, intracranial bleeding)
- Caution in hemostatic disorders/history of bleeding
- Potential interaction with anticoagulants (warfarin), aspirin, NSAIDs, antiplatelet agents
- Discontinue use prior to dental or surgical procedures (14 days before)

Black Cohosh

- Contraindicated in pregnancy and breast-feeding
- Use caution in individuals with allergies to salicylates, with a history of estrogen-dependent tumors, endometrial cancer, thromboembolic disease, or stroke
- May cause nausea, vomiting, headache and hypotension (at higher dosages)
- Monitoring of serum hormone levels is recommended after 6 months of treatment
- Potential interaction with oral contraceptives, hormonal replacement therapy

Chromium – Caution in individuals receiving oral hypoglycemics or insulin; monitor blood glucose closely and coordinate with prescriber

Progesterone – May alter hormonal regulation; not to be used with oral contraceptives without medical supervision

Isoflavones

- Caution in estrogen-dependent tumors, endometrial cancer; women who are taking estrogen-containing medications (oral contraceptives, hormonal replacement) should consult their physician prior to use

Fish Oils

- High doses may cause GI upset, loose stools, nausea
- May alter glucose regulation; use with caution in diabetes
- Caution in individuals receiving oral hypoglycemics or insulin; monitor blood glucose closely and coordinate with prescriber
- Potential interaction with anticoagulants (warfarin), aspirin, NSAIDs, antiplatelet agents

Flaxseed Oil – No reported toxicity in humans at normal intakes

Magnesium

- Use caution in renal impairment
- May cause diarrhea at high intakes

Vitamin B₆ – No reported toxicity in humans at normal intakes

Vitamin E

- Use with caution when taking anticoagulants (vitamin E ≥200 int. units increases prothrombin times)
- Interrupt or reduce dosage one week prior to dental or surgical procedures

PSORIASIS

Psoriasis is a common skin disease that produces thick patches of reddened skin covered by silvery, scaly patches. This benign proliferation of the skin affects as much as 2% of the general population. Its development appears to be multifactorial, caused by both genetic and environmental factors. One-third of individuals develop symptoms before age 19; however, the mean age of onset is 27. Exacerbating factors include lack of sun exposure, infections, medications, local trauma, nutritional deficiencies or imbalances, and psychological stress.

In psoriasis, new skin cells are being produced about ten times faster than normal, but old skin on the surface continues to shed at its normal rate. Thus, new cells being formed have difficulty reaching the surface, which causes the newly developing live skin cells to bunch and form the characteristic thickened patches. The silvery scales are batches of dead and dying cells that have not been shed.

The disease often persists throughout the individual's life, with episodes of exacerbation and remission. Symptoms of the disease are usually limited to cosmetic inconvenience; however, there may occasionally be a severe form, which is disfiguring and debilitating. Severe symptoms or systemic involvement should prompt medical evaluation and treatment coordination.

LIFESTYLE RECOMMENDATIONS

- Increase consumption of raw foods, such as fruits, vegetables, grains, and fibers

- Decrease consumption of fats

- Spend more time in the sun and use a mild-to-moderate sunscreen to prevent sunburn

- Use skin creams that provide moisturizers

- Use OTC products sparingly and under a physician's supervision

- Stress management is important

PSORIASIS DECISION TREE

1. Client with psoriasis is interested in using natural products (NP) to support this condition

2. Healthcare provider requests basic background information. The following issues are addressed with the client:
   * Allergies?
   * Prescription (Rx)/OTC meds?
   * Natural products?
   * Other medical conditions?
   * Nutrition/diet program?
   * Exercise program?

3. Above data reviewed; if **yes** to Rx/OTC meds, review **Drug-Induced Nutrient Depletion Chart** in Appendix

4A. Client is a candidate for natural products

   * An appropriate homeopathic remedy can be used at any time

4B. Client's case is too complicated at this point; needs additional support from MD before initiating NP program

5. Condition-specific questions:
   * Diagnosed by MD? If **yes**, what was the recommended treatment plan? Effective?
   * Triggers for condition/symptom onset? Worsening?
   * How often does client have flare-ups? Triggers?
   * Is client taking any meds that might aggravate, such as beta-blockers, antimalarials, lithium? If **yes**, refer to MD for evaluation
   * Does client have recurrent infections? If **yes**, refer to MD so a plan can be developed to try and prevent these from occurring so often.

6. See table on following page

PSORIASIS *(Continued)*

PSORIASIS*

Category	Natural Products to Consider	DOC
Herb	Coleus *on page 413*	PA
	Milk Thistle *on page 479*	PA, HE
	Gotu Kola (Topical) *on page 449*	HD
	Evening Primrose *on page 430*	PA
Vitamin/Mineral/ Trace Element/ Nutraceutical	Zinc *on page 534* Condition-specific dosage: 50 mg plus 2 mg of copper daily	HT
	Fish Oils *on page 434* Condition-specific dosage: 750 mg 2-3 times/day	HT
	Flaxseed Oil *on page 435* Condition-specific dosage: 1 Tbsp/day	PA
Homeopathic Remedy	Homeopathic combination formulas are available for many conditions. Listed below are some of the most common single homeopathic remedies for psoriasis. Also see **Homeopathic Quick Reference Chart for Common Complaints** *on page 587*	
	Arsenicum album	PD
	Graphites	PD
	Sulphur	PD
Additional supplements to consider	Vitamin A *on page 518* Condition-specific dosage: 10,000 int. units/day	PA
	Vitamin C *on page 526* Condition-specific dosage: 1000 mg twice daily	PA
	Vitamin E *on page 529* Condition-specific dosage: 800 int. units/day	PA

*Refer to **Introduction to Conditions** *on page 41* for more details on how to apply the information in this table to individuals with this condition.

SPECIAL CONSIDERATIONS

Coleus
- Contraindicated in active bleeding (eg, peptic ulcer, intracranial bleeding)
- May cause hypotension; use caution in cerebrovascular or cardiovascular disease
- Caution in hemostatic disorders/history of bleeding
- Potential interaction with anticoagulants (warfarin), aspirin, NSAIDs, antiplatelet agents
- Potential interaction with antihistamines, decongestants, anticoagulants, antihypertensives
- Discontinue use prior to dental or surgical procedures (14 days before)

Milk Thistle
- No reported toxicity in humans at normal intakes

Gotu Kola
- Topical application may cause contact dermatitis

Evening Primrose
- Contraindicated in seizure disorders, schizophrenia, or in persons receiving anticonvulsant or antipsychotic medications
- Contraindicated in active bleeding (eg, peptic ulcer, intracranial bleeding)
- Caution in hemostatic disorders/history of bleeding
- Potential interaction with anticoagulants (warfarin), aspirin, NSAIDs, antiplatelet agents
- Discontinue use prior to dental or surgical procedures (14 days before)

Zinc
- Prolonged intake at levels >150 mg/day may be associated with toxicity

Fish Oils
- High doses may cause GI upset, loose stools, nausea
- May alter glucose regulation; use with caution in diabetes
- Caution in individuals receiving oral hypoglycemics or insulin; monitor blood glucose closely and coordinate with prescriber
- Potential interaction with anticoagulants (warfarin), aspirin, NSAIDs, antiplatelet agents

Flaxseed Oil
- No known toxicity or serious side effects

Vitamin A
- Contraindicated in pregnancy or in women who may become pregnant

Vitamin C
- Excess intake in diabetics may give falsely elevated blood glucose readings

Vitamin E
- Use with caution when taking anticoagulants (vitamin E ≥200 int. units increases prothrombin times)
- Interrupt or reduce dosage one week prior to dental or surgical procedures

ROSACEA

Rosacea is an inflammatory skin disorder of unknown etiology that resembles, and is often referred to as, adult acne. This condition predominantly affects the skin in and around the center portion of the face. The areas of the face that are normally affected include the nose, cheeks, chin, and forehead. Eye involvement is also found in as many as 50% of cases. Rosacea produces redness, swelling, bumps, and pimples that resemble acne. However, this condition is characterized by the dilation of small blood vessels, just below the surface of the skin, which become visible reddish blotches known as telangiectasia. If left untreated, its progression can result in permanent thickening and reddish discoloration of the skin, especially around the nose. Although it resembles acne, rosacea does not produce blackheads or whiteheads as does true acne. Rosacea has been estimated to affect approximately 13 million people in the United States. The development peaks between 40-50 years of age and affects men and women equally.

Rosacea may be associated with a genetic predisposition, gastrointestinal diseases, gallbladder disease, hypotension, or mite infestation. Exacerbating factors include alcohol, hot liquids, caffeine, spicy foods, or any factor that promotes facial flushing. Niacin may exacerbate this problem due to its vasodilating properties.

LIFESTYLE RECOMMENDATIONS

- Avoid tobacco, alcohol, high humidity, major temperature changes, caffeine, hot beverages, eggs, chocolate, spicy foods, excess sunlight, stress, intense exercise, fatty foods
- Use sunscreen
- Do not use OTC steroid creams or ointments
- Women should avoid using makeup whenever possible
- Emphasize whole food diet

ROSACEA DECISION TREE

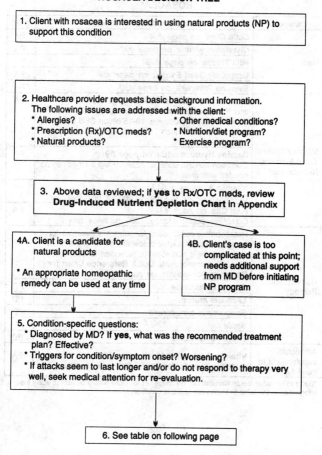

1. Client with rosacea is interested in using natural products (NP) to support this condition

2. Healthcare provider requests basic background information. The following issues are addressed with the client:
   * Allergies?
   * Prescription (Rx)/OTC meds?
   * Natural products?
   * Other medical conditions?
   * Nutrition/diet program?
   * Exercise program?

3. Above data reviewed; if **yes** to Rx/OTC meds, review **Drug-Induced Nutrient Depletion Chart** in Appendix

4A. Client is a candidate for natural products

   * An appropriate homeopathic remedy can be used at any time

4B. Client's case is too complicated at this point; needs additional support from MD before initiating NP program

5. Condition-specific questions:
   * Diagnosed by MD? If **yes**, what was the recommended treatment plan? Effective?
   * Triggers for condition/symptom onset? Worsening?
   * If attacks seem to last longer and/or do not respond to therapy very well, seek medical attention for re-evaluation.

6. See table on following page

ROSACEA *(Continued)*

ROSACEA*

Category	Natural Products to Consider	DOC
Herb	Cat's Claw *on page 404*	PA
	Chasteberry/Vitex *on page 408*	PA
	Milk Thistle *on page 479*	PA
	Grapefruit Seed Extract *on page 450*	PA
	Evening Primrose *on page 430*	PA
Vitamin/Mineral/ Trace Element/ Nutraceutical	**Lactobacillus acidophilus** *on page 467* and **Bifidobacterium bifidum** *on page 391* Condition-specific dosage: 10-15 billion CFU twice daily for 2 weeks, then 1-2 billion CFU twice daily (dairy free)	PA
	Betaine Hydrochloride *on page 391* Condition-specific dosage: 325-650 mg 3 times/day as needed with meals	PA
	Vitamin A *on page 518* Condition-specific dosage: 10,000 int. units/day	PA
	Fish Oils *on page 434* Condition-specific dosage: 1000 mg twice daily	PA
Homeopathic Remedy	Homeopathic combination formulas are available for many conditions. Listed below are some of the most common single homeopathic remedies for rosacea. Also see **Homeopathic Quick Reference Chart for Common Complaints** *on page 587*	
	Atropa belladonna	PD
	Lachesis mutus	PD
	Sanguinaria canadensis	PD
	Sepia	PD
	Thuja occidentalis	PD
Additional supplements to consider	**Vitamin B Complex-25** *on page 526* Condition-specific dosage: 25-50 mg twice daily	PA

*Refer to **Introduction to Conditions** *on page 41* for more details on how to apply the information in this table to individuals with this condition.

SPECIAL CONSIDERATIONS

Cat's Claw
- Contraindicated in transplant recipients, individuals receiving I.V. immuno-globulins or immunosuppressants
- Contraindicated in active bleeding (eg, peptic ulcer, intracranial bleeding)
- Caution in hemostatic disorders/history of bleeding
- Potential interaction with anticoagulants (warfarin), aspirin, NSAIDs, anti-platelet agents
- Discontinue use prior to dental or surgical procedures (14 days before)

Chasteberry/Vitex
- Contraindicated in pregnancy
- Potential interaction with hormonal replacements or oral contraceptives

Milk Thistle
- No reported toxicity in humans at normal intakes

Grapefruit Seed Extract
- Grapefruit seed extract is not equivalent to grapefruit juice/pulp. Juice/pulp has been associated with many drug interactions; see Grapefruit Seed *on page 450*
- Until further information is available, it is reasonable to avoid some medications (terfenadine, astemizole, cisapride). Use other medications metabolized by CYP3A4 with caution.

Evening Primrose
- Contraindicated in seizure disorders, schizophrenia, or in persons receiving anticonvulsant or antipsychotic medications
- Contraindicated in active bleeding (eg, peptic ulcer, intracranial bleeding)
- Caution in hemostatic disorders/history of bleeding
- Potential interaction with anticoagulants (warfarin), aspirin, NSAIDs, anti-platelet agents
- Discontinue use prior to dental or surgical procedures (14 days before)

Lactobacillus acidophilus
- No known toxicity or serious side effects

Bifidobacterium bifidum
- No known toxicity or serious side effects

Betaine Hydrochloride
- Do not use in individuals with ulcers
- High doses may cause gastric irritation

Vitamin A
- Contraindicated in pregnancy or in women who may become pregnant

Fish Oils
- High doses may cause GI upset, loose stools, nausea
- May alter glucose regulation; use with caution in diabetes
- Caution in individuals receiving oral hypoglycemics or insulin; monitor blood glucose closely and coordinate with prescriber
- Potential interaction with anticoagulants (warfarin), aspirin, NSAIDs, anti-platelet agents

Vitamin B Complex-25
- No side effects at the RDI or ODA doses

SCLERODERMA

Scleroderma is a rare, chronic autoimmune disease of unknown origin that primarily attacks the skin and connective tissue. There are two main types of scleroderma, localized and systemic. The localized forms affect only the skin (and sometimes the underlying tissues), sparing the internal organs. Systemic forms may cause fibrosis of the internal organs. Fibrosis eventually causes the involved skin or organs to harden and lose normal function.

As this condition progresses, the skin becomes taut, firm, and edematous. The skin also becomes increasingly bound to subcutaneous tissue, which causes it to develop a tough, leathery feeling. Hyperpigmentation may result in skin darkening. These changes may affect large areas of the body or only the fingers and hands.

Scleroderma has no known cause; however, potential contributing factors include a genetic predisposition, environmental exposures, and viruses. Some cases have been attributed to chemical exposures. Scleroderma is not contagious – contact with an affected individual or with blood or body fluids does not transmit the disease. In addition, there is no known association with cancer. The disease tends to cause progressive deformity and dysfunction.

A related or potentially overlapping syndrome is referred to as CREST syndrome. It is characterized by calcinosis (calcium deposits which usually occur in the fingers), Raynaud's syndrome, esophageal dysmotility, sclerodactyly (a deformity of the bones of the fingers), and telangiectasia (small red spots on the skin of the fingers, face, or inside of the mouth). Only two of the five CREST symptoms are required for diagnosis. To date, it is not possible to predict whether this constellation of symptoms will progress to scleroderma in any given individual.

Scleroderma is estimated to affect 150,000-500,000 Americans. The disease typically has its onset between 30-50 years of age. Women are affected at a ratio of 4:1.

Metabolic lab assessments for scleroderma include heavy metal analysis and organic acids. A complete case history is essential in evaluating all potential xenobiotic and xenotoxic exposures, in addition to bioclinical parameters.

LIFESTYLE RECOMMENDATIONS

- Increase whole food consumption (fruits, vegetables, grains, and seafoods)

- Drink at least 8-10 glasses of water per day

- Avoid red meat, dairy products, processed foods, sugar, alcohol, fried foods, caffeine, tobacco, and gluten-containing foods

- Screen for food intolerances

SCLERODERMA DECISION TREE

1. Client with scleroderma is interested in using natural products (NP) to support this condition

2. Healthcare provider requests basic background information. The following issues are addressed with the client:
   * Allergies?
   * Prescripton (Rx)/OTC meds?
   * Natural products?
   * Other medical conditions?
   * Nutrition/diet program?
   * Exercise program?

3. Above data reviewed; if **yes** to Rx/OTC meds, review **Drug-Induced Nutrient Depletion Chart** in Appendix

4A. Client is a candidate for natural products

   * An appropriate homeopathic remedy can be used at any time

4B. Client's case is too complicated at this point; needs additional support from MD before initiating NP program

5. Condition-specific questions:
   * Diagnosed by MD? If **yes,** what was the recommended treatment plan? Effective?
   * Triggers for condition/symptom onset? Worsening?
   * Specific organ involvement - skin, gastrointestinal system, lungs, joints, kidneys, heart - each must be addressed by MD

6. See table on following page

SCLERODERMA *(Continued)*

SCLERODERMA*

Category	Natural Products to Consider	DOC
Herb	Olive Leaf *on page 483*	PA
	Evening Primrose *on page 430*	PA
	Horse Chestnut *on page 458*	PA
	Bilberry *on page 392* OR Grape Seed *on page 451*	PA
Vitamin/Mineral/ Trace Element/ Nutraceutical	**N-Acetyl Cysteine (NAC)** *on page 482* Condition-specific dosage: 500 mg 2-3 times/day	PA
	Para-Aminobenzoic Acid (PABA) *on page 485* Condition-specific dosage: 100-400 mg/day	HT
	Fish Oils *on page 434* Condition-specific dosage: 750 mg twice daily	HT
	Vitamin E *on page 529* Condition-specific dosage: 200-400 int. units/day	PA
Homeopathic Remedy	Homeopathic combination formulas are available for many conditions. Listed below are some of the most common single homeopathic remedies for scleroderma. Also see **Homeopathic Quick Reference Chart for Common Complaints** *on page 587*	
	Rhododendron chrysanthum	PD
	Sulphur	PD
	Thuja occidentalis	PD
Additional supplements to consider	No recommendations	

*Refer to **Introduction to Conditions** *on page 41* for more details on how to apply the information in this table to individuals with this condition.

SPECIAL CONSIDERATIONS

Olive Leaf
- No reported toxicity in humans at normal intakes

Evening Primrose
- Contraindicated in seizure disorders, schizophrenia, or in persons receiving anticonvulsant or antipsychotic medications
- Contraindicated in active bleeding (eg, peptic ulcer, intracranial bleeding)
- Caution in hemostatic disorders/history of bleeding
- Potential interaction with anticoagulants (warfarin), aspirin, NSAIDs, anti-platelet agents
- Discontinue use prior to dental or surgical procedures (14 days before)

Horse Chestnut
- Contraindicated in active bleeding (eg, peptic ulcer, intracranial bleeding)
- Caution in hemostatic disorders/history of bleeding
- Potential interactions with anticoagulants (warfarin), aspirin, NSAIDs, anti-platelet agents
- Caution in hepatic or renal impairment
- Discontinue use prior to dental or surgical procedures (14 days before)

Bilberry
- Consult physician if pregnant or breast-feeding
- Contraindicated in active bleeding, including peptic ulcer
- Caution in hemostatic disorders/history of bleeding
- Potential interaction with anticoagulants (warfarin), aspirin, NSAIDs, anti-platelet agents
- Potential interaction with insulin, oral hypoglycemics
- Discontinue prior to dental or surgical procedures (14 days before)

Grape Seed
- Contraindicated in active bleeding (eg, peptic ulcer, intracranial bleeding)
- Caution in hemostatic disorders/history of bleeding
- Potential interaction with anticoagulants (warfarin), aspirin, NSAIDs, anti-platelet agents, methotrexate
- Discontinue use prior to dental or surgical procedures (14 days before)

N-Acetyl Cysteine
- No known toxicity or serious side effects

Para-Aminobenzoic Acid (PABA)
- No known toxicity or serious side effects

Fish Oils
- High doses may cause GI upset, loose stools, nausea
- May alter glucose regulation; use with caution in diabetes
- Caution in individuals receiving oral hypoglycemics or insulin; monitor blood glucose closely and coordinate with prescriber
- Potential interaction with anticoagulants (warfarin), aspirin, NSAIDs, anti-platelet agents

Vitamin E
- Use with caution when taking anticoagulants (vitamin E ≥200 int. units increases prothrombin times)
- Interrupt or reduce dosage one week prior to dental or surgical procedures

SEXUAL VITALITY (FEMALES)

Many people believe that a woman's sexual vitality naturally declines as she reaches menopause. This is a common misconception that is not supported by the psychological and gynecological literature. It is important to realize that a decline in reproductive capacity is not related to a decline in sexual capacity. While some women do experience a decline in their libido at menopause, many others find that the postmenopausal period is a time in their lives when they develop an increased interest in sexual activity.

The production of estrogen declines in all women as they reach menopause. Vaginal dryness is one of the primary symptoms that occurs as estrogen levels decline. This can certainly make intercourse painful and decrease a woman's interest in having sex. However, this condition is easily corrected with the use of either vaginal or oral natural estrogen.

Testosterone is also a critical regulator of a woman's libido. If a woman's sex drive has declined because her body is not producing enough testosterone, providing supplemental testosterone can work wonders in terms of renewing an interest in sex. Testosterone prescription is especially critical for women who have had a total hysterectomy. The ovaries produce both estrogen and testosterone. Doctors routinely prescribe estrogen replacement for women who have had a hysterectomy, but if testosterone is not also replaced, a woman's sex drive may suffer.

Natural progesterone is another hormone that can influence a woman's sexual vitality. Many women who have severe symptoms during menopause actually have a greater need for progesterone supplementation than estrogen.

Dehydroepiandrosterone (DHEA) is a precursor to the sexual hormones. It has also been used successfully to restore women's sexual drive. Some women who do not respond to progesterone alone find that the combination of DHEA and progesterone works well.

Fortunately, relatively inexpensive saliva tests are now available to measure a woman's hormone levels. This helps doctors determine which hormones and what dosages should be used to help restore a woman's normal sexual function and desire.

Nonhormonal factors that could affect a woman's sexual vitality include excess alcohol, various medications, being overweight and/or out of shape physically, and depression.

LIFESTYLE RECOMMENDATIONS

- Continuation/initiation of diet and exercise program

- Avoid alcohol

- Avoid tobacco; if a smoker, consider enrolling in a smoking cessation program

- Avoid drugs of abuse

- Consider stress management counseling if this is a contributing factor

SEXUAL VITALITY (FEMALES) DECISION TREE

1. Female client with an interest in improving sexual vitality is interested in using natural products (NP) to support this condition

2. Healthcare provider requests basic background information. The following issues are addressed with the client:
   * Allergies?
   * Prescription (Rx)/OTC meds?
   * Natural products?
   * Other medical conditions?
   * Nutrition/diet program?
   * Exercise program?

3. Above data reviewed; if **yes** to Rx/OTC meds, review **Drug-Induced Nutrient Depletion Chart** in Appendix

4A. Client is a candidate for natural products

   * An appropriate homeopathic remedy can be used at any time

4B. Client's case is too complicated at this point; needs additional support from MD before initiating NP program

5. Condition-specific questions:
   * Diagnosed by MD? If **yes**, what was the recommended treatment plan? Effective?
   * Triggers for condition/symptom onset? Worsening?
   * Recent lifestyle changes, such as new job, relocation, additional stress at work/home, additional fatigue? This may be the cause of less than desired performance
   * Any conditions that may contribute to decreased sex drive such as diabetes, hormonal changes, hypertension, circulation problems, recent cardiovascular event (ie, MI)?
   * Any medications that may contribute to decreased sex drive such as antihypertensives, antidepressants, antipsychotics, antiandrogenic agents?
   * Are anxiety, depression, or relationship issues a concern? Counseling may be the first choice
   * Is intercourse painful for individual or partner? If **yes**, explore options to reduce or eliminate the problem

6. See table on following page

SEXUAL VITALITY (FEMALES) *(Continued)*

SEXUAL VITALITY (FEMALES)*

Category	Natural Products to Consider	DOC
Herb	**Wild Yam** *on page 532*	PA
	Yohimbe *on page 533*	HE
	Saw Palmetto *on page 500*	HE
	Cordyceps *on page 417*	HT
	Ashwaganda *on page 387*	PA
Vitamin/Mineral/ Trace Element/ Nutraceutical	**Arginine** *on page 385* Condition-specific dosage: 1500–4000 mg/day	HT
Homeopathic Remedy	Homeopathic combination formulas are available for many conditions. Listed below are some of the most common single homeopathic remedies for sexual vitality (females). Also see **Homeopathic Quick Reference Chart for Common Complaints** *on page 587*	
	Agnus castus	PD
	Conium maculatum	PD
	Natrum muriacticum	PD
	Sepia	PD
Additional supplements to consider	No recommendations	

*Refer to **Introduction to Conditions** *on page 41* for more details on how to apply the information in this table to individuals with this condition.

SPECIAL CONSIDERATIONS

Wild Yam
- Potential interactions with steroidal agents
- Use with caution in individuals on hormone replacement therapy or oral contraceptives
- Contraindicated in history of estrogen-dependent tumors or endometrial cancer

Yohimbe
- Contraindicated in hypertension and in individuals taking MAO inhibitors
- Contraindicated in cardiovascular disease and in individuals taking alpha$_2$ blockers

Saw Palmetto
- Caution in individuals receiving alpha-adrenergic blocking agents, finasteride

Cordyceps
- Caution if allergic to molds or fungi
- Theoretical interaction in individuals receiving MAO inhibitors
- Contraindicated in active bleeding (eg, peptic ulcer, intracranial bleeding)
- Caution in hemostatic disorders/history of bleeding
- Potential interaction with anticoagulants (warfarin), aspirin, NSAIDs, antiplatelet agents
- Discontinue use prior to dental or surgical procedures (14 days before)

Ashwaganda
- Contraindicated in pregnancy and breast-feeding

Arginine
- No known toxicity or serious side effects
- Avoid use with sildenafil or vasodilators (nitroglycerin)

SEXUAL VITALITY (MALES)

A number of factors influence male sexual vitality as men age. One of the main factors is the gradual and continual decline in testosterone levels. Studies have reported that there is a gradual reduction in a man's testosterone level, and his sexual performance parallels this decline.

Smoking is known to cause a decline in testosterone levels and reduce male sexual vitality. Smoking is also known to increase the incidence of atherosclerosis. Thus, as plaque begins to build up throughout the vascular system, it will begin to block the small penile arteries at an early stage. This will decrease the amount of blood that is able to flow into the penis, which will gradually inhibit a man's ability to have a satisfactory erection.

Other conditions that are known to reduce a man's sexual performance are depression, excessive ingestion of alcohol, antihypertensive drugs, and diseases such as diabetes, benign prostatic hypertrophy (BPH), cardiovascular disease, and cancer.

Studies have shown that most men who are impotent or who have a low sex drive also have low testosterone levels. Testosterone production is highest at about age 25. By the age of 80, testosterone levels fall from 40.8% to 72.8%, with the average decline being 56.8%.

Hormonal precursors such as dehydroepiandrosterone (DHEA) have been reported to boost testosterone levels and male sexual performance. Testosterone is also available, but requires a prescription. There is still some debate over whether the best results in increasing male sexual vitality are obtained by using testosterone directly or by supplying optimal levels of precursors, such as DHEA and letting the body synthesize testosterone naturally.

LIFESTYLE RECOMMENDATIONS

- Continuation/initiation of diet and exercise program

- Avoid alcohol

- Avoid tobacco; if a smoker, consider enrolling in a smoking cessation program

- Avoid drugs of abuse

- Consider stress management counseling if this is a contributing factor

SEXUAL VITALITY (MALES) DECISION TREE

1. Male client with an interest in improving sexual vitality is interested in using natural products (NP) to support this condition

2. Healthcare provider requests basic background information. The following issues are addressed with the client:
   * Allergies?
   * Prescription (Rx)/OTC meds?
   * Natural products?
   * Other medical conditions?
   * Nutrition/diet program?
   * Exercise program?

3. Above data reviewed; if **yes** to Rx/OTC meds, review **Drug-Induced Nutrient Depletion Chart** in Appendix

4A. Client is a candidate for natural products

* An appropriate homeopathic remedy can be used at any time

4B. Client's case is too complicated at this point; needs additional support from MD before initiating NP program

5. Condition-specific questions:
   * Diagnosed by MD? If **yes**, what was the recommended treatment plan? Effective?
   * Triggers for condition/symptom onset? Worsening?
   * Recent lifestyle changes, such as new job, relocation, additional stress at work/home, additional fatigue? This may be the cause of less than desired performance
   * Any conditions that may contribute to decreased sex drive such as diabetes, hypertension, recent cardiovascular event (ie, MI), circulation problems prostate problems?
   * Any medications that may contribute to decreased sex drive such as antihypertensives, antidepressants, antipsychotics, antiandrogenic agents?
   * Are anxiety, depression, or relationship issues a concern? Counseling may be the first choice
   * Is intercourse painful for individual or partner? If **yes**, explore options to reduce or eliminate the problem

6. See table on following page

SEXUAL VITALITY (MALES) *(Continued)*

SEXUAL VITALITY (MALES)*

Category	Natural Products to Consider	DOC
Herb	**Muira Puama** *on page 481*	HD
	Yohimbe *on page 533*	HT†
	Gingko *on page 441*	HT
	Ashwaganda *on page 387*	PA
	Cordyceps *on page 417*	HT
	Tribulus *on page 511*	PA
Vitamin/Mineral/ Trace Element/ Nutraceutical	**Vitamin C** *on page 526* Condition-specific dosage: 500-1000 mg twice daily	HT
	Vitamin B₁₂ *on page 524* Condition-specific dosage: 1000-6000 mcg/day	HT
	Zinc *on page 534* Condition-specific dosage: 60 mg/day for 45 days **WITH** **Copper** *on page 416* Condition-specific dosing: 4 mg/day	HD
	Arginine *on page 385* Condition-specific dosage: 1500-4000 mg/day	HT
Homeopathic Remedy	Homeopathic combination formulas are available for many conditions. Listed below are some of the most common single homeopathic remedies for sexual vitality (males). Also see **Homeopathic Quick Reference Chart for Common Complaints** *on page 587*	
	Graphites	PD
	Lycopodium clavatum	PD
	Phosphoricum acidum	PD
	Sabal serrulata	PD
Additional supplements to consider	No recommendations	

*Refer to **Introduction to Conditions** *on page 41* for more details on how to apply the information in this table to individuals with this condition.

†Constituent "yohimbine" used in studies.

SPECIAL CONSIDERATIONS

Muira Puama
- No reported toxicity in humans at normal intakes

Yohimbe
- Contraindicated in hypertension and in individuals taking MAO inhibitors
- Contraindicated in cardiovascular disease and in individuals taking alpha$_2$ blockers

Gingko
- Contraindicated in active bleeding (eg, peptic ulcer, intracranial bleeding)
- Caution in hemostatic disorders/history of bleeding
- Potential interaction with anticoagulants (warfarin), aspirin, NSAIDs, anti-platelet agents
- Theoretical interaction with MAO inhibitors, acetylcholinesterase inhibitors (tacrine, donepezil)
- Discontinue use prior to dental or surgical procedures (14 days before)

Ashwaganda
- Contraindicated in pregnancy and breast-feeding

Cordyceps
- Caution if allergic to molds or fungi
- Theoretical interaction in individuals receiving MAO inhibitors
- Contraindicated in active bleeding (eg, peptic ulcer, intracranial bleeding)
- Caution in hemostatic disorders/history of bleeding
- Potential interactions with anticoagulants (warfarin), aspirin, NSAIDs, anti-platelet agents
- Discontinue use prior to dental or surgical procedures (14 days before)

Tribulus
- Caution in individuals taking steroidal medications

Vitamin C
- Excess intake in diabetics may give falsely elevated blood glucose readings

Vitamin B$_{12}$
- No known toxicity or serious side effects

Zinc
- No reported toxicity in humans at normal intakes

Copper
- Contraindicated in Wilson's disease

Arginine
- No known toxicity or serious side effects
- Avoid use with sildenafil or vasodilators (nitroglycerin)

SINUSITIS

Sinusitis is an acute inflammation or infection of the sinus (nasal) passages. The sinuses are lined with mucous membranes which warm, moisten, and filter air that is inhaled into the trachea and lungs. When these membranes become inflamed or infected, swelling inhibits sinus drainage. This causes pressure or pain behind the eyes or temples. Sinus pain may also be referred to the back of the neck. Fever, fatigue, and/or malaise often accompany sinusitis.

Potential factors that may contribute to the development of sinusitis include anatomic barriers to drainage or inflammation from allergic reactions. Bacterial, viral, and fungal organisms may initially colonize and later infect tissues lining the nasal passages. Infrequently, long-term inflammation may lead to destruction of some structures, bacterial seeding of the bloodstream, or spread to closely associated structures including the orbit of the eye and lower brain regions, leading to meningitis.

LIFESTYLE RECOMMENDATIONS

- Avoid use of OTC medicated nasal sprays for more than 3 days; these may actually worsen condition (saline sprays are the exception)

- Do not blow nose too hard; may aggravate sinuses

- Increase water consumption

- Reduce consumption of sugars and dairy products

- Avoid irritants such as tobacco, alcohol, excess dust

- Focus on aerobic exercise; if symptoms worsen, stop until cleared up; if symptoms stay the same or improve, continue

- If related to allergies, seek possible options for allergy issue

- Inhaling steam from a shower may open sinus passages

- If planning to fly, the change in air pressure may aggravate condition

- Wash hands thoroughly and do not share utensils, towels, other items that may facilitate transfer of bacteria or viruses

SINUSITIS DECISION TREE

1. Client with sinusitis is interested in using natural products (NP) to support this condition

2. Healthcare provider requests basic background information. The following issues are addressed with the client:

   * Allergies?   * Other medical conditions?
   * Prescription (Rx)/OTC meds?   * Nutrition/diet program?
   * Natural products?   * Exercise program?

3. Above data reviewed; if **yes** to Rx/OTC meds, review **Drug-Induced Nutrient Depletion Chart** in Appendix

4A. Client is a candidate for natural products

   * An appropriate homeopathic remedy can be used at any time

4B. Client's case is too complicated at this point; needs additional support from MD before initiating NP program

5. Condition-specific questions:
   * Diagnosed by MD? If **yes,** what was the recommended treatment plan? Effective?
   * Triggers for condition/symptom onset? Worsening?
   * Accompanying symptoms/severity - fever, breathing problems?
   * Recent dental procedure?
   * Cold or flu?
   * Secretion color? Monitor during first week of condition; if yellow/green and stays that way, or becomes yellow or green, may indicate worsening condition - refer to MD

6. See table on following page

335

SINUSITIS (Continued)

SINUSITIS*

Category	Natural Products to Consider	DOC
Herb	**Grapefruit Seed Extract** *on page 450*	PA
	Golden Seal *on page 448*	PA, HE
	Bromelain *on page 399*	PA
	Stinging Nettle (Leaf) *on page 505*	PA
	Elderberry *on page 428*	PA, HE
Vitamin/Mineral/ Trace Element/ Nutraceutical	**Quercetin** *on page 494* Condition-specific dosage: 300-400 mg 3 times/day	PA
	Thymus Extract *on page 510* Condition-specific dosage: 250 mg 3 times/day	PA
	Lactobacillus acidophilus *on page 467* and *Bifidobacterium bifidum* *on page 391* Condition-specific dosage: 10-15 billion CFU twice daily (dairy free)	HE
	Vitamin C *on page 526* Condition-specific dosage: 500-1000 mg twice daily	HD
Homeopathic Remedy	Homeopathic combination formulas are available for many conditions. Listed below are some of the most common single homeopathic remedies for sinusitis. Also see **Homeopathic Quick Reference Chart for Common Complaints** *on page 587*	
	Hepar sulphuris calcareum	
	Hydrastis canadensis	
	Kali bichromium	
	Silicea	
Additional supplements to consider	No recommendations	

*Refer to **Introduction to Conditions** *on page 41* for more details on how to apply the information in this table to individuals with this condition.

SPECIAL CONSIDERATIONS

Grapefruit Seed Extract

- Grapefruit seed extract is not equivalent to grapefruit juice/pulp. Juice/pulp has been associated with many drug interactions; see Grapefruit Seed *on page 450*
- Until further information is available, it is reasonable to avoid some medications (terfenadine, astemizole, cisapride). Use other medications metabolized by CYP3A4 with caution.

Golden Seal

- Contraindicated in pregnancy

Bromelain

- Contraindicated in active bleeding (eg, peptic ulcer, intracranial bleeding)
- Potential interaction with anticoagulants (warfarin), aspirin, NSAIDs, anti-platelet agents
- Use with caution in individuals with GI ulceration and/or cardiovascular disorders (hypertension)
- Caution in hemostatic disorders/history of bleeding
- Discontinue use prior to dental or surgical procedures (14 days before)

Stinging Nettle

- Contraindicated in pregnancy

Elderberry

- No reported toxicity in humans at normal intakes

Quercetin

- No known toxicity or serious side effects

Thymus Extract

- No known toxicity or serious side effects

Lactobacillus acidophilus

- No known toxicity or serious side effects

Bifidobacterium bifidum

- No known toxicity or serious side effects

Vitamin C

- Excess intake in diabetics may give falsely elevated blood glucose readings

SORE THROAT

The medical term for the most common form of sore throat is pharyngitis (inflammation of the pharynx, the part of the throat between the tonsils and the larynx). Less frequently, sore throats are due to laryngitis (inflammation of the larynx) or tonsillitis (inflammation of the tonsils).

Pharyngitis is most often caused by infection, either viral/chlamydial (95%) or bacterial (5%). Strep throat is a subset of pharyngitis that is caused by Group A *Streptococcus*. Although viral causes are more frequent, the diagnosis of viral pharyngitis is made only after excluding bacterial infection, particularly after screening or culture for Group A strep. It is extremely important for this screening to occur, since complications from untreated streptococcal pharyngitis include rheumatic fever.

Treatment of viral pharyngitis is directed toward symptom relief. Antibiotics are not effective and may lead to the increased resistance of some bacteria in the community. Gargling with warm salt water (one-half teaspoon of salt in a glass of warm water) several times a day may be soothing, or gargling with 4 drops of grapefruit seed extract, and then swallowing. Pain relief may be facilitated by over-the-counter medications. However, it should be noted that antiseptic lozenges and sprays may aggravate this condition and should be avoided.

Bacterial pharyngitis requires antibiotic treatment. While symptom improvement is only marginally affected by antibiotics, the potential for serious sequelae, such as rheumatic fever, is substantially reduced. The full course of antibiotics should be taken, even if symptoms improve before completion. Use *Lactobacillus acidophilus* concurrently with antibiotics and for 1 week after.

Chronic pharyngitis may be caused by a chronic infection of the sinuses, lungs, or mouth, or by constant irritation from environmental irritants, smoking, or by exposure to swallowed substances that scald, corrode, or scratch the throat. Chronic pharyngitis requires treatment of the underlying cause.

Pharyngitis usually resolves over a 7- to 10-day period.

LIFESTYLE RECOMMENDATIONS

- Increase consumption of quality water

- If symptom does not resolve within 2 weeks, contact physician; if not tested for allergies, discuss this option with physician at this point

- Avoid tobacco, alcohol, spicy foods, and anything else that may aggravate the throat area

SORE THROAT DECISION TREE

---

1. Client with sore throat is interested in using natural products (NP) to support this condition

↓

2. Healthcare provider requests basic background information. The following issues are addressed with the client:
   * Allergies?
   * Prescription (Rx)/OTC meds?
   * Natural products?
   * Other medical conditions?
   * Nutrition/diet program?
   * Exercise program?

↓

3. Above data reviewed; if **yes** to Rx/OTC meds, review **Drug-Induced Nutrient Depletion Chart** in Appendix

↓

4A. Client is a candidate for natural products

   * An appropriate homeopathic remedy can be used at any time

4B. Client's case is too complicated at this point; needs additional support from MD before initiating NP program

↓

5. Condition-specific questions:
   * Evaluated by MD? If **yes,** what was the recommended treatment plan? Effective? Reinforce adherence to present therapy
   * Triggers for condition/symptom onset? Worsening?
   * Acute onset should be evaluated by MD to rule-out streptococcal infection
   * If rapid onset with fever ≥102°F may signal bacterial infection and require assessment by MD
   * Recent dental procedure?
   * Recent exposure to someone with a cold, flu, viral illness?
   * Other symptoms: Redness in throat, fever, nausea, diarrhea, vomiting, congestion, watery eyes, headache? May need to refer depending on duration, severity, and number of symptoms
   * Any concomitant conditions that would cause significant concern, such as malignancies, immunologic conditions?

↓

6. See table on following page

SORE THROAT *(Continued)*

SORE THROAT*

Category	Natural Products to Consider	DOC
Herb	**Marshmallow** *on page 476*	PA, HE
	Elderberry *on page 428*	PA
	Golden Seal *on page 448*	PA, HE
	Grapefruit Seed Extract (Leaf) *on page 450*	HT
Vitamin/Mineral/ Trace Element/ Nutraceutical	**Zinc** *on page 534* Condition-specific dosage: Lozenge: Dissolve 1 lozenge every 2-3 hours	PA
Homeopathic Remedy	Homeopathic combination formulas are available for many conditions. Listed below are some of the most common single homeopathic remedies for sore throat. Also see **Homeopathic Quick Reference Chart for Common Complaints** *on page 587*	
	Apis mellifica	PD
	Atropa belladonna	PD
	Crotalus horridus	PD
	Mercurius corrosivus	PD
	Phosphorus	PD
Additional supplements to consider	**Vitamin A** *on page 518* Condition-specific dosage: 10,000-35,000 int. units/day	PA
	Vitamin C *on page 526* Condition-specific dosage: 250-1000 mg/day	HT

*Refer to **Introduction to Conditions** *on page 41* for more details on how to apply the information in this table to individuals with this condition.

SPECIAL CONSIDERATIONS

Marshmallow
- May alter blood glucose; monitor blood sugar closely in diabetics or those predisposed to hypoglycemia
- Potential interactions with insulin, oral hypoglycemic agents

Elderberry
- No reported toxicity in humans at normal intakes

Golden Seal
- Contraindicated in pregnancy

Grapefruit Seed Extract
- Grapefruit seed extract is not equivalent to grapefruit juice/pulp. Juice/pulp has been associated with many drug interactions; see Grapefruit Seed *on page 450*
- Until further information is available, it is reasonable to avoid some medications (terfenadine, astemizole, cisapride). Use other medications metabolized by CYP3A4 with caution.

Zinc Lozenges
- No reported toxicity in humans at normal intakes

Vitamin A
- Contraindicated in pregnancy or in women who may become pregnant

Vitamin C
- Excess intake in diabetics may give falsely elevated blood glucose readings

STRESS / ANXIETY

A number of factors that initiate a distinct collective spectrum of physiologic and psychological responses are referred to as "stress." The neuroendocrine system, in particular, is activated in situations that are perceived as threatening or challenging. This is an adaptive response in the short-term that may become detrimental if sustained.

Catecholamines, or stress response hormones, result in sympathetic activation, causing decreased sweating, increased heart rate, bronchodilation, muscle tension, and increased sensory activation. Increased cortisol release increases mobilization of glucose and alteration of salt and water excretion. Collectively, this is referred to as the "fight-or-flight" response. Sustained responses eventually lead to fatigue and depression as well as physiologic consequences that include hyperlipidemia, hypothyroidism, neurological complications, and hyperinsulinemia.

Anxiety is a psychological state that often accompanies anticipated or actual stressful situations. In some cases, it may lead to avoidance. Environmental factors, exposure to stimulants, and emotional and psychological composition help to define an individual's ability to accommodate and adapt to stress. In particular, repetitive exposure may diminish the ability to adapt to stress.

LIFESTYLE RECOMMENDATIONS

- Continuation/initiation of diet and exercise program

- Consider enrolling in a stress management program

- Establish a support network

- Find activities that help reduce stress, focusing on activities that bring pleasure to everyday living and contribute to positive feelings and self-worth

- Avoid or reduce alcohol, caffeine, dairy products, tobacco, coffee, tea, foods high in fat or sugar content

- Increase consumption of vegetables and fruits

- Attempt to achieve consistent sleep patterns and eating habits

- Keep a diary of symptoms, feelings, responses to various changes, and interventions; attempt to pinpoint what helps and what does not

STRESS / ANXIETY DECISION TREE

1. Client with stress or anxiety is interested in using natural products (NP) to support this condition

2. Healthcare provider requests basic background information. The following issues are addressed with the client:

   * Allergies?
   * Prescription (Rx)/OTC meds?
   * Natural products?
   * Other medical conditions?
   * Nutrition/diet program?
   * Exercise program?

3. Above data reviewed; if **yes** to Rx/OTC meds, review **Drug-Induced Nutrient Depletion Chart** in Appendix

4A. Client is a candidate for natural products

   * An appropriate homeopathic remedy can be used at any time

4B. Client's case is too complicated at this point; needs additional support from MD before initiating NP program

5. Condition-specific questions:
   * Diagnosed by MD? If **yes**, what was the recommended treatment plan? Effective?
   * Triggers for condition/symptom onset? Worsening?
   * Effect of condition on quality of life, daily activities, such as sleep, family life, occupation, eating habits?
   * Recently entered into behavior modification program, such as smoking cessation or weight loss program? Additional stress may be contributing to new symptoms
   * Diagnosed with mitral valve prolapse? May be related; discuss with MD
   * There are many specific anxiety disorders - make sure client understands importance of seeking medical attention to obtain accurate diagnosis, if client has not done so already

6. See table on following page

STRESS / ANXIETY (Continued)

STRESS / ANXIETY*

Category	Natural Products to Consider	DOC
Herb	Kava Kava on page 466	HT
	Valerian on page 515	HT
	Chamomile on page 407	HD
	St John's Wort on page 506	HD
Vitamin/Mineral/ Trace Element/ Nutraceutical	Adrenal Extract on page 380 Condition-specific dosage: 150-200 mg 3 times/day	PA
	Magnesium Malate on page 473 Condition-specific dosage: 400-600 mg 3 time/day	HT
	Vitamin C on page 526 Condition-specific dosage: 500-1000 mg twice daily	HD
Homeopathic Remedy	Homeopathic combination formulas are available for many conditions. Listed below are some of the most common single homeopathic remedies for stress/ anxiety. Also see **Homeopathic Quick Reference Chart for Common Complaints** on page 587	
	Aconitum napellus	PD
	Ignatia amara	PD
	Phosphoricum acidum	PD
Additional supplements to consider	Vitamin B Complex-25 on page 526 Condition-specific dosage: 25-50 mg twice daily	PA

*Refer to **Introduction to Conditions** on page 41 for more details on how to apply the information in this table to individuals with this condition.

SPECIAL CONSIDERATIONS

Kava Kava
- Contraindicated in pregnancy and breast-feeding, or Parkinson's disease
- May cause drowsiness or sedation (higher doses); caution when driving/performing hazardous tasks
- Potential interactions with ethanol, CNS depressants

Valerian
- May cause drowsiness; caution when driving/performing hazardous tasks
- Effects do not appear to be potentiated by ethanol
- Do not use in children <3 years of age; use only valepotriate and baldrinal-free in children <12 years of age
- Increased effect/toxicity: CNS depressants, sedative-hypnotics (barbiturates), antidepressants, anxiolytics, antihistamines

Chamomile
- Avoid use in individuals with allergies to *Asteraceae/Compositae* family (chrysanthemum, daisy) or ragweed pollens
- May cause drowsiness; caution in driving/performing hazardous tasks

St John's Wort
- Contraindicated in pregnancy
- Not for use in severe depression
- May cause drowsiness (mild); caution in driving/performing hazardous tasks
- May cause photosensitivity (rare) at high intakes
- Potential interactions with antidepressants (including SSRIs, tricyclics, MAO inhibitors), narcotics, other CNS depressants, reserpine, digoxin

Adrenal Extract
- May cause excitability when taken in large doses

Magnesium Malate
- Use caution in renal impairment
- May cause diarrhea at high intakes

Vitamin C
- Excess intake may give falsely elevated blood glucose readings

Vitamin B Complex-25
- No side effects at the RDI or ODA doses

SUNBURN

Sunburn is a common affliction resulting from prolonged exposure to ultraviolet light. Its severity depends on the skin type, duration of exposure, and intensity of the ultraviolet light, particularly in the UVB range (290-320 nm). Absorption of this wavelength by melanocytes promotes the production of melanin, deepening the pigmentation of the skin. However, it also promotes damage to other cellular structures and prompts an erythematous inflammatory reaction. The inflammatory reaction begins 1-24 hours after exposure. Erythema appears to be mediated by prostaglandins and possibly other inflammatory mediators.

The initial stage of sunburn is a minor first-degree burn that only involves the epidermis or outer layer of skin. Symptoms of simple sunburn are pain and tenderness. If the sunburn causes blistering and swelling of the skin, a second-degree burn has occurred. Severe sunburn over an extensive surface area can cause a systemic inflammatory response including fever and weakness. Shock may occur and hospitalization may be required.

In minor sunburns, the intensity of inflammation usually subsides within 72 hours and the increased melanin results in tanning of the skin. Increased turnover of epithelial cells results in skin peeling after several days. Epidermal hyperplasia may occur with repeated exposures.

Long-term effects include changes in the appearance of the skin (thickening and wrinkling), as well as an increased risk of basal cell carcinoma and squamous cell melanoma. Ultraviolet light may also cause retinal damage and contribute to cataract formation. A number of medications, including fluoroquinolones, tetracyclines, phenothiazines, tricyclic antidepressants, sulfonamides, and nitrofurantoin may result in photosensitization. Avoidance of exposure to sunlight is prudent. Individuals should be evaluated for potential photosensitizing factors when the degree of inflammation appears to be disproportionate to the exposure.

LIFESTYLE RECOMMENDATIONS

- Use sunscreen with a high SPF on skin and lips as a preventive measure, and reapply moderate amounts frequently, especially if swimming. Suggest sunscreens labeled with the "waterproof" designation; they offer the best protection when swimming, but still must reapply every 60-90 minutes if in the water. Use extreme caution when applying near the eyes.

- Increase consumption of quality water

- Wear loose protective clothing, including a hat

- Avoid exposure to the sun during the hours of 10 AM to 3 PM

- Cool compresses may help relieve pain

SUNBURN DECISION TREE

1. Client with sunburn is interested in using natural products (NP) to support this condition

2. Healthcare provider requests basic background information. The following issues are addressed with the client:

   * Allergies?
   * Prescription (Rx)/OTC meds?
   * Natural products?
   * Other medical conditions?
   * Nutrition/diet program?
   * Exercise program?

3. Above data reviewed; if **yes** to Rx/OTC meds, review **Drug-Induced Nutrient Depletion Chart** in Appendix

4A. Client is a candidate for natural products

   * An appropriate homeopathic remedy can be used at any time

4B. Client's case is too complicated at this point; needs additional support from MD before initiating NP program

5. Condition-specific questions:
   * Condition reviewed by MD? If **yes,** what was the recommended treatment plan? Effective?
   * Triggers for symptoms worsening?
   * Is the client taking any meds that might cause sensitivity to light, photosensitivity? Pharmacist can review med list and assess this on an individual basis
   * Skin blistered? If **yes,** keep clean, prevent infection
   * Accompanying symptoms: Fever, chills, confusion; if **yes** to fever or confusion, refer to MD

6. See table on following page

SUNBURN *(Continued)*

SUNBURN*

Category	Natural Products to Consider	DOC
Herb	**Aloe** *on page 381*	HD
	Lavender (Topical) *on page 468*	HE
	St John's Wort *on page 506*	HE
Vitamin/Mineral/ Trace Element/ Nutraceutical	**Vitamin C** *on page 526* Condition-specific dosage: 2000 mg/day	HD
	Vitamin E *on page 529* Condition-specific dosage: 800 int. units/day	PA
Homeopathic Remedy	Homeopathic combination formulas are available for many conditions. Listed below are some of the most common single homeopathic remedies for sunburn. Also see **Homeopathic Quick Reference Chart for Common Complaints** *on page 587*	
	Apis mellifica	PD
	Atropa belladonna	PD
	Calendula officinalis (Topical)	PD
	Hypericum	PD
Additional supplements to consider	No recommendations	

*Refer to **Introduction to Conditions** *on page 41* for more details on how to apply the information in this table to individuals with this condition.

SPECIAL CONSIDERATIONS

Aloe
- No known toxicity or serious side effects

Lavender
- For topical or inhalation use only

St John's Wort
- Contraindicated in pregnancy
- Not for use in severe depression
- May cause drowsiness (mild); caution in driving/performing hazardous tasks
- May cause photosensitivity (rare) at high dosages
- Potential interactions with antidepressants (including SSRIs, tricyclics, MAO inhibitors), narcotics, other CNS depressants, digoxin, reserpine
- Topically, no reported toxicity

Vitamin C
- Excess intake in diabetics may give falsely elevated blood glucose readings

Vitamin E
- Use with caution when taking anticoagulants (vitamin E ≥200 int. units increases prothrombin times)
- Interrupt or reduce dosage one week prior to dental or surgical procedures

SYSTEMIC LUPUS ERYTHEMATOSUS (SLE)

Systemic lupus erythematosus (SLE), also known as lupus, is a chronic autoimmune inflammatory disease of the connective tissue. The prevalence of lupus ranges from 40-50 individuals per 100,000 population. It is 2-3 times as prevalent in African-Americans, Hispanics, and Asians. Women are up to ten times more likely to be affected with this condition and women of child-bearing age are most likely to be affected.

Although a specific cause has not been identified, the disease has been linked to a genetic predisposition plus possible viral, environmental, or digestive system triggers. Based on the observed differences in men and women, a hormonal influence may also play a role. It has been estimated that 3-4 distinct genes are responsible for a genetic predisposition to lupus.

Lupus is a multisystem inflammatory disorder. Symptoms depend on the involvement and degree of inflammation in a particular organ system. General symptoms of lupus include skin rash, joint pain, malaise, weakness, fatigue, and weight loss. Joint involvement usually includes the knees, ankles, or wrists. The joint inflammation is usually nondeforming. Kidney damage is common, resulting from inflammatory reaction to glomerular components. In addition, respiratory complications may occur in up to 50% of individuals including pleurisy, coughing, and/or dyspnea. Cardiovascular complications include pericarditis, coronary artery disease, hypertension, and anemia. Neurologic symptoms include depression, anxiety, psychosis, headaches, seizures, and neuropathies.

Lupus tends to flare episodically. The prognosis is dependent upon involvement of specific organ systems (renal, central nervous system, and cardiac) and the aggressiveness of the inflammatory process.

LIFESTYLE RECOMMENDATIONS

- Continuation/initiation of diet and exercise program

- Increase consumption of whole foods

- Lupus increases risk of infection, bleeding - take necessary precautions

- Avoid dairy products, red meat, caffeine, alcohol, salt, tobacco, sugar, peppers, tomatoes, white potatoes

- Avoid prolonged exposure to the sun - may require a vitamin D supplement

- Oral contraceptives or hormonal replacement therapy may exacerbate condition - consult with physician before using

LUPUS DECISION TREE

1. Client with lupus is interested in using natural products (NP) to support this condition

2. Healthcare provider requests basic background information. The following issues are addressed with the client:
   * Allergies?
   * Prescription (Rx)/OTC meds?
   * Natural products?
   * Other medical conditions?
   * Nutrition/diet program?
   * Exercise program?

3. Above data reviewed; if **yes** to Rx/OTC meds, review **Drug-Induced Nutrient Depletion Chart** in Appendix

4A. Client is a candidate for natural products

   * An appropriate homeopathic remedy can be used at any time

4B. Client's case is too complicated at this point; needs additional support from MD before initiating NP program

5. Condition-specific questions:
   * Diagnosis by MD? Treatment plan?
   * Precipitating factors that make condition worse?
   * Any interventions that improve symptoms?

6. See table on following page

SYSTEMIC LUPUS ERYTHEMATOSUS (SLE) *(Continued)*

LUPUS*

Category	Natural Products to Consider	DOC
Herb	Cat's Claw *on page 404*	PA
	Bupleurum *on page 400*	PA
	Rehmannia *on page 497*	PA
Vitamin/Mineral/ Trace Element/ Nutraceutical	**Dehydroepiandrosterone (DHEA)** *on page 421* Determined by clinician	HT
	Lactobacillus acidophilus *on page 467* and **Bifidobacterium bifidum** *on page 391* Condition-specific dosage: 2-5 billion CFU twice daily (dairy free)	PA
	N-Acetyl Cysteine *on page 482* Condition-specific dosage: 200-1200 mg/day	PA
	Thymus Extract *on page 510* Condition-specific dosage: 250 mg 3 times/day	HT
	Vitamin E *on page 529* Condition-specific dosage: 400-800 int. units/day	HD
Homeopathic Remedy	Homeopathic combination formulas are available for many conditions. Listed below are some of the most common single homeopathic remedies for lupus. Also see **Homeopathic Quick Reference Chart for Common Complaints** *on page 587*	
	Apis mellifica	PD
	Arsenicum album	PD
	Causticum	PD
	Rhus toxicodendron	PD
	Ruta graveolens	PD
	Thuja occidentalis	PD
Additional supplements to consider	**Flaxseed Oil** *on page 435* Condition-specific dosage: 1 Tbsp/day	PA

*Refer to **Introduction to Conditions** *on page 41* for more details on how to apply the information in this table to individuals with this condition.

SPECIAL CONSIDERATIONS

Cat's Claw
- Contraindicated in transplant recipients, individuals receiving I.V. immuno-globulins or immunosuppressants
- Contraindicated in active bleeding (eg, peptic ulcer, intracranial bleeding)
- Caution in hemostatic disorders/history of bleeding
- Potential interaction with anticoagulants (warfarin), aspirin, NSAIDs, anti-platelet agents
- Discontinue use prior to dental or surgical procedures (14 days before)

Bupleurum
- Use with caution in diabetes, hypertension, edema
- Theoretical interaction with corticosteroids, diuretics, antihypertensives, anti-diabetic agents

Rehmannia
- Caution in organ transplant and individuals taking immunosuppressants

Dehydroepiandrosterone (DHEA)
- Contraindicated in individuals with a history of prostate or breast cancer
- Potential interaction with hormonal agents, hypoglycemics, insulin
- Contraindicated in hypertension
- Caution in congestive heart failure

Lactobacillus acidophilus
- No known toxicity or serious side effects

Bifidobacterium bifidum
- No known toxicity or serious side effects

N-Acetyl Cysteine
- No known toxicity or serious side effects

Thymus Extract
- No known toxicity or serious side effects

Vitamin E
- Use with caution when taking anticoagulants (vitamin E ≥200 int. units increases prothrombin times)
- Interrupt or reduce dosage one week prior to dental or surgical procedures

Flaxseed Oil
- No known toxicity or serious side effects

TEETHING

Teething usually starts between 5-7 months of age. Typically, the two bottom front teeth appear first, followed by the four upper front teeth. Approximately one month later, the bottom incisors appear. The first molars appear next, followed by the canines. The ages at which teeth appear is highly variable, and parents should not be alarmed if the child does not begin this process until later.

Teething may result in irritability, crying, low-grade fever, excessive drooling, and a desire to chew on something hard. Many parents report episodes of loose stools in association with teething. The gums around the new teeth are often swollen and tender. Fever >100°F, persistent fever, or significant discomfort should prompt evaluation of other causes.

LIFESTYLE RECOMMENDATIONS

- Continue same feeding schedule whenever possible
- If child has teething objects, ensure that they are safe, will not break and have no small pieces that might break off and could be swallowed.
- Massage child's gums
- Clean teeth and gums frequently with a moist, soft cloth
- Reassure first-time parents that this is only temporary, and when a tooth breaks through the gum line, symptoms usually resolve quickly.

TEETHING DECISION TREE

1. Client with teething child is interested in using natural products (NP) to support this condition

2. Healthcare provider requests basic background information. The following issues are addressed with client:

* Allergies?
* Prescription (Rx)/OTC meds?
* Natural products?

* Other medical conditions?
* Nutrition/diet program?
* Exercise program?

3. Above data reviewed; if **yes** to Rx/OTC meds, review **Drug-Induced Nutrient Depletion Chart** in Appendix

4A. Client is a candidate for natural products

* An appropriate homeopathic remedy can be used at any time

4B. Client's case is too complicated at this point; needs additional support from MD before initiating NP program

5. Condition-specific questions:
* Evaluation by MD? If **yes,** what was the recommended treatment plan? Effective?
* Triggers for condition/symptom onset? Worsening?
* Other symptoms, such as fever or malaise? Seek medical attention
* How does this situation affect feeding? Sleep?

6. See table on following page

TEETHING *(Continued)*

TEETHING*

Category	Natural Products to Consider	DOC
Herb	**Tea Tree** (Topical) *on page 509* (Apply to gums)	HE
	Clove (Topical) *on page 411* (Apply to gums)	HE
	Chamomile (Tea form) *on page 407*	HE
	Lemon Balm/Melissa *on page 469*	PA
Vitamin/Mineral/ Trace Element/ Nutraceutical	No recommendations	
Homeopathic Remedy	Homeopathic combination formulas are available for many conditions. Listed below are some of the most common single homeopathic remedies for teething. Also see **Homeopathic Quick Reference Chart for Common Complaints** *on page 587*	
	Calcarea fluorica	PD
	Calcarea phosphorica	PD
	Chamomilla	PD
	Mercurius corrosivus	PD
Additional supplements to consider	No recommendations	

*Refer to **Introduction to Conditions** *on page 41* for more details on how to apply the information in this table to individuals with this condition.

SPECIAL CONSIDERATIONS

Tea Tree
- May cause allergic dermatitis in sensitive individuals
- Not for ingestion

Clove
- For topical application only
- Do not use for >48 hours; may cause gingival damage

Chamomile
- Avoid use in individuals with allergies to *Asteraceae/Compositae* family (chrysanthemum, daisy) or ragweed pollens
- May cause drowsiness; caution in driving/performing hazardous tasks

Lemon Balm/Melissa
- No reported toxicity in humans at normal intakes

ULCER (APHTHOUS)

Often referred to as canker sores, these ulcerations are painful, shallow, rounded areas that generally occur on the cheek, inside lip, or tongue. They are extremely common with >20% of the U.S. population experiencing at least one episode. They begin as small red spots and progress to shallow ulcerations in 4-7 days. The ulcer is coated by a white pseudomembrane that gradually heals. Small ulcers heal in 7-14 days, while larger ulcers may require weeks. The main feature of canker sores is pain – they hurt. Pain is exacerbated by physical contact as well as acidic foods and liquids. Recurrence is common, particularly in immunosuppressed individuals. Lesions may be single or multiple.

Individuals with specific systemic diseases may be prone to multiple and severe occurrences (Crohn's disease, HIV, and inflammatory bowel disease). Females and nonsmokers are at greater risk. Viruses, bacteria, hormonal and gluten sensitivity have been associated, but the cause has not been determined. Nutritional deficiencies have been documented in many individuals, including a deficiency of iron, folate, and vitamin B_{12}.

Canker sores should not be confused with cold sores. Cold sores are caused by the herpes virus, are highly contagious, and usually reappear in the same place. Canker sores are not contagious and occur in different locations in the mouth.

LIFESTYLE RECOMMENDATIONS

- Increase consumption of water
- Avoid triggers
- Prepare for possible outbreak when exposed to triggers
- Avoid spicy foods, chocolate, sweets, sugar
- Keep lips and mouth clean - wash carefully
- Use ice wrapped in washcloth to ease pain
- Use sunblock on lips when outside in the sun

APHTHOUS ULCER (CANKER SORE) DECISION TREE

1. Client with aphthous ulcer (canker sore) is interested in using natural products (NP) to support this condition

2. Healthcare provider requests basic background information. The following issues are addressed with the client:

   * Allergies?
   * Prescription (Rx)/OTC meds?
   * Natural products?
   * Other medical conditions?
   * Nutrition/diet program?
   * Exercise program?

3. Above data reviewed; if **yes** to Rx/OTC meds, review **Drug-Induced Nutrient Depletion Chart** in Appendix

4A. Client is a candidate for natural products

   * An appropriate homeopathic remedy can be used at any time

4B. Client's case is too complicated at this point; needs additional support from MD before initiating NP program

5. Condition-specific questions:
   * Diagnosed by MD? If **yes,** what was the recommended treatment plan? Effective?
   * Triggers for condition/symptom onset? Worsening?
   * Client taking immunosuppressant therapy? May contribute to condition onset and/or duration; discuss with healthcare provider

6. See table on following page

ULCER (APHTHOUS) *(Continued)*

APHTHOUS ULCER (CANKER SORE)*

Category	Natural Products to Consider	DOC
Herb	**Tea Tree** (Topical) *on page 509*	PA
	Chamomile (Oral Rinse) *on page 407*	HD
Vitamin/Mineral/ Trace Element/ Nutraceutical	**Zinc** *on page 534* Condition-specific dosage: 15-35 mg/day	HD
	Lysine *on page 473* Condition-specific dosage: 500 mg 3 times/day	PA
	Lactobacillus acidophilus *on page 467* and ***Bifidobacterium bifidum*** *on page 391* Condition-specific dosage: 2-5 billion CFU twice daily (dairy free) **AND/OR** Empty 2 capsules into a cup of water and swish as a mouthwash twice daily (dairy free)	HD
	Folic Acid *on page 435* Condition-specific dosage: 800 mcg/day	HD
Homeopathic Remedy	Homeopathic combination formulas are available for many conditions. Listed below are some of the most common single homeopathic remedies for aphthous ulcer (canker sore). Also see **Homeopathic Quick Reference Chart for Common Complaints** *on page 587*	
	Borax	PD
	Kali muriaticum	PD
	Natrum muriaticum	PD
Additional supplements to consider	No recommendations	

*Refer to **Introduction to Conditions** *on page 41* for more details on how to apply the information in this table to individuals with this condition.

SPECIAL CONSIDERATIONS

Tea Tree
- May cause allergic dermatitis in sensitive individuals
- Not for ingestion

Chamomile
- Avoid use in individuals with allergies to *Asteraceae/Compositae* family (chrysanthemum, daisy) or ragweed pollens
- May cause drowsiness; caution in driving/performing hazardous tasks

Zinc
- No reported toxicity in humans at normal intakes

Lysine
- No known toxicity or serious side effects

Lactobacillis acidophilus
- No known toxicity or serious side effects

Bifidobacterium bifidum
- No known toxicity or serious side effects

Folic Acid
- No known toxicity or serious side effects

ULCER (DUODENAL AND PEPTIC)

Peptic ulcers are disruptions in the protective layer of the stomach or duodenum, which is the first part of the gastrointestinal tract. Approximately 10% of Americans will develop some form of peptic ulcer disease. It has recently been determined that the majority of ulcers are due to bacteria known as *Helicobacter pylori* (*H. pylori*). It is estimated that over 90% of duodenal ulcers, and from 70% to 75% of gastric ulcers, are caused by *H. pylori*. Most of the ulcers not caused by *H. pylori* are believed to result from irritations and ulcerations from medications such as aspirin and nonsteroidal anti-inflammatory drugs (NSAIDs).

Normally, the gastrointestinal tract is uniquely designed to harbor digestive enzymes and acidic secretions, which maintain a protective barrier of mucus and buffering agents for the inner surfaces. When these protective mechanisms are overwhelmed due to underproduction of protective components, overproduction of irritating substances, or erosion of the protective barrier by *H. pylori*, inflammation of the lining may occur. Symptoms include a burning, gnawing abdominal pain and upset stomach. Some ulcer pain may be relieved by food. Symptoms may last for hours. Associated symptoms may include bloating, anorexia, weight loss, nausea, or vomiting.

With severe erosion of the surface, inflammation may extend deeper into the tissue and potentially result in deep ulceration and/or perforation. Blood loss may be significant, possibly resulting in hematemesis or black, tarry melanotic stools. The presence of postural hypotension is particularly significant, indicating a substantial loss of blood. Perforation may be life-threatening, resulting in sepsis or shock.

Foods that are extremely spicy or high in fat can also cause irritation and should be avoided. Eating small, frequent meals, and taking aluminum-free antacids may relieve pain in some individuals.

Ulcers usually heal with treatment, but a high rate of relapse has been noted, particularly if an ulcer is caused by *H. pylori* and the organism is not eradicated. Diet and lifestyle modifications are usually required in order to accomplish complete and long-term eradication of *H. pylori*. Amino acids such as L-glutamine are conditionally essential due to the need for glutamine in rebuilding healthy surface cells of the intestines and stomach.

LIFESTYLE RECOMMENDATIONS

- Increase consumption of vegetables, fruits, soft foods, and fiber

- Avoid triggers, including foods or behaviors, that contribute to worsening of symptoms

- If a smoker, consider enrolling in a smoking cessation program

- Avoid alcohol, caffeine, spicy foods, citrus fruits, sugar, fats

- If using OTC medication for symptom relief, make sure physician is aware

- May want to consider increasing number of meals, decreasing meal size

- Increase clear fluid consumption

ULCER (DUODENAL / PEPTIC) DECISION TREE

1. Client with duodenal or peptic ulcer disease is interested in using natural products (NP) to support this condition

2. Healthcare provider requests basic background information. The following issues are addressed with the client:

   * Allergies?
   * Prescription (Rx)/OTC meds?
   * Natural products?
   * Other medical conditions?
   * Nutrition/diet program?
   * Exercise program?

3. Above data reviewed; if **yes** to Rx/OTC meds, review **Drug-Induced Nutrient Depletion Chart** in Appendix

4A. Client is a candidate for natural products

   * An appropriate homeopathic remedy can be used at any time

4B. Client's case is too complicated at this point; needs additional support from MD before initiating NP program

5. Condition-specific questions:
   * Diagnosed by MD? If **yes,** what was the recommended treatment plan? Effective?
   * Triggers for condition/symptom onset? Worsening?
   * Any new meds? Meds that may contribute include NSAIDs, hormones, tricyclic antidepressants, calcium channel blockers, corticosteroids, narcotics
   * Tested for *Helicobacter pylori*?
   * Severity of pain? Cause awakening at night?
   * Other symptoms?
   * Blood in stool or vomitus? If **yes,** refer to MD

6. See table on following page

ULCER (DUODENAL AND PEPTIC) *(Continued)*

ULCER (DUODENAL / PEPTIC)*

Category	Natural Products to Consider	DOC
Herb	Licorice (DGL) *on page 470*	HT
	Mastic *on page 477*	PA
	Marshmallow *on page 476*	PA
Vitamin/Mineral/ Trace Element/ Nutraceutical	Glutamine *on page 446* Condition-specific dosage: 2000-3000 mg 3 times/day	HT
	Bismuth *on page 393* Condition-specific dosage: 120 mg 4 times/day for no longer than 6-8 weeks	HD
	Vitamin C (Buffered) *on page 526* Condition-specific dosage: 250-1000 mg/day	PA
Homeopathic Remedy	Homeopathic combination formulas are available for many conditions. Listed below are some of the most common single homeopathic remedies for ulcer (duodenal/peptic). Also see **Homeopathic Quick Reference Chart for Common Complaints** *on page 587*	
	Bismuthum oxydatum	
	Hydrastis canadensis	
	Nux vomica	
Additional supplements to consider	Vitamin B₆ *on page 523* Condition-specific dosage: 10-20 mg/day	PA
	Vitamin E *on page 529* Condition-specific dosage: 200-400 int. units/day	PA

*Refer to **Introduction to Conditions** *on page 41* for more details on how to apply the information in this table to individuals with this condition.

SPECIAL CONSIDERATIONS

Licorice (DGL)
- Contraindicated in pregnancy and breast-feeding
- Potential interaction with nitrofurantoin

Mastic
- No known toxicity or serious side effects

Marshmallow
- May alter blood glucose; monitor blood sugar closely in diabetics or those predisposed to hypoglycemia
- Potential interactions with insulin, oral hypoglycemic agents

Glutamine
- No known toxicity or serious side effects

Bismuth
- Possible neurological toxicity with long-term use
- Treatment should not last longer than 6-8 weeks

Vitamin C
- Excess intake in diabetics may give falsely elevated blood glucose readings

Vitamin B$_6$
- No reported toxicity in humans at normal intakes

Vitamin E
- Use with caution when taking anticoagulants (vitamin E $\geq$200 int. units increases prothrombin times)
- Interrupt or reduce dosage one week prior to dental or surgical procedures

ULCERATIVE COLITIS

Ulcerative colitis is a chronic inflammation of colonic mucosa. It differs from Crohn's disease in that it exclusively affects the colon, and the inflammatory changes are limited to colonic mucosa, rather than encompassing the entire thickness of the bowel wall. Systemic symptoms of fatigue, malaise, and fever are less common.

Ulcerative colitis is associated with abdominal cramping, urgency, frequent defecation, diarrhea, and bloody stools. Long remissions are possible between flare-ups of the disease. Ulcerative colitis develops in less than 1 in 10,000 individuals. Individuals are typically between 15-35 years of age. It is most common among Caucasians and a strong genetic predisposition may be observed in specific ethnic groups, such as Ashkenazi Jews.

Systemic effects such as arthritis, skin rashes, or eye inflammation may occur, but these are less common than in Crohn's disease. Fistula formation is rare, and nutritional compromise is less extreme than in Crohn's disease. Severe colitis, toxic megacolon, fever, and abdominal swelling and pain should prompt emergent evaluation. Ulcerative colitis has been associated with an increased risk for colon cancer. The risk increases with the duration of affliction. Surgical colectomy is curative.

LIFESTYLE RECOMMENDATIONS

- Avoid sugar, dairy products, caffeine, alcohol, tobacco, other irritating foods

- Eat soft foods, vegetables, greens, juices, fiber

- Investigate stress reduction techniques

- Monitor nutrition intake; work with a healthcare provider (ie, dietician) for specific meal planning to ensure adequate caloric consumption

ULCERATIVE COLITIS DECISION TREE

1. Client with ulcerative colitis is interested in using natural products (NP) to support this condition

2. Healthcare provider requests basic background information. The following issues are addressed with the client:

   * Allergies?
   * Prescription (Rx)/OTC meds?
   * Natural products?
   * Other medical conditions?
   * Nutrition/diet program?
   * Exercise program?

3. Above data reviewed; if **yes** to Rx/OTC meds, review **Drug-Induced Nutrient Depletion Chart** in Appendix

4A. Client is a candidate for natural products

   * An appropriate homeopathic remedy can be used at any time

4B. Client's case is too complicated at this point; needs additional support from MD before initiating NP program

5. Condition-specific questions:
   * MD treatment plan in place? Is there a plan to support client during emergency situation? Ensure this is in place; review meds and other interventions
   * Precipitating factors? Work to minimize exposure to them
   * Any contributing factors: Environment, medications (antidepressants, benzodiazepines), and discuss with client and work to minimize

6. See table on following page

ULCERATIVE COLITIS *(Continued)*

ULCERATIVE COLITIS*

Category	Natural Products to Consider	DOC
Herb	**Grapefruit Seed Extract** *on page 450*	PA
	Olive Leaf *on page 483*	PA
Vitamin/Mineral/ Trace Element/ Nutraceutical	**Glutamine** *on page 446* Condition-specific dosage: 5 g twice daily for 2 months, then maintenance dose of 500 mg 3 times/day	HD
	Lactobacillus acidophilus *on page 467* and ***Bifidobacterium bifidum*** *on page 391* Condition-specific dosage: 10-15 billion CFU twice daily (dairy free)	PA
	Vitamin C (Buffered) *on page 526* Condition-specific dosage: 250-1000 mg twice daily	PA
Homeopathic Remedy	Homeopathic combination formulas are available for many conditions. Listed below are some of the most common single homeopathic remedies for ulcerative colitis. Also see **Homeopathic Quick Reference Chart for Common Complaints** *on page 587*	
	Aloe socotrina	HD
	Antimonium crudum	HD
	Cichona officinalis (China)	HD
	Colocynthis	HD
Additional supplements to consider	**Selenium** *on page 502* Condition-specific dosage: 200 mcg/day	PA
	Vitamin A *on page 518* Condition-specific dosage: 10,000-35,000 int. units/day	HD
	Vitamin E *on page 529* Condition-specific dosage: 50-400 int. units/day	PA
	Zinc *on page 534* Condition-specific dosage: 15-35 mg/day	PA

*Refer to **Introduction to Conditions** *on page 41* for more details on how to apply the information in this table to individuals with this condition.

SPECIAL CONSIDERATIONS

Grapefruit Seed Extract
- Grapefruit seed extract is not equivalent to grapefruit juice/pulp. Juice/pulp has been associated with many drug interactions; see Grapefruit Seed *on page 450*
- Until further information is available, it is reasonable to avoid some medications (terfenadine, astemizole, cisapride). Use other medications metabolized by CYP3A4 with caution.

Olive Leaf
- No reported toxicity in humans at normal intakes

Glutamine
- No known toxicity or serious side effects

Lactobacillis acidophilus
- No known toxicity or serious side effects

Bifidobacterium bifidum
- No known toxicity or serious side effects

Vitamin C
- Excess intake in diabetics may give falsely elevated blood glucose readings

Selenium
- No reported toxicity in humans at normal intakes

Vitamin A
- Contraindicated in pregnancy or in women who may become pregnant

Vitamin E
- Use with caution when taking anticoagulants (vitamin E ≥200 int. units increases prothrombin times)
- Interrupt or reduce dosage one week prior to dental or surgical procedures

Zinc
- No reported toxicity in humans at normal intakes

URINARY TRACT INFECTION (UTI)

Urinary tract infections can affect the bladder, urethra, or kidneys. Bacterial invasion usually causes urinary frequency, urgency, and burning on passage of urine. These infections may also be termed cystitis. Risk factors include age and gender (occurs more frequently in the young or in females). In addition, trauma to the urethra, sexual activity, and pregnancy increase the potential for organisms to ascend the lower urinary tract. This process may also be influenced by a person's normal protective mechanisms – cleansing properties of urine flow, urinary acidity, immune cells, and the secretions of the urinary tract. Importantly, because of abnormalities in sensation or immune function, typical symptoms may be absent in some populations (the elderly, individuals with diabetes, and immunosuppressed individuals).

Most cases of urinary tract infection are caused by a small number of specific serotypes of *E. coli* bacteria. The infections do not normally cause significant complications. However, if the infection extends upward into the kidneys or if bacterial products seed the bloodstream, systemic complications, including high fever, headache, backache, hypotension, and shock may occur. Repeated infections may lead to scarring or fibrosis of the urinary tract or bladder. In addition, repeated infections may require additional investigation to rule out congenital abnormalities or immune compromise.

LIFESTYLE RECOMMENDATIONS

- Adherence to treatment plan is critical
- If taking antibiotics, use *L. acidophilus/B. bifidus*
- Drink as much water as possible, at least 6-10 glasses per day
- Empty the bladder when you feel the urge to urinate; delaying may increase the risk of infection
- Practice preventive hygiene: Wash genital area thoroughly, do not use feminine sprays or scented douches

URINARY TRACT INFECTION DECISION TREE

1. Client with urinary tract infection is interested in using natural products (NP) to support this condition

2. Healthcare provider requests basic background information. The following issues are addressed with the client:
   * Allergies?   * Other medical conditions?
   * Prescription (Rx)/OTC meds?   * Nutrition/diet program?
   * Natural products?   * Exercise program?

3. Above data reviewed; if **yes** to Rx/OTC meds, review **Drug-Induced Nutrient Depletion Chart** in Appendix

4A. Client is a candidate for natural products

   * An appropriate homeopathic remedy can be used at any time

4B. Client's case is too complicated at this point; needs additional support from MD before initiating NP program

5. Condition-specific questions:
   * Diagnosed by MD? If **yes,** what was the recommended treatment plan? Effective?
   * Is this the client's first UTI? If **no,** what is the history of infection, response to therapy, trigger(s) for onset?
   * Pregnant? Make sure client has been evaluated by a physician
   * Blood in urine? If **yes,** make sure client has been evaluated by a physician
   * If female, what type of birth control is being used? If a diaphragm, this may be contributing to the problem.

6. See table on following page

URINARY TRACT INFECTION (UTI) *(Continued)*

URINARY TRACT INFECTION (UTI)*

Category	Natural Products to Consider	DOC
Herb	Cranberry *on page 418*	HT
	Grapefruit Seed Extract *on page 450*	PA
	Golden Seal *on page 448*	PA
	Olive Leaf *on page 483*	PA
	Uva Ursi *on page 515*	HD
Vitamin/Mineral/ Trace Element/ Nutraceutical	Vitamin C *on page 526* Condition-specific dosage: 5 g/day for 7 days	HD
Homeopathic Remedy	Homeopathic combination formulas are available for many conditions. Listed below are some of the most common single homeopathic remedies for urinary tract infection. Also see **Homeopathic Quick Reference Chart for Common Complaints** *on page 587*	
	Benzoicum acidum	PD
	Cantharis	PD
	Mercurius corrosivus	PD
	Nitricum acidum	PD
	Staphysagria	PD
	Sulphur	PD
Additional supplements to consider	Vitamin A *on page 518* Condition-specific dosage: 10,000-35,000 int. units/day	PA

*Refer to **Introduction to Conditions** *on page 41* for more details on how to apply the information in this table to individuals with this condition.

SPECIAL CONSIDERATIONS

Cranberry
- No known toxicity, contraindications, or serious side effects

Grapefruit Seed Extract
- Grapefruit seed extract is not equivalent to grapefruit juice/pulp. Juice/pulp has been associated with many drug interactions; see Grapefruit Seed *on page 450*
- Until further information is available, it is reasonable to avoid some medications (terfenadine, astemizole, cisapride). Use other medications metabolized by CYP3A4 with caution.

Golden Seal
- Contraindicated during pregnancy

Olive Leaf
- No reported toxicity in humans at normal dosages

Uva Ursi
- Contraindicated in pregnancy and breast-feeding
- Contraindicated in renal failure
- May cause green-brown discoloration of urine

Vitamin C
- Excess intake in diabetics may give falsely elevated blood glucose readings

Vitamin A
- Contraindicated in pregnancy or in women who may become pregnant

WEIGHT MANAGEMENT

In the United States population, up to one-half of individuals may be classified as overweight. Obesity may be defined as a body mass index (BMI) >30 kg/m^2, while an individual is considered overweight when the BMI is 25-29.9 kg/m^2. These values should be interpreted with some degree of caution, however, since individuals with high composition of muscle (bodybuilders, for example) may be overweight despite a very low percentage of body fat.

The health consequences of obesity range from increased osteoarthritis to a significantly increased risk of diabetes and cardiovascular disease. Hyperinsulinemia, dyslipidemia, hypothyroidism, gallstone formation, hypertension, thromboembolism, and an increased risk of some forms of cancer have been associated with obesity.

Fat accumulation results from a variety of metabolic problems including hypothyroidism, hyperinsulinemia, and excessive caloric intake. The degree of excess may not be striking. It has been estimated that a significant annual weight gain (10-20 pounds) may result from an intake that exceeds expenditures by an average of only 100 calories per day. Because intake is normally matched to expenditures, a variety of psychosocial, endocrine, and metabolic factors may contribute to the development of obesity. Genetic predisposition is present, but may be modified by a number of environmental and behavioral factors. A sedentary lifestyle and ready access to high-calorie foods contribute to the extraordinarily high incidence of obesity in the United States.

Weight reductions of as little as 5% to 10% have been demonstrated to result in reduced risk of serious complications. However, weight loss programs should be carefully designed, as rapid loss of weight may deplete lean body mass (usually at the expense of muscle). The goal should be to lose fat and retain lean muscle tissue.

A comprehensive interview needs to be done, taking into account nutrient intake, metabolic profile, detoxification, stress, digestive competence, and elimination function. Endocrine function will assure best results. However, there are several nutritional agents that may help begin the process of weight loss.

LIFESTYLE RECOMMENDATIONS

- Continuation/initiation of diet and exercise program
- Weight management is a multi-dimensional issue to address
- Avoid gimmick products/programs that make promises too good to be true
- Avoid products with stimulants, such as Ma Huang or ephedra, even if they are reported to be "all natural" and safe
- Join a support group for positive reinforcement of steps being taken to control weight; behavior modification is important
- Work with a healthcare professional to design a nutrition program to meet weight goals and caloric needs; "dieting" is more than just reducing fat and/or calories
- Increase consumption of fruits and vegetables, fiber, and grains
- Document important information, such as food intake, exercise, and weight; monitor progress, look for opportunities for positive feedback
- Avoid snacking
- Replace less nutritious snacks with more nutritious ones
- Do not eat after last meal of the day, which should be at least 3 hours before retiring
- Eat slowly and chew food thoroughly

WEIGHT MANAGEMENT DECISION TREE

1. Client who is interested in weight management is interested in using natural products (NP) to support this condition

2. Healthcare provider requests basic background information. The following issues are addressed with the client:
   * Allergies?
   * Prescription (Rx)/OTC meds?
   * Natural products?
   * Other medical conditions?
   * Nutrition/diet program?
   * Exercise program?

3. Above data reviewed; if **yes** to Rx/OTC meds, review **Drug-Induced Nutrient Depletion Chart** in Appendix

4A. Client is a candidate for natural products

   * An appropriate homeopathic remedy can be used at any time

4B. Client's case is too complicated at this point; needs additional support from MD before initiating NP program

5. Condition-specific questions:
   * Assessed by a physician? If YES, what was the recommended treatment plan? Targets/goals set? How is this working? Effective?
   * Has the client had a BMI (body mass index) established? % body fat? These should also be used to set goals
   * Does the client have any health risks that should be considered? Diabetes, thyroid disease? Hypertension, heart disease?
   * Has the client had their blood pressure, lipid panel checked recently? These data would assist in overall plan establishment

6. See table on following page

375

WEIGHT MANAGEMENT *(Continued)*

WEIGHT MANAGEMENT*

Category	Natural Products to Consider	DOC
Herb	Chitosan *on page 409*	PA
	Garcinia *on page 437*	HT
	Guggul *on page 454*	PA
Vitamin/Mineral/ Trace Element/ Nutraceutical	Chromium *on page 410* Condition-specific dosage: 400 mcg/day	HT
	Conjugated Linoleic Acid (CLA) *on page 415* Condition-specific dosage: 1000 mg 3 times/day	PA
	5-Hydroxytryptophan (5-HTP) *on page 461* Condition-specific dosage: 100 mg 1-3 times/day	HT
	Pyruvate *on page 494* Condition-specific dosage: 500-750 mg 3 times/day with food	HT
Homeopathic Remedy	Homeopathic combination formulas are available for many conditions. Listed below are some of the most common single homeopathic remedies for weight management. Also see **Homeopathic Quick Reference Chart for Common Complaints** *on page 587*	
	Calcarea carbonica	PD
	Graphites	PD
	Growth Hormone	PD
	Picricum acidum	PD
	Thyroidinum	PD
Additional supplements to consider	No recommendations	

*Refer to **Introduction to Conditions** *on page 41* for more details on how to apply the information in this table to individuals with this condition.

SPECIAL CONSIDERATIONS

Chitosan
- May inhibit absorption of fat-soluble dietary supplements - should not be taken at the same time as lipid-soluble or lipid-dispersible dietary supplements

Garcinia
- Weight loss efforts should emphasize moderation of caloric intake and appropriate activity
- Monitor blood sugar; caution in individuals with diabetes
- Potential interaction with insulin, oral hypoglycemics

Guggul
- Contraindicated during pregnancy and breast-feeding
- Contraindicated in active bleeding (eg, peptic ulcer, intracranial bleeding)
- Caution in individuals with thyroid disease
- Caution in hemostatic disorders/history of bleeding
- Potential interaction with anticoagulants (warfarin), aspirin, NSAIDs, antiplatelet agents
- Discontinue use prior to dental or surgical procedures (14 days before)
- Potential interactions with antihypertensives (serum levels of propranolol and diltiazem may be increased)

Chromium
- Caution in individuals receiving oral hypoglycemics or insulin; monitor blood glucose closely and coordinate with prescriber

Conjugated Linoleic Acid (CLA)
- No known toxicity or serious side effects

5-Hydroxytryptophan (5-HTP)
- May have additive effects with antidepressants (including SSRIs, MAO inhibitors, and tricyclic antidepressants)
- 5-HTP, St John's wort, tryptophan, or SAMe may have additive effects
- May cause mild-moderate gastrointestinal distress

Pyruvate
- Large doses may cause gas, bloating, and diarrhea

PART III.
ALPHABETICAL LISTING
OF NATURAL PRODUCTS

♦ **Acetylcysteine** *see N*-Acetyl Cysteine (NAC) *on page 482*

Acetyl-L-Carnitine (ALC)

Related Information
Nutraceutical Chart *on page 573*
Organ System Support Using Natural Products *on page 660*

Natural Product Category Nutraceutical

Dosage Oral: Range: 500-2000 mg/day in divided doses

Active Forms Acetyl-L-carnitine

Reported Uses
Alzheimer's disease (Spagnoli, 1991)
Depression (Tempesta, 1987)
Diabetic peripheral neuropathy (Lowitt, 1995)

Summary Acetyl-L-carnitine is an important transport molecule in mitochondrial energy production. Enhanced activity of ALC may be beneficial in the preservation and enhancement of neuronal function, both peripherally and within the central nervous system.

Pharmacology Acetyl-L-carnitine (ALC) is the acetylated ester of the amino acid L-carnitine. ALC facilitates the production of energy from long chain fatty acids. Supplementation is believed to enhance mitochondrial energy production, which is claimed to improve cellular oxygenation and prevent hypoxic damage to cells. In addition, ALC facilitates and enhances the activity of cholinergic and dopaminergic neurons in the CNS. It increases the synthesis of nerve growth factor (NGF) as well as the expression of receptors for this hormone.

Toxicities, Warnings, and Interactions Occasionally, mild abdominal discomfort, restlessness, vertigo, and headache have been reported.

Symptoms of Deficiency Acetyl-L-carnitine is synthesized normally in the human body. No specific symptoms have been identified with a deficiency. It has been speculated that relative deficiency could result in decreased energy production and age-related cognitive decline.

Reported Interactions
Drug/Nutrient Interactions: None known
Nutrient/Nutrient Interactions: None known

References
Lowitt S, Malone JI, Salem AF, et al, "Acetyl-L-Carnitine Corrects the Altered Peripheral Nerve Function of Experimental Diabetes," *Metabolism*, 1995, 44(5):677-80.

Spagnoli A, Lucca U, Menasce G, et al, "Long-Term Acetyl-L-Carnitine Treatment in Alzheimer's Disease," *Neurology*, 1991, 41(11):1726-32.

Tempesta E, Casella L, Pirrongelli C, et al, "L-Acetylcarnitine in Depressed Elderly Subjects. A Cross-Over Study vs Placebo," *Drugs Exp Clin Res*, 1987, 13(7):417-23.

♦ **Acne Vulgaris** *see page 44*

Adrenal Extract

Related Information
Nutraceutical Chart *on page 573*
Organ System Support Using Natural Products *on page 660*

Natural Product Category Nutraceutical, Glandular

Dosage Oral: RDA: None established; dosage range: 100-200 mg 1-3 times/day

Active Forms Adrenal glandular extract

Reported Uses Fatigue, stress (Haas, 1992)

Summary Adrenal products provide rich concentrations of various nutrients that help supplement adrenal function. The quality of a glandular product is variable, so only the most reliable sources should be considered.

Pharmacology Adrenal extracts help support adrenal function. The adrenals secrete hormones, including epinephrine and norepinephrine ("fight or flight" response), as well as corticosteroids (mineralocorticoids, glucocorticoids, and 17-ketosteroids/gonadotropic hormones). They are used to promote energy production, improve an individual's ability to handle stress, and support immune function.

Toxicities, Warnings, and Interactions Adrenal extract may cause excitability when taken in large doses.

Symptoms of Deficiency Deficiency studies in humans have not been conducted.

References

Haas EM, *Staying Healthy With Nutrition: The Complete Guide to Diet and Nutritional Medicine*, Berkeley, CA: Celestial Arts, 1992, 284.

♦ **Adrenal Glandular Extract** see Adrenal Extract *on page 380*

♦ *Aesculus hippocastanum* see Horse Chestnut *(Aesculus hippocastanum)* on page 458

♦ **ALA** see Flaxseed Oil *on page 435*

♦ **ALC** see Acetyl-L-Carnitine (ALC) *on page 380*

♦ **Allergies / Hay Fever** see page 48

♦ *Allium sativum* see Garlic *(Allium sativum)* on page 438

Aloe (*Aloe* spp)

Related Information

Herb/Drug Potential Interactions *on page 642*
Herb Quick Reference Chart *on page 538*

Natural Product Category Herb

Plant Part Leaf

Dosage and Standardization Topical: Apply topical gel 3-4 times/day to affected area

Reported Uses Healing agent in wounds, minor burns, and other minor skin irritations (Davis, 1989; Heggers, 1996)

Summary Aloe has long been used as a topical application for minor cuts and burns. In India, it was historically used to treat intestinal infections, as a laxative, and for suppressed menses, with the root having been used for colic. Aloe gel is used as an emollient, moisturizer, and wound-healing agent in various pharmaceutical and cosmetic formulations.

Pharmacology Aloe promotes wound healing. It is of therapeutic value in thermal injuries and a wide variety of soft tissue injuries, preventing progressive dermal ischemia following thermal injury, frostbite, and electrical injury. Aloe penetrates injured tissues, relieves pain, is anti-inflammatory, and dilates capillaries, thereby increasing blood flow to the injury. Aloe has an antithromboxane activity, yet maintains prostaglandin ratio without causing injured blood vessels to collapse.

Theoretical Cautions and Contraindications Based on animal/*in vitro* studies, some wound healing may be delayed when using topical aloe vera gel (Schmidt, 1991).

General Warnings Caution should be used in individuals having known allergies to plants.

Theoretical Interactions None known

References

Davis RH, Leitner MG, Russo JM, et al, "Wound Healing. Oral and Topical Activity of Aloe Vera," *J Am Podiatr Med Assoc*, 1989, 79(11):559-62.

Heggers JP, Kucukcelebi A, Listengarten D, et al, "Beneficial Effect of Aloe on Wound Healing in an Excisional Wound Model," *J Altern Complement Med*, 1996, 2(2):271-7.

Schmidt JM and Greenspoon JS, "Aloe Vera Dermal Wound Gel is Associated With a Delay in Wound Healing," *Obstet Gynecol*, 1991, 78(1):115-7.

♦ *Aloe* spp see Aloe *(Aloe* spp) *on page 381*

♦ **Alpha-linolenic Acid** see Flaxseed Oil *on page 435*

♦ **Alpha-lipoate** see Alpha-Lipoic Acid *on page 381*

Alpha-Lipoic Acid

Related Information

Nutraceutical Chart *on page 573*

Natural Product Category Nutraceutical

Dosage Oral: Range: 20-600 mg/day; common dosage: 25-50 mg twice daily

Active Forms Alpha-lipoic acid

(Continued)

Alpha-Lipoic Acid (Continued)

Reported Uses

Diabetes, diabetic neuropathy (Borcea, 1999; Kishi, 1999; Zeigler, 1997; Ziegler, 1997; Nagamatsu, 1995)

Glaucoma (Filina, 1995)

Prevention of cataracts (Packer, 1995)

Prevention of neurologic disorders, including stroke (Packer, 1997)

Summary Alpha-lipoic acid is one of the most potent known antioxidants. It is both fat-soluble and water-soluble, facilitating transfer to a variety of physiologic environments. Some to refer to it as the "universal" antioxidant. Alpha-lipoic acid also functions as a cofactor in key energy-producing metabolic reactions. It has been investigated for its ability to limit oxidative damage resulting in diabetic neuropathy, improve glucose utilization, block viral transcription, and in the treatment of ophthalmologic conditions (cataracts and glaucoma).

Pharmacology Alpha-lipoic acid is a sulfur-containing cofactor which is normally synthesized in humans. Synonyms include alpha-lipoate or thioctic acid. Alpha-lipoic acid functions as a potent antioxidant. Its physico-chemical properties facilitate diffusion into lipophilic and hydrophilic environments. In addition, it may improve recycling of additional antioxidant compounds (vitamin C, vitamin E, glutathione, and coenzyme Q_{10}). Alpha-lipoic acid is metabolized to dihydrolipoic acid (DHLA), which also demonstrates antioxidant properties. Alpha-lipoic acid also serves as a cofactor for two enzymes in the energy-producing Krebs cycle: Pyruvate dehydrogenase (PDH) and alpha-ketoglutarate dehydrogenase.

Alpha-lipoic acid increases muscle cell glucose uptake and increases insulin sensitivity in individuals with type 2 diabetes. In addition, the antioxidant activity may limit the development of diabetic complications, including neuropathy. In experimental models, alpha-lipoic acid increased neuronal blood flow, reduced oxidative stress, and improved distal nerve conduction. Alpha-lipoic acid blocks activation of NF-kappa B, which is required for HIV virus transcription. Supplementation with alpha-lipoic acid was noted to improve antioxidant status, T-helper lymphocytes, and the T-helper/suppressor cell ratio in HIV-infected individuals. Alpha-lipoic acid demonstrates antioxidant activity and may improve regeneration of glutathione, potentially limiting damage leading to the cataract formation. Individuals with stage II open angle glaucoma exhibited significant improvement after alpha-lipoic acid supplementation (150 mg daily) for a period of 2 months.

Toxicities, Warnings, and Interactions Use with caution in individuals who may be predisposed to hypoglycemia (including individuals receiving antidiabetic agents). Dermatologic reactions (rashes) have been reported with alpha-lipoic acid.

Symptoms of Deficiency There is no deficiency syndrome associated with alpha-lipoic acid. Since it may be synthesized in the human body, it is not classified as an essential nutrient.

Reported Interactions

Drug/Nutrient Interactions: Theoretically, oral hypoglycemics, insulin

Nutrient/Nutrient Interactions: None known

References

Borcea V, Nourooz-Zadeh J, Wolff SP, et al, "Alpha-Lipoic Acid Decreases Oxidative Stress Even in Diabetic Patients With Poor Glycemic Control and Albuminuria," *Free Radic Biol Med*, 1999, 26(11-12):1495-500.

Filina AA, Davydova NG, Endrikhovskii SN, et al, "Lipoic Acid as a Means of Metabolic Therapy of Open-Angle Glaucoma," *Vestn Oftalmol*, 1995, 111(4):6-8.

Kishi Y, Schmelzer JD, Yao JK, et al, "Alpha-Lipoic Acid: Effect on Glucose Uptake, Sorbitol Pathway, and Energy Metabolism in Experimental Diabetic Neuropathy," *Diabetes*, 1999, 48(10):2045-51.

Nagamatsu M, Nickander KK, Schmelzer JD, et al, "Lipoic Acid Improves Nerve Blood Flow, Reduces Oxidative Stress, and Improves Distal Nerve Conduction in Experimental Diabetic Neuropathy," *Diabetes Care*, 1995, 18(8):1160-7.

Packer L, Tritschler HJ, Wessel K, et al, "Neuroprotection by the Metabolic Antioxidant Alpha-Lipoic Acid," *Free Radic Biol Med*, 1997, 22(1-2):359-78.

Packer L, Witt EH, Tritschler HJ, et al, "Alpha-Lipoic Acid as a Biological Antioxidant," *Free Radic Biol Med*, 1995, 19(2):227-50.

Ziegler D and Gries FA, "Alpha-Lipoic Acid in the Treatment of Diabetic Peripheral and Cardiac Autonomic Neuropathy," *Diabetes*, 1997, 46(Suppl 2):S62-6.

Ziegler D, Schatz H, Conrad F, et al, "Effects of Treatment With the Anti-oxidant Alpha-Lipoic Acid on Cardiac Autonomic Neuropathy in NIDDM Patients. A 4-Month Randomized Controlled Multicenter Trial (DEKAN Study)," *Diabetes Care*, 1997, 20(3):369-73.

- ♦ *Althaea officinalis* see Marshmallow *(Althaea officinalis)* on page 476
- ♦ **Alzheimer's Disease / Senility** see page 52
- ♦ **Amenorrhea** see page 56
- ♦ **American Elder** see Elder *(Sambucus nigra, Sambucus canadensis)* on page 428
- ♦ *Anas comosus* see Bromelain *(Anas comosus)* on page 399

Androstenedione

Related Information

Nutraceutical Chart *on page 573*

Natural Product Category Nutraceutical

Dosage Oral: 50-100 mg/day, usually about 1 hour before exercising

Active Forms Androstenedione (androstene, adriol), 4-androstenediol (4-AD, androdiol), 5-androstenediol (5-AD, 5-androdiol), norandrostenediol (norandrostene), 19-norandrostenedione (19-nordione), 19-nor-androstenediol (19-nordiol)

Reported Uses

Increase strength and muscle mass (Kreider, 1999; King, 1999)

Contradictory study (King, 1999)

Summary Androstenedione is claimed to produce transient increases in testosterone levels for 1 to 1½ hours following ingestion. It has been used to enhance athletic performance, improve recovery from strenuous workouts, and improve the efficiency of physical training. The FDA does not regulate androstenedione and it is legal for OTC purchase. However, androstenedrione is considered unsafe by many in the medical community. In addition, it has been banned by many amateur and professional athletic organizations. The FDA requires specific labeling on this supplement regarding hormonal effects (See Toxicities, Warnings and Interactions).

Pharmacology Androstenedione is a weak androgenic steroid hormone. It is a product of natural gonadal and adrenal synthesis. As a precursor to testosterone; converted in the body to testosterone. Testosterone regulates the development and function of the reproductive organs, enhances development of muscle and bone mass, and increases muscular strength. Androstenedione is believed to facilitate faster recovery from exercise and to promote muscle development in response to training.

Toxicities, Warnings, and Interactions Use with caution in individuals with congestive heart failure; not to be used in individuals with hypertension. The potential toxicity and side effects are controversial. It is reasonable to expect that adverse effects would be similar to testosterone excess (see FDA warning, below). However, some claim that the majority of androstenedione absorbed after oral administration is metabolized by the liver. The remainder which reaches the systemic circulation may not be sufficient to cause toxicity. Since the testosterone concentrations are transiently elevated, suppression of pituitary function is not believed to be affected, and normal testosterone synthesis is unimpaired. However, caution should be used in prostate conditions and hormone-sensitive tumors.

Despite this controversy, the FDA requires specific labeling on this supplement, noting that these supplements "contain steroid hormones that may cause breast enlargement, testicular shrinkage, and infertility in males, and increased facial and body hair, voice deepening and clitoral enlargement in females".

Symptoms of Deficiency Deficiency studies in humans have not been conducted.

Reported Interactions

Drug/Nutrient Interactions: Estrogens and androgenic drugs

(Continued)

Androstenedione *(Continued)*

Nutrient/Nutrient Interactions: Adequate levels of zinc, cobalt, and calcium are needed for dependent enzymes in the conversion of androstenedione to testosterone. Selenium and zinc are needed for detoxification and excretion of excess testosterone.

References

Kreider RB, "Dietary Supplements and the Promotion of Muscle Growth With Resistance Exercise," *Sports Med*, 1999, 27(2):97-110.

King DS, Sharp RL, Vukovich MD et al, "Effect of Oral Androstenedione on Serum Testosterone and Adaptations to Rresistance Training," *JAMA*, 1999, 281(21):2020-8.

♦ ***Angelica sinensis*** *see* Dong Quai *(Angelica sinensis) on page 425*

Aortic Extract

Related Information

Nutraceutical Chart *on page 573*

Natural Product Category Nutraceutical, Glandular

Dosage Oral: 200 mg 1-3 times/day

Active Forms Aortic extract

Reported Uses Enhancement of the function, structure, and integrity of arteries and veins (Mansi, 1988); helps to protect against various forms of vascular disease, including atherosclerosis, cerebral and peripheral arterial insufficiency, varicose veins, hemorrhoids, and vascular retinopathies such as macular degeneration (Laurora, 1993)

Pharmacology Studies report that extracts rich in aortic glycosaminoglycans improve arterial function and blood flow, which helps reduce the risks of atherosclerosis. Other aspects of glycosaminoglycans that help to interfere with the progression of atherosclerosis include their ability to help prevent damage to the surface of arteries, reduce the formation of blood clots, inhibit the migration of smooth muscle cells into the intima, and lower total cholesterol levels while raising HDL cholesterol.

Toxicities, Warnings, and Interactions No known toxicity or serious side effects reported.

Symptoms of Deficiency No deficiency conditions exist since the ingredients in aortic extracts are not essential nutrients for humans.

Reported Interactions

Drug/Nutrient Interactions: None known

Nutrient/Nutrient Interactions: None known

References

Laurora G, Cesarone MR, De Sanctis MT, et al, "Delayed Arteriosclerosis Progression in High Risk Subjects Treated With Mesoglycan. Evaluation of Intima-Media Thickness," *J Cardiovasc Surg (Torino)*, 1993, 34(4):313-8.

Mansi D, Sinisi L, De Michele G, et al, "Open Trial of Mesoglycan in the Treatment of Cerebrovascular Ischemic Disease," *Acta Neurol (Napoli)*, 1988, 10(2):108-12.

♦ **Aotic Glandular Extract** *see* Aortic Extract *on page 384*

Arabinoxylane

Related Information

Herb Quick Reference Chart *on page 538*

Natural Product Category Herb

Plant Part Isolated from *Ganoderma lucidum*

Dosage Oral: Initially, 12 capsules (250 mg each) daily (5-14 days depending on individual's condition), then decrease to 4 capsules daily

Reported Uses

Decreases chemotherapy-induced leukopenia (Ghoneum, 1998)

Immune system enhancement: Antiviral and anticancer activity (Ghoneum, 1998)

Reported useful in HIV infection (Ghoneum, 1998)

Summary Using a patented proprietary extraction process, arabinoxylane compound is produced by an enzymatic hydrolysis process that integrates an extract from the outer shell of rice bran with the extracts from three different mushrooms. The mushroom extracts used in the preparation of MGN-3, a proprietary form of arabinoxylane compound, are grown in a rice bran media and enzymatically modified by *Hyomycetes mycelia*. The patented process seems to enhance systemic absorption of the active constituents and produce strong immune-enhancing effects.

Pharmacology Arabinoxylane reportedly triples natural killer cell activity and enhances the activity of other important immune cells such as B cells (+200%) and T cells (+250%). Arabinoxylane provides additional immune system enhancement by increasing the production of tumor necrosis factor (proteins help destroy cancer cells) and interferon levels (antiviral activity). It also reduces chemotherapy-induced leukopenia.

Toxicities, Warnings, and Interactions No significant side effects have been noted. Use with caution in individuals with renal failure due to relatively high phosphorus content.

Symptoms of Deficiency Since arabinoxylane does not occur naturally in humans, no deficiency condition exists.

Theoretical Interactions May enhance the effects of immune stimulants; may limit the effects of immune suppressants

References

Ghoneum, M, "Anti-HIV Activity *In Vitro* of MGN-3, an Activated Arabinoxylane from Rice Bran," *Biochem Biophys Res Commun*, 1998, 243(1):25-9.

Ghoneum M, "Enhancement of Human Natural Killer Cell Activity by Modified Arabinoxylane from Rice Bran (MGN-3)," *Int J Immunotherapy*, XIV, 1998.

♦ **Arabinoxylane Compound** see Arabinoxylane on page 384

♦ **Arctostaphylos uva-ursi** see Uva Ursi *(Arctostaphylos uva-ursi)* on page 515

Arginine

Related Information

Vitamins/Minerals/Trace Elements/Amino Acids Chart *on page 604*

Natural Product Category Amino Acid

Dosage Oral: RDI: None established; most people do not need arginine supplementation because the body makes ample quantities; Dosage range: 3-6 g/day

Active Forms L-arginine

Reported Uses

Helps lower elevated cholesterol (Rajamohan, 1997)
Improvement in circulation (Kakumitsu, 1998)
Increases lean body mass (Elam, 1989)
Inflammatory bowel disease (Tomita, 1998)
Immune enhancement (Sax, 1994)
Male infertility (Scibona, 1994; De Aloysio, 1982)
Surgery and wound healing (Kirk, 1993)
Sexual vitality and enhancement (Melman, 1997)

Summary Arginine is a nonessential amino acid that is produced in the body from glutamic acid. However, it is sometimes referred to as a "semi-essential amino acid" because under some conditions the body might not be able to manufacture sufficient arginine. Arginine's primary function in the body is the detoxification of urea.

Pharmacology Arginine plays a key role in the urea cycle, which is the biochemical pathway that metabolized protein and other nitrogen-containing compounds. Arginine is also necessary for the synthesis of polyamines, creatine, and quanidinoacetic acid. More recently, it has been elucidated that arginine is also the precursor to nitric oxide, which is a neurotransmitter that relaxes blood vessels and improves circulation.

Toxicities, Warnings, and Interactions Caution in individuals with herpes simplex since arginine can stimulate the growth of this virus, especially in persons having low lysine levels

Symptoms of Deficiency Arginine deficiency is seldom a problem because sufficient amounts are usually made in the body. However, when arginine deficiency does occur, it causes symptoms of poor wound healing, hair loss, skin rash, constipation, and fatty liver.

Reported Interactions

Drug/Nutrient Interactions: Theoretically: Nitroglycerin, sildenafil
(Continued)

Arginine *(Continued)*

Nutrient/Nutrient Interactions: None known

References

De Aloysio D, Mantuano R, Mauloni M, et al, "The Clinical Use of Arginine Aspartate in Male Infertility," *Acta Eur Fertil*, 1982, 13(3):133-67.

Elam RP, Hardin DH, Sutton RA, et al, "Effects of Arginine and Ornithine on Strength, Lean Body Mass and Urinary Hydroxyproline in Adult Males," *J Sports Med Phys Fitness*, 1989, 29(1):52-6.

Kakumitsu S, Shijo H, Yokoyama M, et al, "Effects of L-Arginine on the Systemic, Mesenteric, and Hepatic Circulation in Patients With Cirrhosis," *Hepatology*, 1998, 27(2):377-82.

Kirk SJ, Hurson M, Regan MC, et al, "Arginine Stimulates Wound Healing and Immune Function in Elderly Human Beings," *Surgery*, 1993, 114(2):155-9.

Melman A, "This Month in Investigative Urology. L-Arginine and Penile Erection," *J Urol*, 1997,158:686.

Rajamohan T and Kurup PA, "Lysine: Arginine Ratio of a Protein Influences Cholesterol Metabolism. Part 1-Studies on Sesame Protein Having Low Lysine: Arginine Ratio," *J Exp Biol*, 1997, 35(11):1218-23.

Sax HC, "Arginine Stimulates Wound Healing and Immune Function in Elderly Human Beings," *JPEN J Parenter Enteral Nutr*, 1994, 18(6):559-60.

Scibona M, Meschini P, Capparelli S, et al, "L-Arginine and Male Infertility," *Minerva Urol Nefrol*, 1994, 46(4):251-3.

Tomita R and Tanjoh K, "Role of Nitric Oxide in the Colon of Patients With Ulcerative Colitis," *World J Surg*, 1998, 22(1):88-91.

♦ **Arthritis (Osteo)** *see page 60*

♦ **Arthritis (Rheumatoid)** *see page 64*

Artichoke *(Cynara scolymus)*

Related Information

Herb/Drug Potential Interactions *on page 642*

Herb Quick Reference Chart *on page 538*

Organ System Support Using Natural Products *on page 660*

Natural Product Category Herb

Plant Part Leaf

Dosage and Standardization Oral: 250 mg (standardized extract) 2-3 times/day, standardized to contain 15% chlorogenic acid, or 2% to 5% cynarin per dose

Reported Uses

Eczema and other dermatologic problems; hepatic protection/stimulation (Khadzhai, 1971; Maros, 1968)

Hypercholesterolemia (Kirchhoff, 1994)

Improvement in bile flow (Kirchhoff, 1994)

Summary The flower head of the globe artichoke has been used as a food and medicinal agent for centuries. In medicine, the globe artichoke has historically been used for poor digestion, along with "sluggish" liver, atherosclerosis, elevated cholesterol levels, and as a mild diuretic. It has reportedly been used in Europe since Roman times as a choleretic and diuretic. In addition, it has been reported to have hepatoprotective and regenerating effects.

Pharmacology Active constituents: Caffeic acid, caffeoylquinic acids (chlorogenic acid and cynarin), flavone glycosides, and phytosterols. The primary pharmacological activity of artichoke has been attributed to cynarin. However, chlorogenic acid has also been reported to demonstrate antioxidant properties. Artichoke was protective against the hepatotoxic effects of tetracholoromethane. In addition, cynarin is claimed to restore healthy growth and reproduction of hepatocytes.

Artichoke products have been reported to lower blood cholesterol and triglyceride levels in humans and animals. Cynarin reportedly decreases the rate of cholesterol synthesis in the liver, enhances biliary excretion of cholesterol, and increases conversion towards the bile acids. Artichoke is also reported to stimulate bile production (choleretic action). In addition, it is claimed to have antioxidant properties.

Theoretical Cautions and Contraindications Use with caution in individuals with allergies to members of the *Asteraceae/Compositae* family (chrysanthemum, daisy). Do not use in presence of bile duct obstruction (based on animal or *in vitro* studies, DeSmet, 1993).

General Warnings Use all herbal supplements with extreme caution in children <2 years of age and in pregnancy or lactation. Some herbs are contraindicated in pregnancy or lactation; make sure to observe warnings. Use with caution in individuals on medication and with pre-existing medical conditions. Always review for potential herb-drug interactions (HDIs) and other warnings. Large and prolonged doses may increase the potential for adverse effects. Herbs may cause transient adverse effects such as nausea, vomiting, and GI distress due to a variety of chemical constituents. Caution should be used in individuals having known allergies to plants.

Theoretical Interactions None known. Theoretically, may potentiate effects of lipid-lowering agents.

References

DeSmet PA, Hansel R, Keller K, et al, "Adverse Effects of Herbal Drugs," Vol 2, New York, NY: Springer-Verlag, 1993, 45.

Khadzhai II and Kuznetsova VF, "Effect of Artichoke Extracts on the Liver," *Farmakol Toksikol*, 1971, 34(6):685-7.

Kirchhoff R, et al, "Increase in Choleresis by Means of Artichoke Extract," *Phytomedicine*, 1994, 1:107-15.

Maros T, Seres-Sturm L, Racz G, et al, "Effect of Cynara Scolymus-Extracts on the Regeneration of Rat Liver. 2," *Arzneimittelforschung*, 1968, 18(7):884-6.

♦ **Ascorbic Acid** *see* Vitamin C *on page 526*

Ashwagandha *(Withania somnifera)*

Related Information

Common Herbal Supplements Contraindicated During Pregnancy *on page 656*
Herb/Drug Potential Interactions *on page 642*
Herb Quick Reference Chart *on page 538*
Organ System Support Using Natural Products *on page 660*

Natural Product Category Herb

Plant Part Root

Dosage and Standardization Oral: 450 mg 1-2 times/day, standardized to contain 1.5% withanolides per dose

Reported Uses

Adaptogen (Grandhi, 1994)
Chemotherapy and radiation protection (Kuttan, 1996; Devi, 1996)
General tonic; stress, fatigue, nervous exhaustion (Ziauddin, 1996)

Summary Ashwagandha root, a Ayurvedic (traditional Indian) medicine, helps the body cope with various stresses. It has also been used to enhance mental and physical performance. Ashwagandha helps protect the body during radiation and chemotherapy.

Pharmacology As an adaptogen, ashwagandha helps protect the body against stress. Ashwagandha has antioxidant properties that inhibit lipid peroxidation and increase levels of various enzymes, such as superoxide dismutase (SOD), catalase (CAT), and glutathione peroxidase (GPX). This antioxidant activity may help explain ashwagandha's immunomodulating effects and cognitive-enhancement properties. Ashwagandha may improve hemoglobin and red blood cell counts, because of its high iron content. Ashwagandha also contains two amino acids, arginine and ornithine, which are important for proper nervous system function. Ashwagandha acts as a radiosensitizer when administered with radiation therapy, with heat reportedly enhancing these effects. It is reported to protect against cyclophosphamide-induced leukemia.

Theoretical Cautions and Contraindications Contraindicated in pregnancy and lactation. May be an abortifacient based on *in vitro* or animal studies (Sudhir, 1986). Contraindicated in individuals with hemachromatosis. Use with caution in individuals receiving narcotic analgesics; studies report decreased tolerance to opiates (Kulkami, 1997). Based on animal
(Continued)

Ashwagandha *(Withania somnifera)* (Continued)

studies, there is a potential interaction with sedative medications, including benzodiazepines (Mehta, 1991).

General Warnings Use all herbal supplements with extreme caution in children <2 years of age and in pregnancy or lactation. Some herbs are contraindicated in pregnancy or lactation; make sure to observe warnings. Use with caution in individuals on medication and with pre-existing medical conditions. Always review for potential herb-drug interactions (HDIs) and other warnings. Large and prolonged doses may increase the potential for adverse effects. Herbs may cause transient adverse effects such as nausea, vomiting, and GI distress due to a variety of chemical constituents. Caution should be used in individuals having known allergies to plants.

Theoretical Interactions Barbiturates, benzodiazepines, narcotic analgesics, other sedatives

References

Devi PU, Akagi K, Ostapenko V, et al, "Withaferin A: A New Radiosensitizer From the Indian Medicinal Plant *Withania somnifera*," *Int J Radiat Biol*, 1996, 69(2):193-7.

Grandhi A, Mujumdar AM, and Patwardhan B, "A Comparative Pharmacological Investigation of Ashwagandha and Ginseng," *J Ethnopharmacol*, 1994, 44(3):131-5.

Kulkarni SK and Ninan I, "Inhibition of Morphine Tolerance and Dependence by *Withania somnifera* in Mice," *J Ethnopharmacol*, 1997, 57(3):213-7.

Kuttan G, "Use of *Withania somnifera* Dunal as an Adjuvant During Radiation Therapy," *Indian J Exp Biol*, 1996, 34(9):854-6.

McGuffin M, et al, eds, *American Herbal Products Association's Botanical Safety Handbook*, Boca Raton, FL: CRC Press, 1997, 124.

Praveenkumar V, Kuttan R, and Kuttan G, "Chemoprotective Action of Rasayanas Against Cyclosphamide Toxicity," *Tumori*, 1994, 80(4):306-8.

Sharad AC, Solomon FE, Devi PU, et al, "Antitumor and Radiosensitizing Effects of Withaferin A on Mouse Ehrlich Ascites Carcinoma *In Vivo*," *Acta Oncol*, 1996, 35(1):95-100.

Ziauddin M, Phansalkar N, Patki P, et al, "Studies on the Immunomodulatory Effects of Ashwagandha," *J Ethnopharmacol*, 1996, 50(2):69-76.

♦ **Asian Ginseng** *see* Ginseng, Panax *(Panax ginseng)* on page 442
♦ **Asthma** *see* page 68

Astragalus *(Astragalus membranaceus)* [Milk Vetch]

Related Information
Herb/Drug Potential Interactions *on page 642*
Herb Quick Reference Chart *on page 538*
Organ System Support Using Natural Products *on page 660*

Natural Product Category Herb

Plant Part Root

Dosage and Standardization Oral: 250-500 mg 4 times/day, standardized to a minimum 0.4% 4′-hydroxy-3′ methoxy-isoflavone-7-glycoside per dose

Reported Uses
Adaptogen (tonic-enhanced endurance, stamina) (Chang, 1986)
Improvement in immune function and disease resistance (Geng, 1986)
Improvement in tissue oxygenation (Griga, 1977)
Support for chemotherapy and radiation (Zhao, 1990)

Summary Astragalus has been used in traditional Chinese medicine for centuries due to its potential to enhance immune function and other properties. As an adaptogen, it may improve the response to stress by augmenting adrenal activity. It has been used as an immune stimulant. In contrast to echinacea, astragalus does not appear to suppress immune function in long-term use. Astragalus is also claimed to improve the delivery of oxygen to peripheral tissues. Astragalus has also been reported to be radioprotective.

Pharmacology Astragalus contains isoflavones, triterpenoids, and saponins, including astragalosides I-VIII. Triterpenoids and saponins have a structural similarity to steroid hormone precursors and appear to increase adrenal activity. Polysaccharides contained in astragalus have been shown to stimulate natural killer (NK) cells, augment T-cell function, and increase interferon production. Astragalus administration has been shown to increase phagocytosis by reticuloendothelial cells, decrease T-suppressor cell function, and improve T-killer cell function. Astragalus may decrease cyclophosphamide-induced immune suppression (Chu, 1989) [contradictory study, Khoo, 1995]

Theoretical Cautions and Contraindications None known

General Warnings Use all herbal supplements with extreme caution in children <2 years of age and in pregnancy or lactation. Some herbs are contraindicated in pregnancy or lactation; make sure to observe warnings. Use with caution in individuals on medication and with pre-existing medical conditions. Always review for potential herb-drug interactions (HDIs) and other warnings. Large and prolonged doses may increase the potential for adverse effects. Herbs may cause transient adverse effects such as nausea, vomiting, and GI distress due to a variety of chemical constituents. Caution should be used in individuals having known allergies to plants.

Theoretical Interactions May enhance effects of immune stimulants; may limit effects of immune suppressants.

References

Chang H, *Pharmacology and Application of Chinese Materia Medica*, Philadelphia, PA: World Scientific, 1986, 4.

Chu DT, Sun Y, and Lin JR, "Immune Restoration of Local Xenogeneic Graft-Versus-Host Reaction in Cancer Patients *In Vitro* and Reversal of Cyclophosphamide-Induced Immune Suppression in the Rat *In Vivo* by Fractionated *Astragalus membranaceus*," *Chung Hsi I Chieh Ho Tsa Chih*, 1989, 9(6):326, 351-4.

Geng CS, "Advances in Immuno - Pharmacological Studies on *Astragalus membranaceus*," *Chung Hsi I Chieh Ho Tsa Chih*, 1986, 6(1):62-4.

Griga IV, "Effect of a Summary Preparation of *Astragalus cicer* on the Blood Pressure of Rats With Renal Hypertension and on the Oxygen Consumption by the Tissues," *Farm Zh*, 1977, 6:64-6.

Khoo KS and Ang PT, "Extract of *Astragalus membranaceus* and *Ligustrum lucidum* Does Not Prevent Cyclophosamide-Induced Myelosuppression," *Singapore Med J*, 1995, 36(4):387-90.

Zhao KS, Mancini C, and Doria G, "Enhancement of the Immune Response in Mice by *Astragalus membranaceus* Extracts," *Immunopharmacology*, 1990, 20(3):225-33.

♦ **Astragalus membranaceus** see Astragalus (*Astragalus membranaceus*) [Milk Vetch] *on page 388*

♦ **Athlete's Foot / Jock Itch** *see page 72*

♦ **Attention Deficit Disorder (ADD) / Attention Deficit Hyperactivity Disorder (ADHD)** *see page 76*

Bacopa *(Bacopa monniera)*

Related Information

Herb Quick Reference Chart *on page 538*

Natural Product Category Herb

Plant Part Leaf

Dosage and Standardization Oral: 100 mg 3 times/day, standardized to contain 20% bacosides A and B per dose

Reported Uses Memory enhancement and improvement of cognitive function (Kidd, 1999)

Summary Bacopa has been used in India for centuries as the foremost nerve tonic in Ayurvedic (traditional Indian) medicine. It has been used in epilepsy and insanity and to improve memory and mental capacities. Bacopa is also native to Australia.

Pharmacology Bacopa has been reported to improve learning processes in laboratory animals. It improved performance in the learning phase, but did not improve performance in animals with well-established habits. In another study, bacopa improved learning performance in laboratory animals in brightness-discrimination reaction.

Theoretical Cautions and Contraindications None known

General Warnings Use all herbal supplements with extreme caution in children <2 years of age and in pregnancy or lactation. Some herbs are contraindicated in pregnancy or lactation; make sure to observe warnings. Use with caution in individuals on medication and with pre-existing medical conditions. Always review for potential herb-drug interactions (HDIs) and other warnings. Large and prolonged doses may increase the potential for adverse effects. Herbs may cause transient adverse effects such as
(Continued)

Bacopa *(Bacopa monniera)* *(Continued)*

nausea, vomiting, and GI distress due to a variety of chemical constituents. Caution should be used in individuals having known allergies to plants.

Theoretical Interactions None known

References

Kidd PM, "A Review of Nutrients and Botanicals in the Integrative Management of Cognitive Dysfunction," *Altern Med Rev*, 1999, 4(3):144-61.

♦ *Bacopa monniera* see Bacopa *(Bacopa monniera)* on page 389
♦ **Bearberry** see Uva Ursi *(Arctostaphylos uva-ursi)* on page 515
♦ **Benign Prostatic Hypertrophy (BPH)** see page 80

Beta-Carotene

Related Information

Drug-Induced Nutrient Depletions *on page 625*
Organ System Support Using Natural Products *on page 660*
Pregnancy & Lactation Nutritional Chart *on page 657*
Vitamins/Minerals/Trace Elements/Amino Acids Chart *on page 604*

Natural Product Category Vitamin

Dosage Oral: ODA: 10,000-30,000 int. units/day; no RDI has been established

Active Forms Beta-carotene

Reported Uses

Cancer prevention (Gaby, 1991)
Cervical dysplasia (Muto, 1995)
Immunostimulant (Alexander, 1985)
Photoprotection (erythropoietic protoporphyria) (Matthews-Roth, 1977)

Summary Beta-carotene is the most common carotenoid in the normal human diet and is generally the most important in human physiology. Beta-carotene is present in high quantities in fruits and vegetables. It is an important antioxidant, allowing protection against the cellular oxidative processes which may lead to cancer or damage from ultraviolet light (phototoxicity). In addition, it may enhance immunity.

Pharmacology Beta-carotene, also known as pro-vitamin A, consists of two molecules of vitamin A which are hydrolyzed in the gastrointestinal tract. Vitamin A is critical for the production of visual pigments. In addition, beta-carotene functions as an antioxidant. Beta-carotene is capable of quenching singlet oxygen free radicals, and blocking chain-reaction lipid peroxidation. It serves an important role in both cell-mediated and humoral immunity. Retinoids interact with nuclear receptors, influencing gene expression and apoptosis (cell death). Natural beta-carotene ("cis" form) acts as an antioxidant, whereas the synthetic form ("trans" form) has recently been found to be pro-oxidant (Levin, 1997).

Toxicities, Warnings, and Interactions Ingestion of large doses of beta-carotene can result in carotenosis cutis (orange coloring in the skin). This benign discoloration is most noticeable on the palms of the hands and the soles of the feet. The discoloration is reversible upon dosage reduction or discontinuation.

Symptoms of Deficiency Deficiencies of beta-carotene include increased free radical activity and a weakened immune system. The incidence of some forms of cancer has been correlated to low dietary intake of beta-carotene. The primary cause for a deficiency of beta-carotene is a lack of dietary intake. In addition, some medications may reduce blood levels.

Reported Interactions

Drug/Nutrient Interactions: Drugs which can cause depletion of beta-carotene and/or vitamin A: Cholestyramine, colchicine, colestipol, mineral oil, neomycin; orlistat

Nutrient/Nutrient Interactions: Large doses of beta-carotene may theoretically inhibit the body's ability to utilize other carotenoids.

References

Alexander M, Newmark H, and Miller RG, "Oral Beta-Carotene Can Increase the Number of OKT4+ Cells in Human Blood," *Immunol Lett*, 1985, 9(4):221-4.
Gaby SK, *Vitamin Intake and Health*, New York, NY: Marcel Dekker, Inc, 1991, 36-9.

Levin G, Yeshurun M, and Mokady S, "*In Vivo* Antiperoxidative Effect of 9-Cis Beta-Carotene Compared With That of the All-Trans Isomer," *Nutr Cancer,* 1997, 27(3):293-7.

Mathews-Roth MM, Patrick MA, Fitzpatrick TB, et al, "Beta Carotene Therapy for Erythropoietic Protoporphyria and Other Photosensitivity Diseases," *Arch Dermatol,* 1977, 113(9):1229-32.

Muto Y, Fujii J, Shidoji Y, et al, "Growth Retardation in Human Cervical Dysplasia-Derived Cell Lines by Beta-Carotene Through Down-Regulation of Epidermal Growth Factor Receptor," *Am Clin Nutr,* 1995, 62(6 Suppl): 1535S-40S.

Betaine Hydrochloride

Related Information

Nutraceutical Chart *on page 573*

Natural Product Category Nutraceutical

Dosage Oral: Dosage range: 325-650 mg to be taken with meals that contain protein

Active Forms Betaine hydrochloride

Reported Uses Digestive aid (hypochlorhydria and achlorhydria) (Lipski, 1996)

Summary Betaine hydrochloride is a substance that contains 23% hydrochloric acid. It is primarily obtained from an alkaloid found in beets.

Pharmacology Betaine hydrochloride is used as a digestive aid. It is given orally as a source of hydrochloric acid in treating people who have hypochlorhydria or achlorhydria.

Toxicities, Warnings, and Interactions Do not use in individuals with ulcers. High doses may cause gastric irritation.

References

Lipski E, *Digestive Wellness,* New Canaan, CT: Keats Publishing, Inc, 1996, 201-2.

Bifidobacterium bifidum (bifidus)

Related Information

Drug-Induced Nutrient Depletions *on page 625*

Nutraceutical Chart *on page 573*

Natural Product Category Nutraceutical

Dosage Oral: 5-10 billion colony forming units (CFU) per day (dairy free); refrigerate to maintain maximum potency

Active Forms *Bifidobacterium bifidum*

Reported Uses

Crohn's disease (Favier, 1997)

Diarrhea (Saavedra, 1994)

Maintenance of anaerobic microflora in the colon (Balsari, 1982; Gibson, 1994)

Ulcerative colitis (van der Wiel-Korstanje, 1975)

Summary Bifidobacteria include over 28 species which are a normal component of the bacterial flora of the lower gastrointestinal tract. Their metabolic activity produces a variety of beneficial vitamins, as well as an environment which suppresses the growth of pathogenic species. Broad-spectrum antibiotic use, as well as illness, may disrupt the survival of this normal inhabitant of the colon, altering the gastrointestinal flora and permitting an overgrowth of new species, resulting in adverse gastrointestinal and/or nutritional effects.

Pharmacology Bifidobacteria of the colon digest sugars to acidic shortchain fatty acids, creating a slightly acidic pH, which suppresses the growth of bacteria, yeasts, and other pathogenic organisms. Bifidobacteria may influence the metabolism of fatty acids, bile acids, cholesterol, and steroid hormones in the intestinal tract. In addition, they produce a number of vitamins, including several B vitamins and vitamin K, which are absorbed into the circulation. In addition, the short-chain fatty acids produced by *Bifidobacterium* spp are a primary source of energy for colonic epithelial cells.

Toxicities, Warnings, and Interactions No known toxicity or serious side effects. Refrigerate to maintain maximum potency.

Symptoms of Deficiency Gas, bloating, diarrhea or constipation, bad breath, chronic vaginal yeast infections

(Continued)

Bifidobacterium bifidum (bifidus) (Continued)

Reported Interactions

Drug/Nutrient Interactions: The use of antibiotics may cause a greater need for bifidobacteria

Nutrient/Nutrient Interactions: None known

References

Balsari A, Ceccarelli A, Dubini F, et al, "The Fecal Microbial Population in the Irritable Bowel Syndrome," *Microbiologica*, 1982, 5(3):185-94.

Favier C, Neut C, Mizon C, et al, "Fecal Beta-D-Galactosidase Production and *Bifidobacteria* are Decreased in Crohn's Disease," *Dig Dis Sci*, 1997, 42(4):817-22.

Gibson GR and Wang X, "Regulatory Effects of Bifidobacteria on the Growth of Other Colonic Bacteria," *J Appl Bacteriol*, 1994, 77(4):412-20.

Saavedra JM, Bauman NA, Oung I, et al, "Feeding of *Bifidobacterium bifidum* and *Streptococcus thermophilus* to Infants in Hospital for Prevention of Diarrhoea and Shedding of Rotavirus," *Lancet*, 1994, 344(8929):1046-9.

van der Wiel-Korstanje JA and Winkler KC, "The Faecal Flora in Ulcerative Colitis, *J Med Microbiol*, 1975, 8(4):491-501.

Bilberry (Vaccinium myrtillus)

Related Information

Herb/Drug Potential Interactions *on page 642*
Herb Quick Reference Chart *on page 538*
Organ System Support Using Natural Products *on page 660*

Natural Product Category Herb

Plant Part Berry

Dosage and Standardization Oral: 80 mg 2-3 times/day, standardized to 25% anthocyanosides (calculated as anthocyanidins) per dose

Reported Uses

Ophthalmologic disorders (antioxidant): Myopia, diminished acuity, dark adaptation, macular degeneration, night blindness, diabetic retinopathy, cataracts (Morazonni, 1996)

Vascular disorders: Varicose veins, capillary permeability/stability, phlebitis (Bottecchia, 1977)

Summary Bilberry became popular after British pilots reported an improved ability to adjust to glare, increased visual acuity, and improved night vision during World War II. Investigations have demonstrated a wide variety of pharmacological activities related to antioxidant and collagen-stabilizing effects which have prompted interest in the use of this product as treatment for a number of age-related vascular and ophthalmologic disorders.

Pharmacology Bilberry demonstrates antioxidant activity and is claimed to exert a stabilizing activity on collagen, a major structural component of connective tissue. Bilberry has been reported to strengthen cross-linking in addition to stimulating collagen and mucopolysaccharide production. Bilberry reportedly inhibits a variety of inflammatory mediators, including histamine, proteases, leukotrienes, and prostaglandins. Anthocyanosides contained in bilberry may decrease capillary permeability and reportedly inhibit platelet aggregation. Presumably by virtue of its antioxidant activity and collagen-stabilizing effects, bilberry has been reported to be useful in the prevention and/or treatment of diabetic retinopathy, macular degeneration, and cataracts.

Theoretical Cautions and Contraindications If pregnant or nursing, use caution; based on *in vitro* or animal studies (Morazzoni, 1991). Use bilberry leaf with caution in individuals with diabetes (*in vitro* or animal studies indicate potential to alter glucose regulation).

Based on pharmacological activity, this herb may be contraindicated in individuals with active bleeding (eg, peptic ulcer, intracranial bleeding). Use with caution in individuals with a history of bleeding, hemostatic disorders, or drug-related hemostatic problems. Use with caution in individuals taking anticoagulant medications, including warfarin, aspirin, aspirin-containing products, NSAIDs, or antiplatelet agents (eg, ticlopidine, clopidogrel, dipyridamole). Discontinue use prior to dental or surgical procedures (generally at least 14 days before).

General Warnings Use all herbal supplements with extreme caution in children <2 years of age and in pregnancy or lactation. Some herbs are contraindicated in pregnancy or lactation; make sure to observe warnings. Use with caution in individuals on medication and with pre-existing medical conditions. Always review for potential herb-drug interactions (HDIs) and other warnings. Large and prolonged doses may increase the potential for adverse effects. Herbs may cause transient adverse effects such as nausea, vomiting, and GI distress due to a variety of chemical constituents. Caution should be used in individuals having known allergies to plants.

Theoretical Interactions Insulin and oral hypoglycemic drugs: Effects may be altered with bilberry leaf

References

Bottecchia D, et al, "*Vaccinium myrtillus*," *Fitoterapia*, 1977, 48:3-8.

Morazzoni P and Bombardelli E, "*Vaccinium myrtillus*," *Fitoterapia*, 1996, 67(1):3-29.

Morazzoni P, "*Vaccinium myrtillus* Anthocyanosides Pharmacokinetics in Rats," *Arzneimittelforschung*, 1991, 41(2):128-31.

Biotin

Related Information

Drug-Induced Nutrient Depletions *on page 625*

Pregnancy & Lactation Nutritional Chart *on page 657*

Vitamins/Minerals/Trace Elements/Amino Acids Chart *on page 604*

Natural Product Category Vitamin

Dosage Oral: RDI: 30 mcg/day; ODA: 30-300 mcg/day

Active Forms Biotin

Reported Uses

Brittle nails (Hochman, 1993)

Diabetes (Maebashi, 1983)

Diabetic neuropathy (Koutsikos, 1990)

Seborrheic dermatitis (Bonjour, 1977)

Uncombable hair syndrome (Shelley, 1985)

Summary Biotin is a water-soluble B vitamin which is essential for the activity of many important metabolic reactions. Its activity is required for the maintenance of many tissues, including skin and hair, and is required for normal neuronal and hematopoietic function.

Pharmacology Biotin is a cofactor in four key carboxylase enzymes, with primary activity in the mitochondria. Enzymes are involved in the metabolism of fatty acids, carbohydrates, and proteins. Biotin is important to maintain the health of skin, hair, sweat glands, nerves, and bone marrow.

Toxicities, Warnings, and Interactions No known toxicity or serious side effects

Symptoms of Deficiency Hypercholesterolemia, dermatologic problems, muscular weakness, and hair loss (alopecia)

Reported Interactions

Drug/Nutrient Interactions: Drugs which can cause depletion of biotin: Carbamazepine, primidone, and antibiotics

Nutrient/Nutrient Interactions: None known

References

Bonjour JP, "Biotin in Man's Nutrition and Therapy - A Review," *Int J Vitam Nutr Res*, 1977, 47(2):107-18.

Hochman LG, Scher RK, and Meyerson MS, "Brittle Nails: Response to Daily Biotin Supplementation," *Cutis*, 1993, 51(4):303-5.

Koutsikos D, Agroyannis B, and Tzanatos-Exarchou H, "Biotin for Diabetic Peripheral Neuropathy," *Biomed Pharmacother*, 1990, 44(10):511-4.

Maebashi M, "Therapeutic Evaluation of the Effect of Biotin on Hyperglycemia in Patients With Non-insulin Dependent Diabetes Mellitus," *J Clin Biochem Nutr*, 1983, 14:211-8.

Shelley WB and Shelley ED, "Uncombable Hair Syndrome: Observations on Response to Biotin and Occurrence in Siblings With Ectodermal Dysplasia," *J Am Acad Dermatol*, 1985, 13(1):97-102.

Bismuth

Related Information

Nutraceutical Chart *on page 573*

Natural Product Category Mineral

(Continued)

Bismuth *(Continued)*

Dosage Oral: RDI: None established; dosage range: 120 mg 4 times/day (taken 20 minutes before meals for ulcer therapy)

Active Forms Usually available as bismuth salts such as bismuth subcarbonate, bismuth subgallate, and bismuth subnitrate

Reported Uses Ulcers (Pan, 1991)

Summary Bismuth is a silvery metallic element. Bismuth compounds are used as protective coatings for inflamed surfaces and as opaque media for x-ray visualization.

Pharmacology Bismuth compounds are used to coat, protect, and enhance the healing of inflamed surfaces such as ulcers. Orally ingested bismuth compounds have been reported to suppress the growth of bacteria such as *Campylobacter pylori* and *Helicobacter pylori*.

Toxicities, Warnings, and Interactions Possible neurological toxicity with long-term use; treatment should not last longer than 6-8 weeks

Symptoms of Deficiency Bismuth is not considered to be a nutrient and there is no deficiency condition associated with it.

References

Pan SA, Liao CH, Lien GS, et al, "Histological Maturity of Healed Duodenal Ulcers and Ulcer Recurrence After Treatment With Colloidal Bismuth Subcitrate or Cimetidine," *Gastroenterology*, 1991, 101(5):1187-91.

Bitter Melon *(Momordica charantia)*

Related Information

Common Herbal Supplements Contraindicated During Pregnancy *on page 656*

Herb/Drug Potential Interactions *on page 642*

Herb Quick Reference Chart *on page 538*

Organ System Support Using Natural Products *on page 660*

Natural Product Category Herb

Plant Part Fruit

Dosage and Standardization Oral: 200 mg 2-3 times/day, standardized to contain 5.1% triterpenes per dose

Reported Uses

Antiviral (Lee-Huang, 1995)

Hypoglycemic, impaired glucose tolerance (IGT) (Leatherdale, 1981; Welihinda, 1986)

Summary Bitter melon is a relatively common food item in the tropics. It has been used by natives for various conditions, including infections, cancer, and diabetes. The leaves and fruit have both been used occasionally to make teas and beer or to season soups in the Western world.

Pharmacology Bitter melon fruit is used as a hypoglycemic agent. It has also been reported to potentially inhibit certain viruses, including human immunodeficiency virus (HIV). At least three different groups of constituents in bitter melon are reported to have hypoglycemic (blood sugar lowering) or other actions of potential benefit in diabetes mellitus. These include a mixture of steroidal saponins known as charantin, insulin-like peptides, and alkaloids. It is still unclear which of these is most effective or whether all three work together. Two proteins, known as alpha- and beta-momorcharin, inhibit the acquired immunodeficiency syndrome (AIDS) virus, but this research has only been demonstrated in test tubes and not in humans.

Theoretical Cautions and Contraindications Do not use in pregnancy (*in vitro* or animal data indicate potential emmenagogue and abortifacient). Based on *in vitro* or animal studies, this herb may alter glucose regulation (Sarkar, 1996). Use with caution in individuals with diabetes or in those who may be predisposed to hypoglycemia. Effects of drugs with hypoglycemic activity may be potentiated (including insulin and oral hypoglycemics). The individual's blood sugar should be closely monitored, and the dosage of these agents, including insulin dosage, may require adjustment. This should be carefully coordinated among the individuals' healthcare providers.

General Warnings Use all herbal supplements with extreme caution in children <2 years of age and in pregnancy or lactation. Some herbs are contraindicated in pregnancy or lactation; make sure to observe warnings. Use with caution in individuals on medication and with pre-existing medical conditions. Always review for potential herb-drug interactions (HDIs) and other warnings. Large and prolonged doses may increase the potential for adverse effects. Herbs may cause transient adverse effects such as nausea, vomiting, and GI distress due to a variety of chemical constituents. Caution should be used in individuals having known allergies to plants.

Theoretical Interactions Insulin and oral hypoglycemic agents (effects may be altered)

References

Leatherdale BA, Panesar RK, Singh G, et al, "Improvement in Glucose Tolerance Due to *Momordica charantia* (Karela)," *Br Med J (Clin Res Ed)*, 1981, 282(6279):1823-4.

Lee-Huang S, Huang PL, Chen HC, et al, "Anti-HIV and Anti-tumor Activities of Recombinant MAP30 From Bitter Melon," *Gene*, 1995, 161(2):151-6.

Sarkar S, Pranava M, and Marita R, "Demonstration of the Hypoglycemic Action of *Momordica charantia* in a Validated Animal Model of Diabetes," *Pharmacol Res*, 1996, 33(1):1-4.

Welihinda J, Karunanayake EH, Sheriff MH, et al, "Effect of *Momordica charantia* on the Glucose Tolerance in Maturity Onset Diabetes," *J Ethnopharmacol*, 1986, 17(3):277-82.

Black Cohosh *(Cimicifuga racemosa)*

Related Information

Common Herbal Supplements Contraindicated During Pregnancy *on page 656*

Herb/Drug Potential Interactions *on page 642*

Herb Quick Reference Chart *on page 538*

Natural Product Category Herb

Plant Part Root, rhizome

Dosage and Standardization Oral: 20-40 mg twice daily, standardized to 1 mg triterpene glycosides calculated as 27-deoxyactein per dose

Reported Uses Vasomotor symptoms of menopause; premenstrual syndrome (PMS), mild depression, arthritis (Lieberman, 1998; Shibata, 1980; Jarry, 1985; Newall, 1996)

Summary Black cohosh rhizome has been used for centuries in Chinese medicine as a remedy for conditions such as headache, measles, gingivitis, and uterine and rectal prolapse. Native Americans used black cohosh as a remedy for women's health problems, including painful menses and problems in childbirth. Black cohosh contains phytoestrogens, botanical compounds that mimic estrogens, and has been investigated in a number of disorders related to altered production of these hormones.

Pharmacology Phytoestrogens of black cohosh rhizome have mild estrogenic binding effects. These include formononetin (an isoflavone component of the rhizome) and the triterpenoid 27-deoxyactein. The constituent isoferulic acid has been reported to have anti-inflammatory effects and may decrease muscular spasm. Salicylic acid is also found in small quantities in black cohosh, and it is presumed that the salicylic acid contributes to the anti-inflammatory and analgesic properties of black cohosh. Finally, cimicifugoside contained in black cohosh is believed to affect hypothalamus-pituitary function. Standardized extracts have been demonstrated to improve menopausal and premenopausal symptoms in clinical studies. In addition, due to its anti-inflammatory and spasmolytic properties, black cohosh has been used in the support of rheumatic complaints.

Theoretical Cautions and Contraindications Black cohosh may cause nausea, vomiting, headache and hypotension at higher dosages. Use with caution in individuals allergic to salicylates; it is not known whether the amount of salicylic acid is likely to affect platelet aggregation or have other effects associated with salicylates. Monitoring of serum hormone levels is recommended after 6 months of treatment with black cohosh. Contraindicated in pregnancy (based on *in vitro* or animal studies may stimulate uterine contractions) and lactation (Duker, 1991).

Phytoestrogen-containing herbs have not been associated with the negative health effects seen with synthetic estrogen. However, use with caution in individuals on hormone replacement therapy or oral contraceptives or a (Continued)

Black Cohosh *(Cimicifuga racemosa)* *(Continued)*

history of thromboembolic disease or stroke. Contraindicated in individuals with a history of estrogen-dependent tumors or endometrial cancer.

General Warnings Use all herbal supplements with extreme caution in children <2 years of age and in pregnancy or lactation. Some herbs are contraindicated in pregnancy or lactation; make sure to observe warnings. Use with caution in individuals on medication and with pre-existing medical conditions. Always review for potential herb-drug interactions (HDIs) and other warnings. Large and prolonged doses may increase the potential for adverse effects. Herbs may cause transient adverse effects such as nausea, vomiting, and GI distress due to a variety of chemical constituents. Caution should be used in individuals having known allergies to plants.

Theoretical Interactions Oral contraceptives, hormonal replacement therapy

References

Duker EM, Kopanski L, Jarry H, et al, "Effects of Extracts From *Cimicifuga racemosa* on Gonadotropin Release in Menopausal Women and Ovariectomized Rats," *Planta Med*, 1991, 57(5):420-4.

Jarry H, Harnischfeger G, and Duker E, "The Endocrine Effects of Constituents of *Cimicifuga racemosa* 2. In Vitro Binding of Constituents to Estrogen Receptors," *Planta Med*, 1985, (4):316-9.

Lieberman S, "A Review of the Effectiveness of *Cimicifuga racemosa* (Black Cohosh) for the Symptoms of Menopause," *J Womens Health*, 1998, 7(5):525-9.

Newall CA, Anderson LA, and Phillipson JD, *Herbal Medicines: A Guide for Health Care Professionals*, London, England: The Pharmaceutical Press, 1996, 250-2.

Shibata M, Ikoma M, Onoda M, et al, "Pharmacological Studies on the Chinese Crude Drug "Shoma". III. Central Depressant and Antispasmodic Actions of *Cimicifuga rhizoma, Cimicifuga simplex* Wormsk," *Yakugaku Zasshi*, 1980, 100(11):1143-50.

Bladderwrack *(Fucus vesiculosus)*

Related Information

Herb/Drug Potential Interactions *on page 642*

Herb Quick Reference Chart *on page 538*

Natural Product Category Herb

Plant Part Fronds

Dosage and Standardization Oral: 600 mg 1-3 times/day

Reported Uses Rich source of iodine, potassium, magnesium, calcium, and iron; hypothyroidism; fibrocystic breast disease (Bradley, 1992)

Summary Bladderwrack consists of the dried thallus of marine seaweed. Found in the waters off the North Sea coast, the western Baltic coast, and the Atlantic and Pacific coasts, preparations of bladderwrack have been used for the supportive management of hypothyroidism and obesity. Along with proper exercise and diet, bladderwrack may be effective in aiding weight loss.

Pharmacology Bladderwrack contains iodine and is thought to stimulate the thyroid gland, thus increasing basal metabolism. It also appears to assist the problem of lipid balance associated with obesity. Overdosage (dosages greater than 150 mcg of total iodine/day) may lead to hyperthyroidism, tremor, increased pulse rate, and elevated blood pressure. Bladderwrack usually contains from 0.03% to 1% iodine by weight, so standardized preparations are recommended.

Theoretical Cautions and Contraindications Based on pharmacological activity: Use with caution in individuals taking thyroid agents; do not use in hyperthyroidism; caution for individuals with kidney failure (may alter potassium levels). Avoid use in individuals with iodine sensitivity.

General Warnings Use all herbal supplements with extreme caution in children <2 years of age and in pregnancy or lactation. Some herbs are contraindicated in pregnancy or lactation; make sure to observe warnings. Use with caution in individuals on medication and with pre-existing medical conditions. Always review for potential herb-drug interactions (HDIs) and other warnings. Large and prolonged doses may increase the potential for adverse effects. Herbs may cause transient adverse effects such as nausea, vomiting, and GI distress due to a variety of chemical constituents. Caution should be used in individuals having known allergies to plants.

Theoretical Interactions Thyroid agents, lithium

References

Bradley PR, ed, *British Herbal Compendium*, Vol 1, Bournemouth, England: British Herbal Medicine Association, 1992, 37-9.

Boron

Related Information

Vitamins/Minerals/Trace Elements/Amino Acids Chart *on page 604*

Natural Product Category Mineral

Dosage Oral: RDI: None established; ODA: None established

Active Forms Sodium borate and boron chelates (citrate, aspartate, and glycinate)

Reported Uses

Osteoarthritis (Travers, 1990)

Osteoporosis (Nielsen, 1987)

Rheumatoid arthritis (Newnham, 1991)

Summary Boron is a mineral which has recently been recognized as an essential mineral in humans. Although some information about its physiologic functions are speculative, it has been strongly implicated in bone metabolism. It may be important in the prevention and treatment of a number of bone and joint disorders.

Pharmacology Boron is believed to be an essential mineral with a wide variety of effects. It appears to play an important role in normal bone metabolism, participates in the activation of vitamin D, and plays a role in calcium and magnesium homeostasis. Boron also appears to facilitate hydroxylation reactions critical to the synthesis of estrogen and testosterone.

Toxicities, Warnings, and Interactions

Toxic concentration: 150 mg/L of water

Toxicity symptoms: Nausea, diarrhea, skin rashes, fatigue

Symptoms of Deficiency Increased loss of calcium and bone demineralization, resulting in an increased risk of osteoporosis

Reported Interactions

Drug/Nutrient Interactions: No studies reporting drug-induced boron depletion have been found

Nutrient/Nutrient Interactions: None known

References

Newnham RE, "Arthritis or Skeletal Fluorosis and Boron," *Int Clin Nutr Rev*, 1991, 11(2):68-70.

Nielsen FH, Hunt CD, Mullen LM, et al, "Effect of Dietary Boron on Mineral, Estrogen, and Testosterone Metabolism in Postmenopausal Women," *FASEB J*, 1987, 1(15):394-7.

Travers RL, "Boron and Arthritis: The Results of a Double-Blind Study," *J Nutr Med*, 1990, 1:127-32.

Boswellia *(Boswellia serrata)*

Related Information

Herb Quick Reference Chart *on page 538*

Natural Product Category Herb

Plant Part Gum resin

Dosage and Standardization Oral: 200-400 mg 3 times/day, standardized to contain 65% boswellic acids per dose

Reported Uses

Anti-inflammatory (Ammon, 1991; Ammon, 1996)

Ulcerative colitis, arthritis (*Altern Med Rev*, 1998)

Summary Boswellia, or olibanum, is a close relative of the Biblical incense, frankincense, and has been used historically in the Ayurvedic medical system of India for various conditions, including arthritis and other inflammation.

Pharmacology Boswellia's constituents, termed boswellic acids, have an anti-inflammatory action. Reports suggest that boswellia is effective in the management of arthritis. Boswellia inhibits pro-inflammatory mediators in the body, such as leukotrienes. As opposed to NSAIDs, long-term use of boswellia does not lead to irritation or ulceration of the stomach.

Theoretical Cautions and Contraindications None known

(Continued)

Boswellia *(Boswellia serrata)* *(Continued)*

General Warnings Use all herbal supplements with extreme caution in children <2 years of age and in pregnancy or lactation. Some herbs are contraindicated in pregnancy or lactation; make sure to observe warnings. Use with caution in individuals on medication and with pre-existing medical conditions. Always review for potential herb-drug interactions (HDIs) and other warnings. Large and prolonged doses may increase the potential for adverse effects. Herbs may cause transient adverse effects such as nausea, vomiting, and GI distress due to a variety of chemical constituents. Caution should be used in individuals having known allergies to plants.

Theoretical Interactions None known

References

Ammon HP, "Salai Guggal - *Boswellia serrata*: From an Herbal Medicine to a Non-redox Inhibitor of Leukotriene Biosynthesis," *Eur J Med Res*, 1996, 1(8):369-70.

Ammon HP, Mack T, Singh GB, et al, "Inhibition of Leukotriene B4 Formation in Rat Peritoneal Neutrophils by an Ethanolic Extract of the Gum Resin Exudate of *Boswellia serrata*," *Planta Med*, 1991, 57(3):203-7.

"*Boswellia serrata*," *Altern Med Rev*, 1998, 3(4):306-7.

♦ *Boswellia serrata* see Boswellia *(Boswellia serrata)* on page 397

Branched-Chain Amino Acids (BCAAs)

Related Information

Vitamins/Minerals/Trace Elements/Amino Acids Chart *on page 604*

Natural Product Category Amino Acid

Dosage Oral: Dosage range: Isoleucine: 900 mg/day, leucine: 1200 mg/day, valine: 1050 mg/day

Active Forms L-leucine, L-isoleucine, L-valine

Reported Uses Muscle development and improvement in lean body mass (Braverman, 1997)

Summary BCAAs are a primary component of muscle, accounting for over one-third of all amino acids in muscle protein. Muscle tissue demonstrates an increased need for these amino acids during times of physical stress and intense exercise. In addition, these amino acids may help preserve and/or restore muscle mass in individuals following surgery or trauma.

Pharmacology As with any amino acid, the primary function of the BCAAs is to allow synthesis of proteins. In addition, they may be catabolized to serve as an energy source. In particular, they may be used directly by skeletal muscle, as opposed to other amino acids which require hepatic gluconeogenesis to generate useful metabolic currency. Since branched-chain amino acids may be metabolized by peripheral muscle tissues, supplementation may decrease the rate of protein catabolism under stress (such as in infection and trauma), and maintain a balance between serum concentrations of these agents and aromatic amino acids.

Toxicities, Warnings, and Interactions No known toxicity or serious side effects. BCAAs compete with the aromatic amino acids for entry into the brain. Since aromatic amino acids are used in the synthesis of neurotransmitters, ingesting large doses of BCAAs may result in a decline of brain levels of serotonin and dopamine. Increased mortality has been documented in individuals with ALS (see References).

Symptoms of Deficiency Use with caution in individuals with renal or hepatic failure. Human deficiencies are rare. Severe valine deficiency is reported to cause neurological defects. Isoleucine deficiency may cause muscle tremors. There are no reports of leucine deficiencies.

Reported Interactions

Drug/Nutrient Interactions: None known

Nutrient/Nutrient Interactions: The branched-chain amino acids (leucine, isoleucine, and valine) compete with the aromatic amino acids (phenylalanine, tyrosine, and tryptophan) for transport into the brain.

References

"Branched-Chain Amino Acids and Amyotrophic Lateral Sclerosis: A Treatment Failure? Italian ALS Study Group," *Neurology*, 1993, 43(12):2466-70.

Braverman ER, Pfeiffer C, and Blum K, *The Healing Nutrients Within: Facts, Findings, and New Research on Amino Acids*, New Canaan, CT: Keats Publishing Inc, 1997, 335-6.

♦ Breast-Feeding *see page 84*

Bromelain *(Anas comosus)*

Related Information
Herb Quick Reference Chart *on page 538*

Natural Product Category Herb

Plant Part Enzymes extracted from pineapple

Dosage and Standardization
Digestive enzyme: Oral: 1-2 tablets 3 times/day with meals, standardized to contain at least 2000 MCU/g/dose (MCU = milk clotting units)

Inflammation: Oral: 1 tablet 3 times/day between meals (either 1 hour before meals or 2 hours after meals)

Reported Uses
Digestive enzyme (Barbarino, 1982)
Proteolytic; anti-inflammatory (arthritis) (Taussig, 1980)
Sinusitis (Leung, 1996)

Summary Bromelains are sulfhydryl proteolytic enzymes that are obtained from the pineapple plant and used as an enzyme to aid in digestion. Commercial bromelain is usually derived from the stem. It is a mixture of several proteases, small amounts of several nonproteolytic enzymes (including acid phosphatase, peroxidase, and cellulase), polypeptide protease inhibitors, and organically bound calcium. Bromelain acts primarily to help maintain homeostasis in inflammatory processes.

Pharmacology Bromelain inhibits the enzyme thromboxane synthetase. This enzyme converts prostaglandin H_2 into pro-inflammatory prostaglandins and thromboxanes. Early reports found ingesting bromelain to be beneficial in managing arthritis and inflammatory conditions. Other research using enteric-coated bromelain at low dosages, however, reported no benefit. It is clear that more research is needed.

Theoretical Cautions and Contraindications Use with caution in GI ulceration (based on case reports) and in individuals with hypertension or other cardiovascular disorders (based on case reports and *in vitro* or animal data, Gutfreund, 1978).

Based on *in vitro* or animal studies, may have effects on platelet aggregation (Heinicke, 1972). Contraindicated in individuals with active bleeding (eg, peptic ulcer, intracranial bleeding). Use with caution in individuals with a history of bleeding, hemostatic disorders, or drug-related hemostatic problems. Use with caution in individuals taking anticoagulant medications, including warfarin, aspirin, aspirin-containing products, NSAIDs, antiplatelet agents (eg, ticlopidine, clopidogrel, dipyridamole). Discontinue use prior to dental or surgical procedures (generally at least 14 days before).

General Warnings Use all herbal supplements with extreme caution in children <2 years of age and in pregnancy or lactation. Some herbs are contraindicated in pregnancy or lactation; make sure to observe warnings. Use with caution in individuals on medication and with pre-existing medical conditions. Always review for potential herb-drug interactions (HDIs) and other warnings. Large and prolonged doses may increase the potential for adverse effects. Herbs may cause transient adverse effects such as nausea, vomiting, and GI distress due to a variety of chemical constituents. Caution should be used in individuals having known allergies to plants.

Theoretical Interactions Anticoagulants, aspirin, NSAIDs, antiplatelet drugs (ticlopidine, clopidogrel, dipyridamole)

References
Barbarino F, Szabo P, and Neumann E, "The Influence of Bromelin on Digestion and Absorption in Control Animals and in Methotrexate-Induced 'Cytostatic' Enteropathy," *J Nucl Med Allied Sci,* 1982, 26(2):97-103.

Gutfreund AE, Taussig SJ, and Morris AK, "Effect of Oral Bromelain on Blood Pressure and Heart Rate of Hypertensive Patients," *Hawaii Med J,* 1978, 37(5):143-6.

Heinicke RM, van der Wal L, and Yokoyama M, "Effect of Bromelain (Anase) on Human Platelet Aggregation," *Experientia,* 1972, 28(7):844-5.

Leung AY and Foster S, *Encyclopedia of Common Natural Ingredients Used in Foods, Drugs, and Cosmetics,* New York, NY: Wiley, 1996, 100-3.

Taussig SJ, "The Mechanism of the Physiological Action of Bromelain," *Med Hypotheses,* 1980, 6(1):99-104.

Bupleurum *(Bupleurum falcatum)*

Related Information
Herb Quick Reference Chart *on page 538*

Natural Product Category Herb

Plant Part Root

Dosage and Standardization Oral: 500 mg 3 times/day **or** 30-60 drops of
liquid extract (1:4 w/v) 3 times/day

Reported Uses
Chronic inflammatory disease (Just, 1998)
Liver support (Guinea, 1994)

Summary Bupleurum root has been used in traditional Chinese Medicine as
a bitter and cooling agent that is useful in decreasing inflammation.
Bupleurum has anti-inflammatory and diaphoretic properties. It has been
reported to regulate gastrointestinal function and to maintain proper liver
function.

Pharmacology Bupleurum has been reported to have anti-inflammatory
properties, possibly by adrenocortical stimulation. When exposed to chemical toxins, bupleurum has been reported to be hepatoprotective.

Theoretical Cautions and Contraindications Based on possible adrenal
stimulation, use with caution in individuals with hypertension, diabetes,
edema or receiving diuretics or corticosteroids (Hattori, 1991).

General Warnings Use all herbal supplements with extreme caution in
children <2 years of age and in pregnancy or lactation. Some herbs are
contraindicated in pregnancy or lactation; make sure to observe warnings.
Use with caution in individuals on medication and with pre-existing medical
conditions. Always review for potential herb-drug interactions (HDIs) and
other warnings. Large and prolonged doses may increase the potential for
adverse effects. Herbs may cause transient adverse effects such as
nausea, vomiting, and GI distress due to a variety of chemical constituents.
Caution should be used in individuals having known allergies to plants.

Theoretical Interactions If adrenal stimulation occurs: Corticosteroids,
diuretics, antihypertensives

References
Guinea MC, Parellada J, Lacaille-Dubois MA, et al, "Biologically Active Triterpene Saponins
From *Bupleurum fruticosum*," *Planta Med*, 1994, 60(2):163-7.
Just MJ, Recio MC, Giner RM, et al, "Anti-inflammatory Activity of Unusual Lupane Saponins
From *Bupleurum fruticescens*," *Planta Med*, 1998, 64(5):404-7.

♦ *Bupleurum falcatum* see Bupleurum (*Bupleurum falcatum*) on page 400

Calcium

Related Information
Drug-Induced Nutrient Depletions *on page 625*
Pregnancy & Lactation Nutritional Chart *on page 657*
Vitamins/Minerals/Trace Elements/Amino Acids Chart *on page 604*

Natural Product Category Mineral

Dosage Oral: RDI: 1000 mg/day; ODA: 1000-1500 mg/day

Active Forms Calcium citrate, aspartate, ascorbate, lactate, phosphate,
carbonate, glycinate, malate, amino acid chelates, and microcrystalline
hydroxyapatite compound (MCHC)

Reported Uses
Blood pressure regulation (Cappuccio, 1989)
Cancer prevention (Rozen, 1989)
Elevated cholesterol (Bell, 1992)
Hypertension (Moore, 1989)
Kidney stones (Marshall, 1972)
PMS (Thys-Jacobs, 1998)
Pregnancy (Belizan, 1991)
Prevention of osteoporosis (Dawson-Hughes, 1991)

Summary Calcium is the most abundant mineral in the human body. Of total
body stores, approximately 99% is localized in bones and teeth, while the
remaining 1% participates in the other physiologic functions. The need for
calcium supplementation is greatest during periods of rapid growth,

including childhood and pregnancy. In addition, calcium requirements are increased during periods of increased loss, such as during lactation. Due to its critical role in bone homeostasis, calcium has an important role in the prevention of bone diseases such as osteoporosis. It is also important in maintaining normal cardiovascular function.

Pharmacology Calcium is the primary mineral in the development and maintenance of healthy bones and teeth, where it exists primarily as hydroxyapatite, a crystalline calcium carbonate-phosphate compound. In addition, physiologic roles of calcium include coupling of excitation-contraction within muscle cells, generation of transmembrane action potentials in cardiac pacemaker and conducting fibers, activation of clotting factors, activation of intracellular proteins involved in metabolic reactions, and transmission of impulses by nerve fibers. Calcium is a highly regulated ion maintained within a narrow range of serum concentrations.

Toxicities, Warnings, and Interactions

Toxic dose: Large doses normally show no toxic effects

Toxicity symptoms: With hyperparathyroidism, hyperphosphatemia, magnesium deficiency, or vitamin D overdoses, soft tissue calcification may occur. Calcium supplements may contain lead (check for manufacturers who certify low lead levels)

Symptoms of Deficiency Symptoms of calcium deficiency include muscle cramps, irritability, insomnia, hypertension, and tetany. Long-term calcium deficiency contributes to growth deficiency in children, as well as osteoporosis and osteomalacia, resulting in bone deformities and fragility. Magnesium deficiency causes various abnormalities in calcium metabolism.

Reported Interactions

Drug/Nutrient Interactions: Drugs which can cause depletion of calcium: Loop diuretics, potassium-sparing diuretics, anticonvulsants, barbiturates, phenytoin, corticosteroids, isoniazid, neomycin, H_2-receptor antagonists, digoxin, magnesium and aluminum antacids, aminoglycosides, amphotericin B, foscarnet and tetracycline antibiotics. Calcium supplements may decrease the absorption of some medications, including fluoroquinolone and tetracycline antibiotics, salicylates, iron salts, and atenolol.

Nutrient/Nutrient Interactions: Competitive absorption exists between calcium and magnesium, iron, and zinc. Elevated levels of vitamin D can cause an increased absorption of calcium.

References

Belizan JM, Villar J, Gonzalez L, et al, "Calcium Supplementation to Prevent Hypertensive Disorders of Pregnancy," *N Engl J Med*, 1991, 325(20):1399-405.

Bell L, Halstenson CE, Halstenson CJ, et al, "Cholesterol-Lowering Effects of Calcium Carbonate in Patients With Mild to Moderate Hypercholesterolemia," *Arch Intern Med*, 1992, 152(12):2441-4.

Cappuccio FP, Siani A, and Strazzullo P, "Oral Calcium Supplementation and Blood Pressure: An Overview of Randomized Controlled Trials," *J Hypertens*, 1989, 7(12):941-6.

Dawson-Hughes B, "Calcium Supplementation and Bone Loss: A Review of Controlled Clinical Trials," *Am J Clin Nutr*, 1991, 54(1 Suppl):274S-80S.

Marshall RW, Cochran M, and Hodgkinson A, "Relationships Between Calcium and Oxalic Acid Intake in the Diet and Their Excretion in the Urine of Normal and Renal-Stone-Forming Subjects," *Clin Sci*, 1972, 43(1):91-9.

Moore TJ, "The Role of Dietary Electrolytes in Hypertension," *J Am Coll Nutr*, 1989, 8(Suppl):68S-80S.

Rozen P, Fireman Z, Fine N, et al, "Oral Calcium Suppresses Increased Rectal Epithelial Proliferation of Persons at Risk of Colorectal Cancer," *Gut*, 1989, 30(5):650-5.

Thys-Jacobs S, Starkey P, Bernstein D, et al, "Calcium Carbonate and the Premenstrual Syndrome: Effects on Premenstrual and Menstrual Symptoms. Premenstrual Syndrome Study Group," *Am J Obstet Gynecol*, 1998, 179(2):444-52.

Calendula *(Calendula officinalis)*

Related Information

Herb/Drug Potential Interactions *on page 642*

Herb Quick Reference Chart *on page 538*

Natural Product Category Herb

Plant Part Flower

Dosage and Standardization Topical: Apply to affected area as needed

(Continued)

Calendula *(Calendula officinalis)* (Continued)

Reported Uses

Antibacterial, antifungal, antiviral, antiprotozoal (Klouchek-Popova, 1982; Leung, 1996)

Vulnerary (Leung, 1996)

Wound-healing agent (increases wound healing by stimulating immune system) (Kartikeyan, 1990)

Summary Calendula is used topically to treat minor wounds and other skin problems such as mild burns and sunburn. Calendula compounded with tea tree oil is potentially an effective agent in hard to heal wounds such as pressure ulcers.

Pharmacology Calendula acts as a vulnerary. Topically, It has antibacterial, antifungal, antiviral, and antiprotozoal activity. Calendula has been reported to increase wound healing by stimulating phagocytosis and increasing granulation.

Theoretical Cautions and Contraindications None known

General Warnings Caution should be used in individuals with known allergies to plants.

Theoretical Interactions None known

References

Kartikeyan S, Chaturvedi RM, and Narkar SV, "Effect of Calendula on Trophic Ulcers," *Lepr Rev*, 1990, 61(4):399.

Klouchek-Popova E, Popov A, Pavlova N, et al, "Influence of the Physiological Regeneration and Epithelialization Using Fractions Isolated From *Calendula officinalis*," *Acta Physiol Pharmacol Bulg*, 1982, 8(4):63-7.

Leung AY and Foster S, *Encyclopedia of Common Natural Ingredients Used in Foods, Drugs, and Cosmetics*, New York, NY: Wiley, 1996, 113-5.

♦ *Calendula officinalis* see Calendula *(Calendula officinalis)* on page 401

♦ *Camellia sinensis* see Green Tea *(Camellia sinensis)* on page 452

♦ Candidiasis see page 88

Caprylic Acid

Natural Product Category Nutraceutical

Dosage Oral: 300 mg 1-4 times/day, preferably 30 minutes before meals

Active Forms Caprylic acid

Reported Uses

Antifungal/antiyeast (Tsukahara, 1961)

Dysbiosis (Neuhauser, 1954)

Summary Caprylic acid is commonly found in foods such as coconut milk and milk fat. It is an 8-carbon fatty acid. Caprylic acid is a dietary supplement that helps maintain normal bacterial flora in the gastrointestinal tract.

Pharmacology Studies have reported that dietary caprylic acid helps inhibit the growth of *Candida albicans* and other opportunistic fungi in both the small and the large intestine (Neuhauser, 1954). At the same time, caprylic acid does not seem to adversely affect the growth of beneficial intestinal microflora.

Toxicities, Warnings, and Interactions Caprylic acid is safe and effective. There are no reports of interference with other medications, and no significant side effects have been reported.

Symptoms of Deficiency Since caprylic acid does not occur naturally in humans, there is no human deficiency condition.

Reported Interactions

Reported Drug/Nutrient Interactions: None known

Reported Nutrient/Nutrient Interactions: None known

References

Neuhauser E, Gustus L, "Successful Treatment of Intestinal Moniliasis With Fatty Acid-Resin Complex," *Arch Int Med*, 1954, 93:53-60.

Tsukahara T, "Fungicidal Action of Caprylic Acid for *Candida albicans*," *Japan J Microbiol*, 1961, 5:383-94.

♦ *Capsicum annuum* see Cayenne *(Capsicum annuum, Capsicum frutescens)* on page 405

♦ **Capsicum frutescens** see Cayenne *(Capsicum annuum, Capsicum frutescens) on page 405*

Carnitine

Related Information

Drug-Induced Nutrient Depletions *on page 625*
Organ System Support Using Natural Products *on page 660*
Vitamins/Minerals/Trace Elements/Amino Acids Chart *on page 604*

Natural Product Category Amino Acid

Dosage Oral: RDI: None established; ODA: 500-2000 mg/day in divided doses

Active Forms L-carnitine, L-acetylcarnitine (LAC), L-propionylcarnitine (LPC)

Reported Uses

Congestive heart failure (CHF) (Ghidini, 1988)
Enhanced athletic performance (Giamberardino, 1996)
Hyperlipidemia (Abdel-Azid, 1984)
Male infertility (Costa, 1994)
Weight loss

Summary Because it can be synthesized in the body, L-carnitine is usually not considered to be an essential nutrient. However, it is an important physiologic mediator of fatty acid and protein metabolism. Supplementation may enhance cardiac performance and energy production, with benefits ranging from improved athletic performance to symptomatic improvements in individuals with congestive heart failure. It may also be useful in hyperlipidemias and in some forms of male infertility.

Pharmacology L-carnitine is a normally synthesized in humans from two amino acids, methionine and lysine. Physiologically, carnitine participates in the transport of long-chain fatty acids across mitochondrial membranes to allow energy production. In addition, it assists in the oxidation of branched-chain amino acids (a substrate for muscle during stress) and ketones when necessary. Carnitine may lower serum cholesterol and triglycerides. It has been claimed to improve the efficiency of energy production in muscle tissue, including the myocardium. Improved energy generation has been proposed to improve cardiac performance, and to increase energy and endurance.

Toxicities, Warnings, and Interactions L-carnitine is a normally synthesized in humans from two amino acids, methionine and lysine. Physiologically, carnitine participates in the transport of long-chain fatty acids across mitochondrial membranes to allow energy production. In addition, it assists in the oxidation of branched chain amino acids (a substrate for muscle during stress) and ketones when necessary. Carnitine may lower serum cholesterol and triglycerides. It has been claimed to improve the efficiency of energy production in muscle tissue, including the myocardium.

Symptoms of Deficiency Since the body is capable of synthesizing carnitine, absolute deficiency is unlikely. Symptoms of a relative deficiency may include elevated blood lipids, abnormal liver function, muscle weakness, reduced energy, and impaired glucose control.

Reported Interactions

Drug/Nutrient Interactions: Studies have reported that valproic acid and zidovudine are capable of depleting carnitine in humans.

Nutrient/Nutrient Interactions: None known

References

Abdel-Azid MT, et al, "Effect of Carnitine on Blood Lipid Pattern in Diabetic Patients," *Nutr Rep Internat*, 1984, 29:1071-9.

Costa M, Canale D, Filicori M, et al, "L-Carnitine in Idiopathic Asthenozoospermia: A Multicenter Study. Italian Study Group on Carnitine and Male Infertility," *Andrologia*, 1994, 26(3):155-9.

Ghidini O, Azzurro M, Vita G, et al, "Evaluation of the Therapeutic Efficacy of L-Carnitine in Congestive Heart Failure," *Int J Clin Pharmacol Ther Toxicol*, 1988, 26(4):217-20.

Giamberardino MA, Dragani L, Valente R, et al, "Effects of Prolonged L-Carnitine Administration on Delayed Muscle Pain and CK Release After Eccentric Effort," *Int J Sports Med*, 1996, 17(5):320-4.

Cascara *(Rhamnus persiana)*

Related Information

Common Herbal Supplements Contraindicated During Pregnancy *on page 656*

Herb/Drug Potential Interactions *on page 642*

Herb Quick Reference Chart *on page 538*

Natural Product Category Herb

Plant Part Aged bark

Dosage and Standardization Oral: 100 mg as needed, not to exceed 3 capsules/day or for longer than 2 days, standardized to contain 25% to 30% hydroxyanthracene derivatives per dose

Reported Uses Anthranquinone laxative (Petticrew, 1997)

Summary The aged root bark of cascara is used as a laxative. Cascara has traditionally been used as a bitter tonic and detoxicant.

Pharmacology The anthraglycosides found in cascara bark have cathartic properties. The cascarosides A and B are responsible for most of these properties, causing increased peristalsis in the large intestine.

Theoretical Cautions and Contraindications Avoid use in children <12 years of age. Contraindicated in bowel obstruction, diarrhea, or dehydration. Use with caution in bowel disorders, inflammatory bowel disease (ulcerative colitis, Crohn's disease), and appendicitis. The pharmacological activity of this agent suggests it may may decrease absorption of susceptible oral medications by decreasing bowel transit time; excessive use may lead to potassium loss and other electrolyte disturbances. Use with caution in cardiovascular disease (overuse may cause electrolyte disorders). May potentiate the effects of various pharmaceutical drugs with narrow therapeutic windows (Bradley, 1992); also see Potential Interactions

General Warnings Use all herbal supplements with extreme caution in children <2 years of age and in pregnancy or lactation. Some herbs are contraindicated in pregnancy or lactation; make sure to observe warnings. Use with caution in individuals on medication and with pre-existing medical conditions. Always review for potential herb-drug interactions (HDIs) and other warnings. Large and prolonged doses may increase the potential for adverse effects. Herbs may cause transient adverse effects such as nausea, vomiting, and GI distress due to a variety of chemical constituents. Caution should be used in individuals having known allergies to plants.

Theoretical Interactions Antiarrhythmics, digoxin, phenytoin, laxatives, lithium, theophylline, potassium-depleting diuretics; may alter absorption of oral medications

References

Bradley PR, ed, *British Herbal Compendium*, Vol 1, Bournemouth, England: British Herbal Medicine Association, 1992, 52-4.

Petticrew M, Watt I, and Sheldon T, "Systematic Review of the Effectiveness of Laxatives in the Elderly," *Health Technol Assess*, 1997, 1(13):i-iv,1-52.

♦ *Cassia senna see* Senna *(Cassia senna) on page 503*

♦ *Cataracts see page 92*

Cat's Claw *(Uncaria tomentosa)*

Related Information

Herb/Drug Potential Interactions *on page 642*

Herb Quick Reference Chart *on page 538*

Natural Product Category Herb

Plant Part Root (bark)

Dosage and Standardization Oral: 250-1000 mg (standardized extract) 3 times/day, standardized to contain ≥1.3% pentacyclic oxindole alkaloids and ≤0.06% tetracyclic oxindole alkaloids per dose

Reported Uses

Anti-inflammatory (Aquino, 1991)

Antimicrobial (antibacterial, antifungal, antiviral) (Aquino, 1989; Senatore, 1989)

Antioxidant (Aquino, 1990)

Immunosupportive (Wagner, 1985)

Summary Cat's claw is a rain forest-derived botanical used in traditional medicine, possibly dating to the Incan civilization. Claims related to cat's claw involve activity as an immune modulator and free radical scavenger. It has been studied for a potential role in a variety of inflammatory diseases, infections, and allergic conditions.

Pharmacology Due to the number of potentially active components, the pharmacological activity of cat's claw has been difficult to accurately define. Immunomodulatory activity may be derived from multiple components. Several glycosides are reported to stimulate phagocytosis. Isopteridine is claimed to have immuno-stimulatory properties. Triterpenoid alkaloids and quinovic acid glycosides may inhibit replication of some DNA viruses

The anti-inflammatory activity of cat's claw may also be related to multiple components. Sterols have demonstrated anti-inflammatory activity in animal studies, while glycosidic components may reduce inflammation and edema. Proanthocyanidins (PCOs) appear to be potent antioxidants, improve capillary fragility, and inhibit platelet-activating factor (PAF). Rhynchophylline may inhibit platelet aggregation and thrombus formation.

Theoretical Cautions and Contraindications Do not use during pregnancy. Use with caution in transplant recipients or others taking therapeutic immunosuppression or I.V. immunoglobulin therapy (Aquino, 1990).

Pharmacological activity includes potential antiplatelet effects (Haginiwa, 1973). Contraindicated in individuals with active bleeding (eg, peptic ulcer, intracranial bleeding). Use with caution in individuals with a history of bleeding, hemostatic disorders, or drug-related hemostatic problems. Use with caution in individuals taking anticoagulant medications, including warfarin, aspirin, aspirin-containing products, NSAIDs, or antiplatelet agents (eg, ticlopidine, clopidogrel, dipyridamole). Discontinue use prior to dental or surgical procedures (generally at least 14 days before).

General Warnings Use all herbal supplements with extreme caution in children <2 years of age and in pregnancy or lactation. Some herbs are contraindicated in pregnancy or lactation; make sure to observe warnings. Use with caution in individuals on medication and with pre-existing medical conditions. Always review for potential herb–drug interactions (HDIs) and other warnings. Large and prolonged doses may increase the potential for adverse effects. Herbs may cause transient adverse effects such as nausea, vomiting, and GI distress due to a variety of chemical constituents. Caution should be used in individuals having known allergies to plants.

Theoretical Interactions Anticoagulants, aspirin or aspirin-containing products, antiplatelet agents, NSAIDs. Do not use in individuals receiving immunosuppressant therapy or intravenous immunoglobulin therapy.

References

Aquino R, De Feo V, De Simone F, et al, "Plant Metabolites. New Compounds and Anti-Inflammatory Activity of *Uncaria tomentosa*," *J Nat Prod*, 1991, 54(2):453-9.

Aquino R, De Simone F, Pizza C, et al, "Plant Metabolites. Structure and *In Vitro* Antiviral Activity of Quinovic Acid Glycosides From *Uncaria tomentosa* and *Guettarda platyopda*," *J Nat Prod*, 1989, 52(4):679-85.

Aquino R, De Simone F, Vincieri FF, et al, "New Polyhydroxylated Triterpenes From *Uncaria tomentosa*," *J Nat Prod*, 1990, 53(3):559-64.

Haginiwa J, Sakai S, Aimi N, et al, "Studies of Plants Containing Indole Alkaloids. 2. On the Alkaloids of *Uncaria rhynchophylla* Miq," *Yakugaku Zasshi*, 1973, 93(4):448-52.

Senatore A, Cataldo A, Iaccarino FP, et al, "Phytochemical and Biological Study of *Uncaria tomentosa*," *Boll Soc Ital Biol Sper*, 1989, 65(6):517-20.

Wagner H, Kreutzkamp B, and Jurcic K, "The Alkaloids of *Uncaria tomentosa* and Their Phagocytosis-Stimulating Action," *Planta Med*, 1985, (5):419-23.

Cayenne *(Capsicum annuum, Capsicum frutescens)*

Related Information

Herb/Drug Potential Interactions *on page 642*
Herb Quick Reference Chart *on page 538*
Organ System Support Using Natural Products *on page 660*

Natural Product Category Herb

Plant Part Fruit

(Continued)

Cayenne (Capsicum annuum, Capsicum frutescens) (Continued)

Dosage and Standardization

Oral: 400 mg 3 times/day, standardized to contain ≥0.25% capsaicin content per dose; may also be standardized to Scoville heat units, with 150,000 being average

Topical: Apply as directed by manufacturer

Reported Uses

Cardiovascular circulatory support (Newall, 1996)

Digestive stimulant (Newall, 1996)

Inflammation and pain (topical) (Magnusson, 1996; Rains, 1995; Tandan, 1992; Nagy 1982)

Summary Cayenne pepper (chili pepper) has been used as a spice for foods in many cultures and as a traditional medicine for centuries, especially with the Native American culture. Cayenne is regarded as a digestive aid, carminative, antispasmodic, rubefacient, and counter-irritant. Externally, topical preparations of capsicum oleoresin (0.25% to 0.75%) are used for the pain associated with arthritis, rheumatism, and cold injuries. Internally, capsicum has been reported beneficial in increasing peripheral circulation and improving digestion.

Pharmacology Capsaicin selectively activates certain populations of unmyelinated primary afferent sensory neurons (type "C"). Many of cayenne's positive effects on the cardiovascular system can be attributed to its excitation of a distinct population of these neurons in the vagus nerve. Topically, capsaicin is reportedly effective in postherpetic neuralgia, postmastectomy pain syndrome, osteo and rheumatoid arthritis, painful diabetic neuropathy, psoriasis, and pruritus. Both the gastric and duodenal mucosa are thought to contain capsaicin-sensitive areas that protect against acid and drug induced ulcers when stimulated by capsaicin. It increases mucosal blood flow and/or vascular permeability; may inhibit gastric motility, and may activate duodenal motility.

Theoretical Cautions and Contraindications Use with caution in individuals with GI ulceration (based on case reports). Due to pharmacological activity, may interfere with MAO inhibitors and antihypertensive therapies due to increased catecholamine secretion (Newall, 1996).

General Warnings Use all herbal supplements with extreme caution in children <2 years of age and in pregnancy or lactation. Some herbs are contraindicated in pregnancy or lactation; make sure to observe warnings. Use with caution in individuals on medication and with pre-existing medical conditions. Always review for potential herb-drug interactions (HDIs) and other warnings. Large and prolonged doses may increase the potential for adverse effects. Herbs may cause transient adverse effects such as nausea, vomiting, and GI distress due to a variety of chemical constituents. Caution should be used in individuals having known allergies to plants.

Theoretical Interactions Antihypertensives, aspirin or aspirin-containing compounds, MAO inhibitors

References

Magnusson BM and Kaskinen LD, "Effects of Topical Application of Capsaicin to Human Skin: A Comparison of Effects Evaluated by Visual Assessment, Sensation Registration, Skin Blood Flow and Cutaneous Impedance Measurements," *Acta Derm Venereol*, 1996, 76(2):129-32.

Nagy, JI, et al, "Fluoride-Resistant Acid Phosphatase-Containing Neurones in Dorsal Root Ganglia are Separate from Those Containing Substance P or Somatostatin," *Neuroscience*, 1982, 7(1):89-97.

Newall CA, Anderson LA, and Phillipson JD, *Herbal Medicines: A Guide for Health Care Professionals*, London, England: The Pharmaceutical Press, 1996, 60-61.

Rains C and Bryson HM, "Topical Capsaicin. A Review of Its Pharmacological Properties and Therapeutic Potential in Post-Herpetic Neuralgia, Diabetic Neuropathy and Osteoarthritis," *Drugs Aging*, 1995, 7(4):317-28.

Tandan R, Lewis GA, Krusinski PB, et al, "Topical Capsaicin in Painful Diabetic Neuropathy. Controlled Study With Long-Term Follow-up," *Diabetes Care*, 1992, 15(1):8-14.

♦ **Centella asiatica** see Gotu Kola (Centella asiatica) on page 449
♦ **Cervical Dysplasia** see page 96

Chamomile, German *(Matricaria chamomilla, Matricaria recutita)*

Related Information

Common Herbal Supplements Contraindicated During Pregnancy *on page 656*

Herb/Drug Potential Interactions *on page 642*

Herb Quick Reference Chart *on page 538*

Natural Product Category Herb

Plant Part Flower

Dosage and Standardization

Oral: 400-1600 mg/day in divided doses, standardized to contain 1.2% apigenin and 0.5% essential oil per dose

Tea: 1 heaping teaspoonful of dried flowers in hot water; steep for 10 minutes, drink up to 3 times/day

Topical: Apply to affected area as needed

Reported Uses

Carminative, antispasmotic; mild sedative; anxiolytic (Newall, 1996)

Mouth rinse and gargle (for oral health) (Bradley, 1992)

Topical anti-inflammatory (Bradley, 1992)

Uterine tonic (Shipochiliev, 1981)

Summary Chamomile has been used for centuries as a mild sedative and anxiolytic. In contrast to many anxiolytic agents, generally it does not cause drowsiness or motor impairment. Chamomile also has spasmolytic and anti-inflammatory properties which may contribute to its apparent value in relieving a number of gastrointestinal complaints.

Pharmacology The sedative, spasmolytic, and anti-inflammatory activity of chamomile appear to be related to bisabolols, en-indicycloether, and flavonoids. In addition, azulene is claimed to inhibit histamine and serotonin release, which may decrease inflammation. Chamomile is considered a carminative (antiflatulent) agent. It has been used topically for a number of disorders, including acne, superficial infection, burns, and wounds. Chamomile also has been reported to have antibacterial activity against strains of *Staphylococcus, Streptococcus,* and *Candida* spp.

Theoretical Cautions and Contraindications Avoid use in individuals with allergies to members of the *Asteraceae/Compositae* family (chrysanthemum, daisy) or ragweed pollens (Subiza, 1989). Do not use in pregnancy and lactation (Bradley, 1992). Based on pharmacological activity, may cause drowsiness in some individuals. Caution individuals to avoid hazardous tasks (eg, driving or operating machinery). Caution in individuals taking sedative medications (eg, anxiolytics, benzodiazepines).

General Warnings Use all herbal supplements with extreme caution in children <2 years of age and in pregnancy or lactation. Some herbs are contraindicated in pregnancy or lactation; make sure to observe warnings. Use with caution in individuals on medication and with pre-existing medical conditions. Always review for potential herb-drug interactions (HDIs) and other warnings. Large and prolonged doses may increase the potential for adverse effects. Herbs may cause transient adverse effects such as nausea, vomiting, and GI distress due to a variety of chemical constituents. Caution should be used in individuals having known allergies to plants.

Theoretical Interactions May increase effects of sedative medications (benzodiazepine, anxiolytics)

References

Bradley PR, ed, *British Herbal Compendium*, Vol 1, Bournemouth, England: British Herbal Medicine Association, 1992, 154-7.

Newall CA, Anderson LA, and Phillipson JD, *Herbal Medicines: A Guide for Health Care Professionals*, London, England: The Pharmaceutical Press, 1996, 69-71.

Shipochiliev T, "Extracts From a Group of Medicinal Plants Enhancing Uterine Tonus," *Vet Med Nauk*, 1981, 18:94-8.

Subiza J, Subiza JL, Hinojosa M, et al, "Anaphylactic Reaction After Ingestion of Chamomile Tea: A Study of Cross-Reactivity With Other Composite Pollens," *Clin Immunol*, 1989, 84(3):353-8.

Chasteberry *(Vitex agnus-castus)*

Related Information

Common Herbal Supplements Contraindicated During Pregnancy *on page 656*

Herb/Drug Potential Interactions *on page 642*

Herb Quick Reference Chart *on page 538*

Natural Product Category Herb

Plant Part Berry

Dosage and Standardization Oral: 400 mg/day (in the morning, preferably on an empty stomach), standardized to contain 0.5% agnuside and 0.6% aucubin per dose

Reported Uses

Acne vulgaris (Amann, 1975)

Corpus luteum insufficiency; hyperprolactinemia and insufficient lactation (Milewicz, 1993; Sliutz, 1993)

Menopause (Newall, 1996)

Menstrual disorders, including amenorrhea, endometriosis, premenstrual syndrome (Amann, 1979)

Summary The chasteberry tree is a native Mediterranean plant. It has a long history of use in folk medicine for a variety of women's health problems, including endometriosis, menopause, and symptoms of PMS. It has been used to help regulate hormonal balance after discontinuing oral contraceptives.

Pharmacology Chasteberry's effects may be regulated by several mechanisms. It has been noted to possess significant effect on pituitary function and has been demonstrated to have progesterone-like effects. In addition, it may stimulate luteinizing hormone (LH) and inhibit follicle-stimulating hormone (FSH). Because of these hormonal effects, chasteberry has been recommended for a variety of female complaints related to imbalances in female hormones.

Theoretical Cautions and Contraindications Contraindicated in pregnancy and lactation, based on case reports of uterine stimulation and emmenagogue effects (Newall, 1996). Based on pharmacological activity, may interact with medications that increase dopaminergic activity (metoclopramide, levodopa) or antipsychotic agents. Use with caution in individuals receiving hormonal therapy.

General Warnings Use all herbal supplements with extreme caution in children <2 years of age and in pregnancy or lactation. Some herbs are contraindicated in pregnancy or lactation; make sure to observe warnings. Use with caution in individuals on medication and with pre-existing medical conditions. Always review for potential herb-drug interactions (HDIs) and other warnings. Large and prolonged doses may increase the potential for adverse effects. Herbs may cause transient adverse effects such as nausea, vomiting, and GI distress due to a variety of chemical constituents. Caution should be used in individuals having known allergies to plants.

Theoretical Interactions Hormonal replacement therapy, oral contraceptives, dopamine antagonists such as metoclopramide and antipsychotics

References

Amann W, "Acne Vulgaris and *Agnus castus*," *Z Allgemeinmed*, 1975, 51(35):1645-8.

Amann W, "Premenstrual Water Retention. Favorable Effect of *Agnus castus* (Agnolyt) on Premenstrual Water Retention," *ZFA (Stuttgart)*, 1979, 55(1):48-51.

Milewicz A, Gejdel E, Sworen H, et al, "*Vitex agnus castus* Extract in the Treatment of Luteal Phase Defects Due to Latent Hyperprolactinemia. Results of a Randomized Placebo-Controlled Double-Blind Study," *Arzneimittelforschung*, 1993, 43(7):752-6.

Newall CA, Anderson LA, and Phillipson JD, *Herbal Medicines: A Guide for Health Care Professionals*, London, England: The Pharmaceutical Press, 1996, 19-20.

Sliutz G, Speiser P, Schultz AM, et al, "*Agnus castus* Extracts Inhibit Prolactin Secretion of Rat Pituitary Cells," *Horm Metab Res*, 1993, 25(5):253-5.

Snow JM, "*Vitex agnus-castus* L (Verbenaceae)," *Protocol J Botanical Med*, 1996, 1(4):20-3.

- **Chastetree** *see* Chasteberry *(Vitex agnus-castus) on page 408*
- **Chemotherapy and Radiation** *see page 100*
- **Chinese angelica** *see* Dong Quai *(Angelica sinensis) on page 425*

Chitosan

Related Information
Nutraceutical Chart *on page 573*

Natural Product Category Nutraceutical

Dosage Oral: Dosage range: 750-1500 mg (of a 90% deacetylation product) 2-3 times/day taken ½ hour before meals

Active Forms Chitosan

Reported Uses Weight reduction (Han, 1999); contradictory study: (Pittler, 1999)

Summary Chitosan is a fiber that is extracted from chitin, which is a structural component of crustacean shells, lobsters, shrimps, and crabs. Chitin is a polysaccharide containing numerous acetyl groups. When chitin undergoes a process called deacetylation, chitin becomes chitosan.

Pharmacology The ionic nature of chitosan enables it to effectively bind to fat molecules. In fact, when chitosan is taken orally, it is reportedly capable of absorbing 8-10 times its own weight in fat from food that has been eaten. This prevents fats from being absorbed, which in turn forces the body to burn stored fat, resulting in fat loss and weight reduction. In addition to inhibiting intestinal absorption of dietary fat, chitosan may also chelate heavy metals.

Toxicities, Warnings, and Interactions May inhibit absorption of fat-soluble dietary supplements (vitamins, fatty acids, and lipid-containing herbs); should not be taken at the same time as lipid-soluble or lipid-dispersible dietary supplements are taken

Symptoms of Deficiency Deficiency studies in humans have not been conducted.

References
Han LK, Kimura Y, and Okuda H, "Reduction in Fat Storage During Chitin-Chitosan Treatment in Mice Fed a High-Fat Diet," *Int J Obes Relat Metab Disord*, 1999, 23(2):174-9.

Pittler MH, Abbot NC, Harkness EF, et al, "Randomized, Double-Blind Trial of Chitosan for Body Weight Reduction," *Eur J Clin Nutr*, 1999, 53(5):379-81.

Chlorophyll

Related Information
Nutraceutical Chart *on page 573*

Natural Product Category Nutraceutical

Dosage Oral: One teaspoonful mixed in water or juice, or 2-3 tablets/day

Active Forms Two forms, chlorophyll A and chlorophyll B are known, each having a slightly different structure and activity.

Reported Uses
Absorbs and suppresses odors, which makes it useful in breath fresheners, toothpastes, mouthwashes, and deodorants (Tsunoda, 1981)
Anti-inflammatory, antioxidant, and wound-healing properties (Chernomorsky, 1988)
Exhibits bacteriostatic properties (el-Nakeeb, 1974)
Protects against toxins (Ong, 1986)

Summary Chlorophyll is the generic name for any of several oil-soluble green plant pigments, which function as photoreceptors of light energy for photosynthesis. Chlorophyll is the green pigment in green-colored plants. The chlorophyll molecule in plants, which contains carbon, hydrogen, oxygen, nitrogen, and magnesium, bears close resemblance to the hemoglobin molecule in blood. The difference is that the central element in blood is iron, whereas the central element in chlorophyll is magnesium. In both cases, the large organic portion of the molecule is a porphyrin. In addition to green leafy vegetables, high concentrations of chlorophyll can be obtained from "green" foods such as algae, chlorella, spirulina, barley leaves, alfalfa, and wheatgrass.

Pharmacology Chlorophyll absorbs the sun's energy in the form of photons and transfers this energy to other molecules, which initiates the process of photosynthesis. Chlorophyll's primary nutritional benefit is that it is an excellent source of magnesium.
(Continued)

Chlorophyll (Continued)

Toxicities, Warnings, and Interactions Products containing chlorophyll are generally recognized as being safe and without side effects.

Symptoms of Deficiency Since chlorophyll is not an essential nutrient for humans, no deficiency condition exists.

Reported Interactions

Drug/Nutrient Interactions: None known

Nutrient/Nutrient Interactions: None known

References

Chernomorsky SA and Segelman AB, "Biological Activities of Chlorophyll Derivatives," *N J Med*, 1988, 85(8):669-73.

el-Nakeeb MA and Yousef RT, "Antimicrobial Activity of Sodium Copper Chlorophyllin," *Pharmazie*, 1974, 29(1):48-50.

Ong TM, Whong WZ, Stewart J, et al, "Chlorophyllin: A Potent Antimutagen Against Environmental and Dietary Complex Mixtures," *Mutat Res*, 1986, 173(2):111-5.

Tsunoda M, Sato H, and Ohkushi T, "The Experimental Study for the Effect of Sodium Copper Chlorophyllin in Halitosis," *Nippon Shishubyo Gakkai Kaishi*, 1981, 23(3):490-8.

Chondroitin Sulfate

Related Information

Nutraceutical Chart *on page 573*

Natural Product Category Nutraceutical

Dosage Oral: Dosage range: 300-1500 mg/day

Active Forms Chondroitin sulfate (CS), as chondroitin-4-sulphate and chondroitin-6-sulphate, found naturally combined with type II collagen

Reported Uses Osteoarthritis (Uebelhart, 1998)

Summary Chondroitin sulfate is a natural physiologic compound and is one of the critical compounds in connective tissue (including vessel walls) and joint cartilage. Chondroitin sulfate absorbs water, adding to the cartilage thickness and its capacity to absorb and distribute compressive forces. The ability of cartilage to compress and expand also facilitates distribution to chondrocytes and tissues adjacent to the cartilage. Supplementation of chondroitin sulfate is claimed to support the maintenance of strong, healthy cartilage and maintain joint function.

Pharmacology Cartilage tissue is a mixture of glycosaminoglycans (GAGs). One of the primary GAGs is chondroitin sulfate. Chondroitin sulfate also inhibits synovial enzymes (elastase, hyaluronidase) which may contribute to cartilage destruction and loss of joint function. Although studies are not conclusive, chondroitin has been reported to act synergistically with glucosamine to support the maintenance of joint cartilage in osteoarthritis.

Toxicities, Warnings, and Interactions No known toxicity or serious side effects

Symptoms of Deficiency Synthesized in human body, although synthesis tends to decrease with age, which may decrease ability to maintain normal structure and function of joint cartilage.

Reported Interactions

Drug/Nutrient Interactions: None known

Nutrient/Nutrient Interactions: No adverse interactions have been reported either with CS or in combination with glucosamine/galactosamine

References

Uebelhart D, Thonar EJ, Delmas PD, et al, "Effects of Oral Chondroitin Sulfate on the Progression of Knee Osteoarthritis: A Pilot Study," *Osteoarthritis Cartilage*, 1998, 6(Suppl A):39-46.

Chromium

Related Information

Organ System Support Using Natural Products *on page 660*

Pregnancy & Lactation Nutritional Chart *on page 657*

Vitamins/Minerals/Trace Elements/Amino Acids Chart *on page 604*

Natural Product Category Mineral

Dosage Oral: RDI: None established; ODA: 200-600 mcg/day

Active Forms Chromium picolinate, chromium polynicotinate, chromium chloride

Reported Uses
Atherosclerosis (Newman, 1978)
Elevated cholesterol (Press, 1990)
Elevated triglycerides (Anderson, 1986)
Glaucoma (Lane, 1991)
Hypoglycemia (Anderson, 1987)
Type 1 diabetes (Fox, 1998)
Type 2 diabetes (Anderson, 1987)
Weight loss (Anderson, 1998)

Summary Chromium is an essential trace element. It plays an important role in insulin's regulation of blood glucose and acts as a cofactor for a number of enzymes involved in energy production. It has been claimed to be of value in diseases in which glucose regulation is dysfunctional (diabetes), lipid disorders, and as a supplement to weight loss efforts.

Pharmacology Chromium is biologically active only in the trivalent state. It may form complexes with organic compounds, including niacin, glycine, glutamic acid, and cysteine. This complex is collectively known as glucose tolerance factor (GTF). GTF enhances the blood sugar lowering effects of insulin, which facilitates the uptake of glucose into cells. Chromium is a cofactor in carbohydrate and lipid-metabolizing enzymes, and may play a role in regulating LDL and HDL serum levels.

Toxicities, Warnings, and Interactions Use with caution in individuals receiving oral hypoglycemics or insulin. Blood glucose should be closely monitored, and the dosage of diabetic agents may need to be reduced. This should be carefully coordinated among the individual's healthcare providers. Excess intake can result in tissue accumulation and can inhibit rather than enhance insulin activity. Extreme excesses may be carcinogenic.

Symptoms of Deficiency Blood sugar fluctuations, glucose intolerance, hypercholesterolemia, hypertriglyceridemia

Reported Interactions
Drug/Nutrient Interactions: Corticosteroids have been reported to cause the depletion of chromium. Chromium has been reported to increase the activity of insulin, potentially reducing the amount of insulin or oral hypoglycemic agent required to control blood sugar.
Nutrient/Nutrient Interactions: Zinc (decreased absorption)

References
Anderson RA, "Effects of Chromium on Body Composition and Weight Loss," *Nutr Rev*, 1998, 56(9):266-70.
Anderson RA, "Trace Elements and Cardiovascular Diseases," *Acta Pharmacol Toxicol (Copenh)*, 1986, 59(Supp 7):317-24.
Anderson RA, Cheng N, Bryden NA, et al, "Elevated Intakes of Supplemental Chromium Improve Glucose and Insulin Variables in Individuals With Type 2 Diabetes," *Diabetes*, 1997, 46(11):1786-91.
Anderson RA, Polansky MM, Bryden NA, et al, "Effects of Supplemental Chromium on Patients With Symptoms of Reactive Hypoglycemia," *Metabolism*, 1987, 36(4):351-5.
Fox GN and Sabovic Z, "Chromium Picolinate Supplementation for Diabetes Mellitus," *J Fam Pract*, 1998, 46(1):83-6.
Lane BC, "Diet and the Glaucomas," *J Am Coll Nutr*, 1991, 10(5):536.
Newman HA, Leighton RF, Lanese RR, et al, "Serum Chromium and Angiographically Determined Coronary Artery Disease," *Clin Chem*, 1978, 24(4):541-4.
Press RI, Geller J, and Evans GW, "The Effect of Chromium Picolinate on Serum Cholesterol and Apolipoprotein Fractions in Human Subjects," *West J Med*, 1990, 152(1):41-5.

♦ **Chronic Fatigue Syndrome (CFS)** *see page 106*
♦ *Cimicifuga racemosa* *see* Black Cohosh *(Cimicifuga racemosa) on page 395*
♦ **Circulation (Peripheral) Problems** *see page 110*
♦ *Citrus paradisi* *see* Grapefruit Seed *(Citrus paradisi) on page 450*
♦ **CLA** *see* Conjugated Linoleic Acid (CLA) *on page 415*

Clove *(Syzygium aromaticum)*
Related Information
Herb/Drug Potential Interactions *on page 642*
Herb Quick Reference Chart *on page 538*
Natural Product Category Herb
(Continued)

Clove *(Syzygium aromaticum)* *(Continued)*

Plant Part Oil

Dosage and Standardization Topical: Apply as needed to affected area

Reported Uses Antiseptic; symptomatic relief of toothache and teething problems (Newall, 1996)

Summary Clove has been used a major spice throughout the ages. Clove bud oil is used in the symptomatic relief of toothache and teething problems, by applying the oil directly to the problem area using a cotton swab.

Pharmacology Clove oil has anodyne effects (due to eugenol), producing analgesia when applied to mucous membranes. Clove oil is also antibacterial and antiviral.

Theoretical Cautions and Contraindications NOT FOR INTERNAL USE: For topical application only; do not use for longer than 48 hours (based on case reports of gingival damage, Newall, 1996)

General Warnings Caution should be used in individuals having known allergies to plants.

Theoretical Interactions None known

References

Newall CA, Anderson LA, and Phillipson JD, *Herbal Medicines: A Guide for Health Care Professionals*, London, England: The Pharmaceutical Press, 1996, 69-71.

- ◆ **Cobalamin** *see* Vitamin B_{12} (Cobalamin) *on page 524*
- ◆ **Coenzyme 1** *see* Nicotinamide Adenine Dinucleotide (NADH) *on page 483*

Coenzyme Q_{10}

Related Information

Drug-Induced Nutrient Depletions *on page 625*
Nutraceutical Chart *on page 573*
Organ System Support Using Natural Products *on page 660*

Natural Product Category Nutraceutical

Dosage Oral: Dosage range: 30-200 mg/day

Active Forms Coenzyme Q_{10}

Reported Uses

Angina (Kamikawa, 1985)
Adjunct in chemotherapy (Kokawa, 1983)
Chronic fatigue syndrome (Langsjoen, 1993)
Congestive heart failure (CHF) (Sinatra, 1997)
Hypertension (Langsjoen, 1994)
Muscular dystrophy (Folkers, 1995)
Obesity (van Gaal, 1984)
Periodontal disease (Hansen, 1976)

Summary Coenzyme Q_{10} (CoQ$_{10}$) is a fat-soluble, vitamin-like compound that is also known as ubiquinone. Of the ten forms of coenzyme Q found in nature, only coenzyme Q_{10} is synthesized in humans. Coenzyme Q_{10} is widely used throughout Europe and Asia. It is claimed to be of benefit in a variety of cardiovascular diseases, including angina, CHF, and hypertension, although one small study did not show benefit in individuals with heart failure (Watson, 1999). In addition, it may be of value in musculoskeletal disorders, periodontal disease, diabetes, and in obesity.

Pharmacology Coenzyme Q10 is involved in ATP generation, the primary source of energy in human physiology. Functions as a lipid-soluble antioxidant, providing protection against free radical damage within mitochondria. Dosages in excess of 300 mg per day have been reported to be of benefit in some condition, including breast cancer, diabetes, and cardiovascular diseases.

Toxicities, Warnings, and Interactions May decrease response to warfarin (Landbo, 1998)

Symptoms of Deficiency Hypertension, congestive heart failure, mitral valve prolapse (MVP), and angina pectoris; in addition, deficiency increases the incidence of periodontal disease.

Reported Interactions

Drug/Nutrient Interactions: Drugs which can cause depletion of CoQ_{10}: Hydralazine, thiazide diuretics, HMG-CoA reductase inhibitors, sulfonylureas, beta blockers, tricyclic antidepressants, chlorpromazine, clonidine, methyldopa, diazoxide, biguanides, haloperidol. CoQ_{10} may decrease response to warfarin.

Nutrient/Nutrient Interactions: None known

References

Folkers K and Simonsen R, "Two Successful Double-Blind Trials With Coenzyme Q_{10} (Vitamin Q_{10}) on Muscular Dystrophies and Neurogenic Atrophies," *Biochim Biophys Acta*, 1995, 1271(1):281-6.

Hansen IL, Iwamoto Y, Kishi T, et al, "Bioenergetics in Clinical Medicine. IX. Gingival and Leucocytic Deficiencies of Coenzyme Q_{10} in Patients With Periodontal Disease," *Res Commun Chem Pathol Pharmacol*, 1976, 14(4):729-38.

Kamikawa T, Kobayashi A, Yamashita T, et al, "Effects of Coenzyme Q_{10} on Exercise Tolerance in Chronic Stable Angina Pectoris," *Am J Cardiol*, 1985, 56(4):247-51.

Kishi T, Watanabe T, and Folkers K, "Bioenergetics in Clinical Medicine XV. Inhibition of Coenzyme Q_{10} - Enzymes by Clinically Used Adrenergic Blockers of Beta-Receptors," 1977, 17(1):157-64.

Kokawa T, Shiota K, Oda K, et al, "Coenzyme Q_{10} in Cancer Chemotherapy - Experimental Studies on Augmentation of the Effects of Masked Compounds, Especially in the Combined Chemotherapy with Immunopotentiators," *Gan To Kagaku Ryoho*, 1983, 10(3):768-74.

Landbo C and Almdal TP, "Interaction Between Warfarin and Coenzyme Q_{10}," *Ugeskr Laeger*, 1998, 160(22):3226-7.

Langsjoen PH, Langsjoen PH, and Folkers K, "Isolated Diastolic Dysfunction of the Myocardium and its Response to CoQ_{10} Treatment," *Clin Investig*, 1993, 71(8 Suppl):S140-4.

Langsjoen P, Langsjoen P, Willis R, et al, "Treatment of Essential Hypertension With Coenzyme Q_{10}," *Mol Aspects Med*, 1994, 15(Suppl): S265-72.

Oda T, "Effect of Coenzyme Q_{10} on Stress-Induced Cardiac Dysfunction in Paediatric Patients With Mitral Valve Prolapse: A Study by Stress Echocardiography," *Drugs Exp Clin Res*, 1985, 11(8):557-76.

Sinatra ST, "Coenzyme Q_{10}: A Vital Therapeutic Nutrient for the Heart With Special Application in Congestive Heart Failure," *Conn Med*, 1997, 61(11):707-11.

van Gaal L, Folkers K, and Yamamura Y, eds, *Explotory Study of Coenzyme Q_{10} in Obesity*, Biomedical and Clinical Aspects of Coenzyme Q, Vol 4, Amsterdam: Elsevier Science Publications, 1984, 369-73.

Watson PS, Scalia GM, Galbraith A, et al, "Lack of Effect of Coenzyme Q on Left Ventricular Function in Patients with Congestive Heart Failure," *J Am Coll Cardiol*, 1999, 33(6):1549-52.

♦ **Cold / Flu** see page 114

Coleus *(Coleus forskohlii)*

Related Information

Herb/Drug Potential Interactions on page 642
Herb Quick Reference Chart on page 538

Natural Product Category Herb

Plant Part Root

Dosage and Standardization Oral: 250 mg 1-3 times/day, standardized to contain 1% forskolin per dose **or** 50 mg 1-2 times/day, standardized to contain 18% forskolin per dose

Reported Uses

Asthma, allergies; hypertension, congestive heart failure; eczema (Baumann, 1990; Kreutner 1985; Ammon, 1985)

Psoriasis (Bronczkowita, 1984)

Summary Coleus is a relatively new medicinal herb in the United States, although it has been extensively researched in India over the last twenty years. It has been used primarily for its antiasthmatic, spasmolytic and antihypertensive effects. While the majority of studies have used the isolated forskolin extract, it has been postulated that the whole plant may be more effective, due to the presence of multiple compounds which may act synergistically.

Pharmacology Forskolin derived from coleus is believed to activate adenylate cyclase, increasing intracellular c-AMP concentrations and activating a number of key enzymatic pathways. Forskolin stimulates thyroid function, increases insulin secretion, inhibits histamine release from mast cells, and increases the utilization of fats as an energy source. In addition to the effects mediated by cyclic nucleotides, forskolin may act through direct binding to PAF receptors. This binding may inhibit platelet aggregation in (Continued)

Coleus *(Coleus forskohlii)* *(Continued)*

addition to blocking inflammatory reactions mediated by platelet-derived products. Neutrophil activation, vascular permeability, and smooth muscle contraction are reduced, while coronary blood flow may be increased.

Theoretical Cautions and Contraindications Based on its pharmacological activity, coleus may cause hypotension (Lindner, 1978). Use with caution in individuals at risk of hypotension (receiving antihypertensive medications or agents which predispose to orthostasis) or individuals who would not tolerate transient hypotensive episodes (cerebrovascular or cardiovascular disease). Avoid use in peptic ulcer disease (based on pharmacological activity and/or *in vitro* studies).

May alter platelet aggregation (Christenson, 1995). Contraindicated in individuals with active bleeding (eg, peptic ulcer, intracranial bleeding). Use with caution in individuals with a history of bleeding, hemostatic disorders, or drug-related hemostatic problems. Use with caution in individuals taking anticoagulant medications, including warfarin, aspirin, aspirin-containing products, NSAIDs, or antiplatelet agents (eg, ticlopidine, clopidogrel, dipyridamole). Discontinue use prior to dental or surgical procedures (generally at least 14 days before).

General Warnings Use all herbal supplements with extreme caution in children <2 years of age and in pregnancy or lactation. Some herbs are contraindicated in pregnancy or lactation; make sure to observe warnings. Use with caution in individuals on medication and with pre-existing medical conditions. Always review for potential herb-drug interactions (HDIs) and other warnings. Large and prolonged doses may increase the potential for adverse effects. Herbs may cause transient adverse effects such as nausea, vomiting, and GI distress due to a variety of chemical constituents. Caution should be used in individuals having known allergies to plants.

Theoretical Interactions Antihistamines, decongestants, anticoagulants, antihypertensives

References

Ammon HP and Muller AB, "Forskolin: From an Ayurvedic Remedy to a Modern Agent," *Planta Med*, 1985, (6):473-7.

Baumann G, Felix S, Sattelberger U, et al, "Cardiovascular Effects of Forskolin (HL 362) in Patients With Idiopathic Congestive Cardiomyopathy - A Comparative Study With Dobutamine and Sodium Nitroprusside," *J Cardiovasc Pharmacol*, 1990, 16(1):93-100.

Bronczkowita, H and Methner GF, [Title Unknown], *Akt Dermatol*, 1984, 121.

Christenson JT, Thulesius D, and Nazzal MM, "The Effect of Forskolin on Blood Flow, Platelet Metabolism, Aggregation and ATP Release," *Vasa*, 1995, 24(1):56-61.

Kreutner W, Chapman RW, Gulbenkian A, et al, "Bronchodilator and Anti-allergy Activity of Forskolin," *Eur J Pharmacol*, 1985, 111(1):1-8.

Lindner E, Dohadwalla AN, and Bhattacharya BK, "Positive Inotropic and Blood Pressure Lowering Activity of a Diterpene Derivative Isolated From *Coleus forskohlii*: Forskolin," *Arzneimittelforschung*, 1978, 28(2):284-9.

♦ ***Coleus forskohlii*** see Coleus *(Coleus forskohlii)* on page 413

♦ **Colic** see page 118

Collagen (Type II)

Related Information

Nutraceutical Chart *on page 573*

Natural Product Category Nutraceutical

Dosage Topical: Dosage range: 200-400 mg 3 times/day

Active Forms Type II collagen

Reported Uses

Arthritis (Barnett, 1998)

First- and second-degree burns (Chvapil, 1973)

Pressure ulcers, venous stasis ulcers, diabetic ulcers (those resulting from arterial insufficiencies); surgical and traumatic wounds

Topical application for wound healing

Summary Type II collagen is the primary form of collagen contained in cartilage. Type II collagen extracts contain the amino acids found in the framework of human cartilage. These are also the amino acids that are required for the synthesis and repair of connective tissue throughout the body.

Pharmacology Type II collagen extracts support the production of collagen in the body. These products reportedly aid in reducing the destruction of collagen within the body. They also may provide anti-inflammatory activity and may improve joint flexibility.

Toxicities, Warnings, and Interactions No known toxicity or serious side effects

Symptoms of Deficiency Deficiency studies in humans have not been conducted.

References

Barnett ML, Kremer JM, St Clair EW, et al, "Treatment of Rheumatoid Arthritis With Oral Type II Collagen: Results of a Multicenter, Double-Blind, Placebo-Controlled Trial," *Arthritis Rheum*, 1998; 41(2):290-7.

Chvapil M, Kronenthal L, and Van Winkle W Jr, "Medical and Surgical Applications of Collagen," *Int Rev Connect Tissue Res*, 1973, 6:1-61.

Colostrum

Related Information

Nutraceutical Chart *on page 573*

Natural Product Category Nutraceutical

Dosage Oral: Dosage range: 500-1000 mg 1-3 times/day

Active Forms Colostrum

Reported Uses

Antidiarrheal (Rump, 1992)

Antiviral (Palmer, 1980)

Immunostimulant (Wilson, 1998; Bertotto, 1997)

Summary Colostrum is the liquid that is secreted from a mother's breast during the first 72 hours following the birth of an infant. This "first food of life" actually precedes the production of breast milk. In addition to being rich with nutrients, colostrum contains substances that are important to the development of the infant's immune system.

Pharmacology Colostrum contains substances such as immunoglobulins and lactoferrin that play key roles in the immune system, including fighting viruses, bacteria, fungi, allergens, and toxins. Colostrum also stimulates maturation of white blood cells called B lymphocytes and increases the activity of macrophages, thereby enhancing the immune system. Colostrum's growth and immune factors are reported to be helpful in a wide variety of health conditions, including accelerating wound healing, stimulating fat burning, helping to maintain stable blood glucose levels, and balancing blood sugar.

Toxicities, Warnings, and Interactions No known toxicity or serious side effects. Use with caution in individuals allergic to dairy products.

Symptoms of Deficiency Deficiency studies in humans have not been conducted.

References

Bertotto A, Vagliasindi C, Gerli R, et al, "Soluble CD30 Antigen in Human Colostrum," *Biol Neonate*, 1997, 71(2):69-74.

Palmer EL, Gary GW Jr, Black R, et al, "Antiviral Activity of Colostrum and Serum Immunoglobulins A and G," *J Med Virol*, 1980, 5(2):123-9.

Rump JA, Arndt R, Arnold A, et al, "Treatment of Diarrhea in Human Immunodeficiency Virus-Infected Patients With Immunoglobulins From Bovine Colostrum," *Clin Investig*, 1992, 70(7):588-94.

Wilson DC, et al, "Immune System Breakthrough: Colostrum," *J Longevity*, 1998, 4(2):43-6.

♦ **Commiphora mukul** see Guggul *(Commiphora mukul) on page 454*
♦ **Common Herbal Supplements Contraindicated During Pregnancy** *see page 656*
♦ **Conditions/Decision Trees/Considerations** *see page 44*
♦ **Coneflower** see Echinacea *(Echinacea purpurea, Echinacea angustifolia) on page 426*

Conjugated Linoleic Acid (CLA)

Related Information

Nutraceutical Chart *on page 573*

(Continued)

Conjugated Linoleic Acid (CLA) *(Continued)*

Natural Product Category Nutraceutical

Dosage Oral: Dosage range: 1000-2000 mg 3 times/day in divided doses

Active Forms Conjugate linoleic acid

Reported Uses Increases metabolism, decreases body fat (West, 1998)

Summary CLA is a naturally occurring polyunsaturated fatty acid present in small quantities in many foods, especially meat and dairy products. Although the human body does not make CLA, it is readily absorbed from foods and in supplement form. Changes in the way beef, chickens, and other animals are fed and raised over the past several decades has resulted in a drastic reduction in the amount of CLA in the average American diet.

Pharmacology CLA is essential for the delivery of dietary fat into cells. It transports glucose into cells where it can be used to build muscle and produce energy rather than being converted to fat. This makes CLA a useful supplement in weight loss programs and among bodybuilders. CLA is also a potent antioxidant and exhibits properties which enhance the immune system.

Toxicities, Warnings, and Interactions No known toxicity or serious side effects

Symptoms of Deficiency Deficiency studies in humans have not been conducted; however, weight gain would be a result of deficiency.

References

West DB, Delany JP, Camet PM, et al, "Effects of Conjugated Linoleic Acid on Body Fat and Energy Metabolism in the Mouse," *Am J Physiol,* 1998, 275(3 Pt 2):R667-72.

♦ **Constipation** *see page 122*

♦ **Contact Dermatitis** *see* Eczema *on page 162*

♦ **Contact Dermatitis** *see* Poison Ivy / Poison Oak *on page 306*

Copper

Related Information

Drug-Induced Nutrient Depletions *on page 625*

Vitamins/Minerals/Trace Elements/Amino Acids Chart *on page 604*

Natural Product Category Mineral

Dosage Oral: RDI: 2 mg/day; ODA: 2-3 mg/day

Active Forms Copper gluconate, copper amino acid chelates, copper glycinate, copper lysinate, copper citrate, copper sulfate, and copper sebacate

Reported Uses

Anemia (Gyorffy, 1992)

Osteoporosis (Strain, 1988)

Rheumatoid arthritis (Sorenson, 1977)

Summary Copper is an essential trace mineral which is a cofactor in cuproenzyme systems. It participates in a number of enzymatic reactions with varied physiologic roles. These include melanin production (hair and skin color), wound healing, and red blood cell production. It is an important component of key antioxidant enzymes, preventing damage from inflammatory processes. It appears to be particularly important in the maintenance of connective tissue and joint function, and deficiency may contribute to the development of anemia.

Pharmacology Copper is involved in the maintenance of bone, collagen, and nerve tissue. Copper is a cofactor in a number of antioxidant enzymes, including superoxide dismutase (SOD). It is required for the synthesis and function of hemoglobin and stimulates the intestinal absorption of iron. Copper is involved in the production of elastin and collagen, which contribute to the structural stability of bone, cartilage, skin, and tendons as well as the elasticity of the lungs, blood vessels, and skin. It may play a role in emotional regulation and cognitive function. Some researchers have shown that copper deficiency is associated with elevated cholesterol and triglycerides, and the development of atherosclerosis.

Toxicities, Warnings, and Interactions Hemolytic anemia, hemoglobinuria, jaundice, nausea, vomiting, epigastric pain, headache, dizziness, weakness, diarrhea, and hemochromatosis

Use in Wilson's disease is contraindicated

Symptoms of Deficiency Severe copper deficiency is rare, but since the diet of many Americans only supplies about 50% of the RDA, moderate deficiency is common. The symptoms may include loss of color in the hair and skin, anemia, inflammation, arthritis, connective tissue weakening, cardiovascular damage, and leukocytopenia.

Reported Interactions

Drug/Nutrient Interactions: Drugs which can cause depletion of copper: Zidovudine (AZT) and D-penicillamine. Estrogens have been shown to increase serum copper and ceruloplasmin levels in humans.

Nutrient/Nutrient Interactions: Zinc and iron can both inhibit the absorption of copper. Large doses of vitamin C can lead to a depletion of copper.

References

Gyorffy EJ and Chan H, "Copper Deficiency and Microcytic Anemia Resulting From Prolonged Ingestion of Over-the-Counter Zinc," *Am J Gastroenterol*, 1992, 87(8):1054-5.

Sorenson JR and Hangarter W, "Treatment of Rheumatoid and Degenerative Diseases With Copper Complexes: A Review With Emphasis on Copper-Salicylate," *Inflammation*, 1977, 2(3):217-38.

Strain JJ, "A Reassessment of Diet and Osteoporosis - Possible Role for Copper," *Med Hypotheses*, 1988, 27(4):333-8.

Cordyceps *(Cordyceps sinensis)*

Related Information

Herb/Drug Potential Interactions *on page 642*

Herb Quick Reference Chart *on page 538*

Organ System Support Using Natural Products *on page 660*

Natural Product Category Herb

Plant Part Fungus

Dosage and Standardization Oral: 1050 mg 2-3 times/day, standardized to contain 0.14% adenosine and 5% mannitol per dose

Reported Uses

Adaptogen/tonic (to promote wellness, longevity, and general health) (Bao, 1998)

Adjunct support for chemotherapy and radiation (Xu, 1992; Zhu, 1998)

Antioxidant (Zhu, 1997)

Enhancement in cellular oxygenation during stress; reduction in symptoms of fatigue; immunomodulatory (Chen, 1983)

Enhancement of sexual vitality; males and females (Wan, 1988)

Hepatoprotection (Zhou, 1990)

Improvement in endurance and stamina (Sun, 1985)

Support of lung, liver and kidney function (Lei, 1992)

Summary Cordyceps is a unique black mushroom originally found to grow only on the surface of a caterpillar found in the mountains of Tibet and China. Cordyceps is an important agent in traditional Chinese medicine. It has been employed in treating lung and kidney disorders, as well as a tonic to promote longevity, vitality, and endurance. More recently, cyclosporine was isolated from a species of cordyceps. Large-scale production processes are now available. Cordyceps has been used to improve energy and increase activity levels in individuals with fatigue.

Pharmacology Cordyceps contains a variety of proteins, amino acids, polysaccharides, sterols and fatty acids, nucleosides, vitamins B_1, B_2, B_{12}, E, and K. Its proposed mechanism of action involves improving oxygen utilization and increased tissue "steady state" energy levels. This activity may improve symptoms of various lung and kidney disorders. Cordyceps may modulate immune and endocrine function, which are claimed to result in increased physical strength and endurance. Cordyceps functions as an antioxidant by increasing serum concentrations of superoxide dismutase (SOD), which acts as a free radical scavenger. Effects on sexual vitality may be due to an increase in gonadotropic hormones, or direct actions on the CNS, sex organs, and the hypothalamic-pituitary-adrenocortical axis. (Continued)

Cordyceps (Cordyceps sinensis) (Continued)

Cordyceps has been reported to decrease proliferation and differentiation of cancer cells and has immunomodulatory effects. Cordyceps has been reported to decrease the renal toxicity of aminoglycosides and cyclosporine (Bao, 1994; Zhao, 1993). It increases sex hormone binding capacity. Cordyceps protects stem cells and red blood cells during chemotherapy and radiation. See References.

Theoretical Cautions and Contraindications Use with caution in individuals with allergies to molds or fungi. In addition, based on pharmacological activity, use is contraindicated in individuals receiving MAO inhibitors (Xu, 1988).

May alter platelet aggregation (based on pharmacological activity of some components, Hammerschmidt, 1980). Contraindicated in individuals with active bleeding (eg, peptic ulcer, intracranial bleeding). Use with caution in individuals with a history of bleeding, hemostatic disorders, or drug-related hemostatic problems. Use with caution in individuals taking anticoagulant medications, including warfarin, aspirin, aspirin-containing products, NSAIDs, or antiplatelet agents (eg, ticlopidine, clopidogrel, dipyridamole). Discontinue use prior to dental or surgical procedures (generally at least 14 days before).

General Warnings Use all herbal supplements with extreme caution in children <2 years of age and in pregnancy or lactation. Some herbs are contraindicated in pregnancy or lactation; make sure to observe warnings. Use with caution in individuals on medication and with pre-existing medical conditions. Always review for potential herb-drug interactions (HDIs) and other warnings. Large and prolonged doses may increase the potential for adverse effects. Herbs may cause transient adverse effects such as nausea, vomiting, and GI distress due to a variety of chemical constituents. Caution should be used in individuals having known allergies to plants.

Theoretical Interactions Anticoagulants, antiplatelet drugs, MAO inhibitors

References

Bao TT, Wang GF, and Yang JL, "Pharmacological Actions of *Cordyceps sinensis*," *Chung Hsi I Chieh Ho Tsa Chih*, 1988, 8(6):352-6.

Bao ZD, Wu ZG, and Zheng F, "Amelioration of Aminoglycoside Nephrotoxicity by *Cordyceps sinensis* in Old Patients," *Chung Kuo Chung Hsi I Chieh Ho Tsa Chih*, 1994, 14(5):271-3, 259.

Chen YP, "Studies on Immunological Actions of *Cordyceps sinensis*. I. Effect on Cellular Immunity," *Chung Yao Tung Pao*, 1983, 8(5):33-5.

Hammerschmidt DE, "Szechwan purpura," *N Engl J Med*, 1980, 302(21):1191-3.

Lei J, Chen J, and Guo C, "Pharmacological Study on *Cordyceps sinensis* (Berk.) Sacc. and ze-e Cordyceps," *Chung Kuo Chung Yao Tsa Chih*, 1992, 17(6):364-6, 384.

Sun YH, "*Cordyceps sinensis* and Cultured *Mycelia*," *Chung Yao Tung Pao*, 1985, 10(12):3-5.

Wan F, et al, "Sex Hormone-Like Effects of JinShiuBao Capsule: Pharmacology and Clinical Studies," *Chinese Traditional Patent Medicine*, 1988, 9:29-31.

Xu RH, Peng XE, Chen GZ, et al, "Effects of *Cordyceps sinensis* on Natural Killer Cell Activity and Colony Formation of B16 Melanoma," *Chin Med J (Engl)*, 1992, 105(2):97-101.

Xu WZ, et al, "Effects of *Cordyceps sinensis* on Monoamine Oxidase and Immunity," *Shanghai J Traditional Chinese Med*, 1988, 1:48-9.

Zhao X and Li L, "*Cordyceps sinensis* in Protection of the Kidney From Cyclosporine A Nephrotoxicity," *Chung Hua I Hsueh Tsa Chih*, 1993, 73(7):410-2, 447.

Zhou L, Yang W, Xu Y, et al, "Short-Term Curative Effect of Cultured *Cordyceps sinensis* (Berk.) Sacc. Mycelia in Chronic Hepatitis B," *Chung Kuo Chung Yao Tsa Chih*, 1990, 15(1):53-5, 65.

Zhu J, et al, "CordyMax Cs-4: A Scientific Product Review," *Pharmanex Phytoscience Review Series*, 1997.

Zhu JS, Halpern GM, and Jones K, "The Scientific Discovery of an Ancient Chinese Herbal Medicine: *Cordyceps sinensis*: Part I," *J Altern Complement Med*, 1998, 4(3):289-303.

♦ *Cordyceps sinensis* see Cordyceps (Cordyceps sinensis) on page 417

♦ Cough see page 126

Cranberry (Vaccinium macrocarpon)

Related Information

Herb Quick Reference Chart on page 538

Organ System Support Using Natural Products on page 660

Natural Product Category Herb

Plant Part Berry

Dosage and Standardization Oral: 300-400 mg twice daily, standardized to contain 11% to 12% quinic acid per dose; **or** 8-16 ounces of cranberry juice daily

> **Note**: Cranberry juice cocktails contain sugar and may be diluted by other juices. While cranberry juice cocktail is effective in reducing the frequency and severity of UTI, the use of 100% cranberry juice is recommended.

Reported Uses

Prevention of nephrolithiasis (Leung, 1996)

Urinary tract infection (Zafiri, 1989)

Summary In folk medicine, cranberry fruit juice has been recommended as a treatment for a variety of urinary tract disorders. The cranberry is closely related to the American blueberry and European bilberry. Most urinary tract infections are caused by *E. coli*, and infection is facilitated by the bacterial adherence to the epithelial cells of the urinary tract. Cranberry may alter bacterial adherence and has been reported to be clinically useful in these infections.

Pharmacology Although early research indicated that cranberry worked through urinary acidification, current research indicates that a cranberry-derived glycoprotein inhibits *E. coli* adherence to the epithelial cells of the urinary tract. The urinary acidification achieved by cranberry does not appear to be sufficient to exert antibacterial activity. The alteration in bacterial adherence appears to be most effective against the most virulent strains of *E. coli*. Due to its potential to acidify the urine, cranberry has been used to prevent kidney stones, as well as to remove unwanted toxins from the body.

Theoretical Cautions and Contraindications None known

General Warnings Use all herbal supplements with extreme caution in children <2 years of age and in pregnancy or lactation. Some herbs are contraindicated in pregnancy or lactation; make sure to observe warnings. Use with caution in individuals on medication and with pre-existing medical conditions. Always review for potential herb-drug interactions (HDIs) and other warnings. Large and prolonged doses may increase the potential for adverse effects. Herbs may cause transient adverse effects such as nausea, vomiting, and GI distress due to a variety of chemical constituents. Caution should be used in individuals having known allergies to plants.

Theoretical Interactions None known

References

Leung AY and Foster S, *Encyclopedia of Common Natural Ingredients Used in Foods, Drugs, and Cosmetics*, New York, NY: Wiley, 1996, 198-9.

Zafriri D, Ofek I, Adar R, et al, "Inhibitory Activity of Cranberry Juice on Adherence of Type 1 and Type P Fimbriated *Escherichia coli* to Eucaryotic Cells," *Antimicrob Agents Chemother*, 1989, 33(1):92-8.

♦ *Crataegus oxyacantha* see Hawthorn *(Crataegus oxyacantha)* on page 456

Creatine

Related Information

Nutraceutical Chart *on page 573*

Natural Product Category Nutraceutical

Dosage Oral: Dosage range: 10-20 g/day in divided doses, for 1 week during the loading phase, then 5 g/day during the maintenance phase

Active Forms Creatine

Reported Uses Enhancement of athletic performance: Energy production and protein synthesis for muscle building (Greenhaff, 1995)

Summary Creatine is a substance that occurs in the organs, muscles, and body fluids of animals. It combines readily with phosphate to form phospho-creatine, which serves as a source of high-energy phosphate, that is released during the anaerobic phase of muscle contraction.

Pharmacology Creatine supplements are used to enhance athletic performance. They promote protein synthesis and are a quick source of available energy for muscle contraction. Creatine also enhances the formation of polyamines, which are powerful growth promoting substances. Because it (Continued)

Creatine *(Continued)*

enhances energy production and increases the synthesis of muscle protein, creatine is a favorite supplement of bodybuilders.

Toxicities, Warnings, and Interactions May cause elevation of serum creatinine (not a reflection of renal dysfunction). Use with caution in renal or hepatic disease. No known toxicity or serious side effects.

Symptoms of Deficiency Deficiency studies in humans have not been conducted

Reported Interactions
Drug/Nutrient Interactions: Caffeine may block effects
Nutrient/Nutrient Interactions: None known

References
Greenhaff PL, "Creatine and Its Application as an Erogenic Aid," *Int J Sport Nutr,* 1995, 5(Suppl):S100-10.

♦ **Crohn's Disease** *see page 130*
♦ **Croup** *see page 134*
♦ **Curcuma longa** *see* Turmeric *(Curcuma longa) on page 512*

Cyclo-Hispro

Related Information
Nutraceutical Chart *on page 573*
Natural Product Category Nutraceutical
Dosage Oral: Dosage range: 200-300 mg (of powdered prostate extract containing cyclo-hispro) 2-4 times/day
Active Forms Cyclo-hispro
Reported Uses Type 2 diabetes (Song, 1998)
Summary Cyclo-hispro is a metabolite of a major thyrotropin-releasing hormone, which occurs in larger quantities in the prostate gland than in any other tissue. This newly discovered substance in prostate tissue appears to influence the intestinal absorption of zinc.
Pharmacology Cyclo-hispro enhances the intestinal absorption of zinc. Zinc is a mineral that is involved in more than 200 enzymatic reactions in the body. It is intimately involved in the production of insulin and the regulation of blood sugar. Many diabetics have low zinc levels. Studies report that cyclo-hispro is very effective in helping to control glucose metabolism in individuals with insulin-dependent and noninsulin-dependent diabetes.
Toxicities, Warnings, and Interactions No known toxicity or serious side effects. May alter glucose regulation. Use with caution in individuals with diabetes or in those who may be predisposed to hypoglycemia. Effects of drugs with hypoglycemic activity may be potentiated (including insulin and oral hypoglycemics). The individual's blood sugar should be closely monitored, and the dosage of these agents, including insulin dosage, may require adjustment. This should be carefully coordinated among the individual's healthcare providers.
Symptoms of Deficiency Deficiency studies in humans have not been conducted.
Reported Interactions
Drug/Nutrient Interactions: Theoretically: Insulin, oral hypoglycemics
References
Song MK, Rosenthal MJ, Naliboff BD, et al, "Effects of Bovine Prostate Powder on Zinc, Glucose, and Insulin Metabolism in Old Patients With Non-insulin-Dependent Diabetes Mellitus," *Metabolism,* 1998, 47(1):39-43.

♦ **Cynara scolymus** *see* Artichoke *(Cynara scolymus) on page 386*

Dandelion *(Taraxacum officinale)*

Related Information
Herb/Drug Potential Interactions *on page 642*
Herb Quick Reference Chart *on page 538*
Organ System Support Using Natural Products *on page 660*
Natural Product Category Herb
Plant Part Root, leaf

Dosage and Standardization

Oral:

Root: 250-500 mg 3 times/day standardized to contain 20% taraxisterol per dose **or** 5-10 mL 3 times/day of liquid extract (1:1 w/v fresh root or 1:4 w/v dried root) in water or juice

Leaf: 250-500 mg 2-3 times/day **or** 5-10 mL 2-3 times/day of liquid extract (1:1 w/v fresh leaf or 1:4 w/v dried leaf) in water or juice

Reported Uses

Leaf: Diuretic (Racz-Kotilla, 1974)

Root: Disorders of bile secretion (cholerectic); appetite stimulation; dyspeptic complaints (Newall, 1996)

Summary Dandelion root is used in digestive disorders to increase bile secretion (choleretic), for appetite stimulation, and for dyspeptic complaints. The leaf has been reported to act as a potassium-sparing diuretic.

Pharmacology Dandelion leaf is a diuretic comparing favorably to furosemide in a study. The usual potassium loss seen in many conventional diuretics was not seen in dandelion's use, due to the high potassium content in the leaves. Bitter constituents in the root increase bile and gastric secretions.

Theoretical Cautions and Contraindications Do not use root preparation in biliary obstruction or if gallstones are present (based on pharmacological activity, Bradley, 1992). Due to diuretic properties, use leaf preparation with caution in individuals taking diuretics, lithium, or digoxin; excessive use of leaf may lead to electrolyte imbalances (Racz-Kotilla, 1974). Allergic reaction may develop from contact with plant (Davies, 1986).

General Warnings Use all herbal supplements with extreme caution in children <2 years of age and in pregnancy or lactation. Some herbs are contraindicated in pregnancy or lactation; make sure to observe warnings. Use with caution in individuals on medication and with pre-existing medical conditions. Always review for potential herb-drug interactions (HDIs) and other warnings. Large and prolonged doses may increase the potential for adverse effects. Herbs may cause transient adverse effects such as nausea, vomiting, and GI distress due to a variety of chemical constituents. Caution should be used in individuals having known allergies to plants.

Theoretical Interactions Digoxin, lithium, diuretics

References

Bradley PR, ed, *British Herbal Compendium*, Vol 1, Bournemouth, England: British Herbal Medicine Association, 1992, 76-7.

Davies MG, et al, "Contact Allergy to Yarrow and Dandelion," *Contact Dermatitis*, 1986, 14(4):256-7.

McGuffin M, et al, eds, *American Herbal Products Association's Botanical Safety Handbook*, Boca Raton, FL: CRC Press, 1997, 114.

Newall CA, Anderson LA, and Phillipson JD, *Herbal Medicines: A Guide for Health Care Professionals*, London, England: The Pharmaceutical Press, 1996, 96-7.

Racz-Kotilla E, Racz G, and Solomon A, "The Action of *Taraxacum officina* Extracts on Body Weight and Diuresis of Laboratory Animals," *Planta Med*, 1974, 26(3):212-7.

Dehydroepiandrosterone (DHEA)

Related Information

Nutraceutical Chart *on page 573*

Natural Product Category Nutraceutical

Dosage Oral: Dosage range: 5-50 mg/day; doses of 100 mg/day are sometimes used in elderly individuals

Active Forms Dehydroepiandrosterone, micronized dehydroepiandrosterone

Reported Uses

Antiaging (Yen, 1995)

Depression (Wolkowitz, 1997)

Diabetes (Casson, 1995)

Fatigue (Scott, 1999)

Lupus (Van Vollenhoven, 1996)

Summary Human production of DHEA normally peaks during the mid-20s and then begins a steady, progressive decline. Supplementation with DHEA has been claimed to have antiaging effects, including increased libido, (Continued)

Dehydroepiandrosterone (DHEA) *(Continued)*

enhanced immune function, increased muscle mass, and improvements in energy, mood, and memory. It may be used as a supplement to improve symptoms associated with depression, diabetes, and lupus. Adequate human trials have not been conducted. Although DHEA is available without a prescription, it should be used with caution since it affects the levels of many other hormones in the body.

Pharmacology DHEA is secreted by the adrenal glands, and is the precursor for the synthesis of over 50 additional hormones, including estrogen and testosterone. DHEA has also been shown to stimulate the production of insulin growth factor-1 (IGF-1), a hormone which stimulates anabolic metabolism, accelerates muscle growth, improves insulin sensitivity, and enhances energy production. It has been reported to cause a change in the response to insulin, decreasing the insulin requirement in individuals with diabetes.

Toxicities, Warnings, and Interactions No known toxicity or serious side effects, however, long-term human studies have not been conducted. Use is contraindicated in individuals with a history of prostate or breast cancer. May alter blood glucose regulation. Use with caution in individuals with diabetes or in those who may be predisposed to hypoglycemia, including those receiving insulin or oral hypoglycemics. Blood glucose should be closely monitored in individuals with diabetes, and the dosage of antidiabetic agents should be closely among health care providers. Use with caution in individuals with hepatic dysfunction.

Symptoms of Deficiency Since DHEA is synthesized normally, absolute deficiency does not occur. Blood levels decline steadily with age, and low blood levels have been claimed to be associated with an increased risk for many of the common diseases of aging. These include hypertension, hypercholesterolemia, type 2 diabetes, osteoporosis, and obesity. In addition, low levels have been correlated to a loss of muscle mass, memory problems, and increased thrombogenicity (increased platelet aggregation).

Reported Interactions

Drug/Nutrient Interactions: May interact with androgens, estrogens, corticosteroids, insulin, oral hypoglycemic agents

Nutrient/Nutrient Interactions: None known

References

Casson PR, Faguin LC, Stentz FB, et al, "Replacement of Dehydroepiandrosterone Enhances T-Lymphocyte Insulin Binding in Postmenopausal Women," *Fertil Steril*, 1995, 63(5):1027-31.

Scott, LV, Salahuddin F, Cooney J, et al, "Differences in Adrenal Steroid Profile in Chronic Fatigue Syndrome, In Depression and in Health," *J Affect Disord*, 1999, 54(1-2):129-37.

Van Vollenhoven RF and McGuire JL, "Studies of Dehydroepiandrosterone (DHEA) as a Therapeutic Agent in Systemic Lupus Erythematosus," *Ann Med Interne (Paris)*, 1996, 147(4):290-6.

Wolkowitz OM, Reus VI, Roberts E, et al, "Dehydroepiandrosterone (DHEA) Treatment of Depression," *Biol Psychiatry*, 1997, 41(3):311-8.

Yen SS, Morales AJ, and Khorram O, "Replacement of DHEA in Aging Men and Women. Potential Remedial Effects," *Ann N Y Acad Sci*, 1995, 774:128-42.

♦ **Depression** see page 138

Devil's Claw *(Harpagophytum procumbens)*

Related Information

Herb/Drug Potential Interactions *on page 642*
Herb Quick Reference Chart *on page 538*

Natural Product Category Herb

Plant Part Tuber

Dosage and Standardization Oral: 100-200 mg 1-2 times/day, standardized to contain 5% harpagoside (iridoid glycoside) per dose

Reported Uses

Anti-inflammatory (Erdos, 1978; Lanhers, 1992); contradictory study (Whitehouse, 1983)

Back pain (Chrubasik, 1999)

Osteoarthritis, gout, and other inflammatory conditions (Grahame 1981; Lanhers, 1992)

Summary Historically, devil's claw has been used in a variety of conditions related to the liver and kidneys. However, current use of devil's claw generally focuses on the anti-inflammatory effects of this tuber, including arthritis, tendonitis, and inflammatory conditions.

Pharmacology Anti-inflammatory activity has been reported for two constituents, harpagoside and beta sitosterol. The anti-inflammatory effects of devil's claw have been reported to be comparable to phenylbutazone in animal models. However, some contradictory evidence has been published (Whitehouse, 1983). Devil's claw reportedly improves joint mobility and reduces pain and swelling in arthritis. It may be more effective for osteoarthritis as compared to rheumatoid arthritis. In addition, it may be more effective for chronic, rather than acute, arthritis symptoms.

Theoretical Cautions and Contraindications Use of devil's claw is contraindicated in pregnancy and lactation; case reports indicate potential to stimulate uterine contractions (Newall, 1996). Based on pharmacological activity, use caution in individuals receiving antiarrhythmic medications or cardiac glycosides (Shaw, 1997). Use with caution in GI disorders (De Smet, 1993).

Based on pharmacological activity, may alter hemostasis (Shaw, 1997). Contraindicated in active bleeding (eg, peptic ulcer, intracranial bleeding). Use with caution in individuals with a history of bleeding, hemostatic disorders, or drug-related hemostatic problems. Use with caution in individuals taking anticoagulant medications, including warfarin, aspirin, aspirin-containing products, NSAIDs, or antiplatelet agents (eg, ticlopidine, clopidogrel, dipyridamole). Discontinue use prior to dental or surgical procedures (generally at least 14 days before).

General Warnings Use all herbal supplements with extreme caution in children <2 years of age and in pregnancy or lactation. Some herbs are contraindicated in pregnancy or lactation; make sure to observe warnings. Use with caution in individuals on medication and with pre-existing medical conditions. Always review for potential herb-drug interactions (HDIs) and other warnings. Large and prolonged doses may increase the potential for adverse effects. Herbs may cause transient adverse effects such as nausea, vomiting, and GI distress due to a variety of chemical constituents. Caution should be used in individuals having known allergies to plants.

Theoretical Interactions Antiarrhythmics, anticoagulants, aspirin or aspirin-containing products, NSAIDs, antiplatelet agents, cardiac glycosides, warfarin

References

Chrubasik S, Junck H, Breitschwerdt H, et al, "Effectiveness of Harpagophytum Extract WS 1531 in the Treatment of Exacerbation of Low Back Pain: A Randomized, Placebo-Controlled, Double-Blind Study," *Eur J Anaesthesiol*, 1999, 16(2):118-29.

De Smet PA, Hansel R, Keller K, et al, *Adverse Effects of Herbal Drugs*, Vol 2, New York, NY: Springer-Verlag, 1993.

Erdos A, Fontaine R, Friehe H, et al, "Contribution to the Pharmacology and Toxicology of Different Extracts as Well as the Harpagoside From *Harpagophytum procumbens* DC," *Planta Med*, 1978, 34(1):97-108.

Grahame R and Robinson BV, "Devil's Claw (*Harpagophytum procumbens*): Pharmacological and Clinical Studies," *Ann Rheum Dis*, 1981, 40(6):632.

Lanhers MC, Fleurentin J, Mortier F, et al, "Anti-inflammatory and Analgesic Effects of an Aqueous Extract of *Harpagophytum procumbens*," *Planta Med*, 1992, 58(2):117-23.

Newall CA, Anderson LA, and Phillipson JD, *Herbal Medicines: A Guide for Health Care Professionals*, London, England: The Pharmaceutical Press, 1996, 98-100.

Shaw D, Leon C, Kolev S, et al, "Traditional Remedies and Food Supplements. A 5-Year Toxicological Study (1991-1995)," *Drug Saf*, 1997, 17(5):342-56.

Whitehouse LW, Znamirowska M, and Paul CJ, "Devil's Claw (*Harpagophytum procumbens*): No Evidence for Anti-inflammatory Activity in the Treatment of Arthritic Disease," *Can Med Assoc J*, 1983, 129(3):249-51.

♦ **DHA** see Docosahexaenoic Acid (DHA) *on page 424*
♦ **DHEA** see Dehydroepiandrosterone (DHEA) *on page 421*
♦ **Diaper Rash** see *page 142*
♦ **Diarrhea** see *page 146*

- **Dimethyl Sulfone** *see* Methyl Sulfonyl Methane (MSM) *on page 479*
- **Dioscorea villosa** *see* Wild Yam *(Dioscorea villosa) on page 532*
- **Diverticulitis** *see page 150*
- **DMSO₂** *see* Methyl Sulfonyl Methane (MSM) *on page 479*

Docosahexaenoic Acid (DHA)

Related Information
Nutraceutical Chart *on page 573*

Natural Product Category Nutraceutical

Dosage Oral: Dosage range: 125-250 mg 1-2 times/day

Active Forms Docosahexaenoic acid (DHA)

Reported Uses
Alzheimer's disease (Kyle, 1999)
Attention deficit disorder (ADD) and attention deficit hyperactivity disorder (Stevens, 1995)
Crohn's disease (Belluzzi, 1996)
Diabetes (McManus, 1996)
Eczema (Bjorneboe, 1989)
Elevated triglycerides (Pritchard, 1995)
Hypertension (Morris, 1993)
Psoriasis (Bittiner, 1988)
Rheumatoid arthritis (Kremer, 1991)

Summary DHA is a long-chain unsaturated fatty acid that is a member of the omega-3 family of fatty acids. The primary dietary source of DHA is from cold water or oily fish such as mackerel, salmon, herring, sardines, and tuna. DHA plays a major role in the development of the brain and the retina of the eyes in infants. DHA is also the most abundant unsaturated fatty acid found in the brain.

Pharmacology Alpha-linolenic acid (ALA) is the precursor for all of the other omega-3 fatty acids. However, it is estimated that only a small percentage of ALA gets converted to DHA. DHA is found in high concentration in areas of the brain that require a high degree of electrical activity. For example, large quantities of DHA are concentrated in synaptosomes in the brain, which is the region where nerve cells communicate with each other. It is also concentrated in the photoreceptors, the portion of the retina that receives light stimulation. Other areas with high levels of DHA include the mitochondria and the cerebral cortex. DHA also helps to lower elevated triglyceride levels.

Toxicities, Warnings, and Interactions Contraindicated in individuals with active bleeding (eg, peptic ulcer, intracranial bleeding). Use with caution in individuals with a history of bleeding, hemostatic disorders, or drug-related hemostatic problems. Use with caution in individuals taking anticoagulant medications, including warfarin, aspirin, aspirin-containing products, NSAIDs, or antiplatelet agents (eg, ticlopidine, clopidogrel, dipyridamole). Discontinue use prior to dental or surgical procedures (generally at least 14 days before).

Symptoms of Deficiency Vision problems; lower IQ; slower rate of learning

Reported Interactions Anticoagulants, antiplatelet agents, NSAIDs, aspirin, aspirin-containing products

References
Belluzzi A, Brignola C, Campieri M, et al, "Effect of an Enteric-Coated Fish Oil Preparation on Relapses in Crohn's Disease," *N Engl J Med*, 1996, 334(24):1557-60.

Bittiner SB, Tucker WF, Cartwright I, et al, "A Double-Blind, Randomised, Placebo-Controlled Trial of Fish Oil in Psoriasis," *Lancet*, 1988, 1(8582):378-80.

Bjorneboe A, Soyland E, Bjorneboe GE, et al, "Effect of n-3 Fatty Acid Supplement to Patients With Atopic Dermatitis," *J Intern Med Suppl*, 1989, 225(731):233-6.

Kremer JM, "Clinical Studies of Omega-3 Fatty Acid Supplementation in Patients Who Have Rheumatoid Arthritis," *Rheum Dis Clin North Am*, 1991, 17(2):391-402.

Kyle DJ, Schaefer E, Patton G, et al, "Low Serum Docosahexanoic Acid is a Significant Risk Factor for Alzheimer's Dementia," *Lipids*, 1999, 34(Suppl):S245.

McManus RM, Jumpson J, Finegood DT, et al, "A Comparison of the Effects of n-3 Fatty Acids From Linseed Oil and Fish Oil in Well-Controlled Type II Diabetes," *Diabetes Care*, 1996, 19(5):463-7.

Morris MC, Sacks F, and Rosner B, et al, "Does Fish Oil Lower Blood Pressure? A Meta-Analysis of Controlled Trials," *Circulation,* 1993, 88(2):523-33.

Pritchard BN, Smith CC, Ling KL, et al, "Fish Oils and Cardiovascular Disease," *BMJ,* 1995, 310(6983):819-20.

Song MK, Rosenthal MJ, Naliboff BD, et al, "Effects of Bovine Prostate Powder on Zinc, Glucose, and Insulin Metabolism in Old Patients With Non-insulin-Dependent Diabetes Mellitus," *Metabolism,* 1998, 47(1):39-43.

Stevens LJ, Zentall SS, Deck JL, et al, "Essential Fatty Acid Metabolism in Boys with Attention-Deficit Hyperactivity Disorder," *Am J Clin Nutr,* 1995, 62(4):761-8.

Dong Quai *(Angelica sinensis)*

Related Information

Herb/Drug Potential Interactions *on page 642*

Herb Quick Reference Chart *on page 538*

Natural Product Category Herb

Plant Part Root

Dosage and Standardization Oral: 200 mg twice daily, standardized to contain 0.8% to 1.1% ligustilide per dose

Reported Uses

Anemia (Zhu, 1987)

Hypertension (Zhu, 1987)

Improvement in energy, particularly in females (Zhu, 1987)

Menopause, dysmenorrhea, premenstrual syndrome (PMS), and amenorrhea (Xu, 1981; Hirata, 1977)

Contradictory study (Hirata,1997)

Phytoestrogen (Lin, 1979)

Summary
Dong quai is considered to be one of the most important remedies in traditional Chinese medicine. It has been used for centuries for a variety of female health disorders. It is considered a tonic for women who are tired, recovering from illness, or have low vitality. It has also been used for reduction in smooth muscle spasms.

Pharmacology
Dong quai is rich in phytoestrogens, which may demonstrate similar pharmacological effects, but are less potent than pure estrogenic compounds. However, there are conflicting reports concerning the direct estrogenic effects of dong quai (Hirata, 1997). Theoretically, phytoestrogens demonstrate partial agonist activity, modulating the effect of estrogen in both deficiency and excess. They may act as competitive antagonists to estrogen when concentrations are high (such as in PMS). In contrast, the agonist activity of phytoestrogens may be useful in situations where the estrogen concentrations are low (such as menopause). Dong quai has also been reported to cause vasodilation, contributing to its use in hypertension. Dong quai also reportedly has hematopoietic properties, which may act to stimulate blood cell production and improve energy.

Theoretical Cautions and Contraindications
Based on potential interference with platelet aggregation (observed with related species) may alter hemostasis. Contraindicated in individuals with active bleeding (eg, peptic ulcer, intracranial bleeding). Use with caution in individuals with a history of bleeding, hemostatic disorders, or drug-related hemostatic problems. May potentiate effects of warfarin (Lo, 1995). Use caution in individuals taking anticoagulant medications, including warfarin, aspirin, aspirin-containing products, NSAIDs, or antiplatelet agents (eg, ticlopidine, clopidogrel, dipyridamole). Discontinue use prior to dental or surgical procedures (generally at least 14 days before).

Caution in pregnancy and lactation. May cause photosensitization (Leung, 1996); avoid prolonged exposure to sunlight or other sources of ultraviolet radiation (ie, tanning booths). Based on pharmacological activity (Zhu, 1987), use with caution in individuals at risk of hypotension, or in those who would tolerate hypotension poorly (cerebrovascular or cardiovascular disease). Use with caution in individuals taking antihypertensive medications.

Phytoestrogen-containing herbs have not been associated with the negative health effects seen with synthetic estrogen. However, use with caution in individuals on hormone replacement therapy or oral contraceptives or with a

(Continued)

Dong Quai *(Angelica sinensis)* *(Continued)*

history of estrogen-dependent tumors, endometrial cancer, thromboembolic disease, or stroke.

General Warnings Use all herbal supplements with extreme caution in children <2 years of age and in pregnancy or lactation. Some herbs are contraindicated in pregnancy or lactation; make sure to observe warnings. Use with caution in individuals on medication and with pre-existing medical conditions. Always review for potential herb-drug interactions (HDIs) and other warnings. Large and prolonged doses may increase the potential for adverse effects. Herbs may cause transient adverse effects such as nausea, vomiting, and GI distress due to a variety of chemical constituents. Caution should be used in individuals having known allergies to plants.

Theoretical Interactions Increased effect: Antihypertensives, anticoagulants, antiplatelet drugs, hormonal replacement therapy, oral contraceptives, photosensitizing medications.

References

Hirata JD, Swiersz LM, Zell B, et al, "Does Dong Quai Have Estrogenic Effects in Postmenopausal Women? A Double-Blind, Placebo-Controlled Trial," *Fertil Steril*, 1997, 68(6):981-6.

Leung AY and Foster S, *Encyclopedia of Common Natural Ingredients Used in Foods, Drugs, and Cosmetics*, New York, NY: Wiley, 1996, 32-3.

Lin M, Zhu GD, Sun QM, et al, "Chemical Studies of *Angelica sinensis*," *Yao Hsueh Hsueh Pao*, 1979, 14(9):529-34.

Lo AC, Chan K, Yeung JH, et al, "Danggui (*Angelica sinensis*) Affects the Pharmacodynamics But Not the Pharmacokinetics of Warfarin in Rabbits," *Eur J Drug Metab Pharmacokinet*, 1995, 20(1):55-60.

Xu LN, Ouyang R, Yin ZZ, et al, "The Effect of Dang-gui (*Angelica sinensis*) and Its Constituent Ferulic Acid on Phagocytosis in Mice," *Yao Hsueh Hsueh Pao*, 1981, 16(6):411-4.

Zhu DP, "Dong Quai," *Am J Chin Med*, 1987, 15(3-4):117-25.

♦ **Drug-Induced Nutrient Depletions** *see page 625*

♦ **Dyslipidemia** *see page 154*

♦ **Dysmenorrhea** *see page 158*

♦ ***Echinacea angustifolia*** see Echinacea (*Echinacea purpurea, Echinacea angustifolia*) on page 426

Echinacea *(Echinacea purpurea, Echinacea angustifolia)*

Related Information

Herb/Drug Potential Interactions *on page 642*
Herb Quick Reference Chart *on page 538*
Organ System Support Using Natural Products *on page 660*

Natural Product Category Herb

Plant Part Varies by species: *E. purpurea* - flower, whole plant; *E. angustifolia* - root

Dosage and Standardization Oral:

Capsule: 500 mg 3 times/day on day 1, then 250 mg 4 times/day, standardized to contain 4% echinacosides (*E. angustifolia*) or 4% sesquiterpene esters (*E. purpurea*) per dose

Plant juice: Freshly expressed (*E. purpurea*): 60 drops 3 times/day with food for 1 day, then 40 drops 3 times/day with food for up to 10 days, standardized to contain not less than 2.4% soluble beta-1,2 D-5 fructofuranosides per dose

Topical: Apply to affected area as needed

Reported Uses

Antiviral (Orinda, 1973)
Arthritis (*E. augustifolia*) (Tubaro, 1987)
Immunostimulant (colds and other upper respiratory infection) (Brinkeborn, 1999; Bauer, 1996; Luettig, 1989)
Topical anti-infective (boils, abscesses, tonsillitis) (Leung, 1996)

Summary Echinacea is one of the most popular herbs, and has been extensively studied for its effects on the immune system. It has been used as an immune stimulant for a variety of afflictions, including colds and flu. As opposed to its use during colds and flu, some published trials of this herb in the prevention of colds and upper respiratory infection have failed to demonstrate benefit (Grimm, 1999; Hoheisel, 1997). However, other reports support its use. It has been promoted as a general health measure to improve resistance during seasonal outbreaks, but there is some concern related to the potential immunosuppressive effects of prolonged use. In general, prolonged continuous use is not recommended (see Cautions and Contraindications).

Pharmacology Echinacea appears to have a variety of nonspecific stimulatory effects on the immune system. Echinacea is claimed to stimulate white blood cell function and cell-mediated immunity, including T lymphocytes, macrophages, and natural killer cells. As a consequence of macrophage stimulation, echinacea has been reported to increase the production of interferon, tumor necrosis factor, and interleukin-1. Echinacea activates white blood cells to scavenge for bacteria and cellular debris. In addition, echinacea inhibits the hyaluronidase and stimulates fibroblast production of collagen. Echinacea is reported to have broad antimicrobial activity, including effects on bacteria, fungi, and viruses. It has been used externally for wound cleansing, eczema, burns, herpes, canker sores, and abscesses.

Theoretical Cautions and Contraindications Based on this agent's pharmacological activity, use for more than 10 days in acute infections or in immunosuppressed individuals is not recommended (Bradley, 1992). When used as prophylaxis, ingestion should be cycled for 3 weeks on and 1 week off (Brown, 1999). Use with caution in individuals with renal disease or impairment; may cause electrolyte imbalance (Murray, 1995). Use with caution in individuals allergic to members of the *Asteraceae/Compositae* family (ragweed, daisy, aster, chrysanthemum) and other pollens; rare, but severe reactions have been reported (Mullins, 1998).

General Warnings Use all herbal supplements with extreme caution in children <2 years of age and in pregnancy or lactation. Some herbs are contraindicated in pregnancy or lactation; make sure to observe warnings. Use with caution in individuals on medication and with pre-existing medical conditions. Always review for potential herb-drug interactions (HDIs) and other warnings. Large and prolonged doses may increase the potential for adverse effects. Herbs may cause transient adverse effects such as nausea, vomiting, and GI distress due to a variety of chemical constituents. Caution should be used in individuals having known allergies to plants.

Theoretical Interactions Therapeutic immunosuppressants (cyclosporin, tacrolimus, sirolimus, methotrexate), corticosteroids

References

Bauer R, "Echinacea Drugs - Effects and Active Ingredients," *Z Arztl Fortbild (Jena)*, 1996, 90(2):111-5.

Bradley PR, ed, *British Herbal Compendium*, Vol 1, Bournemouth, England: British Herbal Medicine Association, 1992, 81-3.

Brinkeborn RM, Shah DV, and Degenring FH, "Echinaforce and other Echinacea Fresh Plant Preparations in the Treatment of the Common Cold: A Randomized, Placebo Controlled, Double-Blind Clinical Trial," *Phytomedicine*, 1999, 6:1-5.

Brown D, "Echinacea Root Fails to Prevent Upper Respiratory Tract Infections," *HealthNotes Rev Complement Alternative Med*, 1999, 6(1):6-7.

Grimm W, Müller HH, "A Randomized Controlled Trial of the Effect of Fluid Extract of *Echinacea purpurea* on the Incidence and Severity of Colds and Respiratory Infections," *Am J Med*, 1999, 106(2):138-43.

Hoheisel O, Sandbers M, Bertram S, et al, "Echinacea Root Extracts for the Prevention of Upper Respiratory Tract Infections: A Double-Blind, Placebo Controlled Trial," *Eur J Clin Res*, 1997, 9:261-8.

Leung AY and Foster S, *Encyclopedia of Common Natural Ingredients Used in Foods, Drugs, and Cosmetics*, New York, NY: Wiley, 1996, 216-20.

Luettig B, Steinmuller C, Gifford GE, et al, "Macrophage Activation by the Polysaccharide Arabinogalactan Isolated From Plant Cell Cultures of *Echinacea purpurea*," *Natl Cancer Inst*, 1989, 81(9):669-75.

Mullins RJ, "Echinacea-Associated Anaphylaxis," *Med J Aust*, 1998, 168(4):170-1.

Murray MT, "Echinacea: Pharmacology and Clinical Applications," *Am J Natural Med*, 1995, 2:18-24.

Orinda D, Diederich J, and Wacker A, "Antiviral Activity of Components of *Echinacea purpurea*," *Arzneimittelforschung*, 1973, 23(8):1119-20.

Tubaro A, Tragni E, Del Negro P, et al, "Anti-inflammatory Activity of a Polysaccharidic Fraction of *Echinacea angustifolia*," *J Pharm Pharmacol*, 1987, 39(7):567-9.

◆ **Echinacea purpurea** see Echinacea *(Echinacea purpurea, Echinacea angustifolia)* on page 426

◆ **Eczema** see page 162

◆ **Elderberry** see Elder *(Sambucus nigra, Sambucus canadensis)* on page 428

Elder *(Sambucus nigra, Sambucus canadensis)*

Related Information

Herb/Drug Potential Interactions *on page 642*
Herb Quick Reference Chart *on page 538*

Natural Product Category Herb

Plant Part Flower, berry (see Reported Uses, Dosage and Standardization)

Dosage and Standardization Oral:

Berry: 500 mg 2-3 times/day, standardized to contain 30% anthocyanins with 8% total acids and 7% total phenols per dose **or**

Liquid extract: 15 mL 2-3 times/day for 3-4 days *(Sambucus nigra)*

Flower: 500 mg 2-3 times/day, standardized to contain 5% bioflavonoids per dose

Reported Uses

Berry: Antiviral; antioxidant; influenza (Zakay, 1995)

Flower:

Anti-inflammatory (Yesliada, 1997)

Colds and influenza (Zakay-Rones, 1995)

Diaphoretic (Newall, 1996)

Diuretic (Bradley, 1992)

Summary Although used as a food in ancient times, elder has also been used as a medicinal agent for thousands of years. Elder flowers are thought to possess diuretic, diaphoretic (increase sweating), and anticatarrhal properties. It has been traditionally used in individuals with colds, influenza, chronic nasal catarrh, and sinusitis. A patented liquid extract of the berries has been used in Israel as an effective antiviral agent in the prevention and treatment of colds and influenza.

Pharmacology An extract of the berries of the black elder *(Sambucus nigra)* has been reported to inhibit the ability of several strains of influenza virus to replicate. The antioxidant properties of the berries are related to its flavonoid constituents. Elder flowers have diuretic properties. An infusion of elder flowers has been reported to have anti-inflammatory properties, mainly inhibiting cytokine production.

Theoretical Cautions and Contraindications Short-term use of elder flowers has not been associated with adverse effects. Theoretically, long-term use and/or high doses of elder flowers may alter lithium and/or digoxin levels due to diuretic properties. Use caution with diuretics.

General Warnings Use all herbal supplements with extreme caution in children <2 years of age and in pregnancy or lactation. Some herbs are contraindicated in pregnancy or lactation; make sure to observe warnings. Use with caution in individuals on medication and with pre-existing medical conditions. Always review for potential herb-drug interactions (HDIs) and other warnings. Large and prolonged doses may increase the potential for adverse effects. Herbs may cause transient adverse effects such as nausea, vomiting, and GI distress due to a variety of chemical constituents. Caution should be used in individuals having known allergies to plants.

Theoretical Interactions Diuretics, digoxin, and lithium

References

Bradley PR, ed, *The British Herbal Compendium, Vol 1*, London, England: British Herbal Medicine Association, 1992, 84-6.

Brown D, "Echinacea Root Fails to Prevent Upper Respiratory Tract Infections," *HealthNotes Rev Complement Alternative Med*, 1999, 6(1):6-7.

Newall CA, Anderson LA, and Phillipson JD, *Herbal Medicines: A Guide for Health Care Professionals*, London, England: The Pharmaceutical Press, 1996, 104-5.

Yesilada E, Utson O, Sezik E, et al, "Inhibitory Effects of Turkish Folk Remedies on Inflammatory Cytokines: Interleukin-1Alpha, Interleukin-1Beta and Tumor Necrosis Factor Alpha," *J Ethnopharmacol*, 1997, 58(1):59-73.

Zakay-Rones Z, Varsano N, Zlotnik M, et al, "Inhibition of Several Strains of Influenza Virus In-Vitro and Reduction of Symptoms by an Elderberry Extract *(Sambucus nigra)* During an Outbreak of Influenza B Panama," *J Altern Complement Med*, 1995, 1(4):361-9.

♦ *Eleutherococcus senticosus* see Ginseng, Siberian *(Eleutherococcus senticosus)* on page 444
♦ *Endometriosis* see page 166

Ephedra *(Ephedra sinica)*

Related Information
Herb Quick Reference Chart *on page 538*
Unsafe Herbs *on page 654*

Natural Product Category Herb

Plant Part Stem

Dosage and Standardization No more than 8 mg total ephedra alkaloids per dose **or** no more than 24 mg total ephedra alkaloids per 24 hours

Reported Uses
Bronchodilator in asthma (Redman, 1998)
Decongestant in allergies, sinusitis, hay fever (Langwinski, 1972)
Thermogenic aid in weight loss (Betz, 1997)

Summary The Chinese have used ephedra medicinally for over 5000 years. Ephedra is listed as one of the original 365 herbs from the classical first century A.D. text on Chinese herbalism by Shen Nong. Ephedra's traditional medicinal uses include the alleviation of sweating, lung and bronchial constriction, and water retention. It was not until 1924 that the herb became popular with physicians in the United States for its bronchodilation and decongestant properties.

Pharmacology Ephedra contains the alkaloids ephedrine and pseudoephedrine, which are routinely isolated and used in OTC products as decongestants. Ephedra is a potent sympathomimetic that stimulates alpha-, beta$_1$-, and beta$_2$-adrenergic receptors, and the release of norepinephrine (Langwinski, 1972). Its activity on the sympathetic nervous system causes vasoconstriction and cardiac stimulation. It is a sympathomimetic, and produces a temporary rise in both systolic and diastolic blood pressure, causes mydriasis, produces bronchial muscle relaxation, and is a vasoconstrictor.

Theoretical Cautions and Contraindications Consult a physician before using in individuals with renal impairment (including nephrolithiasis, Powell, 1998), hypertension, cardiovascular disease, thyroid disease, diabetes, prostate disorders; in individuals taking sympathomimetic medications and OTC stimulants, (such as caffeine, phenylpropanolamine, and pseudoephedrine); use is contraindicated in individuals taking MAO inhibitors (Dawson, 1995); use is contraindicated in pregnancy and lactation (Leung, 1996). Some individuals may be sensitive to ephedra and may experience excitability and other complaints. If symptoms do occur and continue for longer than 2 days, discontinue use. Ephedra has many reports of abuse. Use caution when considering this supplement.

Theoretical Interactions MAO inhibitors, sympathomimetic medications, OTC stimulants, thyroid medications, calcium channel blockers, antiarrhythmics, beta-blockers, cardiac glycosides

References
Betz JM, Gay ML, Mossoba MM, et al, "Chiral gas Chromatographic Determination of Ephedrine-Type Alkaloids in Dietary Supplements Containing Ma Huang," *J AOAC Int*, 1997, 80(2):303-15.
Dawson JK, Earnshaw SM, and Graham CS, "Dangerous Monoamine Oxidase Inhibitor Interactions are Still Occurring in the 1990s," *J Accid Emerg Med*, 1995, 12(1):49-51.
Langwinski R, "Central Effects of Ephedrine," *Pol Tyg Lek*, 1972, 27(31):1205-7.
Leung AY and Foster S, *Encyclopedia of Common Natural Ingredients Used in Foods, Drugs, and Cosmetics*, 2nd ed, New York, NY: John Wiley and Sons, Inc, 1996.
Powell T, Hsu FF, Turk J, et al, "Ma-huang Strikes Again: Ephedrine Nephrolithiasis," *Am J Kidney Dis*, 1998, 32(1):153-9.
Redman CM and Druce HM, "Nonprescription Bronchodilator Use in Asthma, *Chest*, 1998, 11(4):657-8.

♦ *Ephedra sinica* see Ephedra *(Ephedra sinica)* on page 429
♦ *Epilepsy* see page 170

- ◆ **Equisetum arvense** see Horsetail (Equisetum arvense) on page 459
- ◆ **Euphrasia officinalis** see Eyebright (Euphrasia officinalis) on page 431
- ◆ **European Elder** see Elder (Sambucus nigra, Sambucus canadensis) on page 428

Evening Primrose (Oenothera biennis)

Related Information

Herb/Drug Potential Interactions on page 642
Herb Quick Reference Chart on page 538

Natural Product Category Herb

Plant Part Seed oil

Dosage and Standardization Oral: 500 mg to 8 g/day, depending on severity of condition, standardized to contain 8% to 9% gamma-linolenic acid and at least 72% linoleic acid per dose

Reported Uses

Attention Deficit Disorder (Colquhoun, 1981)
Diabetic neuropathy (Keen, 1993; Dines, 1995)
Eczema, dermatitis, and psoriasis (Horrobin, 1992; Li Wan Po, 1991)
Endometriosis (Horrobin, 1990)
Hyperglycemia (van Doormaal, 1988)
Irritable bowel syndrome (Cottrell, 1990)
Multiple sclerosis (Dworkin, 1984)
Omega-6 fatty acid supplementation
PMS and menopause (Khoo, 1990)
Rheumatoid arthritis (Li Wan Po, 1991; Horrobin, 1992)

Summary Evening primrose oil is rich in omega-6 fatty acid, an essential fatty acid. Essential fatty acids are compounds which the human body is unable to synthesize, and must be obtained from dietary sources. Humans can synthesize all fatty acids with the exception of two, omega-3 and omega-6 fatty acids. Modern diets tend to be deficient in fatty acids, and fatty acid deficiency has been proposed to contribute to the etiology and morbidity of many diseases. Evening primrose oil has been used to supplement the diet of deficient individuals as well as for a variety of inflammatory, hormonal, and immune diseases.

Pharmacology Evening primrose oil contains high amounts of gamma-linolenic acid, or GLA, which is an essential fatty acid (omega-6 fatty acid). Essential fatty acids are required components of cell membranes and serve as precursors for hormone and prostaglandin synthesis. Symptoms of fatty acid deficiency include fatigue, dry skin and hair, cracked nails, immune deficiency, arthritis, joint "popping", and dry mucous membranes. Omega-6 fatty acids reportedly reduce generation of arachidonic acid metabolites in short-term use, improving symptoms of various inflammatory and immune conditions. The fatty acids found in evening primrose oil also have been reported to stimulate hormone synthesis. The oil has been used for a variety of women's health problems, including PMS and menopausal complaints. Individuals with diabetes, who do not appear to convert linoleic acid to gamma-linolenic acid, are felt to require a supplemental source of GLA. This may be essential to maintain nerve function and prevent diabetic neuropathy. Borage oil presents similar pharmacological activity.

Theoretical Cautions and Contraindications Evening primrose oil may lower seizure threshold (based on animal studies); use is contraindicated in individuals with seizure disorders, schizophrenia, or in individuals receiving anticonvulsant or antipsychotic medications (based on evidence from human studies, Miller, 1998; Vaddadi, 1981; Dines, 1995).

May inhibit platelet aggregation (De La Cruz, 1997). Contraindicated in individuals with active bleeding (eg, peptic ulcer, intracranial bleeding). Use with caution in individuals with a history of bleeding, hemostatic disorders, or drug-related hemostatic problems. Use with caution in individuals taking anticoagulant medications, including warfarin, aspirin, aspirin-containing products, NSAIDs, or antiplatelet agents (eg, ticlopidine, clopidogrel, dipyridamole). Discontinue use prior to dental or surgical procedures (generally at least 14 days before).

General Warnings Use all herbal supplements with extreme caution in children <2 years of age and in pregnancy or lactation. Some herbs are contraindicated in pregnancy or lactation; make sure to observe warnings. Use with caution in individuals on medication and with pre-existing medical conditions. Always review for potential herb-drug interactions (HDIs) and other warnings. Large and prolonged doses may increase the potential for adverse effects. Herbs may cause transient adverse effects such as nausea, vomiting, and GI distress due to a variety of chemical constituents. Caution should be used in individuals having known allergies to plants.

Theoretical Interactions Anticonvulsant medications (seizure threshold decreased); anticoagulants, aspirin, aspirin-containing products, NSAIDs, or antiplatelet agents

References

Colquhoun I and Bunday S, "A Lack of Essential Fatty Acids as a Possible Cause of Hyperactivity in Children," *Med Hypotheses*, 1981, 7(5):673-9.

Cotterell JC, Lee AJ, and Hunter JO, "Double-Blind Cross-Over Trial of Evening Primrose Oil in Women With Menstrually-Related Irritable Bowel Syndrome," *Omega-6 Essential Fatty Acids: Pathophysiology and Roles in Clinical Medicine*, Horrobin DF, ed, New York, NY: Wiley-Liss, 1990, 421-6.

De La Cruz JP, Martin-Romero M, Carmona JA, et al, "Effect of Evening Primrose Oil on Platelet Aggregation in Rabbits Fed an Atherogenic Diet," *Thromb Res*, 1997, 87(1):141-9.

Dines CD, Cotter MA, and Cameron NE, "Nerve Function in Galactosaemic Rats: Effects of Evening Primrose Oil and Doxazosin," *Eur J Pharmacol*, 1995, 281(3):303-9.

Dworkin RH, Bates D, Millar JH, et al, "Linoleic Acid and Multiple Sclerosis: A Reanalysis of Three Double-Blind Trials," *Neurology*, 1984, 34(11):1441-5.

Horrobin DF, "Nutritional and Medical Importance of Gamma-Linoleic Acid," *Prog Lipid Res*, 1992, 31(2):163-94.

Horrobin DF, "Gamma-Linolenic Acid; An Intermediate in Essential Fatty Acid Metabolism With Potential as an Ethical Pharmaceutical and as a Food," *Rev Contemp Pharmacother*, 1990:1-45.

Keen H, Payan J, Allawi J, et al, "Treatment of Diabetic Neuropathy With Gamma-Linolenic Acid. The Gamma-Linolenic Acid Multicenter Trial Group," *Diabetes Care*, 1993, 16(1):8-15.

Khoo SK, Munro C, and Battistutta D, "Evening Primrose Oil and Treatment of Premenstrual Syndrome," *Med J Aust*, 1990, 153(4):189-92.

Li Wan Po A, "Evening Primrose Oil," *Pharm J*, 1991, 246:670-6.

Miller LG, "Herbal Medicinals: Selected Clinical Considerations Focusing on Known or Potential Drug-Herb Interactions," *Arch Intern Med*, 1998, 158(20):2200-11.

Vaddadi KS, "The Use of Gamma-Linolenic Acid and Linoleic Acid to Differentiate Between Temporal Lobe Epilepsy and Schizophrenia," *Prostaglandins Med*, 1981, 6(4):375-9.

van Doormaal JJ, Idema IG, Muskiet FA, et al, "Effects of Short-Term High Dose Intake of Evening Primrose Oil on Plasma and Cellular Fatty Acid Compositions, Alpha-Tocopherol Levels, and Erythropoiesis in Normal and Type 1 (Insulin-Dependent) Diabetic Men," *Diabetologia*, 1988, 31(8):576-84.

♦ **Evening Primrose Oil** *see* Evening Primrose *(Oenothera biennis)* on page 430

Eyebright *(Euphrasia officinalis)*

Related Information

Herb/Drug Potential Interactions *on page 642*
Herb Quick Reference Chart *on page 538*
Organ System Support Using Natural Products *on page 660*

Natural Product Category Herb

Plant Part Whole plant

Dosage and Standardization

Oral: 250 mg twice daily

Compress: Infuse 1-2 teaspoonfuls, apply as a warm compress to eyes 2-3 times/day

Reported Uses Eye fatigue; catarrh of the eyes (Leung, 1996)

Summary Eyebright is used mainly in Europe as a rinse, compress, or patch for eye-related inflammatory conditions, including blepharitis, conjunctivitis, eye fatigue, and catarrh of the eyes.

Pharmacology Eyebright infusions act as an astringent in eye conditions. Eyebright has been reported to provide rapid relief from redness, swelling, and visual disturbances in acute and subacute eye inflammations, particularly conjunctivitis and blepharitis.

(Continued)

Eyebright *(Euphrasia officinalis)* *(Continued)*

Theoretical Cautions and Contraindications In rare instances, may cause itching and redness of eyes with increased lacrimation. If condition fails to improve rapidly (within 24-48 hours), seek medical attention.

General Warnings Use all herbal supplements with extreme caution in children <2 years of age and in pregnancy or lactation. Some herbs are contraindicated in pregnancy or lactation; make sure to observe warnings. Use with caution in individuals on medication and with pre-existing medical conditions. Always review for potential herb-drug interactions (HDIs) and other warnings. Large and prolonged doses may increase the potential for adverse effects. Herbs may cause transient adverse effects such as nausea, vomiting, and GI distress due to a variety of chemical constituents. Caution should be used in individuals having known allergies to plants.

Theoretical Interactions None known

References

Leung AY and Foster S, *Encyclopedia of Common Natural Ingredients Used in Foods, Drugs, and Cosmetics,* New York, NY: Wiley, 1996, 237-8.

♦ **Fatigue** *see page 174*

Fenugreek *(Trigonella foenum-graecum)*

Related Information

Common Herbal Supplements Contraindicated During Pregnancy *on page 656*

Herb/Drug Potential Interactions *on page 642*

Herb Quick Reference Chart *on page 538*

Organ System Support Using Natural Products *on page 660*

Natural Product Category Herb

Plant Part Seed

Dosage and Standardization Oral: 250-500 mg 2-3 times/day

Reported Uses Support of blood sugar regulation (Leung, 1996)

Summary Fenugreek extracts have been used for thousands of years in Egypt, the Middle East, and India as not only a food but as a medicinal agent with a multitude of benefits. Fenugreek seed may have benefits on blood sugar regulation.

Pharmacology Hypoglycemic activity has been reported in laboratory animals and attributed to the trigonelline, nicotinic acid, and coumarin fractions. The high fiber content of the seed may also contribute to the blood sugar regulating effects.

Theoretical Cautions and Contraindications Based on pharmacological activity, may alter insulin and/or oral hypoglycemic needs in diabetic individuals; close monitoring of blood sugar levels is recommended.

General Warnings Use all herbal supplements with extreme caution in children <2 years of age and in pregnancy or lactation. Some herbs are contraindicated in pregnancy or lactation; make sure to observe warnings. Use with caution in individuals on medication and with pre-existing medical conditions. Always review for potential herb-drug interactions (HDIs) and other warnings. Large and prolonged doses may increase the potential for adverse effects. Herbs may cause transient adverse effects such as nausea, vomiting, and GI distress due to a variety of chemical constituents. Caution should be used in individuals having known allergies to plants.

Theoretical Interactions Insulin, oral hypoglycemic agents

References

Leung AY and Foster S, *Encyclopedia of Common Natural Ingredients Used in Foods, Drugs, and Cosmetics,* New York, NY: Wiley, 1996, 237-5.

♦ **Fever** *see page 178*

Feverfew *(Tanacetum parthenium)*

Related Information

Common Herbal Supplements Contraindicated During Pregnancy *on page 656*

Herb/Drug Potential Interactions *on page 642*

Herb Quick Reference Chart *on page 538*

Natural Product Category Herb

Plant Part Leaf

Dosage and Standardization Oral:

Migraine prevention:100-250 mg, standardized to contain 0.2% parthenolide

Anti-inflammatory and rheumatoid arthritis: 250 mg 3 times/day

Reported Uses

Anti-inflammatory, rheumatoid arthritis (Pattrick, 1989)

Prevention of migraine headaches (Johnson, 1985)

Summary Feverfew contains a number of compounds with anti-inflammatory and smooth muscle relaxant activities. It has increased in popularity in recent years, particularly for migraines. Since the effects of this herb may take several weeks of continuous therapy, individuals should be encouraged to use the herb for a minimum of 1 month before determining whether it has been effective.

Pharmacology Feverfew reportedly inhibits the synthesis of leukotrienes, prostaglandins, and thromboxanes which mediate inflammation. In addition, feverfew is claimed to inhibit platelet aggregation and induce smooth muscle relaxation. It has been used most commonly for migraine headaches. Feverfew has been claimed to relax uterine smooth muscle and should be avoided in pregnancy. It also may inhibit platelet aggregation and blood coagulation.

Theoretical Cautions and Contraindications Use of feverfew is contraindicated in pregnancy (animal data suggests emmenagogue activity, Bradley, 1992) or in individuals with allergies to members of the *Asteraceae/ Compositae* family (chrysanthemum, daisy). The onset of feverfew's effects may be delayed for several weeks. Abrupt discontinuation may increase migraine frequency. A "post-feverfew syndrome" has been described, including nervousness, insomnia, joint stiffness and pain which may occur following discontinuation in some individuals.

Pharmacological activity may include inhibition of platelet aggregation (Makheja, 1982). Contraindicated in individuals with active bleeding (eg, peptic ulcer, intracranial bleeding). Use with caution in individuals with a history of bleeding, hemostatic disorders, or drug-related hemostatic problems. Use with caution in individuals taking anticoagulant medications, including warfarin, aspirin, aspirin-containing products, NSAIDs, or antiplatelet agents (eg, ticlopidine, clopidogrel, dipyridamole). Discontinue use prior to dental or surgical procedures (generally at least 14 days before).

General Warnings Use all herbal supplements with extreme caution in children <2 years of age and in pregnancy or lactation. Some herbs are contraindicated in pregnancy or lactation; make sure to observe warnings. Use with caution in individuals on medication and with pre-existing medical conditions. Always review for potential herb-drug interactions (HDIs) and other warnings. Large and prolonged doses may increase the potential for adverse effects. Herbs may cause transient adverse effects such as nausea, vomiting, and GI distress due to a variety of chemical constituents. Caution should be used in individuals having known allergies to plants.

Theoretical Interactions Anticoagulants, aspirin, aspirin-containing products, NSAIDs, or antiplatelet agents

References

Bradley PR, ed, *British Herbal Compendium,* Vol 1, Bournemouth, England: British Herbal Medicine Association, 1992, 96-8.

Johnson ES, Kadam NP, Hylands DM, et al, "Efficacy of Feverfew as Prophylactic Treatment of Migraine," *Br Med J (Clin Res Ed),* 1985, 291(6495):569-73.

Makheja AN and Bailey JM, "A Platelet Phospholipase Inhibitor From the Medicinal Herb Feverfew (*Tanacetum parthenium*)," *Prostaglandins Leukot Med,* 1982, 8(6):653-60.

Newall CA, Anderson LA, and Phillipson JD, *Herbal Medicines: A Guide for Health Care Professionals,* London, England: The Pharmaceutical Press, 1996, 119-21.

Pattrick M, Heptinstall S, and Doherty M, "Feverfew in Rheumatoid Arthritis: A Double-Blind Placebo Controlled Study," *Ann Rheum Dis,* 1989, 48(7):547-49.

♦ **Fibrocystic Breast Disease (FBD)** *see page 182*

♦ **Fibromyalgia** *see page 186*

♦ **Field Horsetail** *see* Horsetail *(Equisetum arvense) on page 459*

Fish Oils

Related Information
  Nutraceutical Chart *on page 573*
  Organ System Support Using Natural Products *on page 660*

Natural Product Category Nutraceutical

Dosage Oral: Dosage range: 750 mg 2-3 times/day

Active Forms Eicosapentaenoic acid (EPA), docosahexaenoic acid (DHA)

Reported Uses
  Crohn's disease (Belluzzi, 1996)
  Diabetes (McManus, 1996)
  Dysmenorrhea (Harel, 1996)
  Eczema, psoriasis (Bjorneboe, 1989)
  Hypertension (Morris, 1993)
  Hypertriglyceridemia (Pritchard, 1995)
  Memory enhancement (Gamoh, 1999)
  Psoriasis (Bittiner, 1988)
  Rheumatoid arthritis (Kremer, 1991)

Summary Fish oils contain eicosapentaenoic acid (EPA) and docosahexaenoic acid (DHA). Both of these fats are omega-3 fatty acids. Although the body can synthesize these fats from alpha-linolenic acid (ALA), this conversion is believed to be inefficient in many people.

Pharmacology The fish oils, EPA and DHA, are important for the production of nervous tissue, hormones, and cellular membranes. EPA is converted into the series 3 prostaglandins, which have anti-inflammatory activity. These fats also help lower high blood pressure, reduce elevated cholesterol and triglycerides, prevent atherosclerotic plaque formation, and improve skin conditions such as eczema and psoriasis.

Toxicities, Warnings, and Interactions High doses may cause gastrointestinal upset, loose stools, and nausea

May alter glucose regulation. Use with caution in individuals with diabetes or in those who may be predisposed to hypoglycemia. Effects of drugs with hypoglycemic activity may be potentiated (including insulin and oral hypoglycemics). The individual's blood sugar should be closely monitored, and the dosage of these agents, including insulin dosage, may require adjustment. This should be carefully coordinated among the individuals' healthcare providers.

Contraindicated in individuals with active bleeding (eg, peptic ulcer, intracranial bleeding). Use with caution in individuals with a history of bleeding, hemostatic disorders, or drug-related hemostatic problems. Use with caution in individuals taking anticoagulant medications, including warfarin, aspirin, aspirin-containing products, NSAIDs, or antiplatelet agents (eg, ticlopidine, clopidogrel, dipyridamole). Discontinue use prior to dental or surgical procedures (generally at least 14 days before).

Symptoms of Deficiency Increased risk of cardiovascular disease, inflammatory problems

Reported Interactions
  Drug/Nutrient Interactions: Theoretically; anticoagulants, aspirin, aspirin-containing products, NSAIDs, antiplatelet agents, insulin oral hypoglycemics
  Nutrient/Nutrient Interactions: None known

References
Belluzzi A, Brignola C, Campieri M, et al, "Effect of an Enteric-Coated Fish Oil Preparation on Relapses in Crohn's Disease," *N Engl J Med*, 1996, 334(24):1557-60.

Bjorneboe A, Soyland E, Bjorneboe GE, et al, "Effect of n-3 Fatty Acid Supplement to Patients With Atopic Dermatitis," *J Intern Med Suppl*, 1989, 225(731):233-6.

Bittiner SB, Tucker WF, Cartwright I, et al, "A Double-Blind, Randomised, Placebo-Controlled Trial of Fish Oil in Psoriasis," *Lancet*, 1988, 1(8582):378-80.

Gamoh S, Hashimoto M, Sugioka K, et al, "Chronic Administration of Docosahexaenoic Acid Improves Reference Memory-Related Learning Ability in Young Rats," *Neuroscience*, 1999, 93(1):237-41.

Harel Z, Biro FM, Kottenhahn RK, et al, "Supplementation With Omega-3 Polyunsaturated Fatty Acids in the Management of Dysmenorrhea in Adolescents," *Am J Obstet Gynecol*, 1996, 174(4):1335-8.

Kremer JM, "Clinical Studies of Omega-3 Fatty Acid Supplementation in Patients Who Have Rheumatoid Arthritis," *Rheum Dis Clin North Am*, 1991, 17(2):391-402.

McManus RM, Jumpson J, Finegood DT, et al, "A Comparison of the Effects of n-3 Fatty Acids From Linseed Oil and Fish Oil in Well-Controlled Type II Diabetes," *Diabetes Care*, 1996, 19(5):463-7.

Morris MC, Sacks F, and Rosner B, et al, "Does Fish Oil Lower Blood Pressure? A Meta-Analysis of Controlled Trials," *Circulation*, 1993, 88(2):523-33.

Prichard BN, Smith CC, Ling KL, et al, "Fish Oils and Cardiovascular Disease," *BMJ*, 1995, 310(6983):819-20.

Flaxseed Oil

Related Information

Nutraceutical Chart *on page 573*

Organ System Support Using Natural Products *on page 660*

Natural Product Category Nutraceutical

Dosage Oral: Dosage range: 1 Tbsp/day which contains ~58% to 60% omega-3 (also available in capsules)

Note: Flaxseed oil must be refrigerated at all times

Active Forms Flaxseed oil

Reported Uses

Source of omega-3 essential fatty acid; integral part of structure of cell walls and cellular membranes; necessary for the transport and oxidation of cholesterol

Precursor for prostaglandins (Sinclair, 1984)

Summary Flaxseed oil is the richest source of the essential fatty acid known as alpha-linolenic acid (ALA) or omega-3 fatty acid. It contains approximately 58% to 60% omega-3 fatty acids and 18% to 20% omega-6 fatty acids. It is estimated that the optimal ratio between omega-3 and omega-6 fatty acids is approximately 1 to 4. Most people are deficient in omega-3 and consume excessive amounts of the omega-6 fats and oils. In fact, studies report that the omega-3/omega-6 ratio for many people in the United States is between 1:20 and 1:30. Flaxseed oil, which contains 3 times more omega-3 than omega-6, may be used to help reverse the imbalance between omega-3 and omega-6.

Pharmacology Flaxseed oil's only health application is as a supplement for the essential fatty acid known as omega-3. The body uses omega-3 to build cell walls and cellular membranes. It is the precursor for the longer chain omega-3 fatty acids known as eicosapentaenoic acid (EPA) and docosahexaenoic acid (DHA).

Toxicities, Warnings, and Interactions No known toxicity or serious side effects

Symptoms of Deficiency Symptoms may include cardiovascular problems, elevated blood pressure, increased platelet stickiness, increased inflammation, asthma, allergies, problems with skin or hair. Other problems can develop from a deficiency because it upsets the synthesis of prostaglandins.

References

Sinclair HM, "Essential Fatty Acids in Perspective," *Hum Nutr Clin Nutr*, 1984, 38(4):245-60.

Folic Acid

Related Information

Drug-Induced Nutrient Depletions *on page 625*

Pregnancy & Lactation Nutritional Chart *on page 657*

Vitamins/Minerals/Trace Elements/Amino Acids Chart *on page 604*

Natural Product Category Vitamin

Dosage Oral: RDI: 400 mcg/day; ODA: 400-1000 mcg/day

Active Forms Folic acid (also known as folate) and folinic acid (also known as 5-methyl tetrahydro-folate)

Reported Uses

Alcoholism (Lindenbaum, 1980)

Anemia (Swain, 1997)

(Continued)

Folic Acid *(Continued)*

Atherosclerosis (Swain, 1997)

Cancer prevention (colon and breast) (Freudenheim, 1991; Zhang, 1999)

Cervical dysplasia (Buckley, 1992)

Crohn's disease (Rath, 1998)

Depression (Godfrey, 1990)

Gingivitis (Pack, 1984)

Osteoporosis (Brattstrom, 1985)

Pregnancy (prevention of birth defects) and lactation (Steegers-Theunissen, 1995)

Summary Folic acid is a water-soluble B vitamin which serves as a cofactor in many enzymatic reactions related to growth and development, neuronal function, and blood cell production. The dietary intakes of many individuals, particularly alcoholics, are known to less than the RDI. Folic acid is an important nutrient which may be useful in the prevention of atherosclerosis and neural tube birth defects. In addition, it has been used for anemias, depression, and osteoporosis.

Pharmacology In humans, folic acid is converted to its biologically active form, tetrahydrofolic acid (THFA). Folic acid participates in methylation reactions, such as the conversion of homocysteine to methionine. Homocysteine is a risk factor for accelerated atherosclerosis in some individuals. Folic acid is also required for the synthesis of amino acids, the precursors to protein synthesis. In addition, folate is necessary for the synthesis of both DNA and RNA. For this reason, it is essential for cellular growth and division. It is required for the formation of all new cells, and is particularly important in the production of red blood cells, hair, and skin. In addition, it is required for proper functioning of the neuronal cells. Folic acid is necessary for closure of the neural tube during pregnancy.

Toxicities, Warnings, and Interactions Large doses can mask symptoms of vitamin B_{12} deficiency.

Symptoms of Deficiency Anemia, heartburn, fatigue, diarrhea, constipation, depression, frequent infections, mental confusion

Reported Interactions

Drug/Nutrient Interactions:

Drugs which can cause depletion of folic acid: Oral contraceptives, potassium-sparing diuretics (triamterene), bile acid sequestrants, anticonvulsants (barbiturates, phenytoin, carbamazepine, primidone, valproate), corticosteroids (prednisone), NSAIDs, sulfasalazine, methotrexate, trimethoprim-containing antibiotics (co-trimoxazole), H_2-receptor antagonists, aspirin, antacids, alcohol, cycloserine, pyrimethamine, antibiotics, biguanides, salsalate

High doses of folic acid may alter the metabolism of phenytoin, phenobarbital, or primidone; may decrease the efficacy of methotrexate (in cancer therapy) and pyrimethamine; cholestyramine, and colestipol may decrease absorption

Nutrient/Nutrient Interactions: There are no known adverse nutrient/nutrient interactions between folic acid and other nutrients. However, folic acid participates with other B vitamins in many biochemical activities and many health professionals suggest that folic acid be taken along with other B vitamins.

References

Brattstrom LE, Hultberg BL, and Hardebo JE, "Folic Acid Responsive Postmenopausal Homocysteinemia," *Metabolism*, 1985, 34(11):1073-7.

Buckley DI, McPherson RS, North CQ, et al, "Dietary Micronutrients and Cervical Dysplasia in Southwestern American Indian Women," *Nutr Cancer*, 1992, 17(2):179-85.

Freudenheim, et al, "Folate Intake and Carcinogenesis of the Colon and Rectum," *Int J Epidemiol*, 1991, 20(2)368-74.

Godfrey PS, Toone BK, Carney MW, et al, "Enhancement of Recovery From Psychiatric Illness by Methylfolate," *Lancet*, 1990, 336(8712):392-5.

Lindenbaum J and Roman MJ, "Nutritional Anemia in Alcoholism," *Am J Clin Nutr*, 1980, 33(12):2727-35.

Rath HC, Caesar I, Roth M, et al, "Nutritional Deficiencies and Complications in Chronic Inflammatory Bowel Diseases, *Med Klin*, 1998, 93(1):6-10.

Steegers-Theunissen RP, "Folate Metabolism and Neural Tube Defects: A Review, *Eur J Obstet Gynecol Reprod Biol*, 1995, 61(1):39-48.

Swain RA and Clair L, "The Role of Folic Acid in Deficiency States and Prevention of Disease," *J Fam Pract*, 1997, 44(2):138-44.

Truswell AS, "ABC of Nutrition. Nutrition for Pregnancy," *Br Med J (Clin Res Ed)*, 1985, 291(6490):263-6.

Zhang S, et al, "A Prospective Study of Folate Intake and the Risk of Breast Cancer," *JAMA*, 1999, 281(17);1632-7.

♦ *Fucus vesiculosus* see Bladderwrack (*Fucus vesiculosus*) on page 396

♦ **Gallbladder / Gallstones** see page 190

♦ *Ganoderma lucidum* see Reishi (*Ganoderma lucidum*) on page 497

♦ *Garcinia cambogia* see Garcinia (*Garcinia cambogia*) on page 437

Garcinia (*Garcinia cambogia*)

Related Information

Herb/Drug Potential Interactions *on page 642*

Herb Quick Reference Chart *on page 538*

Natural Product Category Herb

Plant Part Fruit

Dosage and Standardization Oral: 500-1000 mg 3 times/day, taken on an empty stomach (½ hour before or 1 hour after meals), standardized to contain 50% (-) hydroxy citric acid [(-)HCA] content per dose

Reported Uses

Support of pancreas function and glucose regulation (McCarty, 1995)

Weight reduction protocols (Sergio, 1988; Sullivan, 1977)

Contradictory study, (Kriketos, 1999)

Summary The popularity of *Garcinia cambogia* has been increasing due to a growing emphasis on weight control. As opposed to most anorectic medications, it does not appear to have CNS stimulating effects, but may induce weight loss by an alteration in energy utilization and metabolism. However, a recent study indicated that (-) hydroxy citric acid did not affect energy expenditure in adult males (Kriketos, 1999). Most claims focus on garcinia's ability to modify the storage of carbohydrate as glycogen, rather than fat. It has been noted that obese individuals have less glycogen storage and more triglyceride storage than their thinner counterparts. In addition, glycogen storage may be defective in obese individuals and in individuals with type 2 diabetes. For this reason, Garcinia has gained popularity as a weight-loss agent and for support of individuals with diabetes.

Pharmacology Garcinia is an inhibitor of adenosine triphosphate citrate lyase, an important enzymatic step in the process of converting carbohydrate to fat. Garcinia is claimed to increase glycogen storage in the liver and small intestine. Garcinia may reduce blood lipid concentrations, and may increase energy production and metabolic rate. These effects may lead to weight loss and/or normalization of blood glucose levels.

Theoretical Cautions and Contraindications Weight loss efforts should emphasize proper food selection, moderation of caloric intake, and appropriate activity levels/exercise as directed by a health care practitioner. Based on pharmacological activity, it may alter glucose regulation. Use with caution in individuals with diabetes or in those who may be predisposed to hypoglycemia. Effects of drugs with hypoglycemic activity may be potentiated (including insulin and oral hypoglycemics). The individual's blood sugar should be closely monitored, and the dosage of these agents, including insulin dosage, may require adjustment. This should be carefully coordinated among the individual's healthcare providers. Use with caution in individuals taking hypolipidemic agents (based on pharmacological activity, the effects may be additive).

General Warnings Use all herbal supplements with extreme caution in children <2 years of age and in pregnancy or lactation. Some herbs are contraindicated in pregnancy or lactation; make sure to observe warnings. Use with caution in individuals on medication and with pre-existing medical conditions. Always review for potential herb-drug interactions (HDIs) and other warnings. Large and prolonged doses may increase the potential for adverse effects. Herbs may cause transient adverse effects such as (Continued)

Garcinia *(Garcinia cambogia)* *(Continued)*

nausea, vomiting, and GI distress due to a variety of chemical constituents. Caution should be used in individuals having known allergies to plants.

Theoretical Interactions Insulin, oral hypoglycemics, hypolipidemic agents (including lipase inhibitors)

References

Kriketos AD, Thompson HR, Greene H, et al, "(-)-Hydroxycitric Acid Does Not Affect Energy Expenditure and Substrate Oxidation in Adult Males in a Post-Absorptive State," *Int J Obes Relat Metab Disord*, 1999, 23(8):867-73.

McCarty MF, "Inhibition of Citrate Lyase May Aid Aerobic Endurance," *Med Hypotheses*, 1995, 45(3):247-54.

Sergio W, "A Natural Food, the Malabar Tamarind, May Be Effective in the Treatment of Obesity," *Med Hypotheses*, 1988, 27(1):39-40.

Sullivan C and Triscari J, "Metabolic Regulation as a Control for Lipid Disorders. II. Influence of (-)-Hydroxycitrate on Experimentally Induced Obesity in the Rodent," *Am J Clin Nutr*, 1977, 30(5):767-6.

Garlic *(Allium sativum)*

Related Information

Herb/Drug Potential Interactions *on page 642*
Herb Quick Reference Chart *on page 538*
Organ System Support Using Natural Products *on page 660*

Natural Product Category Herb

Plant Part Bulb

Dosage and Standardization Oral:

400 mg 2-3 times/day, equivalent to 1200 mg of fresh garlic

or 10 mg of alliin standardized to provide 4 mg of total allicin potential (TAP) per dose

or 600 mg of aged extract 1-3 times/day, standardized to contain 1 mg/g S-allyl cysteine (SAC) per dose

Reported Uses

Antimicrobial (bacteria and fungi) (Adetumbi, 1983; Pai, 1995)

Hypertension (Ernst, 1987; Neil, 1996)

May lower cholesterol and blood fats (Agarwal, 1996; Steiner, 1996; Neil, 1996; Bordia, 1981; Simons, 1995)

Contradictory studies: See Summary (Byrne, 1999; Bertold, 1998; Isaacsohn, 1998)

Mild inhibitor of platelet-activating factor (Bordia, 1998)

Practitioners should be aware that aged garlic extracts have been reported to improve the antioxidant benefits (Steiner, 1996; Munday, 1999)

Support of immune function (Salman, 1999)

Summary Garlic is a popular herb which is often used for its flavoring properties in food preparation. As an agent in traditional medicine, it has been used primarily as a digestive aid. Its potential to lower blood cholesterol, a known risk factor for cardiovascular disease, has dramatically increased its popularity. However, conflicting evidence has been reported from clinical trials (Byrne, 1999; Bertold, 1998; Isaacsohn, 1998). The failure to demonstrate efficacy in these trials has been attributed by some to a study design which employed garlic preparations with questionable pharmacological activity.

Pharmacology Garlic ingestion has been shown to lower total cholesterol, LDL cholesterol, and triglycerides, while increasing HDL cholesterol. Garlic has been reported to lower blood pressure, and may be of benefit in the prevention of coronary heart disease. Garlic has been claimed to improve glycemic control, either by increasing the release of insulin or enhancing the response to insulin. Garlic has fibrinolytic activity, may inhibit platelet aggregation, and reduce blood viscosity. This has led to the use of garlic as an agent to prevent thrombotic events, including stroke and myocardial infarction. The sulfur-containing compounds in garlic (alliin and allicin) are believed to be responsible for the lipid-lowering effects and have been reported to have antimicrobial effects against bacteria and fungi. Garlic has been reported to increase the fungicidal amphotericin B against *Cryptococcus neoformans* (Davis, 1994).

Theoretical Cautions and Contraindications Garlic may cause GI distress or irritation in some individuals during the initiation of therapy.

Garlic has *in vitro* effects on platelet aggregation (Kiesewetter, 1993) and has been associated with reports of bleeding. Contraindicated in individuals with active bleeding (eg, peptic ulcer, intracranial bleeding). Use with caution in individuals with a history of bleeding, hemostatic disorders, or drug-related hemostatic problems. Use with caution in individuals taking anticoagulant medications, including warfarin, aspirin, aspirin-containing products, NSAIDs, or antiplatelet agents (eg, ticlopidine, clopidogrel, dipyridamole). Discontinue use prior to dental or surgical procedures (generally at least 14 days before).

Based on pharmacological activity, use caution in individuals at risk of hypotension (including those taking antihypertensive medication or agents that predispose to orthostasis), elderly individuals, or those who would not tolerate transient hypotensive episodes (ie, cerebrovascular or cardiovascular disease). May potentiate effects of antihypertensives.

Pharmacological activity may alter glucose regulation. Use with caution in individuals with diabetes or in those who may be predisposed to hypoglycemia. Effects of drugs with hypoglycemic activity may be potentiated (including insulin and oral hypoglycemics). The individual's blood sugar should be closely monitored, and the dosage of these agents, including insulin dosage, may require adjustment. This should be carefully coordinated among the individual's healthcare providers.

General Warnings Use all herbal supplements with extreme caution in children <2 years of age and in pregnancy or lactation. Some herbs are contraindicated in pregnancy or lactation; make sure to observe warnings. Use with caution in individuals on medication and with pre-existing medical conditions. Always review for potential herb-drug interactions (HDIs) and other warnings. Large and prolonged doses may increase the potential for adverse effects. Herbs may cause transient adverse effects such as nausea, vomiting, and GI distress due to a variety of chemical constituents. Caution should be used in individuals having known allergies to plants.

Theoretical Interactions Anticoagulants, aspirin, aspirin-containing products, NSAIDs, antiplatelet agents, antihypertensives, insulin, oral hypoglycemics

References

Adetumbi MA and Lau BH, "*Allium sativum* (Garlic)-A Natural Antibiotic," *Med Hypotheses* 1983, 12(3):227-37.

Agarwal KC, "Therapeutic Actions of Garlic Constituents," *Med Res Rev*, 1996, 16(1):111-24.

Berthold HK, Sudhop T, and von Bergmann K, "Effect of a Garlic Oil Preparation on Serum Lipoproteins and Cholesterol Metabolism: A Randomized Controlled Trial," *JAMA*, 1998, 279(23):1900-2.

Bordia A, "Effect of Garlic on Blood Lipids in Patients With Coronary Heart Disease," *Am J Clin Nutr*, 1981, 34(10):2100-3.

Bordia A, Verma SK, and Srivastava KC, "Effect of Garlic (*Allium sativum*) on Blood Lipids, Blood Sugar, Fibrinogen and Fibrinolytic Activity in Patients With Coronary Artery Disease," *Prostaglandins Leukot Essent Fatty Acids*, 1998, 58(4):257-63.

Byrne DJ, Neil HA, Vallance DT, et al, "A Pilot Study of Garlic Consumption Shows No Significant Effect on Markers of Oxidation or Sub-fraction Composition of Low-Density Lipoprotein Including Lipoprotein(a) After Allowance for Non-compliance and the Placebo Effect," *Clin Chim Acta*, 1999, 285(1-2):21-33.

Davis LE, Shen J, and Royer RE, "*In Vitro* Synergism of Concentrated *Allium sativum* Extract and Amphotericin B Against *Cryptococcus neoformans*," *Planta Med*, 1994, 60(6):546-9.

Ernst E, "Cardiovascular Effects of Garlic (*Allium sativum*): A Review," *Pharmatherapeutica*, 1987, 5(2):83-9.

Isaacsohn JL, Moser M, Stein EA, et al, "Garlic Powder and Plasma Lipids and Lipoproteins: A Multicenter, Randomized, Placebo-Controlled Trial," *Arch Intern Med*, 1998, 158(11):1189-94.

Munday JS, James KA, Fray LM, et al, "Daily Supplementation With Aged Garlic Extract, But Not Raw Garlic, Protects Low Density Lipoprotein Against *In Vitro*, Oxidation," *Atherosclerosis*, 1999, 143(2):399-404.

Neil HA, Silagy CA, Lancaster T, et al, "Garlic Powder in the Treatment of Moderate Hyperlipidaemia: A Controlled Trial and Meta-Analysis," *J R Coll Physicians Lond*, 1996, 30(4):329-34.

Pai ST and Platt MW, "Antifungal Effects of *Allium sativum* (Garlic) Extract Against the *Aspergillus* Species Involved in Otomycosis," *Lett Appl Microbiol*, 1995, 20(1):14-8.

(Continued)

Garlic *(Allium sativum)* *(Continued)*

Salman H, Beyman M, Bessler H, et al, "Effect of Garlic Derivative (Alliin) on Peripheral Blood Cell Immune Responses," *Int J Immunopharmacol*, 1999, 21(9):589-97.

Simons LA, Balasubramaniam S, von Konigsmark M, et al, "On The Effect of Garlic on Plasma Lipids and Lipoproteins in Mild Cholesterolaemia," *Atherosclerosis*, 1995, 113(2):219-25.

Steiner M, Khan AH, Holbert D, et al, "A Double-Blind Crossover Study in Moderately Hypercholesterolemic Men That Compared the Effect of Aged Garlic Extract and Placebo Administration on Blood Lipids," *Am J Clin Nutr*, 1996, 64(6):866-70.

Ginger *(Zingiber officinale)*

Related Information

Herb/Drug Potential Interactions *on page 642*

Herb Quick Reference Chart *on page 538*

Natural Product Category Herb

Plant Part Root

Dosage and Standardization Oral: 250 mg 3 times/day with food, standardized to contain 4% volatile oils or 5% total pungent compounds (most prominently 6-gingerol and 6-shogaol) per dose

Reported Uses

Antiemetic (Grontved, 1988; Bone, 1990)

Anti-inflammatory (musculoskeletal) (Srivastava, 1992)

GI distress and dyspepsia (Newall, 1996)

Summary Ginger has been used extensively as both a culinary herb and an agent in traditional medicine. In the United States, it has been popularized as a treatment for motion sickness, dyspepsia, and nausea. Its lack of sedative effects may be an advantage over other antiemetic agents.

Pharmacology The antiemetic activity of ginger is believed to be due to shogaol, while gingerol has been shown to stimulate gastric secretions and peristalsis. The antiemetic activity of ginger has been documented to be comparable to several antiemetic medications, having local effects in the gastrointestinal tract and/or activity in the central nervous system. Due to a lack of sedative effects, ginger has been claimed to be superior to antihistamines for motion sickness. Ginger may delay coagulation by an effect on platelet-activating factor. Ginger may decrease nausea associated with radiation and chemotherapy. It also decreases gastric-emptying delays associated with cisplatin (see References).

Theoretical Cautions and Contraindications Pharmacological activity may include alteration of platelet aggregation (Guh, 1995). Contraindicated in individuals with active bleeding (eg, peptic ulcer, intracranial bleeding). Use with caution in individuals with a history of bleeding, hemostatic disorders, or drug-related hemostatic problems. Use with caution in individuals taking anticoagulant medications, including warfarin, aspirin, aspirin-containing products, NSAIDs, or antiplatelet agents (eg, ticlopidine, clopidogrel, dipyridamole). Discontinue use prior to dental or surgical procedures (generally at least 14 days before).

General Warnings Use all herbal supplements with extreme caution in children <2 years of age and in pregnancy or lactation. Some herbs are contraindicated in pregnancy or lactation; make sure to observe warnings. Use with caution in individuals on medication and with pre-existing medical conditions. Always review for potential herb-drug interactions (HDIs) and other warnings. Large and prolonged doses may increase the potential for adverse effects. Herbs may cause transient adverse effects such as nausea, vomiting, and GI distress due to a variety of chemical constituents. Caution should be used in individuals having known allergies to plants.

Theoretical Interactions Anticoagulants, aspirin, aspirin-containing products, NSAIDs, or antiplatelet agents

References

Bone ME, Wilkinson DJ, Young JR, et al, "Ginger Root - A New Antiemetic. The Effect of Ginger Root on Postoperative Nausea and Vomiting After Major Gynaecological Surgery," *Anaesthesia*, 1990, 45(8):669-71.

Grontved A, Brask T, Kambskard J, et al, "Ginger Root Against Seasickness. A Controlled Trial on the Open Sea," *Acta Otolaryngol (Stockh)*, 1988, 105(1-2):45-9.

Guh JH, Kof N, Jong TT, et al, "Antiplatelet Effect of Gingerol Isolated From *Zingiber officinale*," *J Pharm Pharmacol*, 1995, 47(4):329-32.

Meyer K, Schwartz J, Crater D, et al, "*Zingiber officinale* (Ginger) Used to Prevent 8-Mop Associated Nausea," *Dermatol Nurs*, 1995, 7(4):242-4.

Newall CA, Anderson LA, and Phillipson JD, *Herbal Medicines: A Guide for Health Care Professionals*, London, England: The Pharmaceutical Press, 1996, 135-7.

Sharma SS and Gupta YK, "Reversal of Cisplatin-Induced Delay in Gastric Emptying in Rats by Ginger (*Zingiber officinale*)," *J Ethnopharmacol*, 1998, 62(1):49-55.

Srivastava KC and Mustafa T, "Ginger (*Zingiber officinale*) in Rheumatism and Musculoskeletal Disorders," *Med Hypotheses*, 1992, 39(4):342-8.

♦ **Gingivitis** *see page 194*

♦ **Ginkgo biloba** *see Ginkgo (Ginkgo biloba) on page 441*

Ginkgo (Ginkgo biloba)

Related Information

Herb/Drug Potential Interactions *on page 642*

Herb Quick Reference Chart *on page 538*

Organ System Support Using Natural Products *on page 660*

Natural Product Category Herb

Plant Part Leaf

Dosage and Standardization Oral: 40-80 mg 3 times/day, standardized to contain 24% to 27% ginkgo flavone glycosides and 6% to 7% triterpenes per dose

Reported Uses

Alzheimer's disease, dementia (Ernst, 1999; LeBars, 1997; Itil, 1998; Oken, 1998)

Asthma (Braquet, 1987)

Increase peripheral blood flow: Cerebral vascular disease, peripheral vascular insufficiency, impotence, tinnitus, and depression (resistant) (Kleijnen, 1992)

Intermittent claudication (Peters, 1998; Ernst, 1996)

Macular degeneration (Lebuisson, 1986)

Memory enhancement (Allain, 1993; Kleijnen, 1992)

Sexual dysfunction (antidepressant-induced) (Cohen, 1998)

Summary Ginkgo has been used in China for thousands of years and is the most frequently prescribed medicinal herb in Europe. Most uses of ginkgo have centered on improvement in regional (ie, CNS) or peripheral blood flow and oxygen delivery. Claims of benefit range from improved cognitive function in Alzheimer's disease to decreased symptoms of peripheral vascular disease. Other neurologic uses include tinnitus and vertigo. It has also become popular among students who hope to enhance memory during their academic studies.

Pharmacology The primary activity of ginkgo appears to be derived from flavoglycosides. These compounds are potent free radical scavengers and demonstrate a variety of pharmacological activities. Ginkgo has also been reported to inhibit platelet-activating factor (PAF). It may stimulate endothelial releasing factor and prostacyclin. Ginkgo may augment venous tone and improve the clearance of toxins during periods of ischemia. In addition, ginkgo may improve cholinergic neurotransmission. The effect of ginkgo may be to increase cerebral brain flow and, therefore, improve oxygen and nutrient delivery while enhancing the elimination of metabolic end products. Ginkgo may reduce capillary fragility and function as an antioxidant. Ginkgo has been reported to improve circulation in the elderly. This has been proposed to enhance memory, potentially delaying the onset of senile dementia and Alzheimer's.

Theoretical Cautions and Contraindications Ginkgo demonstrates *in vitro* inhibition of platelet aggregation and has been associated with case reports of bleeding (Odawara, 1997; Skogh, 1998; Vale, 1998; Matthews, 1998; Rosenblatt, 1997). Contraindicated in individuals with active bleeding (eg, peptic ulcer, intracranial bleeding). Use with caution in individuals with a history of bleeding, hemostatic disorders, or drug-related hemostatic problems. Use with caution in individuals taking anticoagulant medications, including warfarin, aspirin, aspirin-containing products, NSAIDs, or antiplatelet agents (eg, ticlopidine, clopidogrel, dipyridamole). Discontinue use prior to dental or surgical procedures (generally at least 14 days before). (Continued)

Ginkgo *(Ginkgo biloba)* (Continued)

Based on pharmacological activity, may increase effect or toxicity of monoamine oxidase inhibitors (MAOIs) (White, 1966; Wu 1999).

General Warnings Use all herbal supplements with extreme caution in children <2 years of age and in pregnancy or lactation. Some herbs are contraindicated in pregnancy or lactation; make sure to observe warnings. Use with caution in individuals on medication and with pre-existing medical conditions. Always review for potential herb-drug interactions (HDIs) and other warnings. Large and prolonged doses may increase the potential for adverse effects. Herbs may cause transient adverse effects such as nausea, vomiting, and GI distress due to a variety of chemical constituents. Caution should be used in individuals having known allergies to plants.

Theoretical Interactions Anticoagulants, aspirin, aspirin-containing products, antiplatelet agents, NSAIDs (increased risk of GI bleeding), MAO inhibitors, acetylcholinesterase inhibitors

References

Allain H, Raoul P, Lieury A, et al, "Effect of Two Doses of *Ginkgo biloba* Extract (EGb 761) on the Dual-Coding Test in Elderly Subjects," *Clin Ther*, 1993, 15(3):549-58.

Balon R, "*Ginkgo biloba* for Antidepressant-Induced Sexual Dysfunction," *J Sex Marital Ther*, 1999, 25(1):1-2.

Braquet P, "The Ginkgolides: Potent Platelet-Activating Factor Antagonists Isolated from Ginkgo biloba L.: Chemistry, Pharmacology, and Clinical Applications," *Drugs of the Future*, 1987, 12:643-99.

Cohen AJ and Bartlik B, "*Ginkgo biloba* for Antidepressant-induced Sexual Dysfunction," *J Sex Marital Ther*, 1998, 24(2):139-43.

Ernst E, "*Ginkgo biloba* in Treatment of Intermittent Claudication. A Systematic Research Based on Controlled Studies in the Literature," *Fortschr Med*, 1996, 114(8):85-7.

Ernst E and Pittler MH, "*Ginkgo biloba* for Dementia: A Systematic Review of Double-Blind, Placebo-Controlled Trials," *Clin Drug Invest*, 1999, 17(4):301-8.

Itil TM, Erlap E, Ahmed I, et al, "The Pharmacological Effects of *Ginkgo biloba*, a Plant Extract, on the Brain of Dementia Patients in Comparison With Tacrine," *Psychopharmacol Bull*, 1998, 34(3):391-7.

Kleijnen J and Knipschild P, "*Ginkgo biloba*," *Lancet*, 1992, 340(8828):1136-9.

Le Bars PL, Katz MM, Berman N, et al, "A Placebo-Controlled, Double-Blind, Randomized Trial of an Extract of *Ginkgo biloba* for Dementia. North American EGb Study Group," *JAMA*, 1997, 278(16):1327-32.

Lebuissen DA, Leroy L, and Rigal G, "Treatment of Senile Macular Degeneration with *Ginkgo biloba* Extract. A Preliminary Double-Blind Drug Vs Placebo Study," *Presse Med*, 1986, 15(31):1556-8.

Matthews MK Jr, "Association of *Ginkgo biloba* With Intracerebral Hemorrhage," *Neurology*, 1998, 50(6):1933-4.

Odawara M, Tamaoka A, and Yamashita K, "*Ginkgo biloba*," *Neurology*, 1997, 48(3):789-90.

Oken BS, Storzbach DM, and Kaye JA, "The Efficacy of *Ginkgo biloba* on Cognitive Function in Alzheimer Disease," *Arch Neurol*, 1998, 55(11):1409-15.

Peters H, Kieser M, and Holscher U, "Demonstration of the Efficacy of *Ginkgo biloba* Special Extract EGb 761 on Intermittent Claudication - A Placebo-Controlled, Double-Blind Multicenter Trial," *Vasa*, 1998, 27(2):106-10.

Rosenblatt M and Mindel J, "Spontaneous Hyphema Associated With Ingestion of *Ginko biloba* Extract," *N Engl J Med*, 1997, 336(15):1108.

Skogh M, "Extracts of *Ginkgo biloba*, and Bleeding or Haemorrhage," *Lancet*, 1998, 352(9134):1145-6.

Vale S, "Subarachnoid Haemorrhage Associated With *Ginkgo biloba*," *Lancet*, 1998, 352(9121):36.

White HL, Scates PW, and Cooper BR, "Extracts of *Ginkgo biloba* Leaves Inhibit Monoamine Oxidase," *Life Sci*, 1966, 58(16):1315-21.

Wu WR and Zhu XZ, "Involvement of Monoamine Oxidase Inhibition in Neuroprotective and Neurorestorative Effects of *Ginkgo biloba* Extract Against MPTP-Induced Nigrostriatal Dopaminergic Toxicity in C57 Mice," *Life Sci*, 1999, 65(2):157-64.

Ginseng, Panax *(Panax ginseng)*

Related Information

Herb/Drug Potential Interactions *on page 642*
Herb Quick Reference Chart *on page 538*
Organ System Support Using Natural Products *on page 660*

Natural Product Category Herb

Plant Part Root

Dosage and Standardization Oral: 100-600 mg/day in divided doses, standardized to contain a minimum of 5% ginsenosides per dose. A

regimen of 4 weeks on, followed by 2 weeks off is recommended for maximum benefit.

Reported Uses

Adrenal tonic (Hiai, 1979)

Enhancement of physical and mental performance; enhancement of energy levels; adaptation to stress; supports immune function; adjunct support for chemotherapy and radiation (Chong, 1988; Kim, 1990)

Summary Historically, Panax ginseng has been used primarily for its reported ability to help people during fatigue or stress (adaptogenic properties). It is promoted to enhance wellness, by increasing the ability to cope with physiologic, emotional, and environmental stressors, reducing susceptibility to illness. In addition, it may assist in physiologic adaptation to the stress of illness, including chemotherapeutic regimens or radiation therapy.

Pharmacology The primary active constituents of ginseng are believed to be the ginsenosides, which include over 20 saponin triterpenes similar in structure to steroid hormones. These are believed to act via hormone receptors in the hypothalamus, pituitary glands, and other tissues. Ginsenosides stimulate secretion of adrenocorticotropic hormone (ACTH), leading to production of increased release of adrenal hormones, including cortisol. Ginsenosides reportedly stimulate RNA transcription, protein synthesis, and hepatic cholesterol production. In addition, they may stimulate synthesis of adrenal hormone precursors. Evidence suggests that Panax ginseng lowers cortisol levels in individuals with diabetes, while increasing cortisol levels in nondiabetic individuals.

Specific triterpenoid saponins (diols) are claimed to be mediate improvements in endurance and learning. These compounds are also believed to contribute to sedative and antihypertensive properties. A second group (triols) reportedly increase blood pressure and function as central nervous system stimulants. Ginsenosides and have carbohydrate-sparing and increase muscle stamina.

The effects of Panax ginseng have been reported to be dose-dependent. Low doses increase blood pressure, while high doses exhibit a hypotensive effect. Additionally, Panax ginseng is reported to have immunostimulating effects on the reticuloendothelial system. Panax ginseng has been postulated to decrease weight loss and stabilize white blood cell counts during chemotherapy, and may also accelerate postsurgical recovery. Panax ginseng helps the body adapt to stresses caused by chemotherapy and radiation (Chong, 1988; Kim, 1990)

Theoretical Cautions and Contraindications

Use of Panax ginseng is contraindicated in renal failure, and acute infection. Avoid in pregnancy and lactation (Bradley, 1992). Use with caution in individuals receiving MAO inhibitors (based on pharmacological activity and case reports). Use caution with stimulant medications, including decongestants, caffeine, and caffeine-containing beverages (based on pharmacological activity). May be associated with a syndrome of diarrhea, hypertension, nervousness, dermatologic eruptions, and insomnia (Ginseng Abuse Syndrome) after prolonged use or high dosages (Chen, 1981). May also cause mastalgia in prolonged, high-dose use (case reports, Dukes, 1978). May cause vaginal breakthrough bleeding (case reports, Hopkins, 1988). Due to pharmacological activity, may interfere with hormonal therapy.

May cause palpitations and tachycardia in sensitive individuals or in high doses. Based on pharmacological activity, use with caution in individuals with hypertension or in those receiving antihypertensives (Siegel, 1980). Also use caution in individuals at risk of hypotension (including those taking antihypertensive medication or agents that predispose to orthostasis), elderly individuals, or those who would not tolerate transient hyper- or hypotensive episodes (ie, cerebrovascular or cardiovascular disease).

Based on pharmacological activity and case reports, may alter hemostasis (Teng, 1989; Janetsky, 1997). Contraindicated in individuals with active
(Continued)

Ginseng, Panax *(Panax ginseng)* (Continued)

bleeding (eg, peptic ulcer, intracranial bleeding). Use with caution in individuals with a history of bleeding, hemostatic disorders, or drug-related hemostatic problems. Use with caution in individuals taking anticoagulant medications, including warfarin, aspirin, aspirin-containing products, NSAIDs, or antiplatelet agents (eg, ticlopidine, clopidogrel, dipyridamole). Discontinue use prior to dental or surgical procedures (generally at least 14 days before).

General Warnings Use all herbal supplements with extreme caution in children <2 years of age and in pregnancy or lactation. Some herbs are contraindicated in pregnancy or lactation; make sure to observe warnings. Use with caution in individuals on medication and with pre-existing medical conditions. Always review for potential herb-drug interactions (HDIs) and other warnings. Large and prolonged doses may increase the potential for adverse effects. Herbs may cause transient adverse effects such as nausea, vomiting, and GI distress due to a variety of chemical constituents. Caution should be used in individuals having known allergies to plants.

Theoretical Interactions Antihypertensives, anticoagulants, antiplatelet agents, MAO inhibitors, central nervous stimulants (caffeine), sympathomimetics, and hormonal therapies.

References

Chen KJ, "The Effect and Abuse Syndrome of Ginseng," *J Tradit Chin Med*, 1981, 1(1):69-72.

Chong SK and Oberholzer VG, "Ginseng - Is There a Use in Clinical Medicine?" *Postgrad Med J*, 1988, 64(757):841-6.

Dukes MN, "Ginseng and Mastalgia," *Br Med J*, 1978, 1(6127):1621.

Hiai S, et al, "Stimulation of Pituitary-Adrenocortical System by Ginseng Saponin," *J Endocrinol Jpn*, 1979, 26(6):661-5.

Hopkins MP, Androff L, and Benninghoff AS, "Ginseng Face Cream and Unexplained Vaginal Bleeding," *Am J Obstet Gynecol*, 1988, 159(5):1121-2

Janetzky K and Morreale AP, "Probable Interaction Between Warfarin and Ginseng," *Am J Health Syst Pharm*, 1997, 54(6):692-3.

Jones BD and Runikis AM, "Interaction of Ginseng With Phenelzine," *J Clin Psychopharmacol*, 1987, 7(3):201-2.

Kim JY, Germolec DR, and Luster MI, "*Panax ginseng* As a Potential Immunomodulator: Studies in Mice," *Immunopharmacol Immunotoxicol*, 1990, 12(2):257-76.

Siegel RK, "Ginseng and High Blood Pressure," *JAMA*, 1980, 243(1):32.

Teng CM, Kuo SC, Kof N, et al, "Antiplatelet Actions of Panaxynol and Ginsenosides Isolated From Ginseng," *Biochim Biophys Acta*, 1989, 990(3):315-20.

Ginseng, Siberian *(Eleutherococcus senticosus)*

Related Information

Herb/Drug Potential Interactions *on page 642*

Herb Quick Reference Chart *on page 538*

Organ System Support Using Natural Products *on page 660*

Natural Product Category Herb

Plant Part Root

Dosage and Standardization Oral: 100-200 mg twice daily, standardized to contain 0.8% eleutherosides B and E per dose. A regimen of 4 weeks on, 2 weeks off is recommended for maximum benefit.

Reported Uses

Adaptogen (Brekhman, 1965; Brekhman, 1969)

Beneficial in athletic performance; adaptation to stress (decreased fatigue); support of immune function (Hikino, 1986)

Summary Although Siberian ginseng is a member of the ginseng family, it is of a different genus than the *Panax* or Asian varieties. It has been used for thousands of years in traditional Chinese medicine and in Russia, and has been shown to improve energy and vitality. Siberian ginseng has been reported to increase stamina and endurance, and protect the body systems against stress-induced illness. It is believed to increase the body's ability to adapt to chemical, physical, psychological, and biological stressors (adaptogen). As an aid to general health, it has been used in chronic illnesses such as atherosclerosis, diabetes mellitus, and hypertension.

Pharmacology The eleutheroside content of Siberian ginseng is believed to be responsible for its ability to facilitate adaptation to stress. In addition, polysaccharides in Siberian ginseng appear to act as immune stimulants. Siberian ginseng has been demonstrated to improve adaptation to reduced cellular oxygen levels, thermal changes, radiation and toxic exposures (chemotherapy, alcohol, and environmental). It enhances immunity, leading to resistance against viral and microbial infections. Reported benefits include increased physical endurance, mental alertness, increased amount and quality of work performed, decreased sick days, and enhanced athletic performance.

Theoretical Cautions and Contraindications Based on pharmacological activity, use with caution with stimulant products, including decongestants, caffeine, and caffeine-containing beverages.

Based on pharmacological activity, use with caution in individuals with hypertension or in individuals receiving antihypertensive medications. Caution in individuals at risk of hypotension (including those taking antihypertensive medication or agents that predispose to orthostasis), elderly individuals, or those who would not tolerate transient hyper- or hypotensive episodes (ie, cerebrovascular or cardiovascular disease). May potentiate effects of antihypertensives.

Use with caution in individuals taking barbiturates (based on *in vitro* or animal studies, McRae, 1996; Medon, 1984)

May alter glucose regulation. Use with caution in individuals with diabetes or in those who may be predisposed to hypoglycemia. Effects of drugs with hypoglycemic activity may be potentiated (including insulin and oral hypoglycemics). The individual's blood sugar should be closely monitored, and the dosage of these agents, including insulin dosage, may require adjustment. This should be carefully coordinated among the individual's healthcare providers.

Based on pharmacological activity and case reports, hemostasis may be affected. Contraindicated in individuals with active bleeding (eg, peptic ulcer, intracranial bleeding). Use with caution in individuals with a history of bleeding, hemostatic disorders, or drug-related hemostatic problems. Use with caution in individuals taking anticoagulant medications, including warfarin, aspirin, aspirin-containing products, NSAIDs, or antiplatelet agents (eg, ticlopidine, clopidogrel, dipyridamole). Discontinue use prior to dental or surgical procedures (generally at least 14 days before).

Extensive or prolonged use may heighten estrogenic activity (based on pharmacological activity).

General Warnings Use all herbal supplements with extreme caution in children <2 years of age and in pregnancy or lactation. Some herbs are contraindicated in pregnancy or lactation; make sure to observe warnings. Use with caution in individuals on medication and with pre-existing medical conditions. Always review for potential herb-drug interactions (HDIs) and other warnings. Large and prolonged doses may increase the potential for adverse effects. Herbs may cause transient adverse effects such as nausea, vomiting, and GI distress due to a variety of chemical constituents. Caution should be used in individuals having known allergies to plants.

Theoretical Interactions Barbiturates, antihypertensives, anticoagulants, antiplatelet agents, insulin, oral hypoglycemics, digoxin, stimulants (including OTC stimulants)

References

Brekhman II and Kirillov OI, "Effect of *Eleurococcus* on Alarm-Phase of Stress," *Life Sci*, 1969, 8(3):113-21.

Brekhman II and Maianskii GM, "*Eleutherococcus* - a Means of Increasing the Nonspecific Resistance of the Organism," *Izv Akad Nauk SSSR Biol*, 1965, 5:762-5.

Hikino H, Takahashi M, Otakek, et al, "Isolation and Hypoglycemic Activity of Eleutherans A, B, C, D, E, F and G: Glycans of *Eleutherococcus senticosus* Roots," *J Nat Prod*, 1986, 49(2):293-7.

McRae S, "Elevated Serum Digoxin Levels in a Patient Taking Digoxin and Siberian Ginseng," *CMAJ*, 1996, 155(3):293-5.

Medon PJ, Ferguson PW, and Watson CF, "Effects of *Eleutherococcus senticosus* Extracts on Hexobarbital Metabolism In Vivo and In Vitro," *J Ethnopharmacol*, 1984, 10(2):235-41.

♦ **Glaucoma** see page 198

♦ **Glossary of Natural Medicine Terms** *see page 663*

Glucosamine

Related Information
   Nutraceutical Chart *on page 573*

Natural Product Category Nutraceutical

Dosage Oral: Dosage range: 500 mg 3-4 times/day

Active Forms Glucosamine sulfate, glucosamine hydrochloride

Reported Uses
   Osteoarthritis (Noack, 1994; Müller, 1994; Qiu, 1998; Shankland, 1998; Phillipi, 1999; Pujalte, 1980)
   Rheumatoid arthritis and other inflammatory conditions (McCarty, 1998)

Summary Glucosamine, a precursor molecule, is important for maintaining elasticity, strength, and resiliency of the cartilage in articular (movable) joints. The cartilage pad distributes the force of impact across the broad surface of bone and supporting structures, limiting damage to the joint. In addition, cartilage facilitates frictionless gliding of the joint surfaces. Along with supporting cartilage and other connective tissue, glucosamine has anti-inflammatory properties. It has been used extensively to promote the maintenance of joint function and to decrease pain in individuals suffering from osteoarthritis. Glucosamine may act synergistically with chondroitin sulfate.

Pharmacology Glucosamine is an amino-sugar that is naturally produced in humans. It is the key substrate used in the synthesis of macromolecules which comprise connective tissue. It is involved in the synthesis of glycolipids, glycoproteins, hyaluronic acid, proteoglycans, and glycosaminoglycans. These are the major structural components of cartilage. In addition to structural support, facilitating production of hyaluronic acid enhances the anti-inflammatory effects of this molecule.

Toxicities, Warnings, and Interactions No known toxicity or serious side effects. Occasional reports of mild gastrointestinal discomfort or stomach upset. Based on animal studies, may alter glucose regulation/insulin sensitivity.

Symptoms of Deficiency Synthesized in the human body, absolute deficiency has not been observed. A relative deficiency may accelerate the damage to joints caused by failure of the protective mechanisms in the joint.

Reported Interactions
   Drug/Nutrient Interactions: Theoretically, insulin or oral hypoglycemics may be less effective
   Nutrient/Nutrient Interactions: None known

References
McCarty MF, "Vascular Heparan Sulfates May Limit the Ability of Leukocytes to Penetrate the Endothelial Barrier - Implications for Use of Glucosamine in Inflammatory Disorders," *Med Hypotheses*, 1998, 51(1):11-15.

Muller H, Bach GL, Haase W, et al, "Glucosamine Sulfate Compared to Ibuprofen in Osteoarthritis of the Knee," *Osto and Cart*, 1994, 2:61-9.

Noack W, Fischer M, Forster KK, et al, "Glucosamine Sulfate in Osteoarthritis of the Knee," *Osto and Cart*, 1994, 2:51-9.

Phillipi AF, Leffler CT, Leffler SG, et al, "Glucosamine, Chondroitin, and Manganese Ascorbate for Degenerative Joint Disease of the Knee or Low Back: A Randomized, Double-Blind, Placebo-Controlled Pilot Study," *Military Medicine*, 1999, 164:85-91.

Pujalte JM, Llavore EP, and Ylescupidez FR, "Double-Blind Clinical Evaluation of Oral Glucosamine Sulfate in the Basic Treatment of Osteoarthrosis," *Curr Med Res Opin*, 1980, 7(2):110-14.

Qui GX, Gao SN, Giacovelli G, et al, "Efficacy and Safety of Glucosamine Sulfate Versus Ibuprofen in Patients With Knee Osteoarthritis," *Arzneimittelforschung*, 1998, 48(5):469-74.

Shankland WE 2nd, "The Effects of Glucosamine and Chondroitin Sulfate on Osteoarthritis of the TMJ: A Preliminary Report of 50 Patients," *Cranio*, 1998, 16(4):230-5.

♦ **Glucosamine Hydrochloride** *see* Glucosamine *on page 446*
♦ **Glucosamine Sulfate** *see* Glucosamine *on page 446*

Glutamine

Related Information
   Vitamins/Minerals/Trace Elements/Amino Acids Chart *on page 604*

Natural Product Category Amino Acid

Dosage Oral: RDI: None established; dosage range: 500-4000 mg 3 times/day

Active Forms L-glutamine

Reported Uses

Adjunct therapy for cancer (Decker-Baumann, 1999)

Adjunct therapy for HIV (Rohde, 1995)

Alcoholism (Rogers, 1956)

Catabolic wasting processes (Sacks, 1999)

Immunosupportive (Calder, 1999)

Peptic ulcers (Shive, 1957)

Performance enhancement (Antonio, 1999)

Postsurgical healing (Hammarqvist, 1989)

Ulcerative colitis and other forms of inflammatory bowel disease (Fujita, 1995)

Summary Glutamine is classified as a nonessential amino acid because the body is capable of synthesizing it. However, it is sometimes called a "conditionally essential" amino acid, since it may become essential for some individuals during periods of high stress such as burns, injury, or inflammatory bowel conditions. Glutamine is the most abundant amino acid in the human body.

Pharmacology Glutamine promotes protein synthesis and muscle growth. It is also the primary source of energy for cells in the lining of the gastrointestinal tract. Glutamine also serves as an alternative source of energy for the brain. Glutamine helps block cortisol-induced protein catabolism. Glutamine may become a "conditionally essential" amino acid in conditions such as gastrointestinal disorders and tissue-wasting phenomena.

Toxicities, Warnings, and Interactions No known toxicity or serious side effects

Symptoms of Deficiency Deficiency studies in humans have not been conducted.

References

Antonio J and Street C, "Glutamine: A Potentially Useful Supplement for Athletes," *Can J Appl Physiol*, 1999, 24(1):1-14.

Calder PC, Yaqoob P, "Glutamine and the Immune System," *Amino Acids*, 1999, 17(3):227-41.

Decker-Bauman C, Buhl K, Frohmuller S, et al, "Reduction of Chemotherapy-Induced Side-Effects by Parenteral Glutamine Supplementation in Patients with Metastatic Colorectal Cancer," *Eur J Cancer*, 1999, 35(2):202-7.

Fujita T and Sakurai K, "Efficacy of Glutamine-Enriched Enteral Nutrition in an Experimental Model of Mucosal Ulcerative Colitis," *Br J Surg*, 1995, 82(6):749-51.

Hammarqvist F, Wernerman J, Ali R, et al, "Addition of Glutamine to Total Parenteral Nutrition After Elective Abdominal Surgery Spares Free Glutamine in Muscle, Counteracts the Fall in Muscle Protein Synthesis, and Improves Nitrogen Balance," *Ann Surg*, 1989, 209(4):455-61.

Rogers LL, et al, "Voluntary Alcohol Consumption by Rats Following Administration of Glutamine," *J Biol Chem*, 1956, 220(1):321-3.

Rohde T, Ullum H, Rasmussen JP, et al, "Effect of Glutamine on the Immune System: Influence of Muscular Exercise and HIV Infection," *J Appl Physiol*, 1995, 79(1):146-50.

Sacks GS, "Glutamine Supplementation in Catabolic Patients," *Ann Pharmacother*, 1999, 33(3):348-54.

Shive W, et al, "Glutamine in Treatment of Peptic Ulcer," *Texas State J Med*, 1957, 53:840-3.

Glutathione

Related Information

Nutraceutical Chart *on page 573*

Natural Product Category Nutraceutical

Dosage Oral: Dosage range: 500-3000 mg/day in divided doses

Active Forms L-glutathione

Reported Uses

Hepatoprotection (alcohol-induced liver damage) (Altomare, 1988)

Immune system support (Spallholz, 1990)

Peptic ulcer disease (Hirokawa, 1995)

Summary Glutathione is a part of critical detoxifying and antioxidant enzyme systems. Supplementation may aid in protecting the liver from toxic damage, strengthen the immune system, and protect against oxidative damage to tissues.

(Continued)

Glutathione *(Continued)*

Special note: Glutathione must be in its reduced form to be active. Some manufacturers do not indicate if their product is reduced. In general, the unreduced form is cheaper, but it is not metabolically active.

Pharmacology Glutathione is a sulfur-containing tripeptide that is composed of cysteine, glycine, and glutamic acid. Glutathione participates in the hepatic detoxification of many compounds via glutathione S-transferase. This enzyme participates in the detoxification of compounds from cigarette smoke, ethanol, and overdoses of aspirin or acetaminophen. Glutathione is part of the antioxidant enzyme systems, including glutathione peroxidase. It reduces oxidative damage, particularly in mitochondria and red blood cells, and appears to reduce free radical damage due to radiation. Glutathione is involved in cellular transmembrane amino acid transport systems and is involved in fatty acid synthesis. It facilitates the development and function of a variety of immune cells, including macrophages and lymphoctyes.

Toxicities, Warnings, and Interactions No known toxicity or serious side effects

Symptoms of Deficiency Decreased capacity for hepatic detoxification. Decreased immunity and suppression of macrophage activity. A lack of glutathione may lead to increased free radical damage throughout the body, especially in the membranes of red blood cells and mitochondria. Glutathione deficiency could result in hair loss and baldness.

Reported Interactions

Drug/Nutrient Interactions: None known

Nutrient/Nutrient Interactions: None known

References

Altomare E, Vendemiale G, and Albano O, "Hepatic Glutathione Content in Patients With Alcoholic and Non-alcoholic Liver Diseases," *Life Sci*, 1988, 43(12):991-8.

Hirokawa K and Kawasaki H, "Changes in Glutathione in Gastric Mucosa of Gastric Ulcer Patients," *Res Commun Mol Pathol Pharmacol*, 1995, 88(2):163-76.

Spallholz JE, "Selenium and Glutathione Peroxidase: Essential Nutrient and Antioxidant Component of the Immune System," *Adv Exp Med Biol*, 1990, 262:145-58.

♦ *Glycyrrhiza glabra* see Licorice (Glycyrrhiza glabra) on page 470

Golden Seal *(Hydrastis canadensis)*

Related Information

Common Herbal Supplements Contraindicated During Pregnancy *on page 656*

Herb/Drug Potential Interactions *on page 642*

Herb Quick Reference Chart *on page 538*

Natural Product Category Herb

Plant Part Root, rhizome

Dosage and Standardization Oral: 250 mg (standardized extract), 2-4 times/day, standardized to contain 10% alkaloids or 2.5% berberine and 1.5% to 5% hydrastine per dose

Reported Uses Mucous membrane tonifying (used in inflammation of mucosal membranes); treatment of gastritis; antimicrobial (antibacterial/antifungal); treatment of bronchitis, cystitis, and infectious diarrhea (Bradley, 1992)

Summary Golden seal was initially used by Native Americans. It has been used for GI disturbances and as an anti-infective. It is often used for colds and upper respiratory infections, sometimes in combination with the herb echinacea. It is believed that golden seal may mask urine drug screens, but there has been no evidence to support this claim.

Pharmacology The primary constituents are berberine and hydrastine. Berberine has antimicrobial activity against a broad array of pathogens, including viruses, fungi, parasites, and bacteria. Berberine has also been reported to have antipyretic effects. The alkaloids in golden seal have astringent activity which appears to contribute its anti-inflammatory activity on mucous membranes. Hydrastine has been reported to have antitussive, antiperistaltic and antihypertensive effects. Berberine compounds cause uterine stimulation, and should be avoided in pregnancy. High doses may cause hypotension, and hypoglycemic effects has been observed.

Theoretical Cautions and Contraindications Use of golden seal is contraindicated in pregnancy (based on animal studies, De Smet, 1992). Use with caution in individuals with cardiovascular disease. High doses may cause hypotension or bradycardia (based on animal studies, see Sabir, 1971). Doses in the range of 2-3 g may cause gastrointestinal distress or bradycardia. Extremely high-dose ingestion (18 g) has been reported to induce CNS depression. High-dose hydrastine has been associated with hypertension, hyper-reflexia, and seizures (Genest, 1969). Extended use of high doses has been associated in some reports with neuroexcitation, hallucinations, delirium, and gastrointestinal disorders. Overdose has been associated with myocardial damage and respiratory failure (Genest, 1969).

General Warnings Use all herbal supplements with extreme caution in children <2 years of age and in pregnancy or lactation. Some herbs are contraindicated in pregnancy or lactation; make sure to observe warnings. Use with caution in individuals on medication and with pre-existing medical conditions. Always review for potential herb-drug interactions (HDIs) and other warnings. Large and prolonged doses may increase the potential for adverse effects. Herbs may cause transient adverse effects such as nausea, vomiting, and GI distress due to a variety of chemical constituents. Caution should be used in individuals having known allergies to plants.

Theoretical Interactions None known

References

Bradley PR, ed, *British Herbal Compendium*, Vol 1, Bournemouth, England: British Herbal Medicine Association, 1992, 119-20.

Genest, K et al, "Natural Products in Canadian Pharmaceuticals, *Hydrastis canadensis*," *Can J Pharm Sci*, 1969, 4:41-45.

Newall CA, Anderson LA, and Phillipson JD, *Herbal Medicines: A Guide for Health Care Professionals*, London, England: The Pharmaceutical Press, 1996, 151-2.

Sabir M and Bhide NK, "Study of Some Pharmacological Actions of Berberine," *Indian J Physiol Pharmacol*, 1971, 15(3):111-32.

Gotu Kola *(Centella asiatica)*

Related Information

Common Herbal Supplements Contraindicated During Pregnancy *on page 656*

Herb/Drug Potential Interactions *on page 642*

Herb Quick Reference Chart *on page 538*

Organ System Support Using Natural Products *on page 660*

Natural Product Category Herb

Plant Part Leaf

Dosage and Standardization

Oral: 50-250 mg 2-3 times/day, standardized to contain 10% to 30% asiaticosides and 2% to 4% triterpenes per dose

Topical: Apply a 0.2% to 0.4% preparation topically to wound areas 2-3 times/day

Reported Uses

Hemorrhoids (topical) (Suguna, 1996; Tenni, 1988)

Memory enhancement (Newall, 1996)

Psoriasis (Natarajan, 1973)

Support/modulation of connective tissue synthesis (Newall, 1996)

Venous insufficiency (Cesarone, 1994)

Wound healing (topical) (Suguna, 1996; Tenni, 1988)

Summary Despite its name, gotu kola is not related to the kola nut and does not contain caffeine. It is believed to be useful to promote healing of tissues following damage from trauma, inflammation, or infection.

Pharmacology The primary activity of gotu kola appears to be on the connective tissue. It reportedly stimulates synthesis of hyaluronidase and chondroitin sulfate in connective tissue. Gotu kola is also believed to have an effect on keratinization in areas of infection and to stimulate the reticuloendothelial system. Gotu kola has also been reported to increase superoxide dismutase (SOD) and glutathione peroxidase while decreasing lipid peroxide levels. Topical Gotu kola is claimed to improve tissue healing, (Continued)

Gotu Kola *(Centella asiatica) (Continued)*

particularly in the skin, connective tissue, lymph, and mucous membranes. It also may stabilize connective tissue growth in scleroderma. Gotu kola has been used to treat venous insufficiency, soft tissue inflammation and infection, and has been used as an adjunct for postsurgical wound healing.

Theoretical Cautions and Contraindications Contraindicated during pregnancy (emmenagogue and abortifacient in animal studies, Ramswamy, 1970). Large doses may be sedating (Ramswamy, 1970). Caution individuals to avoid hazardous tasks (eg, driving or operating machinery). Caution in individuals taking sedative medications (eg, anxiolytics, benzodiazepines). Effects may be additive with other CNS depressants. Topical administration may cause contact dermatitis in sensitive individuals (Danese, 1994). High doses of gotu kola may elevate cholesterol levels (Ramswamy, 1970).

General Warnings Use all herbal supplements with extreme caution in children <2 years of age and in pregnancy or lactation. Some herbs are contraindicated in pregnancy or lactation; make sure to observe warnings. Use with caution in individuals on medication and with pre-existing medical conditions. Always review for potential herb-drug interactions (HDIs) and other warnings. Large and prolonged doses may increase the potential for adverse effects. Herbs may cause transient adverse effects such as nausea, vomiting, and GI distress due to a variety of chemical constituents. Caution should be used in individuals having known allergies to plants.

Theoretical Interactions Sedative medications, anxiolytics

References

Cesarone MR, Laurora G, De Santis MT, et al, "The Microcirculatory Activity of *Centella asiatica* in Venous Insufficiency. A Double-blind Study," *Minerva Cardioangiol*, 1994, 42(6):299-304.

Danese P, Carnevali C, and Bertazzoni MG, "Allergic Contact Dermatitis Due to *Centella asiatica* Extract," *Contact Dermatitis*, 1994, 31(3):201.

Natarajan S and Paily PP, "Effect of Topical *Hydrocotyle asiatica* in Psoriasis," *Indian J Dermatol*, 1973, 18(4):82-5.

Newall CA, Anderson LA, and Phillipson JD, *Herbal Medicines: A Guide for Health Care Professionals*, London, England: The Pharmaceutical Press, 1996, 170-2.

Ramswamy AS, et al, "Pharmacological Studies of *Centella asiatica*," *Indian J Med Res*, 1970, 4:160-75.

Suguna L, Sivakumar P, and Chandrakasan G, "Effects of *Centella asiatica* Extract on Dermal Wound Healing in Rats," *Indian J Exp Biol*, 1996, 34(12):1208-11.

Tenni R, Zanaboni G, De Agostini MP, et al, "Effect of the Triterpenoid Fraction of *Centella asiatica* on Macromolecules of the Connective Matrix in Human Skin Fibroblast Cultures," *Ital J Biochem*, 1988, 37(2):69-77.

Grapefruit Seed *(Citrus paradisi)*

Related Information

Herb Quick Reference Chart *on page 538*

Natural Product Category Herb

Plant Part Seed extract

Dosage and Standardization

Oral: 100 mg 1-3 times/day with meals

Drops: 5-10 drops 2-3 times/day

Oral rinse: 5-10 drops diluted in water 2-3 times/day (swish and expectorate)

Reported Uses Antifungal, antibacterial, antiparasitic agent (Ionescu, 1990)

Summary Grapefruit seed extract (GSE) is reported to have antibiotic, antifungal, and antiparasitic effects when used topically and internally. GSE is used in gastrointestinal health (bowel terrain integrity).

Pharmacology Grapefruit seed extract seems to exert its antimicrobial activity in the cytoplasmic membrane of the bacteria. GSE primarily causes an alteration of the cell membrane with inhibition of cellular respiration and a dose dependent inhibition of cellular respiration.

Theoretical Cautions and Contraindications Grapefruit seed extract is not the equivalent of grapefruit juice. Grapefruit juice/pulp has been associated with the inhibition of drug metabolism via cytochrome P450 isoenzyme 3A4 (CYP3A4), resulting in a number of drug interactions. It is not known whether extracts of grapefruit seed share in this potential to alter drug metabolism. Until further information is available, it is reasonable to avoid the concurrent use of grapefruit seed extract in individuals receiving terfenadine, astemizole, and cisapride. In addition, caution is warranted in individuals receiving other medications metabolized by this pathway.

General Warnings Use all herbal supplements with extreme caution in children <2 years of age and in pregnancy or lactation. Some herbs are contraindicated in pregnancy or lactation; make sure to observe warnings. Use with caution in individuals on medication and with pre-existing medical conditions. Always review for potential herb-drug interactions (HDIs) and other warnings. Large and prolonged doses may increase the potential for adverse effects. Herbs may cause transient adverse effects such as nausea, vomiting, and GI distress due to a variety of chemical constituents. Caution should be used in individuals having known allergies to plants.

Theoretical Interactions None known, but theoretically may interact with terfenadine, astemizole, cisapride, and other drugs metabolized by CYP3A4. Refer to Theoretical Cautions and Contraindications

References

Ionescu G, Kiehl R, Wichmann-Kunz F, et al, "Oral Citrus Seed Extract in Atopic Eczema: *In Vitro* and *In Vivo* Studies on Intestinal Microflora," *Journal of Orthomolecular Medicine*, 1990, 5:72-3.

Grape Seed *(Vitis vinifera)*

Related Information

Herb/Drug Potential Interactions *on page 642*
Herb Quick Reference Chart *on page 538*
Organ System Support Using Natural Products *on page 660*

Natural Product Category Herb

Plant Part Seed, skin

Dosage and Standardization Oral: 25-100 mg 1-3 times/day, standardized to contain 40% to 80% proanthocyanidins or 95% polyphenols or a proanthrocyanidolic value of greater than 95% per dose

Reported Uses Antioxidant; treatment of allergies, asthma; improve circulation; antiplatelets (blocks aggregation); improve capillary fragility; anti-inflammatory; arterial/venous insufficiency (intermittent claudication, varicose veins) (Maffei Facino, 1997; Frankel, 1993; Jonadet, 1983)

Summary Grape seed is a source of potent free radical scavengers (antioxidants). It has been used in allergic disorders, including asthma. In addition, it has been used in a variety of vascular complaints such as varicose veins and peripheral vascular disease.

Pharmacology Grape seed is a potent antioxidant. Proanthocyanidins are claimed to neutralize many free radicals, including hydroxyl, lipid peroxides, and iron-induced lipid peroxidation. The antioxidant properties of proanthocyanidins are believed to block lipid peroxidation, stabilizing cell membranes. The constituent proanthocyanidins are also claimed to inhibit the destruction of collagen, possibly by stabilizing 1-antitrypsin, which inhibits the activity of destructive enzymes such as elastin and hyaluronic acid. Stabilization of collagen is claimed to allow red blood cells to traverse the capillaries and prevent fluid exudation. Proanthocyanidins have been reported to inhibit the release of mediators of inflammation, such as histamine and prostaglandins, and have been used in individuals with allergies. Grape seed extract may inhibit platelet aggregation.

Theoretical Cautions and Contraindications Based on pharmacological activity, may inhibit platelet aggregation (Chang, 1989). Grape seed is contraindicated in individuals with active bleeding (eg, peptic ulcer, intracranial bleeding). Use with caution in individuals with a history of bleeding, hemostatic disorders, or drug-related hemostatic problems. Use with caution in individuals taking anticoagulant medications, including warfarin, aspirin, aspirin-containing products, NSAIDs, or antiplatelet agents (eg, ticlopidine, clopidogrel, dipyridamole). Discontinue use prior to dental or surgical procedures (generally at least 14 days before).
(Continued)

451

Grape Seed *(Vitis vinifera) (Continued)*

In vitro studies indicate grape seed may inhibit xanthine oxidase (Bombardelli, 1995). May increase toxicity of methotrexate.

General Warnings Use all herbal supplements with extreme caution in children <2 years of age and in pregnancy or lactation. Some herbs are contraindicated in pregnancy or lactation; make sure to observe warnings. Use with caution in individuals on medication and with pre-existing medical conditions. Always review for potential herb-drug interactions (HDIs) and other warnings. Large and prolonged doses may increase the potential for adverse effects. Herbs may cause transient adverse effects such as nausea, vomiting, and GI distress due to a variety of chemical constituents. Caution should be used in individuals having known allergies to plants.

Theoretical Interactions Anticoagulants, aspirin, aspirin-containing products, NSAIDs, antiplatelet agents, xanthine oxidase inhibitors

References

Bombardelli E, "*Vitus vinifera* L.," *Fitoterapia*, 1995, 66(4):291-7.

Chang WC and Hsu FL, "Inhibition of Platelet Aggregation and Arachidonate Metabolism in Platelets by Procyanidins, *Prostaglandins Leukot Essent Fatty Acids*, 1989, 38(3):181-8.

Frankel EN, Kanner J, German JB, et al, "Inhibition of Oxidation of Human Low-Density Lipoprotein by Phenolic Substances in Red Wine," *Lancet*, 1993, 341(8843):454-7.

Jonadet M, Meunier MT, Bastide J, et al, "Anthocyanosides Extracted From *Vitis vinifera, Vaccinium myrtillus* and *Pinus maritimus*. I. Elastase-Inhibiting Activities *In Vitro*. II. Compared Angioprotective Activities *In Vivo*," *J Pharm Belg*, 1983, 38(1):41-6.

Maffei Facino R, Carini M, Aldini G, et al, "Regeneration of Endogenous Antioxidants, Ascorbic Acid, Alpha Tocopherol, by the Oligomeric Procyanide Fraction of *Vitus vinifera* L: ESR Study," *Boll Chim Farm*, 1997, 136(4):340-4.

Green Tea *(Camellia sinensis)*

Related Information

Herb/Drug Potential Interactions *on page 642*
Herb Quick Reference Chart *on page 538*
Organ System Support Using Natural Products *on page 660*

Natural Product Category Herb

Plant Part Leaf

Dosage and Standardization Oral: 250-500 mg/day, standardized to contain 50% to 97% polyphenols per dose, containing per dose at least 50% (-)epigallocatechin-3-gallate (EGCG); **Note:** Caffeine-free products are recommended

Reported Uses

Anticarcinogenic activity (Snow, 1995)

Antioxidant; Support in cancer prevention and cardiovascular disease (Yokozawa, 1997; Stoner, 1995)

Chemotherapy and radiation; adjunct support for chemotherapy and radiation (Mitscher, 1997)

May lower cholesterol (Yang, 1997)

Platelet-aggregation inhibitor (Sagesake-Mitane, 1990)

Summary Green tea has been used for centuries as a beverage as well as a medicinal agent. Green tea is an antioxidant that is used to reduce serum cholesterol levels. It has also been reported to be of value in cancer treatment, may limit damage from exposure to carcinogens or radiation, and may enhance immunity. Green tea also has diuretic, stimulant, astringent, antifungal, antiviral, and antibacterial properties.

Pharmacology Green tea reportedly has antioxidant properties and protects against oxidative damage to cells and tissues. The primary antioxidant activity appears to be mediated by polyphenols (catechin). Green tea may have an important role in cardiovascular disease. Increased consumption of green tea has been demonstrated to increase HDL cholesterol while decreasing LDL cholesterol and triglycerides. Green tea has also been reported to block the peroxidation of LDL, an important step in atherogenesis; and to inhibit formation of thromboxane formation and block platelet aggregation.

Green tea polyphenolics are claimed to have antimutagenic, anticarcinogenic, and antioxidant effects. A component of green tea, (-)epigallocatechin gallate (EGCG) has been reported to inhibit the growth of cancer cells and metastasis. Human studies have noted a correlation between consumption of green tea and improvement in the extent of metastasis and prognosis in some forms of breast cancer. This may be related to a modification of the characteristics of cancer cells by green tea.

The oral administration of green tea reportedly enhanced the antitumor effects of doxorubicin (Adriamycin®) (Stammeler, 1997; Sadzura, 1996). In addition, green tea's potent antioxidant properties have been reported to limit damage to normal tissues exposed to chemotherapy and ultraviolet radiation-induced carcinogenesis. (See References)

Theoretical Cautions and Contraindications If product is not decaffeinated, caffeine may cause gastric irritation, decreased appetite, insomnia, tachycardia, palpitations, and nervousness in sensitive individuals. Nondecaffeinated products should be used with caution in individuals with peptic ulcer disease or cardiovascular disease. At high doses, caffeine-containing products may interact with many medications.

Based on *in vitro* effects on platelet aggregation (Sagesaka-Mitane, 1990): Contraindicated in individuals with active bleeding (eg, peptic ulcer, intracerebral bleeding). Use with caution in individuals with a history of bleeding, hemostatic disorders, or drug-related hemostatic problems. Use with caution in individuals taking anticoagulant medications, aspirin, aspirin-containing products, NSAIDs, or antiplatelet agents (eg, ticlopidine, clopidogrel, dipyridamole). Discontinue use prior to dental or surgical procedures (generally at least 14 days before). Green tea has also been reported to antagonize the effects of warfarin (Taylor, 1999).

Use with caution when taking other stimulants such as caffeine and decongestants, unless a caffeine-free product is used. It is important to note that the addition of milk to any tea may significantly lower the antioxidant potential of this agent.

General Warnings Use all herbal supplements with extreme caution in children <2 years of age and in pregnancy or lactation. Some herbs are contraindicated in pregnancy or lactation; make sure to observe warnings. Use with caution in individuals on medication and with pre-existing medical conditions. Always review for potential herb-drug interactions (HDIs) and other warnings. Large and prolonged doses may increase the potential for adverse effects. Herbs may cause transient adverse effects such as nausea, vomiting, and GI distress due to a variety of chemical constituents. Caution should be used in individuals having known allergies to plants.

Theoretical Interactions Anticoagulants (including warfarin), aspirin, aspirin-containing products, antiplatelet agents

If caffeinated product is used: Aspirin, acetaminophen, fluoroquinolones (CYP1A inhibitors), oral contraceptives, verapamil, quinidine, fluconazole, theophylline, CNS stimulants, sympathomimetics, MAO inhibitors, adenosine, beta-blockers, clozapine, benzodiazepines, proton pump inhibitors, H-2 antagonists, barbiturates (phenobarbital), phenytoin

References

Mitscher LA, Jung M, Shankel D, et al, "Chemoprotection: A Review of the Potential Therapeutic Antioxidant Properties of Green Tea (*Camellia sinensis*) and Certain of Its Constituents," *Med Res Rev*, 1997, 17(4):327-65.

Sadzuka Y, Sugiyama T, Miyagishima A, et al, "The Effects of Theanine, as a Novel Biochemical Modulator, on the Antitumor Activity of Adriamycin," *Cancer Lett*, 1996, 105(2):203-9.

Sagesaka-Mitane Y, Miwa M, and Okada S, "Platelet Aggregation Inhibitors in Hot Water Extract of Green Tea," *Chem Pharm Bull (Tokyo)*, 1990, 38(3):790-3.

Snow J, "*Camellia sinensis* (L) Kuntze (Theaceae)," *Protocol J Botanical Med*, 1995, 47-51.

Stammler G and Volm M, "Green Tea Catechins (EGCG and EGC) Have Modulating Effects on the Activity of Doxorubicin in Drug-Resistant Cell Lines," *Anticancer Drugs*, 1997, 8(3):265-8.

Stoner GD and Mukhtar H, "Polyphenols as Cancer Chemopreventive Agents," *J Cell Biochem Suppl*, 1995, 22:169-80.

Taylor JR, Wilt VM, "Probable Antagonism of Warfarin by Green Tea," *Ann Pharmacother*, 1999, 33(4):426-8.

(Continued)

Green Tea *(Camellia sinensis)* *(Continued)*

Yang TT and Koo MW, "Hypocholesterolemic Effects of Chinese Tea," *Pharmacol Res*, 1997, 35(6):505-12.

Yokozawa T and Dong E, "Influence of Green Tea and Its Three Major Components Upon Low-Density Lipoprotein Oxidation," *Exp Toxicol Pathol*, 1997, 49(5):329-35.

Ground Ivy *(Hedera helix)*

Related Information

Herb/Drug Potential Interactions *on page 642*
Herb Quick Reference Chart *on page 538*

Natural Product Category Herb

Plant Part Leaf

Dosage and Standardization Oral: 50 mg 3 times/day

Reported Uses Mucolytic action; upper respiratory congestion and cough (Bradley, 1992)

Summary Ivy is one of the top-selling herbal supplements in Germany, used mainly as a mucolytic agent. It is used in upper respiratory congestion and coughs.

Pharmacology The expectorant activity of ivy is attributed to its flavonoids.

Theoretical Cautions and Contraindications Contraindicated in individuals with epilepsy (Bradley, 1992)

General Warnings Use all herbal supplements with extreme caution in children <2 years of age and in pregnancy or lactation. Some herbs are contraindicated in pregnancy or lactation; make sure to observe warnings. Use with caution in individuals on medication and with pre-existing medical conditions. Always review for potential herb-drug interactions (HDIs) and other warnings. Large and prolonged doses may increase the potential for adverse effects. Herbs may cause transient adverse effects such as nausea, vomiting, and GI distress due to a variety of chemical constituents. Caution should be used in individuals having known allergies to plants.

Theoretical Interactions None known

References

Bradley PR, ed, *British Herbal Compendium, Vol 1*, Bournemouth, England: British Herbal Medicine Association, 1992, 121-2.

♦ **GSH** *see* Glutathione *on page 447*

Guggul *(Commiphora mukul)*

Related Information

Common Herbal Supplements Contraindicated During Pregnancy *on page 656*
Herb/Drug Potential Interactions *on page 642*
Herb Quick Reference Chart *on page 538*

Natural Product Category Herb

Plant Part Resin

Dosage and Standardization Oral: 500 mg 3 times/day, standardized to contain 5% guggulsterones per dose

Reported Uses May lower blood cholesterol levels (Singh, 1994; Nityanand, 1989; Agarwal, 1986)

Summary Guggul oleoresin has been used in the Ayurvedic (traditional Indian) medical system for centuries. In 1986, it was approved in India for marketing as a lipid-lowering drug. In India, guggul is also used in the management of a variety of other medical problems, including arthritis and inflammatory conditions. Guggul has been noted to lower total cholesterol, LDL cholesterol, and triglycerides while increasing HDL. Guggul has been reported to demonstrate the most benefit in type IIb hyperlipidemia (increased LDL, VLDL, and triglycerides) as well as type IV hyperlipidemia (increased VLDL and triglycerides).

Pharmacology Four mechanisms have been proposed to explain the effects of guggul. It may 1) block hepatic synthesis of cholesterol, 2) increase biliary and fecal excretion of cholesterol, 3) increase hepatic LDL receptor expression, increasing the uptake of circulating LDL particles, or 4) increase thyroid activity, indirectly stimulating metabolism of LDL particles. In addition, guggul is a potent antioxidant. Guggul has been reported to prevent the formation of atherosclerotic plaques as well as aid regression of pre-existing lesions. It also has been reported to inhibit platelet aggregation and increase fibrinolysis.

Theoretical Cautions and Contraindications Use with caution during pregnancy and lactation due to thyroid-stimulating properties (Tripathi, 1984). May increase thyroid activity; use with caution in individuals with thyroid disease. Adverse effects may include gastrointestinal upset. May decrease metabolism of some hepatically metabolized drugs, including propranolol and diltiazem (Dalvi, 1994).

Based on pharmacological activity, may alter platelet aggregation and/or fibrinolytic activity (Satyavati, 1991). Contraindicated in individuals with active bleeding (eg, peptic ulcer, intracranial bleeding). Use with caution in individuals with a history of bleeding, hemostatic disorders, or drug-related hemostatic problems. Use with caution in individuals taking anticoagulant medications, including warfarin, aspirin, aspirin-containing products, NSAIDs, or antiplatelet agents (eg, ticlopidine, clopidogrel, dipyridamole). Discontinue use prior to dental or surgical procedures (generally at least 14 days before).

General Warnings Use all herbal supplements with extreme caution in children <2 years of age and in pregnancy or lactation. Some herbs are contraindicated in pregnancy or lactation; make sure to observe warnings. Use with caution in individuals on medication and with pre-existing medical conditions. Always review for potential herb-drug interactions (HDIs) and other warnings. Large and prolonged doses may increase the potential for adverse effects. Herbs may cause transient adverse effects such as nausea, vomiting, and GI distress due to a variety of chemical constituents. Caution should be used in individuals having known allergies to plants.

Theoretical Interactions Antihypertensives (serum levels of propranolol and diltiazem may be altered), beta-blockers, calcium channel blockers, anticoagulants, aspirin, aspirin-containing products, antiplatelet agents, thyroid medications

References

Agarwal RC, Singh SP, Saran RK, et al, "Clinical Trial of Gugulipid - A New Hypolipidemic Agent of Plant Origin in Primary Hyperlipidemia," *Indian J Med Res*, 1986, 84:626-34.

Dalvi SS, Nayak VK, Pohujanism, et al, "Effects of Gugulipid on Bioavailability of Diltiazem and Propranolol," *J Assoc Physicians India*, 1994, 42(6):454-5.

Nityanand S, Srivastava JS, and Asthana DP, "Clinical Trials With Gugulipid. A New Hypolipidaemic Agent," *J Assoc Physicians India*, 1989, 37(5):323-8.

Satyavati GV, et al, "Guggulipid: A Promising Hypolipidemic Agent From Gum Guggul (*Commiphora wightii*)," *Econ Med Plant Res*, 1991, 5:48-82.

Singh RB, Niazm A, and Ghosh S, "Hypolipidemic and Antioxidant Effects of *Commiphora mukul* as an Adjunct to Dietary Therapy in Patients With Hypercholesterolemia," *Cardiovasc Drugs Ther*, 1994, 8(4):659-64.

Gymnema *(Gymnema sylvestre)*

Related Information

Herb/Drug Potential Interactions *on page 642*
Herb Quick Reference Chart *on page 538*

Natural Product Category Herb

Plant Part Leaf

Dosage and Standardization Oral: 250-500 mg 1-3 times/day, standardized to contain 25% gymnemic acids per dose

Reported Uses Diabetes, supports regulation of blood sugar levels (Baskarran, 1990)

Summary Gymnema is derived from a vine found in the Central and Southern Indian rain forest. It has a long tradition of use in individuals with diabetes. Its use has been documented in Ayurvedic (traditional Indian) medical texts for over 2000 years. The use of gymnema is increasing as a natural therapy protocols to improve control of blood sugar. A reduction in glycosylated hemoglobin and glycosylated plasma proteins have also been reported. In addition, the dosage of conventional hypoglycemic agents may be reduced, and in some cases control of blood sugar has been sufficient (Continued)

Gymnema *(Gymnema sylvestre)* (Continued)

with gymnema alone. Individuals must be warned about the possibility of enhanced effects of other hypoglycemic agents, since hypoglycemia may be life-threatening.

Pharmacology Gymnema is believed to increase insulin secretion by pancreatic beta cells, resulting in improved control of hyperglycemia. Gymnema also has been reported to stimulate enzyme activity in insulin-dependent metabolic pathways, leading to an increased utilization of glucose, and may result in weight loss. Gymnemic acids may inhibit intestinal glucose uptake, and have been reported to suppress the sensation of sweetness on the tongue.

Theoretical Cautions and Contraindications Based on pharmacological activity, may alter glucose regulation. Use with caution in individuals with diabetes or those predisposed to hypoglycemia. Effects of drugs with hypoglycemic activity may be potentiated (including insulin and oral hypoglycemics). The individual's blood sugar should be closely monitored, and the dosage of these agents, including insulin dosage, may require adjustment. This should be carefully coordinated among the individual's healthcare providers.

General Warnings Use all herbal supplements with extreme caution in children <2 years of age and in pregnancy or lactation. Some herbs are contraindicated in pregnancy or lactation; make sure to observe warnings. Use with caution in individuals on medication and with pre-existing medical conditions. Always review for potential herb-drug interactions (HDIs) and other warnings. Large and prolonged doses may increase the potential for adverse effects. Herbs may cause transient adverse effects such as nausea, vomiting, and GI distress due to a variety of chemical constituents. Caution should be used in individuals having known allergies to plants.

Theoretical Interactions Insulin, oral hypoglycemics

References

Baskaran K, Kizar Ahamath B, Radha Shanmugasundaram K, "Antidiabetic Effect of a Leaf Extract From *Gymnema sylvestre* in Non-insulin-Dependent Diabetes Mellitus Patients," *J Ethnopharmacol*, 1990, 30(3):295-300.

♦ *Gymnema sylvestre* see Gymnema *(Gymnema sylvestre)* on page 455

♦ *Halitosis* see page 202

♦ *Harpagophytum procumbens* see Devil's Claw *(Harpagophytum procumbens)* on page 422

Hawthorn *(Crataegus oxyacantha)*

Related Information

Herb/Drug Potential Interactions *on page 642*
Herb Quick Reference Chart *on page 538*
Organ System Support Using Natural Products *on page 660*

Natural Product Category Herb

Plant Part Flower, leaf, berry

Dosage and Standardization Oral: 250 mg 1-3 times/day, standardized to contain at least 2% vitexin and/or 20% procyanidins per dose

Reported Uses Angina, hypotension, hypertension, peripheral vascular disease, tachycardia; cardiotonic; congestive heart failure (Schussler, 1995; Weihmayr, 1996)

Summary Hawthorn is a vasodilator and cardiotonic with a variety of applications in the support of cardiovascular function. It has been used in both hypertension and hypotension, and is used in mild heart failure, angina, and peripheral vascular disorders.

Pharmacology The effect of hawthorn as an antihypertensive may be mediated by several mechanisms. Hawthorn bioflavonoids reportedly cause dilation of both peripheral and coronary vessels. Hawthorn is also believed to inhibit angiotensin-converting enzyme and demonstrates a modest diuretic effect. In addition, hawthorn-derived glycosides reportedly increase vagal tone.

The vasodilating properties have been noted to improve the symptoms of angina and peripheral vascular disease. Proanthocyanidins of hawthorn are claimed to have spasmolytic effects and have been reported to reverse atherosclerotic process in laboratory studies.

Hawthorn has been reported to improve cardiac performance without affecting or increasing coronary blood flow. Flavonoid compounds in hawthorn are reported to have a variety of positive effects on collagen structure in blood vessels.

Theoretical Cautions and Contraindications Contraindicated in pregnancy (based on animal studies and human case reports, Ammon, 1981). Due to pharmacological activity, use with caution in individuals receiving antihypertensive medications, including vasodilators and angiotensin converting enzyme inhibitors (Ammon, 1981), and in individuals receiving cardiac glycosides. It has been used in Europe to decrease the need for digoxin. May cause dizziness, headache, or hypotension. Caution in individuals at risk of hypotension including those taking antihypertensive medication or agents that predispose to orthostasis, elderly individuals, or those who would not tolerate transient hypotensive episodes (ie, cerebrovascular or cardiovascular disease).

Theoretically, based on its proposed pharmacological activity, hawthorn has the potential to share some effects associated with ACE inhibitors. Cough is frequently associated with ACE inhibition and serious, rare reactions (including angioedema and renal impairment) have been attributed to these agents. However, these have not been reported with hawthorn despite broad experience.

General Warnings Use all herbal supplements with extreme caution in children <2 years of age and in pregnancy or lactation. Some herbs are contraindicated in pregnancy or lactation; make sure to observe warnings. Use with caution in individuals on medication and with pre-existing medical conditions. Always review for potential herb-drug interactions (HDIs) and other warnings. Large and prolonged doses may increase the potential for adverse effects. Herbs may cause transient adverse effects such as nausea, vomiting, and GI distress due to a variety of chemical constituents. Caution should be used in individuals having known allergies to plants.

Theoretical Interactions Antiarrhythmics, antihypertensives (vasodilators, ACE inhibitors, angiotensin receptor blockers), cardiac glycosides (digoxin)

References

Ammon HP and Handel M, "Crataegus, Toxicology and Pharmacology, Part I: Toxicity," *Plant Med*, 1981, 43(2):105-20.

McGuffin M, et al, eds, *American Herbal Products Association's Botanical Safety Handbook*, Boca Raton, FL: CRC Press, 1997, 37.

Schussler M, Holzl J, and Fricke U, "Myocardial Effects of Flavonoids From *Crataegus* Species," *Arzneimittelforschung*, 1995, 45(8):842-5.

Weihmayr T and Ernst E, "Therapeutic Effectiveness of *Crataegus*," *Fortschr Med*, 1996, 114(1-2):27-9.

+ **Headache / Migraine Headache** *see page 206*
+ *Hedera helix* see Ground Ivy (*Hedera helix*) *on page 454*
+ **Hemorrhoids** *see page 210*
+ **Herbal Medicine Use In Pediatrics** *see page 641*
+ **Herb/Drug Potential Interactions** *see page 642*
+ **Herb Quick Reference Chart** *see page 538*
+ **Herpes Simplex 1** *see page 214*
+ **Herpes Simplex 2** *see page 218*
+ **HMB** see Hydroxymethyl Butyrate (HMB) *on page 461*
+ **Homeopathic Quick Reference Chart for Common Complaints** *see page 587*

Hops *(Humulus lupulus)*
Related Information
Herb/Drug Potential Interactions *on page 642*
Herb Quick Reference Chart *on page 538*
Natural Product Category Herb
(Continued)

Hops (Humulus lupulus) (Continued)

Plant Part Strobiles

Dosage and Standardization Oral: 100 mg twice daily as needed, standardized to contain 5.2% bitter acids and 4% flavonoids per dose

Reported Uses Mild sedative and hypnotic (Wohlfart, 1983; Hansel, 1980)

Summary Hops have been used for centuries in brewing and as a traditional nerve and sedative tonic. Hops are thought to possess sedative and hypnotic properties. Traditional uses of hops include neuralgia, insomnia, excitability, and, primarily, for the restlessness associated with nervous tension.

Pharmacology The sedative effect of hops is not fully understood. Hops is reported to improve sleep disturbances when given in combination with other sedative herbs such as valerian root and passion flower. The constituent 2-methyl-3-buten-2-ol may have central nervous system depressant activity. It is usually formed *in vivo* through metabolism of the α-bitter acids, humulone and lupulone. This may explain part of the sedative action of hops. Hops is generally combined with valerian for sedative effects.

Theoretical Cautions and Contraindications Use with caution in individuals on the following medications (action may be potentiated): Antianxiety agents, antidepressants, antipsychotics, alcohol, hypnotics, sedatives. Use with caution when driving an automobile or operating heavy machinery. Use with caution while taking sedative medications (reported to increase sleeping time induced by pentobarbital, Hansel, 1980).

General Warnings Use all herbal supplements with extreme caution in children <2 years of age and in pregnancy or lactation. Some herbs are contraindicated in pregnancy or lactation; make sure to observe warnings. Use with caution in individuals on medication and with pre-existing medical conditions. Always review for potential herb-drug interactions (HDIs) and other warnings. Large and prolonged doses may increase the potential for adverse effects. Herbs may cause transient adverse effects such as nausea, vomiting, and GI distress due to a variety of chemical constituents. Caution should be used in individuals having known allergies to plants.

Theoretical Interactions Antianxiety agents, antidepressants, antipsychotics, ethanol, hypnotics, pentobarbital, sedatives

References

Hansel R, Wohlfart R, and Coper H, "Sedative-Hypnotic Compounds in the Exhalation of Hops, II," *Z Naturforsch [C]*, 1980, 35(11-12):1096-7.

Lee KM, et al, "Effects of *Humulus lupulus* Extract on the Central Nervous System in Mice," *Planta Med*, 1993, 59(Suppl):A691.

Wohlfart R, Wurm G, Hansel R, et al, "Detection of Sedative-Hypnotic Active Ingredients in Hops. 5. Degradation of Bitter Acids to 2-Methyl-3-Buten-2-Ol, a Hop Constituent With Sedative-Hypnotic Activity," *Arch Pharm (Weinheim)*, 1983, 316(2):132-7.

Horse Chestnut (Aesculus hippocastanum)

Related Information

Herb/Drug Potential Interactions *on page 642*
Herb Quick Reference Chart *on page 538*

Natural Product Category Herb

Plant Part Seed

Dosage and Standardization

Oral: 300 mg 1-2 times/day, standardized to 50 mg escin per dose
Topical: Apply 2% escin gel 1-2 times/day to affected area

Reported Uses Oral and topical: Varicose veins, hemorrhoids, other venous insufficiencies; deep venous thrombosis, lower extremity edema (Pittler, 1998; Simini, 1996)

Summary Horse chestnut seed extract has been reported to have value in venous disorders such as varicose veins and hemorrhoids. Improvements in subjective symptoms, as well as objective measures have been reported. Horse chestnut has been suggested as an economical alternative to compression stocking therapy.

Pharmacology The components of horse chestnut exhibit a variety of actions on the vasculature. Horse chestnut reportedly inhibits platelet aggregation and contains proanthocyanidins, which are free radical scavengers. A component of horse chestnut, aescin, is reported to be more powerful than the bioflavonoids as an anti-inflammatory, reducing edema lowering fluid exudation by decreasing capillary permeability. It is also reported to support collagen structures and to facilitate red blood cells passage through the capillaries. Horse chestnut contains coumarin glycosides (aesculin and aesculetin) which are believed to improve lymphatic drainage and to exert anti-inflammatory effects.

Horse chestnut's activity as an anti-inflammatory agent may also be related to quercetin's reported ability to inhibit cyclo-oxygenase and lipoxygenase, the enzymes which form inflammatory prostaglandins and leukotrienes. Quercetin is also an inhibitor of phosphodiesterase, which has been correlated to cardiotonic, hypotensive, spasmolytic, antiplatelet, and sedative actions.

Note: The saponins of the horse chestnut extract (aescin) are hemolytic, but they are harmless when taken orally.

Theoretical Cautions and Contraindications Based on pharmacological activity (inhibition of platelet aggregation, Urbaniuk, 1967), may be contraindicated in individuals with active bleeding (eg, peptic ulcer, intracranial bleeding). Use with caution in individuals with a history of bleeding, hemostatic disorders, or drug-related hemostatic problems. Use with caution in individuals taking anticoagulant medications, including warfarin, aspirin, aspirin-containing products, NSAIDs, or antiplatelet agents (eg, ticlopidine, clopidogrel, dipyridamole). Discontinue use prior to dental or surgical procedures (generally at least 14 days before).

May cause gastrointestinal upset. Use with caution in individuals with hepatic or renal impairment.

General Warnings Use all herbal supplements with extreme caution in children <2 years of age and in pregnancy or lactation. Some herbs are contraindicated in pregnancy or lactation; make sure to observe warnings. Use with caution in individuals on medication and with pre-existing medical conditions. Always review for potential herb-drug interactions (HDIs) and other warnings. Large and prolonged doses may increase the potential for adverse effects. Herbs may cause transient adverse effects such as nausea, vomiting, and GI distress due to a variety of chemical constituents. Caution should be used in individuals having known allergies to plants.

Theoretical Interactions Anticoagulants, aspirin, aspirin-containing products, NSAIDs, or antiplatelet agents

References

Pittler MH and Ernst E, "Horse-Chestnut Seed Extract for Chronic Venous Insufficiency. A Criteria-Based Systematic Review," *Arch Dermatol* 1998, 134(11):1356-60.

Simini B, "Horse-Chestnut Seed Extract for Chronic Venous Insufficiency," *Lancet*, 1996, 347(9009):1182-3.

Urbaniuk KG and Gorelov KP, "The Anticoagulant Action of Horse Chestnut and Eskuzan," *Klin Med (Mosk)*, 1967, 45(2):129-33.

Horsetail (Equisetum arvense)

Related Information

Herb/Drug Potential Interactions *on page 642*
Herb Quick Reference Chart *on page 538*

Natural Product Category Herb

Plant Part Shoots

Dosage and Standardization Oral: 300 mg 3 times/day as needed, standardized to contain 10% silica per dose

Reported Uses

Diuretic (Tiktinskii, 1983)

High mineral content (including silicic acid); used to support bone and connective tissue strengthening, including osteoporosis (Harmon, 1992)

Summary Horsetail spring shoots are traditionally used as a diuretic. The high mineral content (including silicic acid) makes horsetail useful in bone and connective tissue strengthening, including osteoporosis.

(Continued)

Horsetail *(Equisetum arvense)* *(Continued)*

Pharmacology Mild diuretic activity has been reported, attributed to the flavonoid content in horsetail. The effects of strengthening and regenerating connective tissues have been attributed to the silicic acid content.

Theoretical Cautions and Contraindications Diuretic effect may cause electrolyte disturbances and may potentiate certain pharmaceutical drugs with narrow therapeutic windows (see Potential Interactions); may deplete thiamine (vitamin B_1) from the body due to thiaminase activity (Meyer, 1989)

General Warnings Use all herbal supplements with extreme caution in children <2 years of age and in pregnancy or lactation. Some herbs are contraindicated in pregnancy or lactation; make sure to observe warnings. Use with caution in individuals on medication and with pre-existing medical conditions. Always review for potential herb-drug interactions (HDIs) and other warnings. Large and prolonged doses may increase the potential for adverse effects. Herbs may cause transient adverse effects such as nausea, vomiting, and GI distress due to a variety of chemical constituents. Caution should be used in individuals having known allergies to plants.

Theoretical Interactions Antiarrhythmics, digoxin, phenytoin, diuretics, lithium, theophylline, vitamin B_1

References

Harmon NW, "*Equisetum arvense*," *Pharm J*, 1992, 399:413-5.

Meyer P, "Thiaminase Activities and Thiamine Content of *Pteridium aquilinum*, *Equisetum ramosissimum*, *Malva parviflora*, *Pennisetum clandestinum*, and *Medicago sativa*," *Onderstepoort J Vet Res*, 1989, 56(2):145-6.

Tiktinskii OL and Bablumian IuA, "Therapeutic Action of Java Tea and Field Horsetail in Uric Acid Diathesis," *Urol Nefrol (Mosk)*, 1983, (1):47-50.

♦ **5-HTP** *see* 5-Hydroxytryptophan (5-HTP) *on page 461*
♦ **Humulus lupulus** *see* Hops (Humulus lupulus) *on page 457*
♦ **Huperzia serrata** *see* HuperzineA (Huperzia serrata) *on page 460*

HuperzineA *(Huperzia serrata)*

Related Information

Herb Quick Reference Chart *on page 538*
Organ System Support Using Natural Products *on page 660*

Natural Product Category Herb

Plant Part Isolated from *Huperzia serrata* (Chinese club moss)

Dosage and Standardization Oral: 50 mcg 1-3 times/day

Reported Uses Acetylcholinesterase inhibitor in senile dementia and Alzheimer's disease (Wang, 1998)

Summary Huperzia (Chinese club moss) has been used for centuries in various problems including memory and alertness. The isolated constituent, huperzineA, is currently used as an acetylcholinesterase (AChE) inhibitor in senile dementia and Alzheimer's disease.

Pharmacology In the 1980s, scientists demonstrated that purified huperzineA kept AChE from breaking down into acetylcholine.

Theoretical Cautions and Contraindications Based on pharmacological activity, use with caution in individuals taking other acetylcholinesterase inhibitors

General Warnings Use all herbal supplements with extreme caution in children <2 years of age and in pregnancy or lactation. Some herbs are contraindicated in pregnancy or lactation; make sure to observe warnings. Use with caution in individuals on medication and with pre-existing medical conditions. Always review for potential herb-drug interactions (HDIs) and other warnings. Large and prolonged doses may increase the potential for adverse effects. Herbs may cause transient adverse effects such as nausea, vomiting, and GI distress due to a variety of chemical constituents. Caution should be used in individuals having known allergies to plants.

Theoretical Interactions Acetylcholinesterase inhibitors (tacrine, donepezil)

References

Wang H and Tang XC, "Anticholinesterase Effects of HuperzineA, E2020, and Tacrine in Rats," *Chung Kuo Yao Li Hsueh Pao*, 1998, 19(1):27-30.

♦ **Hydrastis canadensis** see Golden Seal (Hydrastis canadensis) on page 448

Hydroxymethyl Butyrate (HMB)

Related Information
  Nutraceutical Chart on page 573

Natural Product Category Nutraceutical

Dosage Oral: Dosage range: 500-1000 mg 3 times/day

Active Forms Hydroxymethyl butyrate

Reported Uses Increases muscle mass during intense exercise (Nissen, 1996)

Summary HMB (β-hydroxy β-methylbutyrate) is a metabolite of the essential amino acid leucine. It is produced naturally in the human body. Its use results in increased lean muscle mass and strength in athletes who are on intense training programs. Some studies suggest that HMB may accelerate fat loss following strenuous exercise. It is primarily a supplement for bodybuilders and other highly trained athletes.

Pharmacology HMB is an anticatabolic agent that may reduce protein/muscle breakdown by shifting protein turnover in favor of new muscle growth, which results in greater gains in muscle size and strength. HMB increases the body's ability to build muscle and burn fat during intense exercise, and HMB increases endurance.

Toxicities, Warnings, and Interactions No known toxicity or serious side effects

Symptoms of Deficiency Deficiency studies in humans have not been conducted.

References
  Nissen S, Sharp R, Ray M, et al, "Effect of Leucine Metabolite Beta-Hydroxy-Beta-Methylbutyrate on Muscle Metabolism During Resistance-Exercise Training," J Appl Physiol, 1996, 81(5):2095-104.

5-Hydroxytryptophan (5-HTP)

Related Information
  Nutraceutical Chart on page 573

Natural Product Category Nutraceutical

Dosage Oral: 50-100 mg 1-3 times/day

Active Forms 5-hydroxytryptophan

Reported Uses
  Anxiety (Kahn, 1985)
  Depression (comparable to fluvoxamine) (Poldinger, 1991)
  Depression (comparable to tricyclic antidepressents) (van Praag, 1974)
  Fibromyalgia (Caruso, 1990)
  Headache (De Benedittis, 1985)
  Migraine (Titus, 1986)
  Obesity (Cangiano, 1992)
  Sleep disorders, insomnia (stimulates the production of melatonin) (den Boer, 1990)

Summary 5-Hydroxytryptophan is a precursor molecule in the synthesis of neurotransmitters which regulate mood and behavior. It may be useful in depression, anxiety, impulse control (obsessive behavior, aggression), appetite, pain, and sleep disturbances.

Pharmacology As the immediate precursor for serotonin, 5-hydroxytryptophan may influence concentrations of this neurotransmitter, which regulates mood and emotions. As an antidepressant, its effectiveness has been claimed to be comparable to tricyclic antidepressants and fluvoxamine. 5-HTP is also the precursor for melatonin, which determines sleep cycles. It has been reported to decrease dopamine and norepinephrine concentrations in the CNS, which may impact on behavioral processes.

Toxicities, Warnings, and Interactions Avoid use with antidepressant medications (SSRIs, tricyclics, MAO inhibitors). Concurrent use of 5-HTP and these medications should be conducted only under the supervision of a physician. May cause mild-moderate gastrointestinal distress.
(Continued)

5-Hydroxytryptophan (5-HTP) *(Continued)*

Symptoms of Deficiency Humans are capable of synthesizing 5-HTP, therefore no deficiency syndrome has been described. However, diets low in tryptophan may result in reduced production of serotonin and melatonin, which have been related to symptoms of depression and sleep disorders.

Reported Interactions

Drug/Nutrient Interactions: None known; however, 5-HTP may have additive effects with antidepressants (including SSRIs, MAO inhibitors, and tricyclic antidepressants)

Nutrient/Nutrient Interactions: None known; however, 5-HTP may have additive effects with St John's wort, tryptophan, and SAMe

References

Cangiano C, Ceci F, Cascino A, et al, "Eating Behavior and Adherence to Dietary Prescriptions in Obese Adult Subjects Treated With 5-Hydroxytryptophan," *Am J Clin Nutr*, 1992, 56(5):863-7.

Caruso I, Sarzi Puttini P, Cazzola M, et al, "Double-Blind Study of 5-Hydroxytryptophan Versus Placebo in the Treatment of Primary Fibromyalgia Syndrome," *J Int Med Res*, 1990, 18(3):201-9.

De Benedittis G and Massei R, "Serotonin Precursors in Chronic Primary Headache. A Double-Blind Cross-Over Study With L-5-Hydroxytryptophan vs. Placebo," *J Neurosurg Sci*, 1985, 29(3):239-48.

den Boer JA and Westenberg HG, "Behavioral, Neuroendocrine, and Biochemical Effects of 5-Hydroxytryptophan Administration in Panic Disorder," *Psychiatry Res*, 1990, 31(3):267-78.

Kahn RS and Westenberg HG, "L-5-Hydroxytryptophan in the Treatment of Anxiety Disorders," *J Affect Disord*, 1985, 8(2):197-200.

Poldinger W, Calachini B, and Schwarz W, "A Functional-Dimensional Approach to Depression: Serotonin Deficiency as a Target Syndrome in a Comparison of 5-Hydroxytryptophan and Fluvoxamine," *Psychopathology*, 1991, 24(2):53-81.

Titus F, Davalos A, Alom J, et al, "5-Hydroxytryptophan Versus Methysergide in the Prophylaxis of Migraine. Randomized Clinical Trial," *Eur Neurol*, 1986, 25(5):327-9.

van Praag HM, van den Burg W, Bos ER, et al, "5-Hydroxytryptophan in Combination With Clomipramine in Therapy-Resistant Depression," *Psychopharmacologia*, 1974, 38(3):267-9.

- **Hyperglycemia / Diabetes / Insulin Resistance** *see page 222*
- ***Hypericum perforatum*** *see* St John's Wort *(Hypericum perforatum) on page 506*
- **Hypertension (High Blood Pressure)** *see page 226*
- **Hyperthyroidism** *see page 230*
- **Hypoglycemia** *see page 234*
- **Hypothyroidism** *see page 238*
- **Indigestion / Heartburn** *see page 242*

Inositol Hexaphosphate (IP-6)

Related Information

Drug-Induced Nutrient Depletions *on page 625*

Nutraceutical Chart *on page 573*

Natural Product Category Nutraceutical

Dosage Oral: 600-800 mg 3-4 times/day, taken with 200-250 mg inositol

Active Forms Inositol hexaphosphate

Reported Uses Anticancer agent (Shamsuddin, 1995)

Summary IP-6 is a safe, natural compound found in grains and soybeans, and is essential for healthy cell function throughout the body. It consists of inositol with a phosphate group attached to each of the six sites on inositol's hexagonal ring structure.

Pharmacology IP-6 seems to be able to inhibit the growth of cancer cells, and also causes the differentiation of malignant cells, which often results in transforming them back to their normal phenotype. Preliminary evidence suggests that IP-6 exerts its anticancer activity by helping to regulate signal transduction pathways, cell cycle regulatory genes, differentiation genes, oncogenes, and tumor suppressor genes.

Toxicities, Warnings, and Interactions There are no warnings or toxic effects associated with IP-6.

Symptoms of Deficiency Because IP-6 is not an essential nutrient, no deficiency condition has been identified.

Reported Interactions
Drug/Nutrient Interactions: None known
Nutrient/Nutrient Interactions: None known
References
Shamsuddin AM and Yang GY, "Inositol Hexaphosphate Inhibits Growth and Induces Differentiation of PC-3 Human Prostate Cancer Cells," *Carcinogenesis*, 1995, 16(8):1975-9.

- **Insomnia** see page 246
- **Introduction to Conditions** see page 41
- **Introduction to Glandular Extracts** see page 36
- **Introduction to Herbs** see page 11
- **Introduction to Homeopathy** see page 31
- **Introduction to Natural Medicine** see page 9
- **Introduction to Nutrition** see page 19

Iodine

Related Information
Pregnancy & Lactation Nutritional Chart *on page 657*
Vitamins/Minerals/Trace Elements/Amino Acids Chart *on page 604*
Natural Product Category Mineral
Dosage Oral: RDI: 150 mcg/day; ODA: 250 mcg/day
Active Forms Potassium iodide (SSKI/saturated solution of potassium iodide), sodium iodide, iodine caseinate, aqueous (diatomic) iodine, kelp
Reported Uses
Fibrocystic breast disease (Eskin, 1988)
Goiter prevention
Mucolytic agent

Summary Iodine's only known function is the role it plays in the production of thyroid hormones. Since thyroid hormone is a key regulator of energy production and cellular activity in all tissues, the effects of deficiency are widespread, including disturbances in metabolism and the function of key organ systems. Iodine deficiency has also been associated with severe developmental defects. Supplementation helps to avoid symptoms of thyroid deficiency.

Pharmacology Iodine's primary physiologic role is in the production of thyroid hormones, triiodothyronine (T_3) and thyroxine (T_4). The synthesis of thyroid hormone is dependent on the availability of iodine. Thyroid hormone regulates many facets of cellular metabolism and energy production throughout the body. Thyroid hormone controls body temperature, physical growth, reproduction, neuromuscular function, protein synthesis, and the growth of skin and hair. In the absence of thyroid hormone, the basal metabolic rate can decline to 55% of normal, while it may increase to as much as 160% of normal in excess, causing tachycardia, nervousness and excitability.

Toxicities, Warnings, and Interactions
Toxic dose: Iodine toxicity is rare except in cases of existing hyperthyroidism where doses as small as 1 mg can result in cessation of thyroid hormone production and thyrotoxicosis
Toxicity symptoms: Rashes, nausea, headaches; extensive long-term intake can result in thyroid goiter

Symptoms of Deficiency A deficiency of iodine results in the enlargement of the thyroid gland, a condition known as goiter. The introduction of iodized salt has made iodine deficiency and the development of goiters uncommon in the United States and other developed countries.

Reported Interactions
Drug/Nutrient Interactions: Antithyroid drugs, lithium
Nutrient/Nutrient Interactions: None known
References
Eskin B and Ghent W, reported in *Medical World News*, 1988, 25.
Truswell AS, "ABC of Nutrition. Nutrition for Pregnancy," *Br Med J (Clin Res Ed)*, 1985, 291(6490):263-6.

- **IP-6** see Inositol Hexaphosphate (IP-6) *on page 462*

Ipriflavone

Related Information
Nutraceutical Chart *on page 573*

Natural Product Category Herb

Dosage Oral: 200 mg 3 times/day

Active Forms Ipriflavone or 7-isopropoxyisoflavone

Reported Uses Prevention of and use in osteoporosis (men and women) (Agnusdei, 1997)

Summary Ipriflavone is a synthetic isoflavone. Like many other isoflavones, it has a structure similar to estrogen. However, ipriflavone does not produce the usual "estrogenic" effects such as stimulating the growth of tissue in the breast and uterus. It has quickly gained wide acceptance as a safe and effective product for osteoporosis because it prevents bone resorption and stimulates new one growth. Animal studies have also reported that ipriflavone causes a substantial increase in stamina and endurance.

Pharmacology Ipriflavone acts in several ways to strengthen bones. Studies indicate that it inhibits the activity of cells known as osteoclasts. Osteoclasts are responsible for degrading bone. Ipriflavone also seems to activate bone-building cells called osteoblasts. It also stimulates the synthesis and secretion of calcitonin, which is a hormone that regulates calcium and influences bone health

Toxicities, Warnings, and Interactions Ipriflavone is safe and effective. There are no reports of it interfering with other medications and no significant side effects have been reported. However, until further research is completed, women with a history of estrogen-positive breast cancer should consult a physician prior to use.

Symptoms of Deficiency Since ipriflavone does not occur naturally in humans, there is no human deficiency condition.

Reported Interactions
Drug/Nutrient Interactions: None known
Nutrient/Nutrient Interactions: None known

References
Agnusdei D and Bufalino L, "Efficacy of Ipriflavone in Established Osteoporosis and Long-term Safety," *Calcif Tissue Int*, 1997, 61(7):23-7.

Iron

Related Information
Drug-Induced Nutrient Depletions *on page 625*
Pregnancy & Lactation Nutritional Chart *on page 657*
Vitamins/Minerals/Trace Elements/Amino Acids Chart *on page 604*

Natural Product Category Mineral

Dosage Oral: RDI: Males and postmenopausal females: 10 mg/day, premenopausal females 15 mg/day; ODA: Specific for each individual

Active Forms Ferrous sulfate, ferrous gluconate, ferrous fumarate, ferrous glycinate, ferric ammonium citrate, and heme iron

Reported Uses
Anemia (Hallberg, 1998)
Menorrhagia (Arvidsson, 1981)
Pregnancy (Doyle, 1990)
Restless legs syndrome (O'Keefe, 1994)

Summary Iron is a critical mineral in human physiology. Iron exists in various forms in the body, in functional forms (hemoglobin and enzymes) and in transport and storage forms. It functions as a cofactor in energy-generating and synthetic reactions and allows the transport and storage of oxygen. Blood loss (including menstruation) is the most common cause of iron deficiency. Iron may be used to treat or prevent anemia and must be present to ensure normal immune, neuronal and metabolic function.

Pharmacology As a component of hemoglobin and myoglobin, iron is critical for the transport and storage of oxygen in the body. Iron is required for normal growth and development and is required for normal immune function. It is a critical component of mitochondrial enzymes responsible for oxidative phosphorylation and ATP generation, as well as cytochromes (such as the P450 system) which mediate metabolism of many drugs. Iron is required for the synthesis of carnitine, a critical factor in fatty acid metabolism. Iron-containing enzymes synthesize both serotonin and dopamine, and the synthesis of collagen and elastin involve iron as a cofactor. Therefore, CNS function and connective tissue maintenance depend upon this metal.

Toxicities, Warnings, and Interactions Symptoms of toxicity depend on the time following ingestion.

Early: Nausea, vomiting, abdominal pain, bloody diarrhea

Late: Weakness, pallor, tachycardia, cardiovascular collapse, cyanosis, convulsions, coma

Note: Iron toxicity is relatively rare, but may occur acutely as a result of overdose. Iron is the most common cause of pediatric poisonings. Iron-containing products must be packaged in child-resistant safety packaging.

Chronic accumulation may occur as a result of a genetic disorder (hemochromatosis) or by iaterogenic excess, resulting in cardiac, hepatic, splenic, and pancreatic damage. Alcoholism can also lead to increased iron absorption and accumulation.

Symptoms of Deficiency Fatigue, anemia, intolerance to cold, intellectual impairment, reduced resistance to colds and infections, spoon-shaped nails, pica

Reported Interactions

Drug/Nutrient Interactions:

Drugs which can cause depletion of iron: Cholestyramine, colestipol, indomethacin, neomycin, H_2-receptor antagonists, quinolone antibiotics, tetracyclines, aspirin. Iron may interfere with the absorption of fluoroquinolones and tetracycline antibiotics

Erythropoietin may increase synthesis of red blood cells, increasing need for iron.

Nutrient/Nutrient Interactions: Several other divalent minerals are capable of interfering with the absorption of iron including calcium, magnesium, manganese, and zinc. Vitamin C increases the absorption of iron. Iron can bind and inactivate vitamin E.

References

Arvidsson B, Ekenved G, Rybo G, et al, "Iron Prophylaxis in Menorrhagia," *Acta Obstet Gynecol Scand*, 1981, 60(2):157-60.

Doyle W, "The Association Between Maternal Diet and Birth Dimensions, *J Nutr Med*, 1990, 1:9-17.

Hallberg L, "Combating Iron Deficiency: Daily Administration of Iron Is Far Superior to Weekly Administration," *Am J Clin Nutr*, 1998, 68(2):213-7.

O'Keefe ST, Gavin K, and Lavan JN, "Iron Status and Restless Legs Syndrome in the Elderly," *Age Ageing*, 1994, 23(3):200-3.

♦ **Irritable Bowel Syndrome (IBS)** *see page 250*

Isoflavones (Soy)

Related Information

Nutraceutical Chart *on page 573*

Natural Product Category Nutraceutical

Dosage Oral: Dosage range: 500-1000 mg of soy extract daily (13% to 17% genistein) containing a minimum of 100 mg of total isoflavones per 1000 mg

Active Forms Genistein, daidzein, daidzin, glycitin, glycetein

Reported Uses

Cancer prevention (Messina, 1994)

Chemotherapy support (Lei, 1999)

Decreased bone loss (Schreiber, 1999)

Hypercholesterolemia (Crouse, 1999; Devi, 1972)

Menopausal symptoms (Duncan, 1999)

Summary Soy contains a number of isoflavones, which are phytoestrogens. These weak estrogens are chemically similar in structure to naturally produced estrogen hormones. They appear to be capable of lowering serum lipid levels in some individuals, potentially lowering the risk of coronart heart disease, and may have some benefit in osteoporosis. Although the original interest in isoflavones was due to their estrogenic

(Continued)

Isoflavones (Soy) *(Continued)*

activity, isoflavones also have been reported to exhibit a variety of effects that are not related to estrogen activity, including antitumor effects.

The FDA has authorized the use of health claims about the role of soy protein (25 g/day), in conjunction with a diet low in saturated fat and cholesterol, to reduce the risk of coronary heart disease.

Pharmacology Isoflavones contain plant-derived estrogenic compounds. However, the estrogenic potency has been estimated to be only 1/1000 to 1/100,000 that of estradiol. They have been claimed to inhibit bone resorption in postmenopausal women. In addition, isoflavones in soy have been reported to lower serum lipids, including LDL cholesterol and triglycerides, along with increases in HDL cholesterol. The antitumor effect of isoflavones may be due to a regulation of the enzyme activity related to the control of cell replication.

Toxicities, Warnings, and Interactions Women who are taking estrogen-containing medications or estrogen-dependent tumors (including breast cancer) should consult their physician prior to use.

Symptoms of Deficiency Deficiency studies have not been conducted.

Reported Interactions

Drug/Nutrient Interactions: Soy isoflavones have a weak estrogenic effect. Though no drug interactions have been identified with estrogen-containing medications, close monitoring is recommended.

Nutrient/Nutrient Interactions: None known

References

Crouse JR, Morgan T, Terry JG, et al, "A Randomized Trial Comparing the Effect of Casein with that of Soy Protein Containing Varying Amounts of Isoflavones on Plasma Concentrations of Lipids and Lipoproteins," *Arch Intern Med,* 1999; 159(17):2070-6.

Devi KS and Kurup PA, "Hypolipaemic Activity of *Phaseolus Mungo* (Blackgram) in Rats Fed a High-Fat, High-Cholesterol Diet. Isolation of a Protein and Polysaccharide Fraction," *Atherosclerosis,* 1972, 15(2):223-30.

Duncan AM, Underhill KE, Xu X, et al, "Modest Hormonal Effects of Soy Isoflavones in Postmenopausal Women," *J Clin Endocrinol Metab,* 1999, 84(10):3479-84.

Lei W, Mayotte JE, Levitt ML, et al "Enhancement of Chemosensitivity and Programmed Cell Death by Tyrosine Kinase Inhibitors Correlates With EGFR Expression in Non-small Cell Lung Cancer Cells," *Anticancer Res,* 1999, 19:221-8.

Messina M, Messina V, and Setchell K, *The Simple Soybean and Your Health,* Garden City Park, NY: Avery Publishing Group, 1994, 75-6.

Schreiber MD and Rebar RW, "Isoflavones and Postmenopausal Bone Health: A Viable Alternative to Estrogen Therapy?" *Menopause,* 1999, 6(3):233-41.

Kava Kava *(Piper methysticum)*

Related Information

Common Herbal Supplements Contraindicated During Pregnancy *on page 656*

Herb/Drug Potential Interactions *on page 642*

Herb Quick Reference Chart *on page 538*

Natural Product Category Herb

Plant Part Root, rhizome

Dosage and Standardization Oral:

Children: Attention deficit disorder/attention deficit hyperactivity disorder: Liquid extract (1:1 w/v fresh plant or 1:4 w/v dry plant): 5-15 drops diluted in favorite beverage 2-3 times/day

Adult:

Anxiety: 100-250 mg 1-3 times/day as needed, standardized to contain 30% kavalactones per dose

Sedation: 250-500 mg at bedtime, standardized to contain 30% kavalactones per dose

Reported Uses Anxiety, sedation, skeletal muscle relaxation, postischemic episodes (Singh, 1992; Davies, 1992)

Summary Kava kava is a unique plant which is native to the South Pacific. It has gained popularity as an anxiolytic and sleep aid. It appears to act through a unique mechanism, and is claimed to induce relaxation without impairment in memory or motor function. In fact, cognitive function improvement and sharpened awareness have been claimed to accompany relaxation induced by this product. It is available as capsules or in teas. Individuals should be warned against overindulgence in tea consumption, in particular.

Pharmacology Kava kava appears to act on the amygdala complex in the limbic system (which moderates many emotional processes). In contrast to benzodiazepines and barbiturates, it is not believed to exhibit significant binding or influence on gamma-aminobutyric acid (GABA). Kava kava is claimed to protect against CNS ischemia. Tolerance to the effects of kava kava has not been described. The whole plant extract appears to exhibit more activity than the isolated kavalactones.

Theoretical Cautions and Contraindications Use of kava kava is contraindicated in pregnancy and lactation (based on case reports, Meyer). Due to the potential for dopamine antagonism (Schelosky, 1995), use is also contraindicated in Parkinson's disease. Use with caution in individuals receiving antianxiety agents (ie, alprazolam), antidepressants, antipsychotics, or other agents which cause CNS depression such as sedative/hypnotics (based on pharmacological activity and case reports - Almeida, 1996). May potentiate the effects of concurrent ethanol (Jamieson, 1990). Some conflicting evidence concerning effects with ethanol have been published (Herberg, 1993). May cause drowsiness or sedation in higher doses; use caution when performing tasks which require alertness (driving or operating heavy machinery). Long-term use of high doses may cause rash.

General Warnings Use all herbal supplements with extreme caution in children <2 years of age and in pregnancy or lactation. Some herbs are contraindicated in pregnancy or lactation; make sure to observe warnings. Use with caution in individuals on medication and with pre-existing medical conditions. Always review for potential herb-drug interactions (HDIs) and other warnings. Large and prolonged doses may increase the potential for adverse effects. Herbs may cause transient adverse effects such as nausea, vomiting, and GI distress due to a variety of chemical constituents. Caution should be used in individuals having known allergies to plants.

Theoretical Interactions Ethanol, CNS depressants (including alprazolam and other benzodiazepines, antidepressants, and sedative-hypnotics), antipsychotics, levodopa

References
Almeida JC and Grimsley EW, "Coma From the Health Food Store: Interaction Between Kava and Alprazolam," *Ann Intern Med*, 1996, 125(11):940-1.

Davies LP, Drew CA, Duffield P, et al, "Kava Pyrones and Resin: Studies on GABAA, GABAB and Benzodiazepine Binding Sites in Rodent Brain," *Pharmacol Toxicol*, 1992, 71(2):120-6.

Herberg KW, "Effect of Kava-Special Extract WS 1490 Combined With Ethyl Alcohol on Safety-Relevant Performance Parameters," *Blutalkohol*, 1993, 30(2):96-105.

Jamieson DD and Duffield PH, "Positive Interaction of Ethanol and Kava Resin in Mice," *Clin Exp Pharmacol Physiol*, 1990, 17(7):509-14.

Meyer JJ, "Pharmacology of Kava," Ethnopharmacologic Search for Psychoactive Drugs, U.S. Dept Health, Education, and Welfare, Pub No 1645, Washington, DC: Government Printing Office, 133-40.

Schelosky L, Raffauf C, Jendroska K, et al, "Kava and Dopamine Antagonism," *J Neurol Neurosurg Psychiatry*, 1995, 58(5):639-40.

Singh YN, "Kava: An Overview," *J Ethnopharmacol*, 1992, 37(1):13-45.

Lactobacillus acidophilus

Related Information
Drug-Induced Nutrient Depletions *on page 625*
Nutraceutical Chart *on page 573*

Natural Product Category Nutraceutical

Dosage Oral: Dosage range: 5-10 billion colony forming units (CFU) per day (dairy free); refrigerate to maintain optimum potency

Active Forms *Lactobacillus acidophilus*

Reported Uses
Constipation (Alm, 1984)
Enhance immunity (Schiffrin, 1997)
Hypercholesterolemia (Anderson, 1999)
Infant diarrhea (Michielutti, 1996)
(Continued)

Lactobacillus acidophilus (Continued)

Lactose intolerance (Kim, 1983)

Recolonize the GI tract with beneficial bacteria during and after antibiotic use (Katagiri, 1986)

Vaginal candidiasis (Elmer, 1996)

Summary Lactobacillus acidophilus is a natural colonizing species in the lower gastrointestinal tract of humans. They exist in a symbiotic relationship with the human host, providing resistance to overgrowth of pathogenic bacteria, enhancing digestion and nutrient absorption, blocking cholesterol absorption, and strengthening immune function. Maintaining the intestinal microflora with beneficial bacteria such as L. acidophilus has been claimed to be critical to an individual's overall health. It is believed to be particularly important to restore this flora after exposure to broad-spectrum antibiotics. The most common cause of a deficiency of L. acidophilus bacteria is the use of antibiotic drugs. Other factors that can cause a reduction of L. acidophilus include the use of drugs that increase intestinal pH, stress, diarrhea, intestinal infections, and the presence of toxins in the intestine.

Pharmacology L. acidophilus produces a variety of proteases, lipases, and lactase, which may aid in the digestion of proteins, fats, and milk products. These organisms produce natural antibiotics (acidophilin, lactocidin, lactobicillin, lactobreven), and acidify the colonic environment which may inhibit the growth of pathogenic and toxin-producing organisms. In addition, they produce hydrogen peroxide, which has a wide range of activity against yeasts, molds, and bacteria. The slightly acidic pH caused by these organisms may also enhance the gastrointestinal absorption of minerals such as calcium and iron. L. acidophilus may support immune responses by helping to activate macrophages. In addition, these organisms convert cholesterol to coprostanol, inhibiting its absorption from the gastrointestinal tract.

Toxicities, Warnings, and Interactions No known toxicity or serious side effects. Refrigerate to maintain optimum potency.

Symptoms of Deficiency Gas, bloating, diarrhea or constipation, halitosis, and chronic vaginal yeast infections

Reported Interactions

Drug/Nutrient Interactions: Antibiotics eliminate L. acidophilus from the gastrointestinal flora

Nutrient/Nutrient Interactions: None known

References

Alm L, "Acidophilus Milk for Therapy in Gastrointestinal Disorders," *Nahrung*, 1984, 28(6-7):683-4.

Anderson JW and Gilliland SE, "Effect of Fermented Milk (Yogurt) Containing *Lactobacillus acidophilus* L1 on Serum Cholesterol in Hypercholesterolemic Humans," *J Am Coll Nutr*, 1999, 18(1):43-50.

Elmer GW, Surawicz CM, and McFarland LV, "Biotherapeutic Agents. A Neglected Modality for the Treatment and Prevention of Selected Intestinal and Vaginal Infections," *JAMA*, 1996, 275(11):870-6.

Katagiri S, "Study on the Anti-diarrhea Effect-Combined Use of Augmentin and Lactic Acid Bacteria Product of Multiple Resistance," *Basics and Clinics*, 1986, 20(17):651-3.

Kim HS and Gilliland SE, "*Lactobacillus acidophilus* as a Dietary Adjunct for Milk to Aid Lactose Digestion in Humans," *J Dairy Sci*, 1983, 66(5):959-66.

Michielutti F, Bertini M, Presciuttini B, et al, "Clinical Assessment of a New Oral Bacterial Treatment for Children With Acute Diarrhea," *Minerva Med*, 1996, 87(11):545-50.

Schiffrin EJ, Brassart D, Servin AL, et al, "Immune Modulation of Blood Leukocytes in Humans by Lactic Acid Bacteria: Criteria for Strain Selection," *Am J Clin Nutr*, 1997, 66(2):515S-20S.

♦ **L-Arginine** *see* Arginine *on page 385*

Lavender (Lavendula officinalis)

Related Information

Herb Quick Reference Chart *on page 538*

Natural Product Category Herb

Plant Part Oil

Dosage and Standardization Topical: Apply to affected area, either diluted or undiluted, 2-4 times/day

Reported Uses Wound-healing agent (topical), minor burns (topical) (Schultz, 1996)

Summary Lavender oil has been used for centuries as a fragrance and medicinal agent. It is used topically as a wound-healing agent and on minor burns.

Pharmacology Lavender oil is nonirritating and nonsensitizing to human skin. Lavender oil aids in normal wound-healing processes, is antibacterial, and may decrease scarring in burns and other wounds.

Theoretical Cautions and Contraindications For topical or inhalation use only

General Warnings Caution should be used in individuals having known allergies to plants.

Theoretical Interactions None known

References

Schulz V, Hansel R, and Tyler VE, *Rational Phytotherapy: A Physicians' Guide to Herbal Medicine,* New York, NY: Springer-Verlag, 1996, 84-5.

♦ *Lavendula officinalis* see Lavender *(Lavendula officinalis)* on page 468

♦ **L-Carnitine** see Carnitine on page 403

Lemon Balm/Melissa *(Melissa officinalis)*

Related Information
Common Herbal Supplements Contraindicated During Pregnancy on page 656

Herb Quick Reference Chart on page 538

Natural Product Category Herb

Plant Part Whole plant

Dosage and Standardization
Topical: Apply a 70:1 w/v concentrated product to the affected area, 2-4 times/day at the first signs of a cold sore or fever blister (burning, itching, tingling)

Internal dosage: For teething, use 2-5 drops of a (1:1 w/v) fresh plant or a dried (1:4 w/v) plant extract diluted in liquid 3 times/day as needed

Reported Uses
Antiviral agent (oral herpes virus) (Dimitrova, 1993)

Sedative agent (in pediatrics) (Leung, 1996)

Summary Among its many uses in herbal medicine, an extract of lemon balm has been reported to be effective as a topical agent for oral herpes simplex. The cream is a highly concentrated (70:1 w/v) dry extract.

Pharmacology A significant improvement in symptoms of oral herpes simplex has been reported when using melissa topically. Use in herpes infection of the skin and transitional mucosa is effective, possibly due to the polyphenols in melissa. The extract also showed no induction of viral resistance.

Theoretical Cautions and Contraindications None known

General Warnings Use all herbal supplements with extreme caution in children <2 years of age and in pregnancy or lactation. Some herbs are contraindicated in pregnancy or lactation; make sure to observe warnings. Use with caution in individuals on medication and with pre-existing medical conditions. Always review for potential herb-drug interactions (HDIs) and other warnings. Large and prolonged doses may increase the potential for adverse effects. Herbs may cause transient adverse effects such as nausea, vomiting, and GI distress due to a variety of chemical constituents. Caution should be used in individuals having known allergies to plants.

Theoretical Interactions None known

References

Dimitrova Z, Dimov B, Manolova N, et al, "Antiherpes Effect of *Melissa officinalis* L. Extracts," *Acta Microbiol Bulg,* 1993, 29:65-72.

Leung AY and Foster S, *Encyclopedia of Common Natural Ingredients Used in Foods, Drugs, and Cosmetics,* New York, NY: Wiley, 1996, 57-58.

♦ **L-Glutamine** see Glutamine on page 446

Licorice *(Glycyrrhiza glabra)*

Related Information
Common Herbal Supplements Contraindicated During Pregnancy *on page 656*

Herb/Drug Potential Interactions *on page 642*

Herb Quick Reference Chart *on page 538*

Organ System Support Using Natural Products *on page 660*

Natural Product Category Herb

Plant Part Root

Dosage and Standardization Oral:
Licorice: 250-500 mg 3 times/day, standardized to contain 20% glycyrrhizinic acid **or** 15-30 drops of liquid extract (1:4 w/v) dried root 3 times/day in juice or other beverage

Deglycyrrhizinated (DGL) licorice: 250 mg 3 times/day chewed either 1 hour before or 2 hours after meals and at bedtime, standardized to contain no more than 2% glycyrrhizin per dose

Reported Uses
Adrenal insufficiency (licorice) (Davis, 1991)

Expectorant and antitussive (licorice) (Bradley, 1992)

GI ulceration (DGL chewable products) (Dehpour, 1994; Balakrishnan, 1978)

Summary Although licorice is most recognized as a flavoring agent, it has a long history of use as a medicinal herb. It has been used to relieve symptoms in individuals with adrenal insufficiency and as a treatment for upper respiratory symptoms (antitussive and expectorant). DGL licorice chewable tablets may be beneficial in a variety of gastrointestinal disorders, particularly in peptic ulcer disease and inflammatory disorders.

Pharmacology Licorice reportedly inhibits adrenal and thymic atrophy. It has demulcent activity, which serves to protect irritated mucosal surface membranes (upper respiratory tract and gastrointestinal), and reportedly stimulates the production of mucus, which may cause symptomatic improvements. Licorice reportedly inhibits prostaglandin and leukotriene synthesis. Licorice is also reported to have weak phytoestrogenic activity and stimulates the adrenocortical axis.

Theoretical Cautions and Contraindications May alter platelet aggregation (Tawata, 1990). Contraindicated in individuals with active bleeding (eg, peptic ulcer, intracranial bleeding). Use with caution in individuals with a history of bleeding, hemostatic disorders, or drug-related hemostatic problems. Use with caution in individuals taking anticoagulant medications, including warfarin, aspirin, aspirin-containing products, NSAIDs, or antiplatelet agents (eg, ticlopidine, clopidogrel, dipyridamole). Discontinue use prior to dental or surgical procedures (generally at least 14 days before).

Licorice: Contraindicated in pregnancy and lactation. Based on pharmacological activity, use is contraindicated in individuals with hepatic or renal impairment. Avoid use in hypertension, arrhythmias, congestive heart failure, or edematous states; may cause sodium and water retention (based on human studies and case reports, de Klerk, 1997; Stormer, 1993). Do not use in individuals receiving antihypertensives, diuretics, digoxin, or potassium supplements (due to mineralocorticoid effects, licorice may deplete potassium). Avoid use in hypokalemic states. High doses may cause pseudoaldosteronism.

Phytoestrogen-containing herbs have not been associated with the negative health effects seen with synthetic estrogen. However, use with caution in individuals on hormone replacement therapy or oral contraceptives or with a history of estrogen-dependent tumors, endometrial cancer, thromboembolic disease, or stroke.

DGL Licorice: Use DGL licorice with caution in individuals receiving nitrofurantoin (increases excretion).

General Warnings Use all herbal supplements with extreme caution in children <2 years of age and in pregnancy or lactation. Some herbs are contraindicated in pregnancy or lactation; make sure to observe warnings.

Use with caution in individuals on medication and with pre-existing medical conditions. Always review for potential herb-drug interactions (HDIs) and other warnings. Large and prolonged doses may increase the potential for adverse effects. Herbs may cause transient adverse effects such as nausea, vomiting, and GI distress due to a variety of chemical constituents. Caution should be used in individuals having known allergies to plants.

Theoretical Interactions

Licorice: Laxatives (potential for electrolyte disturbances), corticosteroids, cardiac glycosides (risk of hypokalemia), anticoagulants, antiplatelet agents, NSAIDs, aspirin, aspirin-containing products, antihypertensives, diuretics, hormonal therapy, oral contraceptives, potassium-depleting medications

DGL Licorice: Nitrofurantoin (may alter kinetics)

References

Balakrishnan V, Pillai MV, Raveendran PM, et al, "Deglycyrrhizinated Liquorice in the Treatment of Chronic Duodenal Ulcer," *J Assoc Physicians India*, 1978, 26(9):811-4.

Bradley PR, ed, *British Herbal Compendium*, Vol 1, Bournemouth, England: British Herbal Medicine Association, 1992, 145-8.

Davis EA and Morris DJ, "Medicinal Uses of Licorice Through the Millennia: The Good and Plenty of It," *Mol Cell Endocrinol*, 1991, 78(1-2):1-6.

Dehpour AR, Zolfaghari ME, Samadian T, et al, "The Protective Effect of Liquorice Components and Their Derivatives Against Gastric Ulcer Induced by Aspirin in Rats," *J Pharm Pharmacol*, 1994, 46(2):148-9.

de Klerk GJ, Nieuwenhuis MG, and Beutler JJ, "Hypokalaemia and Hypertension Associated With Use of Liquorice Flavoured Chewing Gum," *BMJ*, 1997, 314(7082):731-2.

Newall CA, Anderson La, and Phillipson JD, *Herbal Medicines: A Guide for Health Care Professionals*, London, England: The Pharmaceutical Press, 1996, 183-6.

Stormer FC, Reistad R, and Alexander J, "Glycyrrhizic Acid in Liquorice-Evaluation of Health Hazard," *Food Chem Toxicol*, 1993, 31(4): 303-12.

Tawata M, Yoda Y, Aida K, et al, "Anti-platelet Action of GU-7, a 3-Arylcoumarin Derivative, Purified from *Glycyrrhizae radix*." *Planta Med*, 1990, 56(3):259-63.

♦ **Lipoic Acid** *see* Alpha-Lipoic Acid *on page 381*

Liver Extract

Related Information

Nutraceutical Chart *on page 573*

Organ System Support Using Natural Products *on page 660*

Natural Product Category Nutraceutical, Glandular

Dosage Oral: RDA: None established; dosage range: 500 mg 1-3 times/day

Active Forms Liver extract

Reported Uses Liver tonic

Summary Liver extracts contain small amounts of the nutrients, enzymes, and other components of liver tissue. The best source for liver glandular products is from New Zealand, where the extracts are free of pesticides, antibiotics, or growth-stimulating hormones. Numerous studies report the efficacy of liver extracts in fat utilization, promotion of tissue regeneration, prevention of liver damage, and performance enhancement.

Pharmacology Liver extract products are used to support liver function. They are a rich source of the antioxidant superoxide dismutase (SOD), and they help build red blood cells.

Toxicities, Warnings, and Interactions Do not use in iron storage disorders (hemochromatosis). No known toxiicty or serious side effects reported.

Symptoms of Deficiency Deficiency studies in humans have not been conducted.

References

Haas EM, *Staying Healthy With Nutrition: The Complete Guide to Diet and Nutritional Medicine*, Berkeley, CA: Celestial Arts, 1992, 286.

♦ **L-Lysine** *see* Lysine *on page 473*

♦ **L-Methionine** *see* Methionine *on page 478*

♦ **L-Phenylalanine** *see* Phenylalanine *on page 487*

♦ **L-Taurine** *see* Taurine *on page 508*

♦ **L-Tyrosine** *see* Tyrosine *on page 514*

Lutein

Related Information
Nutraceutical Chart *on page 573*
Organ System Support Using Natural Products *on page 660*

Natural Product Category Nutraceutical

Dosage Oral: Dosage range: 2-6 mg/day

Reported Uses
Cataracts (Lyle, 1999)
Macular degeneration (Hammond, 1997)

Summary Lutein is an antioxidant pigment which concentrates in the eyes. It appears to serve a filtering and protective role in the visual apparatus and its vascular supply. Lutein may be associated with protection from age-related macular degeneration.

Pharmacology Lutein is a carotenoid which is present in high concentrations in the eye. Within the eye, this pigment filters out blue light and has been claimed to prevent macular degeneration. In addition, it functions as an antioxidant, protecting the visual structures from oxygen free radicals and singlet oxygen. Bioflavonoids such as lutein are known to strengthen capillaries. Since lutein concentrates in the macula, it may protect the vessels responsible for nutrient supply to this region.

Toxicities, Warnings, and Interactions No known toxicity or serious side effects

Symptoms of Deficiency Cataract development, macular degeneration, capillary fragility, and easy bruising

Reported Interactions
Drug/Nutrient Interactions: None known
Nutrient/Nutrient Interactions: Lutein inhibits the availability of beta-carotene

References
Hammond BR Jr, Johnson EJ, Russell RM, et al, "Dietary Modification of Human Macular Pigment Density," *Invest Ophthalmol Vis Sci*, 1997, 38(9):1795-801.
Lyle BJ, Mares-Perlman JA, Klein BE, et al, "Antioxidant Intake and Risk of Incident Age-Related Nuclear Cataracts in the Beaver Dam Eye Study," *Am J Epidemiol*, 1999, 149(9):801-9.

Lycopene

Related Information
Nutraceutical Chart *on page 573*

Natural Product Category Nutraceutical

Dosage Oral: Dosage range: 5 mg 1-3 times/day

Active Forms Lycopene

Reported Uses
Atherosclerosis (Agarwal, 1998)
Cancer prevention, especially prostate (Giovannucci, 1999)
Macular degeneration (Mares-Perlman, 1995)

Summary Lycopene is a carotenoid, one of a family of compounds which function as natural pigments (lending color to carrots and tomatoes) and antioxidants. Supplementation has been reported to protect against macular degeneration, atherosclerosis, and several types of cancer, especially prostate cancer.

Pharmacology Lycopene is a carotenoid pigment and functions as a free radical scavenger. This antioxidant property may prevent oxidative damage to subcellular components, protecting from degenerative changes and carcinogenesis.

Toxicities, Warnings, and Interactions No known toxicity or serious side effects

Symptoms of Deficiency Deficiency symptoms have not been defined (not an essential nutrient). Low levels have been correlated to an increased risk of atherosclerosis and some forms of cancer (prostate).

Reported Interactions
Drug/Nutrient Interactions: None known
Nutrient/Nutrient Interactions: Beta-carotene may increase absorption

References
Agarwal S and Rao AV, "Tomato Lycopene and Low Density Lipoprotein Oxidation: A Human Dietary Intervention Study," *Lipids*, 1998, 33(10):981-4.

Giovannucci E, "Tomatoes, Tomato-Based Products, Lycopene, and Cancer: Review of the Epidemiologic Literature," *J Natl Cancer Inst*, 1999, 91(4):317-31.

Mares-Perlman JA, Brady WE, Klein R, et al, "Serum Antioxidants and Age-Related Macular Degeneration in a Population-Based Case-Control Study," *Arch Ophthalmol*, 1995, 113(12):1518-23.

Lysine

Related Information
Vitamins/Minerals/Trace Elements/Amino Acids Chart *on page 604*

Natural Product Category Amino Acid

Dosage Oral: RDI: None established; dosage range: 500-1000 mg/day

Active Forms L-lysine

Reported Uses
Angina pectoris (Pauling, 1991)

Herpes simplex (Griffith, 1987)

Osteoporosis (Civitelli, 1992)

Summary Lysine is an essential amino acid necessary for the synthesis of protein as well as the metabolism of carbohydrates and fatty acids. It may improve energy production and calcium utilization. In addition, it appears to slow replication and improve healing of lesions caused by herpes simplex. Evidence suggests that supplementation may improve the symptoms of angina in some individuals.

Pharmacology Lysine is an essential amino acid required for normal growth and development. It may be used to synthesize proteins, connective tissue, and neurotransmitters. Lysine may augment calcium absorption and enhances calcium deposition into the bone matrix. Lysine is required to produce acetyl CoA, a critical component in the metabolism of carbohydrates to yield energy. Lysine is also required, along with methionine, to form the dipeptide carnitine, which assists in the mitochondrial metabolism of long-chain fatty acids. Lysine competes for transport with the amino acid arginine, and may limit the availability of this amino acid in Herpesvirus-infected cells, slowing replication. Lysine has been claimed to bind with and remove lipoprotein(a) from atherosclerotic plaques, resulting in a widening of the vessel lumen and increasing blood flow.

Toxicities, Warnings, and Interactions Rare association with interstitial nephritis (Lo, 1996)

Symptoms of Deficiency Human deficiency has not been defined.

Reported Interactions
Drug/Nutrient Interactions: None known

Nutrient/Nutrient Interactions: Arginine and lysine share a common cellular transport pathway. Therefore, excess arginine may compete for transport and lower lysine levels, potentially resulting in deficiency. May increase calcium absorption and decrease renal loss.

References
Civitelli R, Villareal DT, Agnusdei D, et al, "Dietary L-Lysine and Calcium Metabolism in Humans," *Nutrition*, 1992, 8(6):400-5.

Griffith RS, Walsh DE, Myrmel KH, et al, "Success of L-Lysine Therapy in Frequently Recurrent Herpes Simplex Infection. Treatment and Prophylaxis," *Dermatologica*, 1987, 175(4):183-90.

Lo JC, Chertow GM, Rennke H, et al, "Fanconi's Syndrome and Tubulointerstitial Nephritis in Association with L-Lysine," *Am J Kidney Dis*, 1996, 28(4):614-7.

Pauling L, "Case Report: Lysine/Ascorbate-Related Amelioration of Angina Pectoris," *J Orthomolecular Med*, 1991, 6:144-6.

♦ **Macular Degeneration** *see page 254*

Magnesium

Related Information
Drug-Induced Nutrient Depletions *on page 625*
Organ System Support Using Natural Products *on page 660*
Pregnancy & Lactation Nutritional Chart *on page 657*
Vitamins/Minerals/Trace Elements/Amino Acids Chart *on page 604*

(Continued)

Magnesium *(Continued)*

Natural Product Category Mineral

Dosage Oral: RDI: 400 mg/day; ODA: 400-600 mg/day

Active Forms Magnesium oxide, hydroxide, gluconate, glycinate, sulfate, chloride, aspartate, malate, succinate, fumarate, ascorbate, and citrate

Reported Uses

Asthma (Skotnicki, 1997)
Attention deficit hyperactivity disorder (Starobrat-Hermelin, 1997)
Cardiovascular disease (Gaby, 1986)
Congestive heart failure (CHF) (Gottlieb, 1990)
Diabetes (Elamin, 1990)
Epilepsy (Gupta, 1994)
Fatigue (Cox, 1991)
High blood pressure (Moore, 1989)
Kidney stones (Johansson, 1982)
Migraine headaches (Weaver, 1990)
Mitral valve prolapse (MVP) (Galland, 1986)
Muscle cramps (Riss, 1983)
Nervousness (Langley, 1991)
Osteoporosis (Angus, 1988)
Premenstrual syndrome (PMS) (Facchinetti, 1991)

Summary Magnesium is a critical mineral in multiple aspects of human physiology. It is a cofactor in energy-producing reactions, including mitochondrial oxidative phosphorylation. Magnesium regulates muscle and nerve function, and is an important component of bone and tooth structure. Supplementation may augment the management of a variety of diseases, including cardiovascular disorders (hypertension, CHF, dysrhythmia), diabetes, migraines, asthma, and muscle cramps. In addition, it may be necessary to replace depletions caused by medications.

Pharmacology Magnesium is a cofactor in over 300 enzymatic reactions in human physiology. It participates in neuromuscular activity, including excitation-contraction coupling, temperature regulation, detoxification reactions, synthetic activity (including DNA and RNA synthesis), and energy production through carbohydrate metabolism. It is also necessary for the formation of healthy bones and teeth. It may inhibit platelet aggregation and influences calcium metabolism.

Toxicities, Warnings, and Interactions

Toxic dose: Single doses ≥1000 mg may cause diarrhea; use caution in renal impairment (magnesium supplements, antacids, or laxatives)

Toxicity symptoms: Diarrhea, drowsiness, weakness, lethargy

Symptoms of Deficiency Muscle cramps and weakness, insomnia, anorexia, gastrointestinal disorders, kidney stones, osteoporosis, arrhythmias, personality changes, nervousness, restlessness, irritability, fear, anxiety, confusion, depression

Reported Interactions

Drug/Nutrient Interactions: Drugs which can cause depletion of magnesium: Oral contraceptives, estrogens, loop diuretics, thiazide diuretics, digoxin, tetracycline antibiotics, aminoglycosides, pentamidine, amphotericin B, foscarnet and cyclosporine. Magnesium supplements may decrease absorption of fluoroquinolone or tetracycline antibiotics.

Nutrient/Nutrient Interactions: A high intake of calcium or phosphate may inhibit the absorption of magnesium.

References

Angus RM, Sambrook PN, Pocock NA, et al, "Dietary Intake and Bone Mineral Density," *Bone Miner,* 1988, 4(3):265-77.

Cox IM, Campbell MJ, and Dowson D, "Red Blood Cell Magnesium and Chronic Fatigue Syndrome," *Lancet,* 1991, 337(8744):757-60.

Elamin A and Tuvemo T, "Magnesium and Insulin-Dependent Diabetes Mellitus," *Diabetes Res Clin Pract,* 1990, 10(3):203-9.

Facchinetti F, Borella P, Sances G, et al, "Oral Magnesium Successfully Relieves Premenstrual Mood Changes," *Obstet Gynecol,* 1991, 78(2):177-81.

Gaby AR, "Magnesium: An Inexpensive, Safe, and Effective Treatment for Cardiovascular Disease," *J Advancement Med,* 1986, 1:179-81.

Galland LD, Baker SM, and McLellan RK, "Magnesium Deficiency in the Pathogenesis of Mitral Valve Prolapse," *Magnesium*, 1986, 5(3-4):165-74.

Gottlieb SS, Baruch L, Kukin MK, et al, "Prognostic Importance of the Serum Magnesium Concentration in Patients With Congestive Heart Failure," *J Am Coll Cardiol*, 1990, 16(4):827-31.

Gupta SK, Manhas AS, Gupta VK, et al, "Serum Magnesium Levels in Idiopathic Epilepsy," *J Assoc Physicians India*, 1994, 42(6):456-7.

Johansson G, Backman U, Danielson BG, et al, "Effects of Magnesium Hydroxide in Renal Stone Disease," *J Am Coll Nutr*, 1982, 1(2):179-85.

Langley WF and Mann D, "Central Nervous System Magnesium Deficiency," *Arch Intern Med*, 1991, 151(3):593-6.

Moore TJ, "The Role of Dietary Electrolytes in Hypertension," *J Am Coll Nutr*, 1989, 8(Suppl):68S-80S.

Riss P, Bartl W, and Jelincic D, "Clinical Aspects and Treatment of Calf Muscle Cramps During Pregnancy," *Geburtshilfe Frauenheilkd*, 1983, 43(5):329-31.

Skotnicki AB, Jablonski MJ, Musial J, et al, "The Role of Magnesium in the Pathogenesis and Therapy of Bronchial Asthma," *Przegl Lek*, 1997, 54(9):630-3.

Starobrat-Hermelin B and Kozielec T, "The Effects of Magnesium Physiological Supplementation on Hyperactivity in Children With Attention Deficit Hyperactivity Disorder (ADHD). Positive Response to Magnesium Oral Loading Test," *Magnes Res* 1997, 10(2):149-56.

Weaver K, "Magnesium and Migraine," *Headache*, 1990, 30(3):168.

Malic Acid

Related Information
Nutraceutical Chart *on page 573*

Natural Product Category Nutraceutical

Dosage Oral: Dosage range: 500 mg 3-4 times/day with food

Active Forms Malic acid, magnesium malate

Reported Uses
Aluminum toxicity (Domingo, 1988)
Fibromyalgia (Abraham, 1992)

Summary Malic acid is a naturally occurring organic acid found in some fruits such as apples. It plays a role in the Krebs cycle, which is the complex process of deriving ATP, the body's primary unit of energy, from food.

Pharmacology Malic acid promotes the production of cellular energy via the Krebs cycle. Malic acid also facilitates delivery of lactic acid into the Krebs cycle, which helps clear lactic acid and prevent its build-up. Some research has reported that malic acid in combination with magnesium is beneficial for individuals with fibromyalgia.

Toxicities, Warnings, and Interactions No known toxicity or serious side effects; occasionally produces gastrointestinal (GI) disturbance

Symptoms of Deficiency Deficiency studies in humans have not been conducted.

References

Abraham GE, et al, "Management of Fibromyalgia: Rationale for the Use of Magnesium and Malic Acid," *J Nutri Med*, 1992, 3:49-50.

Domingo JL, Gomez M, Llobet JM, et al, "Citric, Malic, and Succinic Acids as Possible Alternatives to Deferoxamine in Aluminum Toxicity," *J Toxicol Clin Toxicol*, 1988, 26 (1-2):67-79.

Manganese

Related Information
Vitamins/Minerals/Trace Elements/Amino Acids Chart *on page 604*

Natural Product Category Mineral

Dosage Oral: RDA: None established; ODA: None established

Active Forms Manganese aspartate, arginate, citrate, chloride, gluconate, glycinate, picolinate, and sulfate

Reported Uses
Diabetes (Baly, 1990)
Epilepsy (Papavasillous, 1979)
Osteoporosis (Saltman, 1993)

Summary Manganese is a mineral cofactor which participates in a variety of enzymatic reactions in human physiology. Supplementation has been claimed to be useful in a number of disorders, including epilepsy and diabetes. In addition, it has been claimed to be of benefit in the prevention of osteoporosis.
(Continued)

Manganese *(Continued)*

Pharmacology Manganese serves as a cofactor for enzymes which participate in the formation of connective tissue, bone, clotting factors, and other proteins. In addition, manganese-containing enzymes participate in glucose transport systems and the metabolism of lipids. Manganese is known to participate as a cofactor in antioxidant enzymes, including superoxide dismutase (SOD). Manganese is required for protein catabolism and synthesis of mucopolysaccharides.

Toxicities, Warnings, and Interactions

Toxic dose: Toxicity is rare, however toxic industrial exposures (mining) have been reported; liver damage may predispose an individual to toxicity

Toxicity symptoms: Excessive doses can cause nausea. Long-term toxicity can produce dementia, psychiatric disorders resembling schizophrenia, and neurologic disorders resembling Parkinson's disease.

Symptoms of Deficiency Deficiency is seldom seen in humans. Magnesium may substitute in some manganese-containing enzymes. Low manganese levels have been associated with poor glucose regulation, frequency of epileptic seizures, and osteoporosis.

Reported Interactions

Drug/Nutrient Interactions: None known

Nutrient/Nutrient Interactions: Calcium, cobalt and iron compete with manganese for absorption. Therefore, elevated intakes of either of these minerals could inhibit the absorption of manganese.

References

Baly DL, Schneiderman JS, and Garcia-Welsh AL, "Effect of Manganese Deficiency on Insulin Binding, Glucose Transport and Metabolism in Rat Adipocytes," *J Nutr*, 1990, 120(9):1075-9.

Papavasiliou PS, Kutt H, Miller ST, et al, "Seizure Disorders and Trace Metals: Manganese Tissue Levels in Treated Epileptics," *Neurology*, 1979, 29(11):1466-73.

Saltman PD and Strause LG, "The Role of Trace Minerals in Osteoporosis," *J Am Coll Nutr*, 1993, 12(4):384-9.

Marshmallow *(Althaea officinalis)*

Related Information

Herb/Drug Potential Interactions *on page 642*

Herb Quick Reference Chart *on page 538*

Natural Product Category Herb

Plant Part Root

Dosage and Standardization Oral: 500 mg 3 times/day, or as needed

Reported Uses Mucilaginous, demulcent; peptic ulceration (Bradley, 1992)

Summary Marshmallow has been used as a food for centuries. The root of marshmallow is very mucilaginous and is used as a demulcent in peptic ulceration.

Pharmacology The active constituents in marshmallow are large carbohydrate molecules that make up mucilage. This smooth, slippery substance can soothe and protect irritated mucous membranes. Marshmallow has primarily been used for the digestive tract and in cough preparations.

Theoretical Cautions and Contraindications Based on pharmacological activity, use with caution in individuals taking hypoglycemic medications (may further lower blood sugar levels, Tomoda, 1987). May interfere with the absorption of other oral medications.

General Warnings Use all herbal supplements with extreme caution in children <2 years of age and in pregnancy or lactation. Some herbs are contraindicated in pregnancy or lactation; make sure to observe warnings. Use with caution in individuals on medication and with pre-existing medical conditions. Always review for potential herb-drug interactions (HDIs) and other warnings. Large and prolonged doses may increase the potential for adverse effects. Herbs may cause transient adverse effects such as nausea, vomiting, and GI distress due to a variety of chemical constituents. Caution should be used in individuals having known allergies to plants.

Theoretical Interactions Insulin and oral hypoglycemic agents

References

Bradley PR, ed, *British Herbal Compendium*, Vol 1, Bournemouth, England: British Herbal Medicine Association, 1992, 151-3.

Newall CA, Anderson LA, and Phillipson JD, *Herbal Medicines: A Guide for Health Care Professionals*, London, England: The Pharmaceutical Press, 1996, 188.

Tomoda M, Shimizu N, Oshima Y, et al, "Hypoglycemic Activity of Twenty Plant Mucilages and Three Modified Products," *Planta Med*, 1987, 53(1):8-12.

Mastic *(Pistacia lentiscus)*

Related Information
Herb Quick Reference Chart *on page 538*

Natural Product Category Herb

Plant Part Resin

Dosage and Standardization Oral: 1000-2000 mg/day in divided doses

Reported Uses *H. pylori* inhibitor; peptic ulcer disease (Huwez, 1998)

Summary Mastic is a multi-branched shrub rarely growing higher than 12 feet. It is found freely scattered over the Mediterranean region, in Spain, Portugal, France, Greece, Turkey, the Canary Islands, and tropical Africa. Mastic is commonly used for peptic ulcer disease in these areas.

Pharmacology Mastic is reported to inhibit *H. pylori*, a causative agent in peptic ulcer disease.

Theoretical Cautions and Contraindications None known

General Warnings Use all herbal supplements with extreme caution in children <2 years of age and in pregnancy or lactation. Some herbs are contraindicated in pregnancy or lactation; make sure to observe warnings. Use with caution in individuals on medication and with pre-existing medical conditions. Always review for potential herb-drug interactions (HDIs) and other warnings. Large and prolonged doses may increase the potential for adverse effects. Herbs may cause transient adverse effects such as nausea, vomiting, and GI distress due to a variety of chemical constituents. Caution should be used in individuals having known allergies to plants.

Theoretical Interactions None known

References

Huwez FU, Thirlwell D, Cockayne A, et al, "Mastic Gum Kills *Helicobacter pylori*," *N Engl J Med*, 1998, 339(26):1946.

- ◆ *Matricaria chamomilla see* Chamomile, German *(Matricaria chamomilla, Matricaria recutita) on page 407*
- ◆ *Matricaria recutita see* Chamomile, German *(Matricaria chamomilla, Matricaria recutita) on page 407*
- ◆ *MCP see* Modified Citrus Pectin (MCP) *on page 480*
- ◆ *Melaleuca alternifolia see* Tea Tree *(Melaleuca alternifolia) on page 509*

Melatonin

Related Information
Nutraceutical Chart *on page 573*

Natural Product Category Nutraceutical

Dosage Oral: Dosage range: 0.5-6 mg/day taken at night

Reported Uses
Insomnia (Zisapel, 1999)
Recovery from jet lag (Suhner, 1998)

Summary Melatonin appears to be the primary sleep-regulating hormone of the body. It is secreted in concert with normal day/night cycles. Adults experience about a 37% decline in daily melatonin output between 20-70 years of age. It has been used by individuals suffering from insomnia, particularly when adjusting to shift-work cycles or jet lag.

Pharmacology Melatonin is a hormone secreted from the pineal gland in a 24-hour circadian rhythm, regulating the normal sleep/wake cycle. As a supplement, melatonin has both phase-shifting and sleep-promoting properties. In addition to promoting sleep, physiologic roles of melatonin include regulation of the secretion of growth hormone and gonadotropic hormones. It also possesses antioxidant activity.
(Continued)

Melatonin *(Continued)*

Toxicities, Warnings, and Interactions No known toxicity or serious side effects, however, long-term human studies have not been conducted. Excessive dosages may cause morning sedation or drowsiness.

Symptoms of Deficiency Insomnia and other sleep disturbances

Reported Interactions

Drug/Nutrient Interactions: Drugs that deplete vitamin B_6 may inhibit the body's ability to synthesize melatonin from the tryptophan-serotonin-melatonin pathway. These include oral contraceptives, estrogen, hydralazine, loop diuretics, penicillamine, and theophylline. In addition, beta-blockers and benzodiazepines may deplete melatonin by enzyme inhibition. Isoniazid alters B_6 metabolism, limiting formation of melatonin. Theoretically, effects may be additive with medications which cause CNS sedation.

Nutrient/Nutrient Interactions: a deficiency of pyridoxine inhibits the synthesis of melatonin

References
Suhner A, Schlagenhauf P, Johnson R, et al, "Comparative Study to Determine the Optimal Melatonin Dosage Form for the Alleviation of Jet Lag," *Chronobiol Int*, 1998, 15(6):655-66.
Zisapel N, "The Use of Melatonin for the Treatment of Insomnia," *Biol Signals Recept*, 1999, 8(1-2):84-9.

♦ **Melissa** *see* Lemon Balm/Melissa *(Melissa officinalis) on page 469*

♦ *Melissa officinalis see* Lemon Balm/Melissa *(Melissa officinalis) on page 469*

♦ **Memory Problems** *see page 258*

♦ **Menopause** *see page 262*

♦ **Menorrhagia** *see page 266*

♦ *Mentha piperita see* Peppermint *(Mentha piperita) on page 486*

Methionine

Related Information

Vitamins/Minerals/Trace Elements/Amino Acids Chart *on page 604*

Natural Product Category Amino Acid

Dosage Oral: RDI: None established; dosage range: 500-3000 mg/day

Active Forms DL-methionine, L-methionine

Reported Uses

Liver detoxification (Wang, 1997)

Summary Methionine is an amino acid which is required in protein synthesis, detoxification reactions, and synthesis of a number of additional physiologic compounds. An activated form of methionine (S-adenosyl methionine) has been used for depression.

Pharmacology Methionine is an essential amino acid which is the precursor for the synthesis of cystine, cysteine, and taurine. These amino acids are important for the synthesis of structural proteins and enzymes. Methionine is converted into S-adenosyl methionine (SAMe) which participates in many biochemical reactions including detoxification of toxic compounds. Methionine may serve as a precursor for the synthesis of glutathione, which is the substrate for glutathione peroxidase, a crucial antioxidant enzyme. Methionine assists in the metabolism of homocysteine, which may lead to cardiovascular disease in excess. Finally, methionine is one of three amino acids required for the synthesis of creatine, a compound necessary for energy production and formation of muscle.

Toxicities, Warnings, and Interactions Supplementation without adequate intake of folic acid, vitamin B_6, and vitamin B_{12}, can increase the conversion of methionine to homocysteine. This can be a risk factor for cardiovascular disease. Toxicity is rare (generally observed only in excessive dosages). Symptoms of toxicity reportedly may include ataxia, hyperactivity, hemosiderosis, reduced growth, loss of appetite, and suppressed hematocrit. Extremely high doses may increase urinary excretion of calcium and may induce hallucinations.

Symptoms of Deficiency Hair loss, poor skin tone, toxic elevation of metabolic waste products, hepatic dysfunction

Reported Interactions
Drug/Nutrient Interactions: None known
Nutrient/Nutrient Interactions: None known
References

Wang ST, Chen HW, Sheen LY, et al, "Methionine and Cysteine Affect Glutathione Level, Glutathione-Related Enzyme Activities and the Expression of Glutathione S-Transferase Isozymes in Rat Hepatocytes," *J Nutr*, 1997, 127(11):2135-41.

Methyl Sulfonyl Methane (MSM)
Related Information
Nutraceutical Chart *on page 573*
Natural Product Category Nutraceutical
Dosage Oral: Dosage range: 2000-6000 mg/day
Active Forms Methyl sulfonyl methane, also known as dimethyl sulfone ($DMSO_2$)
Reported Uses
Analgesic (Jacob, 1999)
Interstitial cystitis (Childs, 1994)
Lupus (Morton, 1986)
Osteoarthritis (Rizzo, 1995)
Summary MSM is a derivative of DMSO which causes less odor and produces sustained concentrations in the body. Although there is a scarcity of published scientific research on the therapeutic aspects of MSM, it is believed to share some of the anti-inflammatory and analgesic properties which have been claimed for DMSO.
Pharmacology MSM is derived from DMSO. DMSO, or dimethyl sulfoxide, is claimed to be an anti-inflammatory agent, but it produces a disagreeable odor. Roughly 15% of DMSO is converted metabolically to $DMSO_2$ or dimethyl sulfone, which is another name for MSM. MSM is a source of biological sulfur, an important component of proteins, connective tissues, hormones, and enzymes. Hepatic detoxification also requires adequate sulfur stores. MSM is believed to relieve pain by several possible mechanisms. It may inhibit transmission of pain impulses along type C nerve fibers, increase blood flow, and reduce muscular spasm. In addition, MSM appears to act as an anti-inflammatory agent, possibly by limiting the release of inflammatory mediators.
Toxicities, Warnings, and Interactions No known toxicity or serious side effects
Symptoms of Deficiency Deficiency symptoms have not been defined.
Reported Interactions
Drug/Nutrient Interactions: None known
Nutrient/Nutrient Interactions: None known
References

Childs SJ, "Dimethyl Sulfone (DMSO2) in the Treatment of Interstitial Cystitis," *Urol Clin North Am*, 1994, 21(1):85-8.

Jacob SW, *The Miracle of MSM: The Natural Solution for Pain*, New York, NY: Putnam, 1999, 57-8.

Morton JI and Moore RD, "Lupus Nephritis and Deaths Are Diminished in B/W Mice Drinking 3% Water Solutions of Dimethyl Sulfoxide (DMSO) and Dimethyl Sulfone ($DMSO_2$)," *J Leukocyte Biol*, 1986, 40(3):322.

Rizzo R, "Calcium, Sulfur and Zinc Distribution in Normal and Arthritic Articular Equine Cartilage: A Synchrotron Radiation Induced X-Ray Emission Study (SRIXE)," *J Exp Zool*,1995, 273(1):82-6.

♦ **MGN-3 (Proprietary Extraction)** *see* Arabinoxylane *on page 384*

Milk Thistle *(Silybum marianum)*
Related Information
Herb Quick Reference Chart *on page 538*
Organ System Support Using Natural Products *on page 660*
Natural Product Category Herb
Plant Part Seed
Dosage and Standardization Oral: 80-200 mg 1-3 times/day, standardized to contain 80% silymarin per dose
(Continued)

Milk Thistle *(Silybum marianum)* (Continued)

Reported Uses

Antidote: Poisoning by Death Cup mushroom (Vogel, 1984)

Antioxidant, specifically for hepatic cells, liver diseases: Acute/chronic hepatitis, jaundice, and stimulation of bile secretion/cholagogue (Carrescia, 1980; Flora, 1998; Kropacova, 1998)

Hepatoprotective, including drug toxicities (ie, phenothiazines, butyrophenones, ethanol, and acetaminophen) (Morazzoni, 1995)

Summary Historically, milk thistle was used as a digestive tonic; a general tonic for the spleen, stomach and liver; for the gallbladder; to promote bile flow; and as a stimulant for milk flow in nursing mothers. Milk thistle appears to supply important compounds for hepatic detoxification reactions (including drug metabolism) and to block the hepatotoxic effects of some compounds. It has also been used in a variety of liver disorders.

Pharmacology The activity of milk thistle is reported to be derived from silymarin, which is composed of three primary flavonoids (silybin, silydianin, and silychristin). Silymarin reportedly alters the composition of hepatocytes, limiting entry of hepatotoxins, and stimulates protein synthesis as well as hepatic regeneration. Silymarin increases hepatic glutathione by over 35%. Glutathione is an important antioxidant in detoxification reactions, acting as an important sulfhydryl donor in detoxification reactions. Milk thistle is also reported to inhibit inflammatory effects of leukotrienes which could contribute to hepatic damage. Milk thistle is reported to be hepatoprotective against psychotropics (eg, phenothiazines, butyrophenones), ethanol, acetaminophen, and other drugs that modify hepatic function (Morazzoni, 1995).

Theoretical Cautions and Contraindications None known

General Warnings Use all herbal supplements with extreme caution in children <2 years of age and in pregnancy or lactation. Some herbs are contraindicated in pregnancy or lactation; make sure to observe warnings. Use with caution in individuals on medication and with pre-existing medical conditions. Always review for potential herb-drug interactions (HDIs) and other warnings. Large and prolonged doses may increase the potential for adverse effects. Herbs may cause transient adverse effects such as nausea, vomiting, and GI distress due to a variety of chemical constituents. Caution should be used in individuals having known allergies to plants.

Theoretical Interactions None known

References

Carrescia O, Benelli L, Saraceni F, et al, "Silymarin in the Prevention of Hepatic Damage by Psychopharmacologic Drugs. Experimental Premises and Clinical Evaluations," *Clin Ter*, 1980, 95(2):157-64.

Flora K, Hahn M, Rosen H, et al, "Milk Thistle (*Silybum marianum*) for the Therapy of Liver Disease," *Am J Gastroenterol*, 1998, 93(2):139-43.

Kropacova K, Misurova E, and Hakova H, "Protective and Therapeutic Effect of Silymarin on the Development of Latent Liver Damage," *Radiats Biol Radioecol*, 1998, 38(3):411-5.

Morazzoni P, et al, "*Silybum marianum*," *Fitoterapia*, 1995, 66:3-42.

Vogel G, Tuchweber B, Trost W, et al, "Protection by Silibinin Against *Amanita phalloides* Intoxication in Beagles," *Toxicol Appl Pharmacol*, 1984, 73(3):355-62.

♦ **Milk Vetch** *see* Astragalus *(Astragalus membranaceus)* [Milk Vetch] *on page 388*

♦ **Minor Injury / Wound Healing** *see page 270*

Modified Citrus Pectin (MCP)

Related Information

Nutraceutical Chart *on page 573*

Natural Product Category Nutraceutical

Dosage Oral: Suggested dose is 8-15 g/day; take 5-10 capsules (500 mg each) 3 times/day or dissolve ½ to 1 rounded teaspoonful in water or juice 3 times/day

Active Forms Modified citrus pectin

Reported Uses

Anticancer activity (Pienta, 1995)

Lowers cholesterol (Vargo, 1985)

Summary Citrus pectin is a fiber component of citrus fruits and apples that has been found to have health benefits. It is a water-soluble polysaccharide found in the cell walls of these fruits. Citrus pectin products reportedly help stabilize blood sugar levels and remove toxins. They also help lower cholesterol, which reduces the risk of heart disease and gallstones. Research indicates that the lower molecular weight products, called MCP, function effectively as nontoxic products which specifically interfere with metastasis of cancer cells throughout the body.

Pharmacology Modified citrus pectins alter cell surface adhesion properties, which inhibits metastasis by interfering with the interactions required for transport and proliferation of tumor cells to other sites in the body. MCP also reportedly enhances the cytotoxic response of the body's natural killer cells.

Toxicities, Warnings, and Interactions Do not use in individuals who are allergic to citrus. Use with caution in renal failure.

Symptoms of Deficiency Since citrus pectins do not occur naturally in humans, no deficiency condition exists.

Reported Interactions

　Drug/Nutrient Interactions: None known

　Nutrient/Nutrient Interactions: None known

References

Pienta KJ, Naik H, Akhtar A, et al, "Inhibition of Spontaneous Metastasis in a Rat Prostate Cancer Model by Oral Administration of Modified Citrus Pectin," *J Natl Cancer Inst*, 1995, 87(5), 348-53.

Vargo D, Doyle R, and Floch MH, "Colonic Bacterial Flora and Serum Cholesterol: Alterations Induced by Dietary Citrus Pectin," *Am J Gastroenterol*, 1985, 80(5):361-4.

♦ *Momordica charantia see* Bitter Melon *(Momordica charantia) on page 394*

♦ *Monascus purpureus see* Red Yeast Rice *(Monascus purpureus) on page 496*

♦ **Motion Sickness** *see page 274*

♦ **MSM** *see* Methyl Sulfonyl Methane (MSM) *on page 479*

Muira Puama *(Ptychopetalum olacoides)*

Related Information

　Herb/Drug Potential Interactions *on page 642*

　Herb Quick Reference Chart *on page 538*

Natural Product Category Herb

Plant Part Bark, root

Dosage and Standardization Oral: 125-250 mg twice daily

Reported Uses

　Athletic performance enhancement (Auterhoff, 1971)

　Increased sexual vitality of males (Werbach, 1994)

Summary Muira puama is a tree up to 5 meters in height that is native to the Brazilian Amazon and other parts of northern Brazil. Historically, all parts of the plants have been used medicinally, but the bark and roots are the primary parts of the plant utilized. It has long been used in the Amazon by indigenous peoples for a variety of purposes including sexual debility and impotency.

Pharmacology The benefits in treating impotency with muira puama have been reported. Muira puama is said to be effective in improving libido and erectile dysfunction. Muira puama bark and root contain steroid saponins that may be responsible for this action.

Theoretical Cautions and Contraindications Use caution in individuals receiving steroidal medications

General Warnings Use all herbal supplements with extreme caution in children <2 years of age and in pregnancy or lactation. Some herbs are contraindicated in pregnancy or lactation; make sure to observe warnings. Use with caution in individuals on medication and with pre-existing medical conditions. Always review for potential herb-drug interactions (HDIs) and other warnings. Large and prolonged doses may increase the potential for adverse effects. Herbs may cause transient adverse effects such as
(Continued)

Muira Puama *(Ptychopetalum olacoides)* (Continued)

nausea, vomiting, and GI distress due to a variety of chemical constituents. Caution should be used in individuals having known allergies to plants.

Theoretical Interactions steroidal medications

References

Auterhoff H and Momberger B, "Lipophilic Constituent of *Muira puama*," *Arch Pharm Ber Dtsch Pharm Ges*, 1971, 304(3):223-8.

Werbach MR and Murray MT, *Botanical Influences on Illness, a Sourcebook of Clinical Research*, Tarzana, CA: Third Line Press, 1994, 200.

♦ **Multiple Sclerosis (MS)** *see page 278*
♦ **Muscle Soreness / Stiffness** *see page 282*
♦ **NAC** *see N-*Acetyl Cysteine (NAC) *on page 482*

N-Acetyl Cysteine (NAC)

Related Information

Nutraceutical Chart *on page 573*
Organ System Support Using Natural Products *on page 660*

Natural Product Category Nutraceutical

Dosage Oral: Dosage range: 200-500 mg up to 3 times/day

Active Forms *N*-acetyl cysteine

Reported Uses

Acetaminophen toxicity (Perry, 1998)
AIDS (Droge, 1993)
Asthma (mucolytic, antioxidant) (Millman, 1985)
Bronchitis (Hansen, 1994)
Cardioprotection during chemotherapy (Schmitt-Graf, 1986)
Fatigue (Reid, 1994)
Heavy metal detoxification (Ornaghi, 1993)
Increases glutathione production (Urban, 1997)

Summary *N*-acetyl cysteine is a nontoxic derivative of the dietary amino acid L-cysteine. It is a dietary precursor to reduced glutathione (GSH). As such, it helps to increase the body's stores of glutathione.

Pharmacology *N*-acetyl cysteine is a sulfhydryl (-SH) substance that functions as a powerful antioxidant and cellular detoxifying agent, making it a major protector of biological structures and functions. NAC is capable of detoxifying heavy metals such as mercury, cadmium, and lead. NAC functions as an antioxidant in two ways. First, it neutralizes hydrogen peroxide, hypochlorous acid, and the extremely dangerous hydroxyl radical. Secondly, it enhances the production of glutathione. In addition to its antioxidant activities, NAC also functions as an antiviral agent.

Toxicities, Warnings, and Interactions No known toxicity or serious side effects. Large doses (5-6 g/day) have been reported to cause diarrhea. Some antibiotics may become inactivated if taken in conjunction with *N*-acetyl cysteine.

Symptoms of Deficiency Deficiency would compromise the immune system by decreasing liver detoxification capabilities, reducing antioxidant activity, and lowering the body's ability to eliminate heavy metal toxins

References

Droge W, "Cysteine and Glutathione Deficiency in AIDS Patients: A Rationale for the Treatment With N-Acetyl-Cysteine," *Pharmacology*, 1993, 46(2):61-5.

Hansen NC, Shriver A, Brorsen-Riis L, et al, "Orally Administered N-Acetylcysteine May Improve General Well-Being in Patients With Mild Chronic Bronchitis," *Respir Med*, 1994, 88(7):531-5.

Millman M, Millman FM, Goldstein IM, et al, "Use of Acetylcysteine in Bronchial Asthma - Another Look," *Ann Allergy*, 1985, 54(4):294-6.

Ornaghi F, Ferrini S, Prati M, et al, "The Protective Effect of N-Acetyl-L-Cysteine Against Methyl Mercury Embryotoxicity in Mice," *Fundam Appl Toxicol*, 1993, 20(4):437-45.

Perry HE and Shannon MW, "Efficacy of Oral Versus Intravenous N-Acetylcysteine in Acetaminophen Overdose: Results of an Open-Label, Clinical Trial," *J Pediatr*, 1998, 132(1):149-52.

Reid MB, Stokic DS, Koch SM, et al, "N-Acetylcysteine Inhibits Muscle Fatigue in Humans," *J Clin Invest*, 1994, 94(6):2468-74.

Schmitt-Graf A and Scheulen ME, "Prevention of Adriamycin Cardiotoxicity by Niacin, Isocit-rate, or N-Acetyl Cysteine in Mice. A Morphological Study," *Pathol Res Pract*, 1986, 181(2):168-74.

Urban T, Akerlund B, Jarstrand C, et al, "Neutrophil Function and Glutathione-Peroxidase (GSH-px) Activity in Healthy Individuals After Treatment With N-Acetyl-L-Cysteine," *Biomed Pharmacother*, 1997, 51(9):388-90.

♦ **NADH** *see* Nicotinamide Adenine Dinucleotide (NADH) *on page 483*

♦ **Nausea / Vomiting** *see page 286*

♦ **Nettle** *see* Stinging Nettle *(Urtica dioica) on page 505*

Nicotinamide Adenine Dinucleotide (NADH)

Related Information
Nutraceutical Chart *on page 573*

Natural Product Category Nutraceutical

Dosage Oral: Dosage range 2.5-5 mg 1-4 times/day

Active Forms Nicotinamide adenine dinucleotide

Reported Uses
Chronic fatigue (Forsyth, 1999)

Parkinson's disease (Swerdlow, 1998)

Stamina and energy (Forsyth, 1999)

Summary NADH, or coenzyme 1, is called the energy-producing coenzyme because it is necessary for the production of energy in all living cells. Coenzymes are catalysts that enable biochemical reactions to take place. NADH provides the catalyst that enables energy to be created in every cell of the body.

Pharmacology NADH is an essential coenzyme in the production of energy in the mitochondria. NADH facilitates DNA-repair mechanisms and it also functions as an antioxidant. NADH supplementation stimulates the production of dopamine and adrenaline.

Toxicities, Warnings, and Interactions No known toxicity or serious side effects

Symptoms of Deficiency Deficiency studies in humans have not been conducted.

References
Forsyth LM, Preuss HG, MacDowell AL, et al, "Therapeutic Effects of Oral NADH on the Symptoms of Patients With Chronic Fatigue Syndrome," *Ann Allergy Asthma Immunol*, 1999, 82(2):185-91.

Swerdlow RH, "Is NADH Effective in the Treatment of Parkinson's Disease?" *Drugs Aging*, 1998, 13(4):263-8.

♦ **Nutraceutical Chart** *see page 573*

♦ **Nutrient Depletion and Cancer Chemotherapy** *see page 637*

♦ *Oenothera biennis* *see* Evening Primrose *(Oenothera biennis) on page 430*

♦ *Olea europaea* *see* Olive Leaf *(Olea europaea) on page 483*

Olive Leaf *(Olea europaea)*

Related Information
Herb Quick Reference Chart *on page 538*

Natural Product Category Herb

Plant Part Leaf

Dosage and Standardization Oral: 250-500 mg 1-3 times/day, standardized to contain 15% to 23% oleuropein per dose

Reported Uses Antibiotic, antifungal, antiviral; hypoglycemic activity; antihypertensive activity (Gonzalez, 1992; Fehri, 1994)

Summary Olive leaf has been used for centuries as a medicinal agent. Olive leaf is used in infections and to improve natural immunity. It is also used to support normalization of GI flora and immune support.

Pharmacology Olive leaf extract has antibacterial, antifungal, antiviral, and antiparasitic action. Olive leaf interferes with certain amino acid production processes necessary for the vitality of various viruses or bacterium. Olive leaf extract has also been reported to destroy or inhibit the growth of many (Continued)

Olive Leaf *(Olea europaea)* *(Continued)*

parasites, including tapeworm, hookworm, flatworm, and roundworm. Olive leaf may stimulate phagocytosis.

Theoretical Cautions and Contraindications Do not use in individuals with gallstones due to cholagogue effect (Brinker, 1998). Based on pharmacological activities, use with caution in individuals on insulin, hypoglycemic, and/or antihypertensive agents.

General Warnings Use all herbal supplements with extreme caution in children <2 years of age and in pregnancy or lactation. Some herbs are contraindicated in pregnancy or lactation; make sure to observe warnings. Use with caution in individuals on medication and with pre-existing medical conditions. Always review for potential herb-drug interactions (HDIs) and other warnings. Large and prolonged doses may increase the potential for adverse effects. Herbs may cause transient adverse effects such as nausea, vomiting, and GI distress due to a variety of chemical constituents. Caution should be used in individuals having known allergies to plants.

Theoretical Interactions Hypoglycemic agents, antihypertensive agents, insulin

References

Brinker F, *Herb Contraindications and Drug Interactions*, Sandy, OR: Eclectic Medical Publications, 1998, 70.

Fehri B, Aiache JM, Memmi A, et al, "Hypotension, Hypoglycemia and Hypouricemia Recorded After Repeated Administration of Aqueous Leaf Extract of *Olea europaea* L," *J Pharm Belg*, 1994, 49(2):101-8.

Gonzalez M, Zarzuelo A, Gamez MJ, et al, "Hypoglycemic Activity of Olive Leaf," *Planta Med*, 1992, 58(6):513-5.

♦ **Organ System Support Using Natural Products** *see page 660*
♦ **Osteoporosis** *see page 290*
♦ **Otitis Media** *see page 294*
♦ **PABA** *see* Para-Aminobenzoic Acid (PABA) *on page 485*
♦ **Panax ginseng** *see* Ginseng, Panax *(Panax ginseng) on page 442*

Pancreatic Extract

Related Information

Nutraceutical Chart *on page 573*

Natural Product Category Nutraceutical, Glandular

Dosage

Digestive aid: Oral: 500-1000 mg 3 times/day immediately before meals
Anti-inflammatory: Oral: 500-1000 mg 3 times/day 10-20 minutes before meals or on an empty stomach

Active Forms Pancreatic Extract

Reported Uses Digestive disturbances, food allergies, celiac disease, anti-inflammatory, immune complex diseases, adjunct support for cancer therapy

Summary Pancreatic extracts contain pancreatic enzymes, including lipases, amylases, and proteases, which aid in the digestion of fats, starches, and proteins.

Pharmacology In addition to aiding in digestion, pancreatic proteases also provide protection in the gastrointestinal tract against organisms such as bacteria, yeasts, protozoa, and intestinal worms. Proteases also increase the breakdown of fibrin, which reduces inflammation and the formation of blood clots.

Toxicities, Warnings, and Interactions No known toxicity or serious side effects have been reported.

Symptoms of Deficiency Symptoms of pancreatic insufficiency include abdominal gas, bloating, and discomfort.

Reported Interactions

Drug/Nutrient Interactions: None known
Nutrient/Nutrient Interactions: None known

♦ **Pancreatic Glandular Extract** *see* Pancreatic Extract *on page 484*
♦ **Pantothenic Acid** *see* Vitamin B$_5$ (Pantothenic Acid) *on page 522*

Para-Aminobenzoic Acid (PABA)

Related Information
Nutraceutical Chart *on page 573*

Natural Product Category Nutraceutical

Dosage Oral: Dosage range: 100-400 mg/day

Active Forms Para-aminobenzoic acid

Reported Uses
Peyronie's disease (Carson, 1997)
Scleroderma (Zarafonetis, 1988)
Vitiligo (Hughes, 1983)

Summary PABA is not a B vitamin, but it is closely associated with the B vitamin group. Like the other B vitamins, PABA is water-soluble. However, it is unique in that it is a "vitamin within a vitamin" because structurally, PABA is part of the folic acid molecule.

Pharmacology PABA facilitates the breakdown and utilization of proteins, aids in the production of red blood cells, and promotes skin health, hair pigmentation, and intestinal health. PABA may enhance the effects of estrogens, cortisone, and other hormones by slowing their rate of metabolism in the liver.

Toxicities, Warnings, and Interactions No known toxicity or serious side effects at doses <400 mg/day; can cause low blood sugar, rash, fever, and liver damage at high doses

Symptoms of Deficiency PABA deficiency has not been reported in humans.

References
Carson CC, "Potassium Para-Aminobenzoate for the Treatment of Peyronie's Disease: Is It Effective?" *Tech Urol*, 1997, 3(3):135-9.
Hughes CG, "Oral PABA and Vitiligo," *J Am Acad Dermatol*, 1983, 9(5):770.
Zarafonetis CJ, Dabich L, Negri D, et al, "Retrospective Studies in Scleroderma: Effect of Potassium Para-Aminobenzoate on Survival," *J Clin Epidemiol*, 1988, 41(2):193-205.

♦ **Parkinson's Disease** *see page 298*

Parsley *(Petroselinum crispum)*

Related Information
Herb Quick Reference Chart *on page 538*

Natural Product Category Herb

Plant Part Leaf (oil)

Dosage and Standardization Oral: Dilute a few drops of oil in a cup of water, gargle, and expectorate; 1-2 pearls 1-3 times/day

Reported Uses Halitosis; antibacterial, antifungal (Newall, 1996)

Summary Parsley is used as a spice in foods and has also traditionally been used as a medicinal agent. The oil is used in halitosis, having antibacterial and antifungal activity.

Pharmacology Parsley's antibacterial and antifungal activity are attributed to its volatile oils. Usage in halitosis is also attributed to the volatile oil component.

Theoretical Cautions and Contraindications Encapsulated parsley products: Extremely large doses of constituents (apiole and myristicin) have been associated with hematologic, renal, and hepatic toxicity (based on *in vitro* or animal studies, Buchanan, 1978). Use with caution in individuals receiving MAO inhibitors.

General Warnings Use all herbal supplements with extreme caution in children <2 years of age and in pregnancy or lactation. Some herbs are contraindicated in pregnancy or lactation; make sure to observe warnings. Use with caution in individuals on medication and with pre-existing medical conditions. Always review for potential herb-drug interactions (HDIs) and other warnings. Large and prolonged doses may increase the potential for adverse effects. Herbs may cause transient adverse effects such as nausea, vomiting, and GI distress due to a variety of chemical constituents. Caution should be used in individuals having known allergies to plants.

Theoretical Interactions MAO inhibitors. Theoretically, high intake may alter response to warfarin (due to vitamin K content).
(Continued)

Parsley *(Petroselinum crispum)* *(Continued)*

References

Buchanan RL, "Toxicity of Species Containing Methylenedioxygenzene Derivatives," *J Food Safety*, 1978, 1:275-293.

Newall CA, Anderson LA, and Phillipson JD, *Herbal Medicines: A Guide for Health Care Professionals*, London, England: The Pharmaceutical Press, 1996, 203-4.

♦ *Passiflora* spp *see* Passion Flower *(Passiflora* spp) *on page 486*

Passion Flower *(Passiflora spp)*

Related Information

Herb Quick Reference Chart *on page 538*

Natural Product Category Herb

Plant Part Whole plant

Dosage and Standardization Oral:

Anxiety: 100 mg 2-3 times/day, standardized to contain 3.5% isovitexin per dose

Insomnia: 200 mg at bedtime, standardized to contain 3.5% isovitexin per dose

Reported Uses Sedative (Wolfman, 1994; Speroni, 1988)

Summary Passion flower, or maypop, is a common roadside vine in many areas of the United States. It has traditionally been used as a sedative in various nervous conditions.

Pharmacology The constituents, maltol and ethylmaltol, have been shown to produce central nervous system sedation and a reduction in spontaneous motor activity (low doses) in laboratory animals. In humans, passion flower may be effective when used in combination with other sedative and antianxiety herbs such as valerian. These effects may be due to synergism, but also may be due to the potential binding of passion flower constituents to benzodiazepine receptors *in vivo*.

Theoretical Cautions and Contraindications Based on pharmacological effects, may cause drowsiness; use caution when driving an automobile or operating heavy machinery. Use with caution in individuals taking antianxiety agents, antidepressants, hypnotics, or sedatives. Reported in animal studies to increase sleeping time induced by hexobarbital (Aoyagi, 1974).

General Warnings Use all herbal supplements with extreme caution in children <2 years of age and in pregnancy or lactation. Some herbs are contraindicated in pregnancy or lactation; make sure to observe warnings. Use with caution in individuals on medication and with pre-existing medical conditions. Always review for potential herb-drug interactions (HDIs) and other warnings. Large and prolonged doses may increase the potential for adverse effects. Herbs may cause transient adverse effects such as nausea, vomiting, and GI distress due to a variety of chemical constituents. Caution should be used in individuals having known allergies to plants.

Theoretical Interactions Anxiolytics, antidepressants, barbiturates, sedatives

References

Aoyagi N, Kimura R, and Murata T, "Studies on *Passiflora incarnata* Dry Extract, Isolation of Maltol and Pharmacological Action of Maltol and Ethyl Maltol," *Chem Pharm Bull (Tokyo)*, 1974, 22(5):1008-13.

Speroni E and Minghetti A, "Neuropharmacological Activity of Extracts From *Passiflora incarnata*," *Planta Med*, 1988, 54(6):488-91.

Wolfman C, Viola H, Paladini A, et al, "Possible Anxiolytic Effects of Chrysin, a Central Benzodiazepine Receptor Ligand Isolated From *Passiflora coerulea*," *Pharmacol Biochem Behav*, 1994, 47(1):1-4.

♦ *Pausinystalia yohimbe* see Yohimbe *(Pausinystalia yohimbe) on page 533*

♦ *PC see* Phosphatidyl Choline (PC) *on page 488*

Peppermint *(Mentha piperita)*

Related Information

Herb Quick Reference Chart *on page 538*

Natural Product Category Herb

Plant Part Leaf, oil

Dosage and Standardization Oral:

One tablet (enteric coated), 2-3 times/day, containing 0.2 mL oil per tablet
Note: The oil should contain:
- ≥4.5% w/v and ≤10% w/w of esters calculated as menthyl acetate
- ≥44% w/v of free alcohols calculated as menthol
- ≥15% w/v and ≤32% w/v ketones calculated as menthone

Infants and Children ≤6 years of age: Infuse 1 teaspoonful of dried leaf per cup of boiling water; cool before using; give 1-2 teaspoonfuls 1-3 times/day

Reported Uses

Carminative, spasmolytic (Schulz, 1996)
Irritable bowel syndrome (Liu, 1997)

Summary Peppermint oil is used for digestive complaints as a carminative and spasmolytic. It is also used in Irritable Bowel Syndrome (IBS).

Pharmacology Peppermint oil has an antispasmodic action on the ileum. Peppermint oil may block calcium exciting stimuli, with the antispasmodic properties being characteristic of calcium channel blockers. Reports suggest that enteric-coated peppermint oil is effective in relieving symptoms of IBS.

Theoretical Cautions and Contraindications Due to pharmacological activity, do not use in individuals presenting with biliary tract obstruction, cholecystitis, gallstones, hiatal hernia, or severe liver damage (Pittler, 1998). Calcium channel blocking activity has been observed in animal models (Beesley, 1996); use with caution in individuals receiving other calcium channel blockers.

General Warnings Use all herbal supplements with extreme caution in children <2 years of age and in pregnancy or lactation. Some herbs are contraindicated in pregnancy or lactation; make sure to observe warnings. Use with caution in individuals on medication and with pre-existing medical conditions. Always review for potential herb-drug interactions (HDIs) and other warnings. Large and prolonged doses may increase the potential for adverse effects. Herbs may cause transient adverse effects such as nausea, vomiting, and GI distress due to a variety of chemical constituents. Caution should be used in individuals having known allergies to plants.

Theoretical Interactions Calcium channel blocking agents

References

Beesley A, Hardcastle J, Hardcastle PT, et al, "Influence of Peppermint Oil on Absorptive and Secretory Processes in Rat Small Intestine," *Gut*, 1996, 39(2):214-9.

Liu JH, Chen GH, Yeh HZ, et al, "Enteric-Coated Peppermint-Oil Capsules in the Treatment of Irritable Bowel Syndrome: A Prospective, Randomized Trial," *J Gastroenterol*, 1997, 32(6):765-8.

Pittler MH and Ernst E, "Peppermint Oil for Irritable Bowel Syndrome: A Critical Review and Meta-analysis," *Am J Gastroenterol*, 1998, 93(7):1131-5.

Shulz V, Hansel R, and Tyler VE, *Rational Phytotherapy: A Physicians' Guide to Herbal Medicine*, New York, NY: Springer-Verlag, 1996, 187-90.

♦ **Performance Enhancement** see page 302

♦ **Petroselinum crispum** see Parsley (Petroselinum crispum) on page 485

Phenylalanine

Related Information

Vitamins/Minerals/Trace Elements/Amino Acids Chart *on page 604*

Natural Product Category Amino Acid

Dosage Oral: RDI: None established; ODA: 1500 mg/day

Active Forms D-phenylalanine, L-phenylalanine, DL-phenylalanine (DLPA)

Reported Uses

Addiction: Reward deficiency syndrome (Blum, 1987)
Depression (Mann, 1980)
Pain relief (Walsh, 1986)
Vitiligo (Camacho, 1999)

Pharmacology Precursor for tyrosine, epinephrine, norepinephrine, dopamine, thyroxine, and melanin; influences the synthesis of many important brain neuropeptides including vasopressin, ACTH, somatostatin, enkephalin, angiotensin II, and cholecystokinin. Converted to phenylethylamine (a (Continued)

Phenylalanine *(Continued)*

chemical that occurs naturally in the brain) mediating the observed effects of this agent.

Toxicities, Warnings, and Interactions Hyperactive children and individuals who suffer from migraine headaches have been found to have elevated plasma phenylalanine; phenylketonuria (PKU), a genetic abnormality causing toxicity from elevated phenylalanine, results in severe mental retardation. Ingestion of the artificial sweetener aspartame causes a rapid increase in brain levels of phenylalanine.

Symptoms of Deficiency Deficiency rarely occurs in humans; symptoms include behavioral changes, eye disorders, poor vascular health, increase in appetite and weight gain

Reported Interactions Nutrient/nutrient interactions: Branched chain amino acids (leucine, isoleucine, and valine) compete with phenylalanine and other aromatic amino acids for transport into the brain.

References
Blum K, Briggs AH, Trachtenberg MC, et al, "Enkephalinase Inhibition: Regulation of Ethanol Intake in Genetically Predisposed Mice," *Alcohol*, 1987, 4(6):449-56.

Camacho F and Mazuecos J, "Treatment of Vitiligo With Oral and Topical Phenylalanine: 6 Years of Experience," *Arch Dermatol*, 1999, 135(2):216-7.

Mann JJ, Peselow ED, Snyderman S, et al, "D-Phenylalanine in Endogenous Depression," *Am J Psychiatry*, 1980, 137(12):1611-2.

Walsh NE, Ramamurthy S, Schoenfeld L, et al, "Analgesic Effectiveness of D-Phenylalanine in Chronic Pain Patients," *Arch Phys Med Rehabil*, 1986, 67(7):436-9.

♦ **Phosphatidylcholine** *see* Phosphatidyl Choline (PC) *on page 488*

Phosphatidyl Choline (PC)

Related Information
Nutraceutical Chart *on page 573*
Organ System Support Using Natural Products *on page 660*

Natural Product Category Nutraceutical

Dosage Oral: RDI: None established; dosage range: 500-1000 mg 2-3 times/day

Active Forms Phosphatidyl choline and lecithin

Reported Uses
Alcohol-induced liver damage (Chwiecho, 1993)
Alzheimer's disease (may benefit some individuals) (Little, 1985)
gallstones (Tuzhilin, 1976)
Hepatitis (Jenkins, 1982)

Summary In the food industry, the term "lecithin" refers to 100% phosphatidyl choline, which is used as a food emulsifier. In the nutritional supplement industry, the word "lecithin" has traditionally referred to a product that contains only about 10% to 20% of the active PC ingredient. In recent years, high-potency lecithin products that contain higher levels of phosphatidyl choline have become available in the nutritional supplement industry.

Pharmacology Phosphatidyl choline is an important structural component of cellular membranes and aids in the breakdown of fats. Phosphatidyl choline is also a source of choline, which the body can utilize to synthesize the neurotransmitter, acetylcholine.

Toxicities, Warnings, and Interactions No known toxicity or serious side effects

Symptoms of Deficiency Deficiency studies in humans have not been conducted.

References
Chwiecko M, Holownia A, Bielawska A, et al, "Inhibition of Non-enzymatic Lipid Peroxidation by "Essentiale" a Drug Enriched in Phosphatidylcholine in Ethanol-Induced Liver Injury," *Drug Alcohol Depend*, 1993, 33(1):87-93.

Jenkins PJ, Portmann BP, Eddleston AL, et al, "Use of Polyunsaturated Phosphatidylcholine in HB$_s$Ag Negative Chronic Active Hepatitis: Results of Prospective Double-Blind Controlled Trial," *Liver*, 1982, 2(2):77-81.

Little A, Levy R, Chuaqui-Kidd P, et al, "A Double-Blind, Placebo Controlled Trial of High-Dose Lecithin in Alzheimer's Disease," *J Neurol Neurosurg Psychiatry*, 1985, 48(8):736-42.

Tuzhilin SA, Dreiling DA, Narodetskaja RV, et al, "The Treatment of Patients With Gallstones by Lecithin," *Am J Gastroenterol*, 1976, 65(3):231-5.

♦ **Phosphatidylserine** *see* Phosphatidyl Serine (PS) *on page 489*

Phosphatidyl Serine (PS)
Related Information
Nutraceutical Chart *on page 573*
Organ System Support Using Natural Products *on page 660*
Natural Product Category Nutraceutical
Dosage Oral: RDI: None established; dosage range: 100 mg 1-3 times/day
Active Forms Phosphatidylserine
Reported Uses
Alzheimer's disease (Engel, 1992)
Depression (Maggioni, 1990)
Memory enhancement (Crook, 1991)
Summary Phosphatidyl serine belongs to a class of fat-soluble compounds called phospholipids. Phospholipids are essential components of cell membranes, with very high concentrations found in the brain. Phosphatidyl serine is the most abundant phospholipid found in the brain.
Pharmacology Phosphatidyl serine is a substance that helps provide cellular membranes with their fluidity, flexibility, and permeability. PS stimulates the release of various neurotransmitters, such as acetylcholine and dopamine. It enhances ion transport and increases the number of certain neurotransmitter receptor sites in the brain. Phosphatidyl serine reportedly may be used in individuals with depression; it may also help to reduce cortisol levels.
Toxicities, Warnings, and Interactions No known toxicity or serious side effects
Symptoms of Deficiency Depression, loss of memory, cognitive decline
References
Crook TH, Tinklenberg J, Yesavage J, et al, "Effects of Phosphatidylserine in Age-Associated Memory Impairment," *Neurology*, 1991, 41(5):644-9.
Engel RR, Satzger W, Gunther W, et al, "Double-Blind Cross-Over Study of Phosphatidylserine vs. Placebo in Patients With Early Dementia of the Alzheimer Type," *Eur Neuropsychopharmacol*, 1992, 2(2):149-55.
Maggioni M, Picotti GB, Bondiolotti GP, et al, "Effects of Phosphatidylserine Therapy in Geriatric Patients With Depressive Disorders," *Acta Psychiatr Scand*, 1990, 81(3):265-70.

Phosphorus
Related Information
Drug-Induced Nutrient Depletions *on page 625*
Pregnancy & Lactation Nutritional Chart *on page 657*
Vitamins/Minerals/Trace Elements/Amino Acids Chart *on page 604*
Natural Product Category Mineral
Dosage Oral: RDI: None established; ODA: 800-1200 mg/day
Active Forms Dicalcium phosphate, phosphatidyl choline, phosphatidyl serine
Reported Uses No reported therapeutic uses
Summary Phosphorus participates in more biological processes than any other mineral. Approximately 20% of total body phosphorus is metabolically active while 80% is maintained in pools which are relatively stable, such as in bone. Phosphorus is so abundant in foods that it rarely requires therapeutic supplementation.
Pharmacology Phosphate is utilized in a wide array of physiologic roles. Phosphate-containing salts are vital to the structure of bones and teeth. In addition, phospholipids are the primary constituents of cellular membranes. Phosphate is required for the production of ATP, the major physiologic molecule used in the storage and transport of energy. It is also used to activate enzymes systems and facilitate cellular processes. Within the bloodstream, phosphoric acid and its salts are one of the key buffering systems used to ensure acid-base balance. As a component of both DNA and RNA, phosphate is required in all cellular reproduction and protein synthesis.
Toxicities, Warnings, and Interactions Contraindicated in individuals with renal dysfunction
(Continued)

Phosphorus *(Continued)*

Toxic dose: Over-consumption is possible. The typical American diet is high in meats, dairy products, and soda pop, which contain relatively high amounts of phosphorus.

Toxicity symptoms: Excess consumption may influence calcium absorption and utilization, potentially contributing to the development of osteoporosis. Hyperphosphatemia may lead to ectopic calcification (calcium phosphate deposition in soft tissues).

Symptoms of Deficiency Muscle cramps, dizziness, anorexia, weakness, joint stiffness, bone fragility, respiratory distress, cardiopulmonary arrest; not to be used in individuals with renal dysfunction

Reported Interactions

Drug/Nutrient Interactions: Drugs which can cause depletion of phosphorus: Digoxin, magnesium and aluminum-containing antacids, thiazide diuretics, mineral oil, colchicine

Nutrient/Nutrient Interactions: The minerals calcium, magnesium, aluminum, and iron can all interfere with the absorption of phosphorus. Vitamin D can increase the absorption of phosphorus.

- ♦ *Piper methysticum* see Kava Kava *(Piper methysticum)* on page 466
- ♦ *Pistacia lentiscus* see Mastic *(Pistacia lentiscus)* on page 477
- ♦ *Plantago isphagula* see Psyllium *(Plantago ovata, Plantago isphagula)* on page 492
- ♦ *Plantago ovata* see Psyllium *(Plantago ovata, Plantago isphagula)* on page 492
- ♦ **Poison Ivy / Poison Oak** see page 306

Potassium

Related Information

Drug-Induced Nutrient Depletions *on page 625*

Vitamins/Minerals/Trace Elements/Amino Acids Chart *on page 604*

Natural Product Category Mineral

Dosage Oral: RDI: None established; ODA: None established; experts recommend keeping potassium intake <3500 mg/day

Active Forms Ascorbate, aspartate, carbonate, chloride, citrate, iodide, and phosphate

Reported Uses

Cardiac arrhythmias (Motte, 1984)

Congestive heart failure (CHF) (Wester, 1986)

Hypertension (Patki, 1990)

Kidney stones (Curhan, 1993)

Summary Potassium is a key physiologic electrolyte. Serum levels are maintained in an exceptionally narrow range. Potassium is critical to allow normal nervous systems and cardiovascular function. However, potassium excess may be life-threatening. Many medications alter potassium concentrations, and supplementation is often guided by measurement of this electrolyte in the serum.

Pharmacology Potassium is an important physiologic ion. It is the most common intracellular cation, and participates in transmembrane ionic shifts, contributing to neuronal transmission and muscle cell depolarization. This ion is essential to normal cardiac impulse generation and conduction. Potassium is important to the function of renal acid-base regulation.

Toxicities, Warnings, and Interactions Use extreme caution in individuals with renal disease

Toxic dose: If potassium excretion is impaired and potassium chloride, other table salt replacements, or potassium tablets are taken in high dosages, blood levels of potassium can become dangerously high.

Toxicity symptoms: Muscular weakness, vomiting, and cardiac disturbances

Symptoms of Deficiency Muscle fatigue, general fatigue, swelling in extremities, confusion, arrhythmia

Reported Interactions

Drug/Nutrient Interactions: Drugs which can cause depletion of potassium: Aminoglycosides, loop diuretics, thiazide diuretics, corticosteroids, colchicine, aspirin, bisacodyl, cyclosporine, beta-adrenergic agonists, calcium channel blockers, penicillin antibiotics, amphotericin B. Potassium-sparing diuretics and ACE inhibitors may increase serum concentrations of potassium. Hypokalemia exacerbates the toxicity of digitalis glycosides.

Nutrient/Nutrient Interactions: None known

References

Curhan GC, Willett WC, Rimm EB, et al, "A Prospective Study of Dietary Calcium and Other Nutrients and the Risk of Symptomatic Kidney Stones," *N Engl J Med*, 1993, 328(12):833-8.

Motte G, "Arrhythmia Caused by Potassium Deficiency," *Arch Mal Coeur Vaiss*, 1984, 77:17-22.

Patki PS, Singh J, Gokhale SV, et al, "Efficacy of Potassium and Magnesium in Essential Hypertension: A Double-Blind, Placebo Controlled, Crossover Study," *BMJ*, 1990, 301(6751):521-3.

Wester PO and Dyckner T, "Intracellular Electrolytes in Cardiac Failure," *Acta Med Scand Supp*, 1986, 707:33-36.

♦ **Pregnancy & Lactation Nutritional Chart** *see page 657*

Pregnenolone

Related Information

Nutraceutical Chart *on page 573*

Natural Product Category Nutraceutical

Dosage Oral: Dosage range: 5-30 mg/day depending on age and gender

Active Forms Pregnenolone

Reported Uses

Arthritis (Freeman, 1950)

Improved mental performance (Pincus, 1944)

Natural precursor for the production of DHEA, cortisol, progesterone, estrogens, and testosterone in the body

Summary Pregnenolone is one of the hormones naturally produced in the body. It is sometimes referred to as the "mother hormone," because it is the precursor for dehydroepiandrosterone (DHEA) and all of the steroid and sex hormones.

Pharmacology Pregnenolone is primarily produced in the adrenal glands. The mechanism of its production is the conversion of cholesterol into pregnenolone. It has recently been discovered that the brain is also capable of synthesizing pregnenolone. Some studies report that pregnenolone has positive effects on mood. It also seems to increase energy levels, especially during times of stress. This has been referred to as pregnenolone's antifatigue effect.

Toxicities, Warnings, and Interactions No known toxicity or serious side effects. However, caution is advised because pregnenolone may potentiate a variety of hormonal pathways including DHEA, progesterone, estrogen, cortisol, and testosterone.

Symptoms of Deficiency Deficiency studies in humans have not been conducted.

References

Freeman H, et al, "Therapeutic Efficacy of Delta-5-Pregnenolone in Rheumatoid Arthritis," *JAMA*, 1950, 142(15):1124-8.

Pincus G, et al, "Effects of Administered Pregnenolone on Fatiguing Psychomotor Performance," *J Aviat Med*, 1944, 15:98-115.

♦ **Premenstrual Syndrome (PMS)** *see page 310*

Progesterone

Related Information

Nutraceutical Chart *on page 573*

Natural Product Category Nutraceutical

Dosage Topical: Dosage range for topical progesterone depends on the strength of the extract; follow manufacturer's directions

(Continued)

Progesterone (Continued)

Reported Uses
Endometriosis (Lee, 1996)
Menopause symptoms (Lee, 1996)
Osteoporosis (Lee, 1991)
PMS symptoms (Martorano, 1998)
Prevention of breast cancer (Chang, 1995)

Summary Progesterone is produced in the female body in the ovaries and adrenal glands. Progesterone is necessary for proper uterine and breast development and function. Progesterone production is high during the luteal phase of the menstrual cycle and low during the follicular phase, as well as being low before puberty and after menopause.

Pharmacology Natural progesterone is used in hormone replacement therapies. It is often used in PMS and the problems associated with menopause. These problems are frequently due to a condition known as estrogen dominance, which means too much estrogen and/or a deficiency of progesterone. Topically-applied natural progesterone cream reportedly aids in bone remodeling and has been reported to cause ~15% increase in bone density in postmenopausal women with osteoporosis.

Toxicities, Warnings, and Interactions No known toxicity or serious side effects with topical administration: however, hormonal regulation may be disrupted. Not to be used with oral contraceptives or other hormonal products without medical supervision.

Symptoms of Deficiency Increased symptoms of PMS or menopause with edema, weight gain, emotional problems; possible increased risk of breast cancer

Reported Interactions Oral contraceptives

References

Chang KJ, Lee TT, Linares-Cruz G, et al, "Influences of Percutaneous Administration of Estradiol and Progesterone on Human Breast Epithelial Cell Cycle *In Vivo*," *Fertil Steril*, 1995, 63(4):785-91.

Lee JR, *What Your Doctor May Not Tell You About Menopause: The Breakthrough Book on Natural Progesterone*, New York, NY: Warner Books, 1996, 117-28.

Lee JR, "Is Natural Progesterone the Missing Link in Osteoporosis Prevention and Treatment?" *Med Hypotheses*, 1991, 35(4):316-8.

Martorano JT, Ahlgrimm M, and Colbert T, "Differentiating Between Natural Progesterone and Synthetic Progestins: Clinical Implications for Premenstrual Syndrome and Perimenopause Management," *Compr Ther*, 1998, 24(6-7):336-9.

♦ **PS** *see* Phosphatidyl Serine (PS) *on page 489*
♦ **Psoriasis** *see page 314*

Psyllium (Plantago ovata, Plantago isphagula)

Related Information
Herb/Drug Potential Interactions *on page 642*
Herb Quick Reference Chart *on page 538*

Natural Product Category Herb

Plant Part Seed

Dosage and Standardization Oral: 1-3 teaspoonful with 6-8 ounces of water in the morning and evening

Reported Uses Bulk-forming laxative (containing 10% to 30% mucilage) (Leung, 1996)

Summary The ripe seed of psyllium is used as a bulk-forming laxative, which usually contains 10% to 30% mucilage. It is used in many over-the-counter laxative products.

Pharmacology Psyllium is used for habitual constipation and disorders where easy bowel movement with a loose stool is desirable. When used in constipation, psyllium decreases the transit time of the bowel content through increasing the volume of the stool.

Theoretical Cautions and Contraindications Avoid use in bowel obstruction. May cause abdominal cramps, diarrhea, or constipation.

General Warnings Use all herbal supplements with extreme caution in children <2 years of age and in pregnancy or lactation. Some herbs are contraindicated in pregnancy or lactation; make sure to observe warnings. Use with caution in individuals on medication and with pre-existing medical conditions. Always review for potential herb-drug interactions (HDIs) and other warnings. Large and prolonged doses may increase the potential for adverse effects. Herbs may cause transient adverse effects such as nausea, vomiting, and GI distress due to a variety of chemical constituents. Caution should be used in individuals having known allergies to plants.

Theoretical Interactions None known

References

Leung AY and Foster S, *Encyclopedia of Common Natural Ingredients Used in Foods, Drugs, and Cosmetics*, New York, NY: Wiley, 1996, 427-9.

♦ *Ptychopetalum olacoides* see Muira Puama *(Ptychopetalum olacoides)* on page 481

Pygeum *(Pygeum africanum, Prunus africana)*

Natural Product Category Herb

Dosage and Standardization Oral: 50-100 mg twice daily, standardized to contain 12% to 13% phytosterols per dose (β-sitosterol)

Reported Uses Symptoms associated with benign prostatic hypertrophy (Breza, 1998; Mathe, 1995)

Summary Pygeum is a tall evergreen tree that grows mainly in Madagascar, South Africa, and in some areas of Central Africa. The powdered bark was historically used as a tea for relief of urinary disorders. European scientists were so impressed with reports of pygeum's action that they began laboratory investigations into the active constituents in the bark. This led to the development of the modern lipophilic (fat-soluble) extract used today in benign prostatic hypertrophy (BPH).

Pharmacology Chemical analysis and pharmacological studies indicate that the lipophilic extract of pygeum bark has three categories of active constituents. The phytosterols, including beta-sitosterol, have anti-inflammatory effects by interfering with the formation of pro-inflammatory prostaglandins (PGE_2 and $PGF_2\alpha$) that tend to accumulate in the prostate of men with BPH (Clavert, 1986). The pentacyclic terpenes have an antiedema or decongestant effect (Bombardelli, 1997). The ferulic esters of long chain fatty alcohols reduce levels of the hormone prolactin and also block cholesterol in the prostate (Bombardelli, 1997). Prolactin increases uptake of testosterone in the prostate, and cholesterol increases binding sites for testosterone and its more active form dihydrotestosterone. Positive results from using pygeum bark in individuals with symptomatic BPH have been demonstrated in several open and double-blind placebo controlled clinical trials (Bombardelli, 1997). Results from a large multicenter European study found that pygeum significantly increased urine flow and decreased residual urine in 66% of men (Barlet, 1990). Many men using pygeum also experienced substantial improvement in sexual performance. Pygeum is used complementary with stinging nettle root and saw palmetto berry in BPH.

Theoretical Cautions and Contraindications Individuals should have a prostatic exam and laboratory studies (PSA) to rule out cancer prior to use for symptoms of BPH. Based on pharmacological activity, use with caution in individuals receiving treatment for BPH with alpha-blockers or finasteride.

Theoretical Interactions Alpha-adrenergic blockers, finasteride

References

Barlet A, Albrecht J, Aubert A, et al, "Efficacy of *Pygeum africanum* Extract in the Medical Therapy of Urination Disorders Due to Benign Prostatic Hyperplasia: Evaluation of Objective and Subjective Parameters. A Placebo-Controlled Double-blind Multicenter Study," *Wien Klin Wochenschr*, 1990, 102(22):667-73.

Bombardelli E, Morazzoni P, "*Prunus africana, Fitoterapia*, 1997, 68(3): 205-18.

Breza J, Dzurny O, Borowka A, et al, "Efficacy and Acceptability of Tadenan (*Pygeum africanum* Extract) in the Treatment of Benign Prostatic Hyperplasia (BPH): A Multicentre Trial in Central Europe," *Curr Med Res Opin*, 1998, 14(3):127-39.

Clavert A, Cranz C, Riffaud JP, et al, "Effects of an Extract of the Bark of *Pygeum africanum* (V.1326) on Prostatic Secretions in the Rat and in Man," *Ann Urol (Paris)*, 1986, 20(5):341-3.

Mathe G, Hallard M, Bourut CH, et al, "A *Pygeum africanum* Extract With So-Called Phyto-Estrogenic Action Markedly Reduces the Volume of True and Large Prostatic Hypertrophy, *Biomed Pharmacother*, 1995, 49(7-8):341-3.

♦ **Pyridoxine** *see* Vitamin B_6 (Pyridoxine) *on page 523*

Pyruvate

Related Information
Nutraceutical Chart *on page 573*

Natural Product Category Nutraceutical

Dosage Oral: Dosage range: 250-750 mg 3 times/day, preferably with meals; dosages 2500-5000 mg/day have been used for weight loss

Active Forms Salts of pyruvate acid such as magnesium pyruvate

Reported Uses
Enhancement of athletic performance (Stanko, 1990)
Obesity and weight loss (Stanko, 1992)

Summary Pyruvate supplements are used to facilitate the transport of glucose into muscle cells, increasing the energy that is available for muscles. Bodybuilders, people engaging in physical training, or people attempting to lose weight often use these supplements.

Pharmacology Pyruvate is a salt of pyruvic acid. Pyruvic acid is chemically unstable and can cause nausea and GI distress when taken orally. To avoid these problems, manufacturers combine it with minerals such as sodium, potassium, calcium, or magnesium to create a stable salt. When glucose, a 6-carbon molecule, is metabolized in the body, it is split in half, releasing energy and forming two molecules of 3-carbon pyruvate.

Toxicities, Warnings, and Interactions Large doses of pyruvate can cause gastrointestinal disturbances, such as gas, bloating, and diarrhea.

Symptoms of Deficiency Pyruvate is not an essential nutrient. There are no studies reporting a deficiency state associated with pyruvate or pyruvic acid.

References
Stanko RT, Robertson RJ, Spina RJ, et al, "Enhancement of Arm Exercise Endurance Capacity With Dihydroxyacetone and Pyruvate," *J Appl Physiol*, 1990, 68(1):119-24.
Stanko RT, Tietze DL, and Arch JE, "Body Composition, Energy Utilization, and Nitrogen Metabolism With a 4.25-MJ/d Low-Energy Diet Supplemented With Pyruvate," *Am J Clin Nutr*, 1992, 56(4):630-5.

Quercetin

Related Information
Nutraceutical Chart *on page 573*

Natural Product Category Nutraceutical

Dosage Oral: Dosage range: 300-500 mg 1-3 times/day

Active Forms Quercetin

Reported Uses
Allergies (Bronner, 1985)
Atherosclerosis (Negre-Salvayre, 1992)
Cataracts (Beyer-Mears, 1979)
Peptic ulcer (Alarcon, 1994)

Summary Quercetin is one of a number of water-soluble plant pigments called bioflavonoids. They are not synthesized by humans, but have been reported to demonstrate a variety of biological effects. Quercetin has been claimed to be of benefit in symptomatic relief of allergies, atherosclerosis, and cataracts. In addition, it may be useful in some individuals with peptic ulcer disease.

Pharmacology Quercetin is a bioflavonoid which is claimed to strengthen capillaries and regulate permeability. It appears to have anti-inflammatory and antihistaminic effects. Quercetin demonstrates antioxidant activity, specifically preventing the oxidation of LDL cholesterol.

Toxicities, Warnings, and Interactions No known toxicity or serious side effects

Symptoms of Deficiency Quercetin deficiency may result in capillary fragility, resulting in frequent nosebleeds, bruising, and bleeding tendencies.

Reported Interactions
Drug/Nutrient Interactions: None known

Nutrient/Nutrient Interactions: None known

References

Alarcon de la Lastra C, Martin MJ, and Motilva V, "Antiulcer and Gastroprotective Effects of Quercetin: A Gross and Histologic Study," *Pharmacology*, 1994, 48(1):56-62.

Beyer-Mears A and Farnsworth PN, "Diminished Sugar Cataractogenesis by Quercetin," *Exp Eye Res*, 1979, 28(6):709-16.

Bronner C and Landry Y, "Kinetics of the Inhibitory Effect of Flavonoids on Histamine Secretion From Mast Cells," *Agents Actions*, 1985, 16(3-4):147-51.

Negre-Salvayre A and Salvayre R, "Quercetin Prevents the Cytotoxicity of Oxidized LDL on Lymphoid Cell Lines," *Free Radic Biol Med*, 1992, 12(2):101-6.

♦ *Quercus alba* see White Oak *(Quercus alba) on page 531*

Red Clover *(Trifolium pratense)*

Related Information
Herb/Drug Potential Interactions *on page 642*
Herb Quick Reference Chart *on page 538*

Natural Product Category Herb

Plant Part Tops

Dosage and Standardization Oral: 500 mg/day, standardized to contain 40 mg isoflavones per dose **or** 30-60 drops 2-3 times/day of liquid extract (1:1 w/v) in juice or other beverage

Reported Uses
Liquid extract used for liver detoxification and kidney detoxification (Bradley, 1992)

Menopausal symptoms; proprietary extract contains 4 phytoestrogens (Nestell, 1999)

Summary Red clover tops are used for menopausal symptoms such as hot flashes and night sweats. A liquid extract is used for liver detoxification and kidney detoxification.

Pharmacology Red clover contains four phytoestrogen components, biochanin A, formononetin, genistein, and daidzein that have some estrogenic activity in the body. A liquid extract is used in Europe as an "alterative" agent that aids in liver and kidney detoxification.

Theoretical Cautions and Contraindications Contraindicated in pregnancy and lactation (proprietary extract). Based on pharmacological activity, use with caution in individuals taking anticoagulants (Bradley 1992).

May alter platelet aggregation (Tao, 1990); contraindicated in individuals with active bleeding (eg, peptic ulcer, intracranial bleeding). Use with caution in individuals with a history of bleeding, hemostatic disorders, or drug-related hemostatic problems. Use with caution in individuals taking anticoagulant medications, including warfarin, aspirin, aspirin-containing products, NSAIDs, or antiplatelet agents (eg, ticlopidine, clopidogrel, dipyridamole). Discontinue use prior to dental or surgical procedures (generally at least 14 days before).

Phytoestrogen-containing herbs have not been associated with the negative health effects seen with synthetic estrogen. However, use with caution in individuals on hormone replacement therapy or oral contraceptives or with a history of estrogen-dependent tumors, endometrial cancer, thromboembolic disease, or stroke.

General Warnings Use all herbal supplements with extreme caution in children <2 years of age and in pregnancy or lactation. Some herbs are contraindicated in pregnancy or lactation; make sure to observe warnings. Use with caution in individuals on medication and with pre-existing medical conditions. Always review for potential herb-drug interactions (HDIs) and other warnings. Large and prolonged doses may increase the potential for adverse effects. Herbs may cause transient adverse effects such as nausea, vomiting, and GI distress due to a variety of chemical constituents. Caution should be used in individuals having known allergies to plants.

Theoretical Interactions Hormonal replacement therapy, oral contraceptives, anticoagulants, aspirin, aspirin-containing products, antiplatelet agents, NSAIDs
(Continued)

Red Clover *(Trifolium pratense)* *(Continued)*

References

Bradley PR, ed, *The British Herbal Compendium, Vol 1,* London, England: British Herbal Medicine Association, 1992, 183-84.

Nestel PJ, Pomeroy S, Kay S, et al, "Isoflavones From Red Clover Improved Systemic Arterial Compliance But Not Plasma Lipids in Menopausal Women," *J Clin Endocrinol Metab,* 1999, 84(3):895-8.

Newall CA, Anderson La, and Phillipson JD, *Herbal Medicines: A Guide for Health Care Professionals,* London, England: The Pharmaceutical Press, 1996, 227.

Red Yeast Rice *(Monascus purpureus)*

Related Information

Herb Quick Reference Chart *on page 538*

Natural Product Category Herb

Dosage and Standardization Oral: 1200 mg twice daily standardized to 0.4% total HMG-CoA reductase inhibitors per dose

Reported Uses Hypercholesterolemic agent; may lower triglycerides and LDL cholesterol and raise HDL cholesterol (Endo, 1986)

Summary *Monascus purpureus* is a yeast which grows naturally on starch and silage. It is cultivated on rice and ground into a fine powder. Red yeast rice has been used for centuries in traditional Chinese medicine. It has been shown to lower LDL cholesterol and triglycerides while increasing HDL cholesterol.

Pharmacology Eight compounds with HMG-CoA reductase inhibitory activity have been identified, including lovastatin and its active hydroxy acid metabolite. Inhibitors of this enzyme block the rate-limiting step in the synthesis of cholesterol. These agents play a prominent role in the support of individuals with hypercholesterolemia, coronary artery disease, or myocardial infarction. In addition to naturally occurring HMG-CoA reductase inhibitors, red yeast rice contains several other active compounds, including unsaturated fatty acids, amino acids, phytosterols, isoflavone, saponins, and trace elements such as selenium. It has been evaluated in clinical trials as a cholesterol-lowering agent, and found to cause significant reductions in total cholesterol, LDL cholesterol, and triglycerides, as well as causing an increase in HDL cholesterol. The clinical evidence strongly suggests that red yeast rice is an effective natural product for controlling serum cholesterol.

Theoretical Cautions and Contraindications Based on pharmacological activity, use is contraindicated in pregnancy or lactation (or if trying to become pregnant). In addition, the use of red yeast rice is contraindicated in individuals with known hypersensitivity to rice or yeast. Use with caution in individuals currently receiving other cholesterol-lowering medications. Keep out of reach of children, do not use if <20 years of age. Adverse effects include gastrointestinal upset.

HMG-CoA reductase inhibitors have been associated with rare (less than 1% to 2% incidence) but serious adverse effects, including hepatic and skeletal muscle disorders (myopathy, rhabdomyolysis). The risk of these disorders may be increased by concomitant therapy with specific medications. These effects have not been specifically reported for red yeast rice. Do not use in individuals with hepatic disease, a history of liver disease, or in those who may be at risk of liver disease. Do not use in individuals with serious infection, recent major surgery, other serious disease, or organ transplant individuals. Do not use in any individual who consumes more than 1-2 alcohol-containing drinks per day. Discontinue use at the first sign of hepatic dysfunction.

General Warnings Use all herbal supplements with extreme caution in children <2 years of age and in pregnancy or lactation. Some herbs are contraindicated in pregnancy or lactation; make sure to observe warnings. Use with caution in individuals on medication and with pre-existing medical conditions. Always review for potential herb-drug interactions (HDIs) and other warnings. Large and prolonged doses may increase the potential for adverse effects. Herbs may cause transient adverse effects such as nausea, vomiting, and GI distress due to a variety of chemical constituents. Caution should be used in individuals having known allergies to plants.

Theoretical Interactions HMG-CoA reductase inhibitors, other cholesterol-lowering agents, anticoagulants, gemfibrozil, erythromycin, itraconazole, ketoconazole, cyclosporin, niacin, clofibrate, fenofibrate

References

Endo A, Komagata D, and Shimada H, "Monacolin M, a New Inhibitor of Cholesterol Biosynthesis," *J Antibiot (Tokyo)*, 1986, 39(12):1670-3.

♦ *Rehmannia glutinosa* see Rehmannia (Rehmannia glutinosa) on page 497

Rehmannia *(Rehmannia glutinosa)*

Related Information

Herb Quick Reference Chart *on page 538*

Natural Product Category Herb

Plant Part Root (cured)

Dosage and Standardization Oral: 250 mg 1-3 times/day, standardized to contain 1% glutannic acid per dose

Reported Uses Used as an immunosuppressive agent in rheumatoid arthritis (Chang, 1986)

Summary Rehmannia root has been used in traditional Chinese medicine for centuries. The cured root is used as an immunosuppressive agent in rheumatoid arthritis.

Pharmacology The cured root has been reported to have mild immunosuppressive activity, having anticomplementary activity on the immune system. Reports have indicated that rehmannia root is effective in relieving the symptoms of rheumatoid arthritis, an autoimmune disease. Rehmannia has been reported to decrease the toxicity of cyclophosphamide.

Theoretical Cautions and Contraindications Based on pharmacological activity, use is contraindicated in transplant recipients or others taking therapeutic immunosuppression (such as in the treatment of various autoimmune diseases).

General Warnings Use all herbal supplements with extreme caution in children <2 years of age and in pregnancy or lactation. Some herbs are contraindicated in pregnancy or lactation; make sure to observe warnings. Use with caution in individuals on medication and with pre-existing medical conditions. Always review for potential herb-drug interactions (HDIs) and other warnings. Large and prolonged doses may increase the potential for adverse effects. Herbs may cause transient adverse effects such as nausea, vomiting, and GI distress due to a variety of chemical constituents. Caution should be used in individuals having known allergies to plants.

Theoretical Interactions Immune stimulants, immunosuppressants

References

Chang HM and But P, *Pharmacology and Applications of Chinese Materia Medica, Vol 1*, Philadelphia, PA: World Scientific Publications, 1986.

Reishi *(Ganoderma lucidum)*

Related Information

Herb/Drug Potential Interactions *on page 642*

Herb Quick Reference Chart *on page 538*

Organ System Support Using Natural Products *on page 660*

Natural Product Category Herb

Plant Part Mushroom

Dosage and Standardization Oral: 150-300 mg 3-4 times/day, standardized to contain 10% to 12.5% polysaccharides and 4% triterpenes per dose

Reported Uses Used for immunomodulation, fatigue, and hemo- and radioprotection, antihypertensive, anticonvulsive (Jong, 1992)

Summary Reishi mushroom is called the "mushroom of immortality" in China and has been used as a tonic and strengthening supplement for thousands of years. Its many uses in traditional healing include lengthening the life span. Reishi is currently used for immunomodulation, fatigue, chemo- and radioprotection, as an antihypertensive, and as an anticonvulsant.

(Continued)

Reishi *(Ganoderma lucidum)* *(Continued)*

Pharmacology Reishi extracts have been reported to enhance endurance and cellular oxygenation in laboratory animals. Reishi has been reported to inhibit superoxide activity and hydroxyl radical activity *in vitro*, supporting its role as an antioxidant. Immunocompromised individuals showed increased levels of CD4/CD8 ratio and T-cell counts and lowered levels of T-suppressor cell counts. Radio- and chemotherapy intolerance was reduced in cancer individuals on reishi extract. Studies using reishi mushroom have been performed on hypertensive individuals with very positive results. It has been concluded that the mechanism of hypotensive action of reishi is due to its central inhibition of sympathetic nerve activity. Reishi has been reported to be chemoprotective. It may increase the effectiveness of cefazolin as an antimicrobial agent. (Yoon, 1994)

Theoretical Cautions and Contraindications May alter platelet aggregation (Tao, 1990); contraindicated in individuals with active bleeding (eg, peptic ulcer, intracranial bleeding). Use with caution in individuals with a history of bleeding, hemostatic disorders, or drug-related hemostatic problems. Use with caution in individuals taking anticoagulant medications, including warfarin, aspirin, aspirin-containing products, NSAIDs, or antiplatelet agents (eg, ticlopidine, clopidogrel, dipyridamole). Discontinue use prior to dental or surgical procedures (generally at least 14 days before).

Use with caution if taking antihypertensive medications.

General Warnings Use all herbal supplements with extreme caution in children <2 years of age and in pregnancy or lactation. Some herbs are contraindicated in pregnancy or lactation; make sure to observe warnings. Use with caution in individuals on medication and with pre-existing medical conditions. Always review for potential herb-drug interactions (HDIs) and other warnings. Large and prolonged doses may increase the potential for adverse effects. Herbs may cause transient adverse effects such as nausea, vomiting, and GI distress due to a variety of chemical constituents. Caution should be used in individuals having known allergies to plants.

Theoretical Interactions Anticoagulants, aspirin, aspirin-containing products, NSAIDs, or antiplatelet agents, antihypertensives

References

Jong SC and Birmingham JM, "Medicinal Benefits of the Mushroom Ganoderma," Adv Appl Microbiol, 1992, 37:101-34.

Tao J and Feng KY, "Experimental and Clinical Studies on Inhibitory Effect of Ganoderma lucidum on Platelet Aggregation," J Tongii Med Univ, 1990, 10(4):240-3.

Yoon SY, Eo SK, Kim YS, et al, "Antimicrobial Activity of Ganoderma lucidum Extract Alone and in Combination With Some Antibiotics," Arch Pharm Res, 1994, 17(6):438-42.

♦ **Retinol** *see* Vitamin A (Retinol) *on page 518*

♦ **Rhamnus persiana** *see* Cascara (Rhamnus persiana) *on page 404*

♦ **Riboflavin** *see* Vitamin B$_2$ *on page 520*

♦ **Rosacea** *see page 318*

♦ **S-adenosylmethionine** *see* SAMe (S-adenosyl methionine) *on page 498*

♦ **Salix alba** *see* White Willow (Salix alba) *on page 532*

♦ **Sambucus canadensis (American Elder)** *see* Elder (Sambucus nigra, Sambucus canadensis) *on page 428*

♦ **Sambucus nigra (European Elder)** *see* Elder (Sambucus nigra, Sambucus canadensis) *on page 428*

SAMe (S-adenosyl methionine)

Related Information

Nutraceutical Chart *on page 573*

Natural Product Category Nutraceutical

Dosage Oral: Dosage range: 400-1600 mg/day

Active Forms S-adenosyl methionine

Reported Uses

Cardiovascular disease (Loehrer, 1996)

Depression (Kagan, 1990; Fava, 1995; Bressa, 1994; Rosenbaum, 1990)

Fibromyalgia (Jacobsen, 1991)

Insomnia (Sitaram, 1995)
Liver disease (Miglio, 1975)
Osteoarthritis (di Padova, 1987)
Rheumatoid arthritis (Polli, 1975)

Summary SAMe is formed from the essential amino acid methionine. It is a cofactor in three important biochemical pathways, and is synthesized throughout the body. Due to the nature and scope of biochemical reactions that it regulates, SAMe has been investigated for its effects in depression, fibromyalgia, arthritis, and cardiovascular disease.

Pharmacology S-adenosyl methionine is involved in several primary biochemical pathways. It functions as a methyl donor in synthetic pathways which form nucleic acids (DNA and RNA), proteins, phospholipids, and neurotransmitters. SAMe's role in phospholipid synthesis may influence membrane fluidity. It has also been noted to protect neuronal anoxia and promote myelination of nerve fibers. It is involved in trans-sulfuration reactions, regulating formation of sulfur-containing amino acids such as cysteine, glutathione, and taurine. Of note, glutathione is an important antioxidant, involved in the detoxification of a number of physiologic and environmental toxins. SAMe is also a cofactor in the synthesis of polyamines, which include spermidine, puescine, and spermine. Polyamines are essential for cellular growth and differentiation by virtue of their effects on gene expression, protein phosphorylation, neuron regeneration, and the DNA repair.

Toxicities, Warnings, and Interactions Minor side effects, including dry mouth, nausea, and restlessness are occasionally reported. Use caution when combining SAMe with other antidepressants, tryptophan, or 5-HTP. SAMe is not effective in the treatment of depressive symptoms associated with bipolar disorder.

Has been reported to block platelet aggregation *in vitro* (De la Cruz, 1997; De la Cruz, 1997); contraindicated in individuals with active bleeding (eg, peptic ulcer, intracranial bleeding). Use with caution in individuals with a history of bleeding, hemostatic disorders, or drug-related hemostatic problems. Use with caution in individuals taking anticoagulant medications, including warfarin, aspirin, aspirin-containing products, NSAIDs, or antiplatelet agents (eg, ticlopidine, clopidogrel, dipyridamole). Discontinue use prior to dental or surgical procedures (generally at least 14 days before).

Symptoms of Deficiency A specific deficiency syndrome has not been adequately defined. As an essential cofactor in multiple biochemical pathways, a wide variety of symptoms are potentially related to a deficiency in SAMe.

Reported Interactions
Drug/Nutrient Interactions: May potentiate activity and/or toxicities of MAO inhibitors, tricyclic antidepressants, or SSRIs (not documented)
Nutrient/Nutrient Interactions: May potentiate the antidepressant effects of 5-HTP, tryptophan, and St John's wort

References

Bressa GM, "S-Adenosyl-L-Methionine (SAMe) as Antidepressant: Meta-Analysis of Clinical Studies," *Acta Neurol Scand*, Suppl 1994, 154:7-14.

De La Cruz JP, Gonzalez-Correa JA, Martin-Aurioles E, et al, "Effects of S-Adenosyl-L-Methionine on Platelet Thromboxane and Vascular Prostacyclin, *Biochem Pharmacol*, 1997, 53(11):1761-3.

De la Cruz JP, Merida M, Gonzalez-Correa JA, et al, "Effects of S-Adenosyl-L-Methionine on Blood Platelet Activation," *Gen Pharmacol*, 1997, 29(4):651-5.

di Padova C, "S-Adenosylmethionine in the Treatment of Osteoarthritis. Review of the Clinical Studies," *Am J Med*, 1987, 83(5A):60-5.

Fava M, Giannelli A, Rapisarda V, et al, "Rapidity of Onset of the Antidepressant Effect of Parenteral S-Adenosyl-L-Methionine, *Psychiatry Res*, 1995, 56(3):295-7.

Jacobsen S, Danneskiold-Samsoe B, and Anderson BB, "Oral S-Adenosylmethionine in Primary Fibromyalgia. Double-Blind Clinical Evaluation," *Scand J Rheumatol*, 1991, 20(4):294-302.

Kagan BL, Sultzer DL, Rosenlicht N, et al, "Oral S-Adenosylmethionine in Depression: A Randomized, Double-Blind, Placebo-Controlled Trial," *Am J Psychiatry*, 1990, 147(5):591-5.

Loehrer FM, Angst CP, Haefeli WE, et al, "Low Whole-Blood S-Adenosylmethionine and Correlation Between 5-Methyltetrahydrofolate and Homocysteine in Coronary Artery Disease," *Arterioscler Thromb Vasc Biol*, 1996, 16(6):727-33.

(Continued)

SAMe (S-adenosyl methionine) (Continued)

Miglio F, Stefanini GF, Corazza GR, et al, "Double-Blind Studies of the Therapeutic Action of S-Adenosylmethionine (SAMe) in Oral Administration, in Liver Cirrhosis and Other Chronic Hepatitides," *Minerva Med*, 1975, 66(33):1595-9.

Polli E, Cortellareo M, Parrini L, et al, "Pharmacological and Clinical Aspects of S-Adenosylme-thionine (SAMe) in Primary Degenerative Arthropathy," *Minerva Med*, 1975, 66(83):4443-59.

Rosenbaum JF, Fava M, Falk WE, et al, "The Antidepressant Potential of Oral S-Adenosyl-L-Methionine, *Acta Psychiatr Scand*, 1990, 81(5):432-6.

Sitaram BR, Sitaram M, Traut M, et al, "Nyctohemeral Rhythm in the Levels of S-Adenosylme-thionine in the Rat Pineal Gland and Its Relationship to Melatonin Biosynthesis," *J Neurochem*, 1995, 65(4):1887-94.

Saw Palmetto (Serenoa repens)

Related Information

Herb/Drug Potential Interactions *on page 642*
Herb Quick Reference Chart *on page 538*

Natural Product Category Herb

Plant Part Berry

Dosage and Standardization Oral: 160 mg twice daily, standardized to contain at least 80% to 90% fatty acids and sterols per dose

Reported Uses Benign prostatic hypertrophy (BPH) (Plosker, 1996; Strauch, 1994; Braeckman, 1994)

Summary Saw palmetto is used in men to improve symptoms of benign prostatic hyperplasia (BPH). Several studies have reported that the effects of saw palmetto are comparable to symptomatic improvements which result from medications commonly used for this disorder.

Pharmacology Excessive formation of dihydrotestosterone (DHT) is believed to stimulate enlargement of the prostate (hyperplasia). Estrogen inhibits the elimination of DHT. There are three mechanisms by which saw palmetto alters the effects of DHT. It is reported to inhibit production, inhibition receptor binding, and to accelerate the metabolism of DHT. Saw palmetto is reported to exert antiestrogenic effects, which may mediate some of the improvement in symptoms. Saw palmetto has been reported to decrease prostate size, but does not alter PSA levels (Gerber, 1998)

Theoretical Cautions and Contraindications Based on its pharmacological activity, use with caution in individuals receiving treatments for BPH (alpha-adrenergic blocking agents, finasteride) (Goepel, 1999). Individuals should have a prostatic exam and laboratory studies (PSA) to rule out cancer prior to use for symptoms of BPH.

General Warnings Use all herbal supplements with extreme caution in children <2 years of age and in pregnancy or lactation. Some herbs are contraindicated in pregnancy or lactation; make sure to observe warnings. Use with caution in individuals on medication and with pre-existing medical conditions. Always review for potential herb-drug interactions (HDIs) and other warnings. Large and prolonged doses may increase the potential for adverse effects. Herbs may cause transient adverse effects such as nausea, vomiting, and GI distress due to a variety of chemical constituents. Caution should be used in individuals having known allergies to plants.

Theoretical Interactions Oral contraceptives, estrogens, alpha-adrenergic blockers, finasteride

References

Braeckman J, "The Extract of *Serenoa repens* in the Treatment of Benign Prostatic Hyper-plasia: A Multicenter Open Study," *Curr Ther Res*, 1994, 55(7):76-84.

Gerber GS, Zagaja GP, Bales GT, et al, "Saw Palmetto (*Serenoa repens*) in Men in Lower Urinary Tract Symptoms: Effects on Urodynamics Parameters and Voiding Symptoms," *Urology*, 1998, 51(6):1003-7.

Goepel M, Hecker U, Krege S, et al, "Saw Palmetto Extracts Potently and Non-competitively Inhibit Human Alpha 1-Adrenoceptors *In Vitro*," *Prostate*, 1999, 38(3):208-15.

Plosker GL and Brogden RN, "*Serenoa repens* (Permixon). A Review of Its Pharmacology and Therapeutic Efficacy in Benign Prostatic Hyperplasia," *Drugs Aging*, 1996, 9(5):379-95.

Strauch G, Perles P, Vergult G, et al, "Comparison of Finasteride (Proscar) and *Serenoa repens*(Permixon) in the Inhibition of 5-Alpha Reductase in Healthy Male Volunteers," *Eur Urol*, 1994, 26(3):247-52.

Schisandra *(Schizandra chinensis)*

Related Information

Herb/Drug Potential Interactions *on page 642*
Herb Quick Reference Chart *on page 538*
Organ System Support Using Natural Products *on page 660*

Natural Product Category Herb

Plant Part Berry

Dosage and Standardization Oral: 100 mg twice daily, standardized to contain at least 9% schisandrins per dose

Reported Uses

Adaptogen/health tonic; hepatic protection and detoxification (Yamada, 1993; Liu, 1989)

Adjunct support for chemotherapy and radiation (Lin, 1991)

Increased endurance, stamina, and work performance (Volicer, 1965; Fuekawa, 1987)

Summary Schisandra has been used in Chinese medicine for centuries. It has been used as an adaptogen, increasing the body's ability to adapt to stresses from chemical, physical, psychological, and environmental sources. Schisandra has been reported to increase human endurance and mental and physical performance. It is believed to be hepatoprotective and has been reported to have a cardioprotective action during administration of doxorubicin (Adriamycin®).

Pharmacology Schisandra has been demonstrated to stimulate hepatic glycogen synthesis, protein synthesis, and to increase microsomal enzyme activity. In addition, these compounds function as antioxidants and protect hepatocyte cell membranes. Schisandra has been reported to prevent liver damage, stimulate liver repair and stimulate normal liver function. Schisandra has been reported to improve cognitive processes, visual, tactile, and auditory sensitivity. It has also been reported to have cardioprotective action during the administration of adriamycin (Lin, 1991).

Theoretical Cautions and Contraindications Contraindicated in pregnancy due to uterine stimulation in animal studies (Liu 1989). Theoretically, enzyme enhancement may alter metabolism of many drugs; caution with drugs which may have a narrow therapeutic window. Use with caution in individuals on calcium channel blockers (Fuekawa 1987).

General Warnings Use all herbal supplements with extreme caution in children <2 years of age and in pregnancy or lactation. Some herbs are contraindicated in pregnancy or lactation; make sure to observe warnings. Use with caution in individuals on medication and with pre-existing medical conditions. Always review for potential herb-drug interactions (HDIs) and other warnings. Large and prolonged doses may increase the potential for adverse effects. Herbs may cause transient adverse effects such as nausea, vomiting, and GI distress due to a variety of chemical constituents. Caution should be used in individuals having known allergies to plants.

Theoretical Interactions Calcium channel blockers. In addition, cytochrome P450 enzyme induction may alter the metabolism of many drugs.

References

Liu GT, "Pharmacological Actions and Clinical Use of *Fructus schizandrae*," *Chin Med J (Engl)*, 1989, 102(10):740-9.

Lin TJ, "Antioxidation Mechanism of Schizandrin and Tanshinonatic Acid A and Their Effects on the Protection of Cardiotoxic Action of Adriamycin," *Sheng Li Ko Hsueh Chin Chan*, 1991, 22(4):342-5.

Juekawa M, Shiga T, Sone H, "Effects of Gomisin J and Analogous Lignan Compounds in Schisandra Fruits on Isolated Smooth Muscles," *Yakugaku Zasshi*, 1987, 107(9):720-6.

Volicer L, Janku I, Motl O, "The Mode of Action of Schisandra chinensis," in Pharmacology of Oriental Plants (New York: Pergamon Press Books, Macmillan Company, 1965).

Yamada S, Murawaki Y, and Kawasaki H, "Preventive Effect of Gomisin A, a Lignan Component of Shizandra Fruits, on Acetaminophen-Induced Hepatotoxicity in Rats," *Biochem Pharmacol*, 1993, 46(6):1081-5.

♦ *Schisandra chinensis* see Schisandra *(Schizandra chinensis)* on page 501

♦ **Scleroderma** see page 322

Selenium

Related Information

Drug-Induced Nutrient Depletions *on page 625*
Organ System Support Using Natural Products *on page 660*
Pregnancy & Lactation Nutritional Chart *on page 657*
Vitamins/Minerals/Trace Elements/Amino Acids Chart *on page 604*

Natural Product Category Mineral

Dosage Oral: RDI: Males: 70 mcg/day, females: 55 mcg/day; ODA: 200 mcg/day

Active Forms Sodium selenite, selenomethioine, high-selenium yeast

Reported Uses

AIDS (Schrauzer, 1994)
Atherosclerosis (Yegin, 1997)
Bronchial asthma (Kadrabova, 1996)
Cancer prevention (Clark, 1996)
Cardiomyopathy (Huttunen, 1997)
Cataracts (Karakucuk, 1995)
Chemotherapy/radiation support (Sundstrom, 1989)
Eczema (Juhlin, 1982)

Summary Selenium is recognized as an important nutritional trace mineral. Selenium plays important roles in detoxification and antioxidant defense mechanisms in the body. Deficiency of this mineral has been implicated as a cause of cardiomyopathy in some individuals. In addition, low concentrations have been correlated to asthma, cancer incidence, atherosclerosis, and cataracts.

Pharmacology Selenium has been reported to demonstrate antiviral activity, increasing T-lymphocytes and enhancing the activity of natural killer cells. It also participates as a cofactor in glutathione peroxidase, an important antioxidant enzyme. It neutralizes hydrogen peroxide radicals and reduces lipid peroxidation. In addition, selenium potentiates the antioxidant effects of vitamin E. Selenium participates in the detoxification of heavy metals such as mercury and cadmium. It has also been found to serve as a cofactor for deiodinase, which converts thyroxine (T_4) to the more active triiodothyronine (T_3).

Toxicities, Warnings, and Interactions Rare cases of thrombocytopenia and hepatorenal dysfunction
Toxic dose: Intake should be restricted to no more than 700 mcg/day unless supervised by a physician
Toxicity symptoms: Loss of hair and nails, skin lesions, nervous system abnormalities, digestive dysfunction, and a garlic-like breath odor. Although deaths from toxicity have been reported in livestock, no deaths have occurred in humans.

Symptoms of Deficiency Muscle soreness, red blood cell fragility, destructive changes to the heart and pancreas, immune system dysfunction

Reported Interactions

Drug/Nutrient Interactions: High-dose corticosteroid therapy can cause depressed plasma selenium levels in some individuals with rheumatoid arthritis.

Nutrient/Nutrient Interactions: None known

References

Clark LC, Combs GF Jr, Turnbull BW, et al, "Effects of Selenium Supplementation for Cancer Prevention in Patients With Carcinoma of the Skin. A Randomized Controlled Trial. Nutritional Prevention of Cancer Study Group," *JAMA*, 1996, 276(24):1957-63.

Huttunen JK, "Selenium and Cardiovascular Diseases - An Update," *Biomed Environ Sci*, 1997, 10(2-3):220-6.

Juhlin L, Edquist LE, Ekman LG, et al, "Blood Glutathione-Peroxidase Levels in Skin Diseases: Effect of Selenium and Vitamin E Treatment," *Acta Derm Venereol*, 1982, 62(3):211-4.

Kadrabova J, Mad'aric A, Kovacikova Z, et al, "Selenium Status Is Decreased in Patients With Intrinsic Asthma," *Biol Trace Elem Res*, 1996, 52(3):241-8.

Karakucuk S, Ertugrul Mirza G, Faruk Ekinciler O, et al, "Selenium Concentrations in Serum, Lens and Aqueous Humour of Patients With Senile Cataract," *Acta Ophthalmol Scand*, 1995, 73(4):329-32.

Schrauzer GN and Sacher J, "Selenium in the Maintenance and Therapy of HIV-Infected Patients," *Chem Biol Interact*, 1994, 91(2-3):199-205.

Sundstrom H, Korpela H, Sajanti E, et al, "Supplementation With Selenium, Vitamin E and Their Combination in Gynaecological Cancer During Cytotoxic Chemotherapy," *Carcogenogenesis*, 1989, 10(2):273-8.

Yegin A, Yegin H, Aliciguzel Y, et al, "Erythrocyte Selenium-Glutathione Peroxidase Activity Is Lower in Patients With Coronary Atherosclerosis, *Jpn Heart J*, 1997, 38(6):793-8.

Senna *(Cassia senna)*

Related Information

Herb/Drug Potential Interactions *on page 642*
Herb Quick Reference Chart *on page 538*

Natural Product Category Herb

Plant Part Seed

Dosage and Standardization Oral: 15-30 mg of sennosides per dose at bedtime

Reported Uses Anthraquinone laxative (Newall, 1996)

Summary Senna leaf is used in many cultures as a laxative. In the United States, senna is a popular over-the-counter laxative used in constipation.

Pharmacology Senna contains hydroxyanthracene glycosides that are not fully absorbed in the upper intestine, but are converted into active aglycones by the microflora in the large intestine. Senna stimulates colonic motility and influences fluid and electrolyte balance in the colon.

Theoretical Cautions and Contraindications Avoid in children less than 12 years of age. Based on its pharmacological effects, senna may increase potassium loss and may decrease absorption of oral medications by decreasing bowel transit time (Brinker 1997). Contraindicated in bowel obstruction, diarrhea, or dehydration. Use with caution in bowel disorders, inflammatory bowel disease (ulcerative colitis, Crohn's disease), and appendicitis. Use with caution in cardiovascular disease (overuse may cause electrolyte disorders). Excessive use may lead to potassium loss and other electrolyte disturbances, and may potentiate the effects of various drugs with narrow therapeutic windows. Overuse may lead to bowel atony.

General Warnings Use all herbal supplements with extreme caution in children <2 years of age and in pregnancy or lactation. Some herbs are contraindicated in pregnancy or lactation; make sure to observe warnings. Use with caution in individuals on medication and with pre-existing medical conditions. Always review for potential herb-drug interactions (HDIs) and other warnings. Large and prolonged doses may increase the potential for adverse effects. Herbs may cause transient adverse effects such as nausea, vomiting, and GI distress due to a variety of chemical constituents. Caution should be used in individuals having known allergies to plants.

Theoretical Interactions Absorption of oral medications could be altered; antiarrhythmics, digoxin, phenytoin, laxatives, lithium, theophylline, potassium-depleting diuretics

References

Brinker F, *Herb Contraindications and Drug Interactions*, Sandy, OR: Eclectic Medical Publications, 1998, 70.

Newall CA, Anderson La, and Phillipson JD, *Herbal Medicines: A Guide for Health Care Professionals*, London, England: The Pharmaceutical Press, 1996, 243-4.

♦ *Serenoa repens* see Saw Palmetto *(Serenoa repens) on page 500*
♦ **Sexual Vitality (Females)** *see page 326*
♦ **Sexual Vitality (Males)** *see page 330*

Shark Cartilage

Related Information

Nutraceutical Chart *on page 573*

Natural Product Category Nutraceutical

Dosage

Oral: Dosage range: 3000 mg 3 times/day, taken 20 minutes before meals
Rectal: Retention enemas; 15-20 g/day

Active Forms Shark cartilage

Reported Uses

Cancer therapy (Prudden, 1985; Lane, 1992)
Osteoarthritis, rheumatoid arthritis (Lane, 1992)
(Continued)

Shark Cartilage *(Continued)*

Summary Shark cartilage products have become popular as supplement for individuals with cancer and for use in osteoarthritis.

Pharmacology Cartilage tissue contains substances called antiangiogenesis factors that inhibit the growth of new blood vessels. It has been hypothesized that high doses of shark cartilage may prevent tumor growth. The proposed mechanism is that the antiangiogenesis factors prevent tumors from developing the network of blood vessels they need to supply them with nutrients. This reportedly "starves" tumors and causes them to shrink. Cartilage tissue is a mixture of glycosaminoglycans (GAGs). One of the primary GAGs is chondroitin sulfate, which may provide some benefit for people with osteoarthritis.

Toxicities, Warnings, and Interactions May cause gastrointestinal upset (nausea)

Symptoms of Deficiency Deficiency studies in humans have not been conducted

Reported Interactions
  Drug/Nutrient Interactions: None known
  Nutrient/Nutrient Interactions: None known

References
Lane IW, *Sharks Don't Get Cancer*, Garden City Park, New York: Avery Publishing Group, 1992, 107-18.
Prudden JF, "The Treatment of Human Cancer With Agents Prepared From Bovine Cartilage," *J Biol Response Mod*, 1985, 4(6):551-84.

♦ **Siberian Ginseng** *see* Ginseng, Siberian *(Eleutherococcus senticosus)* on page 444
♦ **Silybum marianum** *see* Milk Thistle *(Silybum marianum)* on page 479
♦ **Sinusitis** *see* page 334

Sodium

Related Information
  Drug-Induced Nutrient Depletions *on page 625*
  Vitamins/Minerals/Trace Elements/Amino Acids Chart *on page 604*

Natural Product Category Mineral

Dosage Oral: RDI: None established; ODA: None established; experts recommend keeping sodium intake to <3000 mg/day

Active Forms Sodium chloride

Reported Uses No major reported therapeutic uses

Summary Sodium is one of the body's three major electrolytes (the other two being potassium and chloride). They exist as fully dissociated ions and are the main particles responsible for osmotic pressure in body fluids. Sodium is the primary extracellular electrolyte in body fluids. These substances are called electrolytes because they carry an electronic charge in their dissociated (ionic) state. Their ionic strength enables them to influence the solubility of proteins and other substances throughout the body. Most Americans consume too much sodium.

Most foods are a source of sodium, especially salted foods, soy sauce, cheese, milk, seafood, and water.

Pharmacology Sodium influences blood pressure regulation and also plays a critical role in the transmission of electrochemical impulses for nerve function and muscle contraction. Sodium helps regulate the acid/alkaline balance in the blood and lymphatic fluids. It also plays a role in the transport and excretion of CO_2. Sodium helps control and operate the sodium/potassium pump, which regulates cell wall permeability and facilitates the transport of materials across cell membranes.

Toxicities, Warnings, and Interactions Use with caution in cardiovascular, renal, or hepatic disease.
  Toxic symptoms: Excessive sodium intake is associated with high blood pressure and edema

Symptoms of Deficiency Deficiency is uncommon and usually induced by excessive vomiting, diarrhea, profuse sweating; fainting; intolerance to heat; muscle cramps; swelling in extremities

♦ **Sore Throat** see page 338

♦ **Soy Isoflavones** see Isoflavones (Soy) on page 465

Spleen Extract

Related Information
Nutraceutical Chart on page 573

Natural Product Category Nutraceutical

Dosage Oral: 150-300 mg 2-3 times/day

Active Forms Spleen extract

Reported Uses Support following removal of the spleen or for individuals with weak spleen function

Summary The spleen provides a variety of immune system-related functions in the body, such as producing white blood cells, destroying bacteria and cellular debris, and breaking down and recycling worn-out red blood cells and platelets.

Pharmacology Two compounds produced in the spleen provide profound immune system-enhancing activity. Tuftsin stimulates the production of macrophages, which are cells that destroy and remove foreign particles such as bacteria, cancer cells, and other cellular debris from the body. Splentopentin enhances immune function by increasing the production of compounds like interleukin-3 and by increasing the activity of natural killer cells.

Toxicities, Warnings, and Interactions No known toxicity or serious side effects reported.

Symptoms of Deficiency The ingredients in spleen extracts are not essential nutrients for humans, so no deficiency condition exists. However, people with weak or nonexistent spleen function would be expected to have compromised immune systems.

Reported Interactions
Drug/Nutrient Interactions: None known
Nutrient/Nutrient Interactions: None known

Stinging Nettle (Urtica dioica)

Related Information
Common Herbal Supplements Contraindicated During Pregnancy on page 656
Herb Quick Reference Chart on page 538

Natural Product Category Herb

Plant Part Leaf, root (See Reported Uses)

Dosage and Standardization Oral:
Leaf: 300-1200 mg 2-4 times/day as needed of freeze-dried leaf
Root: 250 mg 1-3 times/day, standardized to contain 1% to 2% plant silica per dose

Reported Uses
Leaf: Allergic rhinitis (Mittman, 1990)
Leaf: Increases uric acid excretion (Bradley, 1992)
Root: Benign prostatic hyperplasia (BPH) (Krzeski, 1993; Wagner, 1989)

Summary Stinging nettle leaf has gained increasing recognition for allergic rhinitis (leaf). Stinging nettle root has also been used for its ability to reduce the symptoms of BPH. Stinging nettle leaf has also been used for gout as a consequence of its reported ability to promote the excretion of uric acid.

Pharmacology

Root: Stinging nettle root is reported to inhibit binding to cytosolic androgen receptors within prostatic tissues. It also inhibits the effects of estrogen and should be avoided in pregnancy due to potential uterine stimulation. Stinging nettle root is claimed to influence the binding of 5 alpha-dihydrotestosterone with its receptors.
(Continued)

Stinging Nettle *(Urtica dioica) (Continued)*

Stinging nettle leaf is used to increase the renal excretion of uric acid and mobilizes tissue stores. Freeze-dried stinging nettle leaf has been reported to have antihistaminic properties and may be useful for symptoms of allergic rhinitis.

Theoretical Cautions and Contraindications Use of stinging nettle is contraindicated in pregnancy (uterine stimulation in animal studies, Brinker, 1997). Use with caution in individuals with renal insufficiency or disease (due to silica content in leaf). Prostate exam and laboratory testing should be performed to rule out cancer prior to use for symptoms of BPH. Based on pharmacological activity, use with caution in individuals with gout or a history of uric acid renal stones.

General Warnings Use all herbal supplements with extreme caution in children <2 years of age and in pregnancy or lactation. Some herbs are contraindicated in pregnancy or lactation; make sure to observe warnings. Use with caution in individuals on medication and with pre-existing medical conditions. Always review for potential herb-drug interactions (HDIs) and other warnings. Large and prolonged doses may increase the potential for adverse effects. Herbs may cause transient adverse effects such as nausea, vomiting, and GI distress due to a variety of chemical constituents. Caution should be used in individuals having known allergies to plants.

Theoretical Interactions None known. At high intakes, may alter response to warfarin (due to vitamin K content).

References

Bradley PR, ed, *The British Herbal Compendium, Vol 1*, London, England: British Herbal Medicine Association, 1992, 166-67.

Brinker F, *Herb Contraindications and Drug Interactions*, Sandy, OR: Eclectic Medical Publications, 1998, 83.

Krzeski T, Kazon M, Borkowski A, et al, "Combined Extracts of *Urtica dioica* and *Pygeum africanum* in the Treatment of Benign Prostatic Hyperplasia: Double-Blind Comparison of Two Doses," *Clin Ther*, 1993, 15(6):1011-20.

Mittman P, "Randomized, Double-blind Study of Freeze-Dried *Urtica dioca* in the Treatment of Allergic Rhinitis," *Planta Med*, 1990, 56(1):44-7.

Wagner H, Willer F, and Kreher B, "Biologically Active Compounds From the Aqueous Extract of *Urtica dioica*," *Planta Med*, 1989, 55(5):452-4.

St John's Wort *(Hypericum perforatum)*

Related Information

Common Herbal Supplements Contraindicated During Pregnancy *on page 656*

Herb/Drug Potential Interactions *on page 642*

Herb Quick Reference Chart *on page 538*

Natural Product Category Herb

Plant Part Flowering buds

Dosage and Standardization Note: Use varies with route of administration; see Reported Uses

Oral: 300 mg 3 times/day, standardized to contain 0.3% to 0.5% hypericin and/or 3% to 5% hyperforin per dose; minimum of 4-6 weeks of therapy is recommended before results may be seen.

Topical: Apply oil extract as needed to affected area

Reported Uses

Antiviral activity in increased doses (Miller, 1998)

Antibacterial, anti-inflammatory; used topically for minor wounds and infections (Newall, 1996)

May be used topically for bruises, muscle soreness, and sprains (Newall, 1996)

Used in mild to moderate depression, melancholia, and anxiety (Cott, 1998; Hippius, 1998; Volz, 1997; Harrer, 1999; Linde, 1996; Vorbach, 1997)

Summary St John's wort has been used in Europe for centuries for mild to moderate depression. It has attracted increased attention as a safe and natural alternative to current prescription therapies in the United States. Comparative trials with tricyclic antidepressants have been favorable, and comparative trials with SSRIs are ongoing. St John's wort has also been used as a topical preparation to accelerate wound and burn healing, and to improve muscle soreness/stiffness and neuralgia.

Pharmacology St John's wort is a perennial flowering plant, which grows in many areas of the world, including Europe and the United States. The activity has been correlated to the hypericin component of the plant. It is believed to act through a variety of mechanisms, including inhibition of cortisol secretion, blockade of catabolic hormones (such as IL-6), and increased concentrations of central nervous system neurotransmitters, including serotonin. It may have mild MAO-inhibiting activity, but this does not appear to be its major mechanism of action. St John's wort may amplify the response to serotonin following receptor binding.

Additionally, hypericin and xanthrones have been claimed to have antiviral activity, including activity in HIV, by stimulating an increase in T killer cell activity.

Theoretical Cautions and Contraindications St. John's wort is contraindicated in pregnancy (based on animal studies, Grush 1998). Use with caution in individual's taking digoxin (may alter levels of this medication, Johne 1999). It is not for use in severe depression. Use with caution in individuals taking other antidepressants (Gordon, 1998). Based on its pharmacological activity, St John's wort may alter the actions of monoamine oxidase (MAO) inhibitors, tricyclic antidepressants, and selective serotonin reuptake inhibitors (SSRIs) (Chatterjee, 1998; Bennett, 1998). May elevate hepatic transaminases (noted animal studies at high doses) (Brockmoller, 1990). May cause photosensitivity (based on animal studies and a human clinical trial) (Brockmoller, 1997). Use with caution in individuals on reserpine (effects may be antagonized by St John's wort) (Okpanyi, 1987). Use with caution in individuals on narcotic medications (based on animal studies, may enhance sedation from these drugs) (Okpanyi, 1987).

May cause drowsiness (mild). Based on pharmacological activity, use with caution while driving or operating machinery. Caution in individuals taking sedative medications (eg, anxiolytics, benzodiazepines). Effects may be additive with other CNS depressants or natural products with sedative properties.

Antidepressant therapy may precipitate a shift to mania or hypomania in individuals with bipolar affective disorder (Schneck, 1998).

General Warnings Use all herbal supplements with extreme caution in children <2 years of age and in pregnancy or lactation. Some herbs are contraindicated in pregnancy or lactation; make sure to observe warnings. Use with caution in individuals on medication and with pre-existing medical conditions. Always review for potential herb-drug interactions (HDIs) and other warnings. Large and prolonged doses may increase the potential for adverse effects. Herbs may cause transient adverse effects such as nausea, vomiting, and GI distress due to a variety of chemical constituents. Caution should be used in individuals having known allergies to plants.

Theoretical Interactions Sedatives, CNS depressants, photosensitizing drugs, antidepressants (including SSRIs and tricyclics), MAO inhibitors, narcotics, narcotic analgesics, digoxin

References

Bennett DA Jr, Phun L, Polk JF, et al, "Neuropharmacology of St John's Wort (*Hypericum*)," *Ann Pharmacother*, 1998, 32(11):1201-8.

Brockmoller J, Reum T, Bauer S, et al, "Hypericin and Pseudohypericin: Pharmacokinetics and Effects of Photosensitivity in Humans," *Pharmacopsychiatry*, 1997, 30(Supp 2):94-101.

Chatterjee SS, Bhattacharya SK, Wonnemann M, et al, "Hyperforin As a Possible Antidepressant Component of *Hypericum* Extracts," *Life Sci*, 1998, 63(6):499-510.

Cott JM and Fugh-Berman A, "Is St John's Wort (*Hypericum perforatum*) an Effective Antidepressant?" *J Nerv Ment Dis*, 1998, 186(8):500-1.

Gordon JB, "SSRIs and St John's Wort: Possible Toxicity?" *Am Fam Physician*, 1998, 57(5):950,953.

Grush LR, Nierenberg A, Keefe B, et al, "St John's Wort During Pregnancy," *JAMA*, 1998, 280(18):1566.

Harrer G, Schmidt U, Kuhn U, et al, "Comparison of Equivalence Between the St John's Wort Extract LoHyp-57 and Fluoxetine," *Arzneimittelforschung*, 1999, 49(4):289-96.

Hippius H, "St John's Wort (*Hypericum perforatum*) - A Herbal Antidepressant," *Curr Med Res Opin*, 1998, 14(3):171-84.

(Continued)

St John's Wort *(Hypericum perforatum)* *(Continued)*

Johne A, Brockmoller J, Bauer S, et al, "Pharmacokinetic Interaction of Digoxin With an Herbal Extract from St John's Wort," *Clin Pharmacol Ther*, 1999, 66(4):338-45.

Linde K, Ramirez G, Mulrow CD, et al, "St John's Wort for Depression—An Overview and Meta-analysis of Randomised Clinical Trials," *BMJ*, 1996 313(7052):253-8.

Miller AL, "St John's Wort *(Hypericum perforatum)*: Clinical Effects on Depression and Other Conditions," *Altern Med Rev*, 1998, 3(1):18-26.

Newall CA, Anderson LA, and Phillipson JD, *Herbal Medicines: A Guide for Health Care Professionals*, London, England: The Pharmaceutical Press, 1996, 250-2.

Okpanyi SN and Weischer ML, "Animal Experiments on the Psychotropic Action of a *Hypericum* Extract," *Arzneimittelforschung*, 1987, 37(1):10-3.

Schneck C, "St John's Wort and Hypomania," *J Clin Psychiatry*, 1998 59(12):689.

Volz HP, "Controlled Clinical Trials of *Hypericum* Extracts in Depressed Patients - An Overview," *Pharmacopsychiatry*, 1997, 30(Suppl 2):72-6.

Vorbach EU, Arnoldt KH, and Hubner WD, "Efficacy and Tolerability of St John's Wort Extract LI 160 Versus Imipramine in Patients With Severe Depressive Episodes According to ICD-10," *Pharmacopsychiatry*, 1997, Suppl 2:81-5.

♦ **Stress / Anxiety** *see page 342*

♦ **Suggested Daily Intake of Nutritional Supplements** *see page 27*

♦ **Sunburn** *see page 346*

♦ **Systemic Lupus Erythematosus (SLE)** *see page 350*

♦ ***Syzygium aromaticum*** *see* Clove *(Syzygium aromaticum) on page 411*

♦ ***Tanacetum parthenium*** *see* Feverfew *(Tanacetum parthenium) on page 432*

♦ ***Taraxacum officinale*** *see* Dandelion *(Taraxacum officinale) on page 420*

Taurine

Related Information
Vitamins/Minerals/Trace Elements/Amino Acids Chart *on page 604*

Natural Product Category Amino Acid

Dosage Oral: RDI: None established; ODA: 1500-3000 mg/day

Active Forms L-taurine

Reported Uses
Congestive heart failure (CHF) (Azuma, 1983)
Diabetes (Franconi, 1995)
Epilepsy (Fukuyama, 1982)
Hypertension (Fujita, 1987)

Summary Although humans can normally synthesize taurine, under certain conditions some individuals are not able to generate enough, making it an essential nutrient for those people. Taurine is essential for preterm and newborn infants because they have not yet developed synthetic capacity for this amino acid. Supplementation may be beneficial in epilepsy, cardiovascular disease (congestive heart failure, hypertension), and diabetes.

Pharmacology As with any amino acid, taurine is required for the synthesis of proteins. In addition, it functions as an inhibitory neurotransmitter, potentially limiting aberrant neuronal discharges. It may assist in the regulation of cardiac conduction and contractility. In addition, it may protect the retinal photoreceptors from damage. Taurine appears to modulate intracellular fluid volume, particularly within the brain and kidneys. As a component of bile salts, it facilitates the emulsification and absorption of fats and fat-soluble vitamins.

Toxicities, Warnings, and Interactions No known toxicity or serious side effects

Symptoms of Deficiency In preterm and term infants, taurine insufficiency results in impaired bile acid secretion, fat malabsorption, vision disturbances, and hepatic dysfunction. These may be reversed by taurine supplementation.

Reported Interactions
Drug/Nutrient Interactions: None known
Nutrient/Nutrient Interactions: None known

References
Azuma J, Hasegawa H, Sawamura A, et al, "Therapy of Congestive Heart Failure With Orally Administered Taurine," *Clin Ther*, 1983, 5(4):398-408.

Franconi F, Bennardini F, Mattana A, et al, "Plasma and Platelet Taurine Are Reduced in Subjects With Insulin-Dependent Diabetes Mellitus: Effects of Taurine Supplementation," *Am J Clin Nutr*, 1995, 61(5):1115-9.

Fujita T, Ando K, Noda H, et al, "Effects of Increased Adrenomedullary Activity and Taurine in Young Patients With Borderline Hypertension," *Circulation*, 1987, 75(3):525-32.

Fukuyama Y and Ochiai Y, "Therapeutic Trial by Taurine for Intractable Childhood Epilepsies," *Brain Dev*, 1982, 4(1):63-9.

Tea Tree *(Melaleuca alternifolia)*

Related Information
Herb Quick Reference Chart *on page 538*

Natural Product Category Herb

Plant Part Volatile oils

Dosage and Standardization
Oral mouthwash: Dilute a few drops of oil in a cup of water, gargle, and expectorate; **Note: Not for ingestion**

Topical: Apply oil (preferably diluted) to affected area as needed

Reported Uses Not for Ingestion: Antifungal, antibacterial; mouthwash for dental and oral health; burns, cuts, scrapes, insect bites (Carson, 1998; Concha, 1998)

Summary Tea tree oil has been used worldwide as an antiseptic. Tea tree oil is used in mouthwash for dental and oral health. It is also used topically for burns, cuts, scrapes, and insect bites.

Pharmacology Tea tree oil has as antifungal and antibacterial activity. It has been reported to be effective against methicillin-resistant *Staphylococcus aureus*. Tea tree oil has been recognized by the Australian dental profession as an antiseptic mouthwash for use in oral problems such as gingivitis.

Theoretical Cautions and Contraindications NOT FOR INGESTION. May cause allergic dermatitis in sensitive individuals (Rubel 1998)

General Warnings Caution should be used in individuals having known allergies to plants.

Theoretical Interactions None known

References
Carson CF, Riley TV, and Cookson BD, "Efficacy and Safety of Tea Tree Oil as a Topical Antimicrobial Agent," *J Hosp Infect*, 1998, 40(3):175-8.

Concha JM, Moore LS, and Holloway WJ, "1998 William J. Stickel Bronze Award. Antifungal Activity of *Melaleuca alternifolia* (Tea-Tree) Oil Against Various Pathogenic Organisms," *J Am Podiatr Med Assoc*, 1998, 88(10):489-92.

Rubel DM, Freeman S, and Southwell IA, "Tea Tree Oil Allergy: What Is the Offending Agent? Report of Three Cases of Tea Tree Oil Allergy and Review of the Literature," *Australas J Dermatol*, 1998, 39(4):244-7.

- Teething *see page 354*
- Thiamin *see* Vitamin B₁ (Thiamine) *on page 519*
- Thiamine *see* Vitamin B₁ (Thiamine) *on page 519*
- Thioctic acid *see* Alpha-Lipoic Acid *on page 381*

Thyme *(Thymus vulgaris)*

Related Information
Herb/Drug Potential Interactions *on page 642*
Herb Quick Reference Chart *on page 538*

Natural Product Category Herb

Plant Part Leaf

Dosage and Standardization Oral: 20-40 drops (liquid extract 1:1 w/v fresh leaf or 1:4 w/v dried leaf) 3 times/day in juice or beverage

Reported Uses
Antifungal (van den Broucke, 1981)

Used in coughs and upper respiratory congestion (Leung, 1996)

Summary Thyme leaf is renowned for its use as a culinary spice. Traditional uses of thyme include coughs and upper respiratory congestion.

Pharmacology Thyme has antifungal and antibacterial activity. The volatile oils of thyme (thymol and others) also have antitussive and expectorant action.

(Continued)

Thyme *(Thymus vulgaris) (Continued)*

Theoretical Cautions and Contraindications Use with caution in individuals with allergy or hypersensitivity to oregano/*Labitae* spp. Based on pharmacological activity, may affect individuals with urinary tract or gastrointestinal inflammation.

General Warnings Use all herbal supplements with extreme caution in children <2 years of age and in pregnancy or lactation. Some herbs are contraindicated in pregnancy or lactation; make sure to observe warnings. Use with caution in individuals on medication and with pre-existing medical conditions. Always review for potential herb-drug interactions (HDIs) and other warnings. Large and prolonged doses may increase the potential for adverse effects. Herbs may cause transient adverse effects such as nausea, vomiting, and GI distress due to a variety of chemical constituents. Caution should be used in individuals having known allergies to plants.

Theoretical Interactions None known

References

Leung AY and Foster S, *Encyclopedia of Common Natural Ingredients Used in Foods, Drugs, and Cosmetics*, New York, NY: Wiley, 1996, 492-5.

van den Broucke CO and Lemli JA, "Pharmacological and Chemical Investigation of Thyme Liquid Extracts," *Planta Med*, 1981, 41(2):129-35.

Thymus Extract

Related Information

Nutraceutical Chart *on page 573*

Organ System Support Using Natural Products *on page 660*

Natural Product Category Nutraceutical, Glandular

Dosage Oral: Dosage range: 250-500 mg 3 times/day

Active Forms Thymus extract

Reported Uses Immunostimulant (Kosmala, 1993)

Summary The thymus gland is one of the most important components of the immune system. Thymic lymphoid cells, or T cells, mature in the thymus gland and enter the circulatory system. T cells are an important part of the body's cellular immune response.

Pharmacology Thymus extracts contain small amounts of all the immune components of the thymus gland. Their purpose is to provide additional support and enhancement for the immune system. Thymus glandular extract has been reported to be useful in chronic viral infections, autoimmune disease, and to support immune function in radiation, chemotherapy, and allergies.

Toxicities, Warnings, and Interactions No known toxicity or serious side effects have been reported.

Symptoms of Deficiency Deficiency studies in humans have not been conducted.

Reported Interactions Immunosuppressants

References

Kosmala M, Oledzka K, Kaszczynska M, et al, "Pharmacological Properties of the Extract of Thymus Gland (Thymomodulin-TFX) and Its Effect on Reproduction," *Acta Pol Pharm*, 1993, 50(6):447-52.

♦ **Thymus Glandular Extract** *see* Thymus Extract *on page 510*

♦ ***Thymus vulgaris*** *see* Thyme *(Thymus vulgaris) on page 509*

Thyroid Extract

Related Information

Nutraceutical Chart *on page 573*

Natural Product Category Nutraceutical, Glandular

Dosage Oral: Dosage range: 60 mg 1-3 times/day

Active Forms Thyroid extract

Reported Uses

Fatigue; immune support (Haas, 1992)

Summary The primary function of the thyroid gland is to secrete thyroid hormones. The thyroid hormones control and regulate metabolism, which in turn regulates growth and development. The best source for thyroid extract products is New Zealand, where the extracts are free of pesticides, growth hormones, or antibiotics.

Pharmacology Thyroid extracts support thyroid activities and help regulate metabolic activities. They may produce a mild increase in energy and stamina.

Toxicities, Warnings, and Interactions Use with caution in individuals taking thyroid medication. Use with caution in individuals with cardiovascular disease (arrhythmia, coronary artery disease, hypertension). Use with caution in individuals with CNS disorders.

Symptoms of Deficiency Deficiency studies in humans have not been conducted.

Reported Interactions Antithyroid drugs, thyroid hormones, lithium; theoretically, thyroid extract may enhance the metabolism of many drugs.

References

Haas EM, *Staying Healthy With Nutrition: The Complete Guide to Diet and Nutritional Medicine*, Berkeley, CA: Celestial Arts, 1992, 285.

♦ **Thyroid Glandular Extract** *see* Thyroid Extract *on page 510*

Tocotrienols

Related Information
Nutraceutical Chart *on page 573*

Natural Product Category Nutraceutical

Dosage Oral: 60-220 mg/day

Active Forms There are four tocotrienols: Alpha, beta, gamma, and delta

Reported Uses Heart disease, high cholesterol; cancer prevention; protection from ultraviolet light, protection of the skin

Summary Tocotrienols are a family of dietary supplements related to vitamin E and are considered to be powerful antioxidants. Tocotrienols are found in the oil derived from rice bran, palm fruit, barley, and wheat germ. Natural sources of tocotrienols, such as rice bran oil, contain a mixture of both tocotrienols and tocopherols (vitamin E). While very similar in structure to vitamin E, tocotrienols contain three double bonds in the carbon side chain of the molecule. Gamma-tocotrienol is the form that is most prevalent in nature, and it also appears to be the form with the strongest potential for health benefits.

Pharmacology Tocotrienols function as cellular antioxidants, and some studies suggest that the antioxidant potential of tocotrienols is even greater than that of vitamin E in certain types of lipid cell membranes and in parts of brain cells. Topical application of tocotrienols has been shown to prevent oxidative damage to the skin and preserves the existing vitamin E level in skin cells. Tocotrienols also suppress the activity of HMG-CoA reductase, which helps to decrease the production of cholesterol in the liver.

Toxicities, Warnings, and Interactions No serious side effects have been reported with their use

Symptoms of Deficiency Weakened immune system with increased risk of cancer or cardiovascular disease

Reported Interactions
Drug/Nutrient Interactions: None known
Nutrient/Nutrient Interactions: None known

♦ ***Tribulus terrestris*** *see* Tribulus (*Tribulus terrestris*) *on page 511*

Tribulus (*Tribulus terrestris*)

Related Information
Herb/Drug Potential Interactions *on page 642*
Herb Quick Reference Chart *on page 538*

Natural Product Category Herb

Plant Part Whole plant

Dosage and Standardization Oral: 250-500 mg 3 times/day, standardized to contain 20% steroidal saponins per dose

Reported Uses Steroidal properties (enhancement of athletic performance, increased sexual vitality) (Seth, 1974)
(Continued)

Tribulus *(Tribulus terrestris)* *(Continued)*

Summary Tribulus has been used in India for centuries for various medical conditions. Tribulus is said to improve vitality and sexual virility.

Pharmacology Tribulus has been used in India for centuries for various medical conditions. Tribulus is said to improve vitality and sexual virility.

Theoretical Cautions and Contraindications Based on pharmacological activity, may potentially affect individuals taking steroidal medications.

General Warnings Use all herbal supplements with extreme caution in children <2 years of age and in pregnancy or lactation. Some herbs are contraindicated in pregnancy or lactation; make sure to observe warnings. Use with caution in individuals on medication and with pre-existing medical conditions. Always review for potential herb-drug interactions (HDIs) and other warnings. Large and prolonged doses may increase the potential for adverse effects. Herbs may cause transient adverse effects such as nausea, vomiting, and GI distress due to a variety of chemical constituents. Caution should be used in individuals having known allergies to plants.

Theoretical Interactions Steroidal agents, estrogens, oral contraceptives, hormone replacement therapy, androgens

References
Seth SD and Prabhakar MC, "Preliminary Pharmacological Investigations of *Tribulus terrestris*, Linn. (Gokhru) Part 1," *Indian J Med Sci*, 1974, 28(9):377-80.

♦ *Trifolium pratense see* Red Clover *(Trifolium pratense) on page 495*
♦ *Trigonella foenum-graecum see* Fenugreek *(Trigonella foenum-graecum) on page 432*

Turmeric *(Curcuma longa)*

Related Information
Herb/Drug Potential Interactions *on page 642*
Herb Quick Reference Chart *on page 538*

Natural Product Category Herb

Plant Part Root

Dosage and Standardization Oral: 300 mg 3 times/day with meals, standardized to contain 95% curcuminoids per dose

Reported Uses
Antioxidant; anti-inflammatory (Ammon, 1993)
Antirheumatic; used in arthritic problems; may lower blood lipid levels (Ammon, 1991)

Summary Turmeric has been reported to be a potent anti-inflammatory and antioxidant which may be of value in the treatment of rheumatic disorders (rheumatoid arthritis). In Ayurvedic (traditional Indian) medicine, turmeric rhizome has been used for centuries as a tonic for gastrointestinal complaints. It has also been used topically in various skin diseases.

Pharmacology The antioxidant activity of turmeric is mainly associated with its phenolic fraction, curcuminoids, which act as free radical scavengers as well as inhibitors of leukotrienes and prostaglandin synthesis. The anti-inflammatory activity has been claimed to be comparable to NSAIDs (such as indomethacin), producing significant improvement in clinical trials involving individuals with rheumatoid arthritis.

Curcuminoids reportedly lowered the levels of blood lipid peroxides, and may decrease total cholesterol and LDL cholesterol, while increasing HDL cholesterol. Turmeric is claimed to inhibit platelet aggregation, warranting caution in some individuals. The anti-inflammatory effects of turmeric are claimed to be comparable to nonsteroidal drugs (such as indomethacin) (Ammon, 1993).

Theoretical Cautions and Contraindications Based on its pharmacological activity, turmeric is contraindicated in biliary obstruction (Ammon, 1991). Use with caution in individuals with gastrointestinal disease (peptic ulcer disease, ulcerative colitis, Crohn's). May potentiate lipid-lowering therapies.

May alter platelet aggregation (Srivastava, 1995). Contraindicated in individuals with active bleeding (eg, peptic ulcer, intracranial bleeding). Use with caution in individuals with a history of bleeding, hemostatic disorders, or drug-related hemostatic problems. Use with caution in individuals taking anticoagulant medications, including warfarin, aspirin, aspirin-containing products, NSAIDs, or antiplatelet agents (eg, ticlopidine, clopidogrel, dipyridamole). Discontinue use prior to dental or surgical procedures (generally at least 14 days before).

General Warnings Use all herbal supplements with extreme caution in children <2 years of age and in pregnancy or lactation. Some herbs are contraindicated in pregnancy or lactation; make sure to observe warnings. Use with caution in individuals on medication and with pre-existing medical conditions. Always review for potential herb-drug interactions (HDIs) and other warnings. Large and prolonged doses may increase the potential for adverse effects. Herbs may cause transient adverse effects such as nausea, vomiting, and GI distress due to a variety of chemical constituents. Caution should be used in individuals having known allergies to plants.

Theoretical Interactions Anticoagulants, aspirin, aspirin-containing products, antiplatelet agents, NSAIDs, antihyperlipidemics

References

Ammon HP and Wahl MA, "Pharmacology of *Curcuma longa*," *Planta Med*, 1991, 57(1):1-7.
Ammon HP, Safayhi H, Mack T, et al, "Mechanism of Anti-inflammatory Actions of Curcumin and Boswellic Acids," *J Ethnopharmacol*, 1993, 38(2-3):113-9.
Snow JM, "*Curcuma Longa* L (Zingiberaceae)," *Protocol J Botanical Med*, 1995, 1(2):43-6.
Srivastava KC, Bordia A, and Verma SK, "A Major Component of Food Spice Turmeric (*Curcuma longa*) Inhibits Aggregation and Alters Eicosanoid Metabolism In Human Blood Platelets," *Prostaglandins Leukot Essent Fatty Acids*, 1995, 52(4):223-7.

♦ *Tylophora asthmatica* see Tylophora *(Tylophora asthmatica)* on page 513

Tylophora *(Tylophora asthmatica)*

Related Information

Herb Quick Reference Chart *on page 538*

Natural Product Category Herb

Plant Part Leaf

Dosage and Standardization Oral: 250 mg 1-3 times/day, standardized to contain 0.1% tylophorine per dose

Reported Uses

Allergies (Shipuri, 1969)

Used in bronchial asthma (Gupta, 1979)

Summary Tylophora has been used in Ayurvedic (traditional Indian) medicine for thousands of years for respiratory disorders. It is currently used in asthma and allergy.

Pharmacology The antiasthmatic effects of tylophora are believed to be related to a suppression of inflammatory responses. This immune supression includes a reported depression of cell-mediated immunity. Tylophora may stimulate phagocytosis while inhibiting humoral immunity. Tylophora has been reported to cause adrenal stimulation, which may increase cortisol secretion. It has also been shown to stimulate adenylate cyclase in the leuckocytes of children with asthma, which would be similar to beta-receptor stimulation. Consistent with this activity, tylophora has been claimed to function as a short-acting bronchodilator.

Theoretical Cautions and Contraindications Use with caution if taking asthma medications (based on pharmacological activity of tylophora, effects of these medications may be altered). Based on pharmacological activity, use with caution in individuals with diabetes, fluid retention, edema, congestive heart failure (CHF), and cardiovascular disease (eg, arrhythmia, hypertension).

Until further studies are conducted, tylophora is contraindicated in individuals with serious infection, organ transplants, major systemic disease, or recent major surgery.

General Warnings Use all herbal supplements with extreme caution in children <2 years of age and in pregnancy or lactation. Some herbs are contraindicated in pregnancy or lactation; make sure to observe warnings. Use with caution in individuals on medication and with pre-existing medical
(Continued)

Tylophora *(Tylophora asthmatica) (Continued)*

conditions. Always review for potential herb-drug interactions (HDIs) and other warnings. Large and prolonged doses may increase the potential for adverse effects. Herbs may cause transient adverse effects such as nausea, vomiting, and GI distress due to a variety of chemical constituents. Caution should be used in individuals having known allergies to plants.

Theoretical Interactions Bronchodilators, beta-blockers, antiarrhythmics, antihypertensives, insulin, oral hypoglycemics

References

Gupta S, George P, Gupta V, et al, "*Tylophora Indica* in Bronchial Asthma - A Double Blind Study," *Indian J Med Res*, 1979, 69:981-9.

Shivpuri DN, Menon MP, and Prakash D, "A Crossover Double-Blind Study on *Tylophora indica* in the Treatment of Asthma and Allergic Rhinitis," *J Allergy*, 1969; 43(3):145-50.

Tyrosine

Related Information
Nutraceutical Chart *on page 573*
Vitamins/Minerals/Trace Elements/Amino Acids Chart *on page 604*

Natural Product Category Amino Acid

Dosage Oral: RDI: None established; ODA: 1000-5000 mg/day

Active Forms L-tyrosine

Reported Uses
Alzheimer's disease (Meyer, 1977)
Depression (Gelenberg, 1984)
Hypothyroidism
Phenylketonuria (PKU) (Rohr, 1998)
Substance abuse (Blum, 1974)

Summary Tyrosine is classified as a nonessential amino acid because it can be synthesized from phenylalanine in the body. However, tyrosine is a very important amino acid, because it is part of the structure of almost all proteins in the body.

Pharmacology Tyrosine plays a very important role in brain nutrition, because it serves as a precursor for the synthesis of several neurotransmitters including dopamine, norepinephrine, and epinephrine. Tyrosine is also necessary for the production of melanin, cholecystokinin (CCK), and the thyroid hormones.

Toxicities, Warnings, and Interactions No known toxicity or serious side effects, however, it is not to be taken by individuals on MAO-inhibiting antidepressants

Symptoms of Deficiency Depression and emotional disturbances; underactive thyroid and disturbed metabolism

Reported Interactions
Drug/nutrient interactions: MAO inhibitors
Nutrient/nutrient interactions: The branched chain amino acids (leucine, isoleucine, and valine), compete with tyrosine and other aromatic amino acids for transport into the brain.

References

Blum K and Wallace JE, "Effects of Catecholamine Synthesis Inhibition on Ethanol-Induced Withdrawal Symptoms in Mice," *Br J Pharmacol*, 1974, 51(1):109-11.

Gelenberg AJ and Gibson CJ, "Tyrosine for the Treatment of Depression," *Nutr Health*, 1984, 3(3):163-73.

Meyer JS, Welch KM, Deshmukh VD, et al, "Neurotransmitter Precursor Amino Acids in the Treatment of Multi-infarct Dementia and Alzheimer's Disease," *J Am Geriatr Soc*, 1977, 25(7):289-98.

Rohr FJ, Lobbregt D, and Levy HL, "Tyrosine Supplementation in the Treatment of Maternal Phenylketonuria," *Am J Clin Nutr*, 1998, 67(3):473-6.

♦ **Ubiquinone** *see* Coenzyme Q10 *on page 412*
♦ **Ulcer (Aphthous)** *see page 358*
♦ **Ulcer (Duodenal and Peptic)** *see page 362*
♦ **Ulcer (Gastric)** *see Ulcer (Duodenal and Peptic) on page 362*
♦ **Ulcerative Colitis** *see page 366*
♦ **Uncaria tomentosa** *see* Cat's Claw *(Uncaria tomentosa) on page 404*

- **Unsafe Herbs** see page 654
- **Urinary Tract Infection (UTI)** see page 370
- **Urtica dioica** see Stinging Nettle (Urtica dioica) on page 505

Uva Ursi (Arctostaphylos uva-ursi)

Related Information
Common Herbal Supplements Contraindicated During Pregnancy on page 656
Herb/Drug Potential Interactions on page 642
Herb Quick Reference Chart on page 538

Natural Product Category Herb

Plant Part Leaf

Dosage and Standardization Oral: 100-200 mg/day, standardized to contain 10% to 25% arbutin per dose

Reported Uses Used in urinary tract infections and kidney stone prevention (Bradley, 1992)

Summary Uva ursi has been used as a diuretic, astringent, and antiseptic for centuries. It may be useful in a variety of renal disorders, including nephritis, nephrolithiasis, and cystitis. It is claimed to have antiseptic activity and may function as a urinary analgesic similar to phenazopyridine.

Pharmacology Uva ursi contains arbutin, a phenolic glycoside that reportedly demonstrates antiseptic and analgesic properties in the urinary tract. The disinfectant properties may be most prominent in alkaline urine. Ingestion of arbutin alone is ineffective due to destruction in the gastrointestinal tract. However, additional plant components appear to block its degradation and enhance absorption when whole plant preparations are ingested. In addition, constituents of the whole plant preparations are believed to enhance efficacy by contributing to urinary alkalinization. May cause green-brown discoloration of urine.

Theoretical Cautions and Contraindications Contraindicated in pregnancy and lactation (based on animal studies, Bradley, 1992). Contraindicated in renal failure (based on pharmacological activity). Anecdotal reports state that drinking 1 teaspoonful of baking soda in water prior to use may promote conversion of hydroquinones to their active form. May cause green-brown discoloration of urine.

General Warnings Use all herbal supplements with extreme caution in children <2 years of age and in pregnancy or lactation. Some herbs are contraindicated in pregnancy or lactation; make sure to observe warnings. Use with caution in individuals on medication and with pre-existing medical conditions. Always review for potential herb-drug interactions (HDIs) and other warnings. Large and prolonged doses may increase the potential for adverse effects. Herbs may cause transient adverse effects such as nausea, vomiting, and GI distress due to a variety of chemical constituents. Caution should be used in individuals having known allergies to plants.

Theoretical Interactions None known

References
Bradley PR, ed, British Herbal Compendium, Vol 1, Bournemouth, England: British Herbal Medicine Association, 1992, 211-13.

- **Vaccinium macrocarpon** see Cranberry (Vaccinium macrocarpon) on page 418
- **Vaccinium myrtillus** see Bilberry (Vaccinium myrtillus) on page 392
- **Valeriana officinalis** see Valerian (Valeriana officinalis) on page 515

Valerian (Valeriana officinalis)

Related Information
Herb Quick Reference Chart on page 538

Natural Product Category Herb

Plant Part Root

Dosage and Standardization Oral: 200 mg 1-4 times/day, standardized to contain 0.8% to 1% valerenic acids per dose. Sedative dose: 200-400 mg at bedtime
(Continued)

Valerian *(Valeriana officinalis) (Continued)*

Reported Uses Use as a sedative or hypnotic (Balderer, 1985); used in nervous tension during PMS, menopause; used in restless motor syndromes and muscle spasms (Houghton, 1988)

Summary Valerian has a long history of use as a sedative and anxiolytic. It is one of the most popular herbal preparations in Europe. It has also been reported that valerian improves sleep quality. It may hjave benefit for individuals with stress caused by a number of factors, and may be useful in premenstrual syndrome (PMS). In addition, it has been used in restless leg syndrome and muscle spasms. When used as a hypnotic, it does not appear to be associated with "hangover" effects, an advantage over many sedative-hypnotic drugs.

Pharmacology Valerian components include valepotriates, valeric acid, and pungent oils. These have a sedative effect on the central nervous system, as well as inducing smooth muscle relaxation in the gastrointestinal tract. Valepotriates and valeric acid are believed to bind to receptor sites which are similar to the benzodiazepines, influencing gamma-aminobutyric acid (GABA) affinity in the CNS.

Theoretical Cautions and Contraindications Based on pharmacological activities, may cause drowsiness or sedation. Use with caution when driving or operating heavy machinery (German Commission E 1985). Use caution in individuals taking medications that cause CNS depression, including sedative-hypnotics, antihistamines, antidepressants, and anxiolytics. May increase sleeping time from hypnotic agents (increased sleeping time reported with pentobarbital in animal studies) (Hendriks 1985). Effects do not appear to be potentiated by ethanol.

Note: Do not use valerian supplements in children <3 years of age. Use only valepotriate and baldrinal-free in children <12 years of age due to potential mutagenic properties.

General Warnings Use all herbal supplements with extreme caution in children <2 years of age and in pregnancy or lactation. Some herbs are contraindicated in pregnancy or lactation; make sure to observe warnings. Use with caution in individuals on medication and with pre-existing medical conditions. Always review for potential herb-drug interactions (HDIs) and other warnings. Large and prolonged doses may increase the potential for adverse effects. Herbs may cause transient adverse effects such as nausea, vomiting, and GI distress due to a variety of chemical constituents. Caution should be used in individuals having known allergies to plants.

Theoretical Interactions CNS depressants, sedative-hypnotics (barbiturates), antidepressants, anxiolytics, antihistamines

References

Balderer G and Borbely AA, "Effect of Valerian on Human Sleep," *Psychopharmacology (Berl)*, 1985, 87(4):406-9.

Hendriks H, Bos R, Woerdenbag, HJ, et al, "Central Nervous Depressant Activity of Valerenic Acid in the Mouse," *Planta Med*, 1985, (1):28-31.

Houghton PJ, "The Biological Activity of Valerian and Related Plants," *J Ethnopharmacol*, 1988, 22(2):121-42.

"Valerianae radix," German Commission E Monograph, Bundesanzeiger, 1985, No 90.

Vanadium

Related Information
Organ System Support Using Natural Products *on page 660*
Vitamins/Minerals/Trace Elements/Amino Acids Chart *on page 604*

Natural Product Category Mineral

Dosage Oral: RDI: None established; ODA: 250 mcg 1-3 times/day

Active Forms Vanadium pentoxide, vanadyl sulfate

Reported Uses
Type 1 diabetes (Badmaev, 1999)
Type 2 diabetes (Boden, 1996)

Summary Vanadium may be an essential trace mineral in humans. It functions as a cofactor in several key enzymes, many of which are involved in the regulation of blood glucose levels. For this reason, it has been claimed to be a useful supplement in individuals with diabetes.

Pharmacology Vanadium functions as a cofactor, facilitating the activity of specific enzymes. It is reported to be a cofactor in nicotinamide adenine dinucleotide phosphate (NADPH) oxidation reactions, lipoprotein lipase activity, amino acid transport, and hematopoiesis. Many of the effects of vanadium improve the physiologic regulation of glucose. Vanadium stimulates glycolysis via glucokinase and phosphofructokinase, and may decrease gluconeogenesis by decreasing the activity of glucose-6-phosphatase. At high doses, it has been claimed to lower serum cholesterol and triglyceride levels.

Toxicities, Warnings, and Interactions No dietary toxicity or serious side effects have been reported, however industrial exposure has resulted in toxicity. May alter glucose regulation. Use with caution in individuals with diabetes or in those who may be predisposed to hypoglycemia. Effects of drugs with hypoglycemic activity may be potentiated (including insulin and oral hypoglycemics). The individual's blood sugar should be closely monitored, and the dosage of these agents, including insulin dosage, may require adjustment. This should be carefully coordinated among the individuals' healthcare providers.

Symptoms of Deficiency Deficiency studies in humans have not been conducted.

Reported Interactions

Drug/Nutrient Interactions: Theoretically, insulin or oral hypoglycemics
Nutrient/Nutrient Interactions: None known

References

Badmaev V, Prakash S, and Majeed M, "Vanadium: A Review of Its Potential Role in the Fight Against Diabetes," *J Altern Complement Med*, 1999, 5(3):273-91.

Boden G, Chen X, Ruiz J, et al, "Effects of Vanadyl Sulfate on Carbohydrate and Lipid Metabolism in Patients With Non-Insulin-Dependent Diabetes Mellitus," *Metabolism*, 1996, 45(9):1130-5.

♦ **Venous Stasis** see Circulation (Peripheral) Problems *on page 110*

♦ *Vinca minor* see Vinpocetine *on page 517*

Vinpocetine

Related Information
Herb Quick Reference Chart *on page 538*
Organ System Support Using Natural Products *on page 660*

Natural Product Category Herb

Plant Part Isolated from *Vinca minor*

Dosage and Standardization Oral: 10-40 mg twice daily

Reported Uses Enhanced cognitive function; increased brain function (cerebral metabolic enhancing agent) (Kidd, 1999)

Summary Vinpocetine is used for memory enhancement and to increase brain function (a cerebral metabolic enhancing agent). Because of its stimulating effect on blood flow, vinpocetine has been used for circulatory problems in the brain and memory problems due to low circulation.

Pharmacology Vinpocetine is derived from vincamine, an extract of the lesser periwinkle plant. It has a stimulating effect on memory. Vinpocetine increases metabolism in the brain by several mechanisms. It increases blood flow; it increases the rate at which brain cells produce adenosine triphosphate (ATP); and it speeds up the use of glucose and oxygen in the brain.

Theoretical Cautions and Contraindications None known

General Warnings Use all herbal supplements with extreme caution in children <2 years of age and in pregnancy or lactation. Some herbs are contraindicated in pregnancy or lactation; make sure to observe warnings. Use with caution in individuals on medication and with pre-existing medical conditions. Always review for potential herb-drug interactions (HDIs) and other warnings. Large and prolonged doses may increase the potential for adverse effects. Herbs may cause transient adverse effects such as
(Continued)

Vinpocetine (Continued)

nausea, vomiting, and GI distress due to a variety of chemical constituents. Caution should be used in individuals having known allergies to plants.

Theoretical Interactions None known

References
Kidd PM, "A Review of Nutrients and Botanicals in the Integrative Management of Cognitive Dysfunction," *Altern Med Rev*, 1999, 4(3):144-61.

Vitamin A (Retinol)

Related Information
Drug-Induced Nutrient Depletions *on page 625*
Organ System Support Using Natural Products *on page 660*
Pregnancy & Lactation Nutritional Chart *on page 657*
Vitamins/Minerals/Trace Elements/Amino Acids Chart *on page 604*

Natural Product Category Vitamin

Dosage Oral: RDI: Males: 5000 int. units/day, females: 4000 int. units/day; ODA: 5000 int. units/day (unless pregnant)

Active Forms Retinol acetate, retinol palmitate

Reported Uses
Acne (Kligman, 1981)
AIDS (Semba, 1993)
Cancer prevention (Werbach, 1993)
Cervical dysplasia (Wylie-Rosett, 1984)
Crohn's disease (Dvorak, 1980)
Measles (Hussey, 1990)
Menorrhagia (Lithgow, 1977)
Night blindness (Lindeboom, 1984)
PMS (Block, 1960)
Ulcerative colitis (Regoly-Merei, 1991)

Summary Vitamin A was the first fat-soluble vitamin to be isolated. It was recognized for its potential to prevent night blindness and xerophthalmia. Vitamin A belongs to a class of compounds called retinoids. Substantial amounts are stored in the liver, and it generally does not need to be consumed on a daily basis. Supplementation has been claimed to be beneficial in a variety of disorders, including diseases of epithelial cells (acne, cervical dysplasia, cancer prevention), viral infections (measles, AIDS), Crohn's disease, and PMS.

Toxicities, Warnings, and Interactions
Toxic dose: Doses >50,000 int. units/day have resulted in toxicity; Pregnant women should not exceed 4000 int. units/day due to risk of birth defects
Toxicity symptoms: Headache, nausea, vomiting, fatigue, weakness, anorexia, weight loss, nosebleeds, blurred vision, bone pain, joint pain, dry skin, rashes, hair loss, amenorrhea, liver and spleen enlargement, transient hydrocephalus, stunted growth

Symptoms of Deficiency Night blindness, vision problems, increased susceptibility to infections, defective tooth and bone formation, reduced synthesis of steroid hormones

Reported Interactions
Drug/Nutrient Interactions: Drugs that decrease the absorption of vitamin A include: Bile acid sequesterants (cholestyramine and colestipol), neomycin, mineral oil, orlistat, and antacids. Concurrent use of vitamin A derivatives such as etretinate and isotretinoin may result in increased toxicity.
Nutrient/Nutrient Interactions: Large doses of vitamin E can interfere with the absorption of vitamin A. Vitamin A antagonizes the action of vitamin D.

References
Block E, "The Use of Vitamin A in Premenstrual Tension," *Acta Obstet Gynecol Scand*, 1960, 39:586-92.
Dvorak AM, "Vitamin A in Crohn's Disease," *Lancet*, 1980, 1(8181), 1303-4.
Hussey GD and Klein M, "A Randomized, Controlled Trial of Vitamin A in Children With Severe Measles," *N Engl J Med*, 1990, 323(3):160-4.
Kligman AM, Mills OH Jr, Leyden JJ, et al, "Oral Vitamin A in Acne Vulgaris. Preliminary Report," *Int J Dermatol*, 1981, 20(4):278-85.

Lindeboom GA, "Historical Milestones in the Treatment of Night Blindness," *Clio Med*, 1984, 19(1-2):40-9.

Lithgow DM and Politzer WM, "Vitamin A in the Treatment of Menorrhagia," *S Afr Med*, 1977, 51(7):191-3.

Regoly-Merei A, Ferencz A, Frenkl R, et al, "Effect of Fat and Retinol Loading on Serum Triglyceride and Retinol Levels in Patients With Ulcerative Colitis," *Nahrung*, 1991, 35(1):21-6.

Semba RD, Graham NM, Caiaffa WT, et al, "Increased Mortality Associated With Vitamin A Deficiency During Human Immunodeficiency Virus Type 1 Infection," *Arch Intern Med*, 1993, 153(18):2149-54.

Werbach MR, *Nutritional Influences on Illness*," 2nd ed, Tarzana, CA: Third Line Press, 1993, 138-40.

Wylie-Rosett JA, Romney SL, Slagle NS, et al, "Influence of Vitamin A on Cervical Dysplasia and Carcinoma *in Situ*," *Nutr Cancer*, 1984, 6(1):49-57.

Vitamin B₁ (Thiamine)

Related Information

Drug-Induced Nutrient Depletions *on page 625*

Pregnancy & Lactation Nutritional Chart *on page 657*

Vitamins/Minerals/Trace Elements/Amino Acids Chart *on page 604*

Natural Product Category Vitamin

Dosage Oral: RDI: 1.5 mg/day; ODA: 5-10 mg/day

Active Forms Thiamine hydrochloride, thiamine mononitrate, tetrahydrofurfuryl disulfide (TTFD)

Reported Uses

Alcoholism (Cook, 1998)

Alzheimer's disease (Meador, 1993)

Anemia (megaloblastic) (Mandel, 1984)

Congestive heart failure (CHF) (Seligmann, 1991)

Diabetes (Saito, 1987)

Insomnia (Crespi, 1982)

Neurological conditions (Bell's palsy, trigeminal neuralgia, sciatica, sensory neuropathies) (Skelton, 1989)

Psychiatric illness (Carney, 1990)

Summary Vitamin B₁, also known as thiamine, exerts metabolic activities which primarily affect the nerves, muscles, and cardiovascular system. Thiamine is a water-soluble vitamin and is not stored in the body. Since thiamine is involved in the maintenance of nerve cell function, it is not surprising that supplementation has been claimed to improve a number of nervous system disorders, including Alzheimer's dementia and many neuropathies. Thiamine is depleted in many psychiatric individuals and alcoholics. In addition, losses may be accelerated by many medications used in the management of heart failure. Supplementation may be beneficial in these disorders.

Toxicities, Warnings, and Interactions No known toxic effects from oral intake

Symptoms of Deficiency Fatigue, memory loss, irritability, depression, loss of reflexes, wasting, weakness, edema, dysrhythmia, cardiomegaly, CHF

Reported Interactions

Drug/Nutrient Interactions: Drugs which can cause depletion of vitamin B₁: Loop diuretics, phenytoin, ethanol, theophylline, antibiotics

Nutrient/Nutrient Interactions: There are no known adverse nutrient/nutrient interactions between thiamine and other nutrients. However, thiamine is intimately involved with other B vitamins in many biochemical activities and many health professionals therefore suggest that vitamin B₁ be taken along with other B vitamins.

References

Carney MW, "Vitamin Deficiency and Mental Symptoms," *Br J Psychiatry*, 1990, 156:878-82.

Cook CC, Hallwood PM, and Thomason AD, "B Vitamin Deficiency and Neuropsychiatric Syndromes in Alcohol Misuse," *Alcohol*, 1998, 33(4):317-36.

Crespi F and Jouvet M, "Sleep and Indolamine Alterations Induced by Thiamine Deficiency," *Brain Res*, 1982, 248(2):275-83.

Mandel H, Berant M, Hazani A, et al, "Thiamine-Dependent Beriberi in the Thiamine-Responsive Anemia Syndrome," *N Engl J Med*, 1984, 311(13):836-8.

(Continued)

Vitamin B₁ (Thiamine) *(Continued)*

Meador K, Loring D, Nichols M, et al, "Preliminary Findings of High-Dose Thiamine in Dementia of Alzheimer's Type," *J Geriatr Psychiatry Neurol*, 1993, 6(4):222-9.

Saito N, Kimura M, Kuchiba A, et al, "Blood Thiamine Levels in Outpatients With Diabetes Mellitus," *J Nutr Sci Vitaminol (Tokyo)*, 1987, 33(6):421-30.

Seligmann H, Halkin H, Rauchfleisch S, et al, "Thiamine Deficiency in Patients With Congestive Heart Failure Receiving Long-Term Furosemide Therapy: A Pilot Study," *Am J Med*, 1991, (2):151-5.

Skelton WP and Skelton NK, "Thiamine Deficiency Neuropathy. It's Still Common Today," *Postgrad Med*, 1989, 85(8):301-6.

Vitamin B₂

Related Information

Drug-Induced Nutrient Depletions *on page 625*
Pregnancy & Lactation Nutritional Chart *on page 657*
Vitamins/Minerals/Trace Elements/Amino Acids Chart *on page 604*

Natural Product Category Vitamin

Dosage Oral: RDI: 1.7 mg/day; ODA: 5-10 mg/day

Active Forms Riboflavin, riboflavin hydrochloride, activated riboflavin (riboflavin-5-phosphate)

Reported Uses

Cataracts (Leske, 1995)
Depression (Carney, 1982)
Migraine (Schoenen, 1998)

Summary Vitamin B₂ (riboflavin) is a water-soluble vitamin essential for normal growth and development. It is a cofactor in a number of essential biochemical reactions, particularly within metabolic pathways which yield energy. Supplementation may be necessary to avoid symptoms of deficiency in the face of inadequate intake or excessive loss (as may be caused by some medications). In addition, supplementation has been claimed to be of therapeutic benefit in individuals with migraines, depression, and cataracts.

Pharmacology Riboflavin is incorporated into flavin coenzymes. These include flavin mononucleotide (FMN) and flavin adenine dinucleotide (FAD). These riboflavin-containing enzymes function as hydrogen carriers involved in many of the oxidation-reduction reactions performed in cells. These have a role in fatty-acid synthesis, beta-oxidation of fatty acids, deamination of amino acids, and conversion of pyruvic acid to acetyl coenzyme A (a critical step in carbohydrate metabolism via the Krebs cycle). In addition, riboflavin may function as an antioxidant, and participates in antioxidant reactions mediated by glutathione reductase. Skin, hair, and nail growth appear to be particularly dependent on adequate supplies of riboflavin.

Toxicities, Warnings, and Interactions No known toxicity or serious side effects

Symptoms of Deficiency Light sensitivity, reddening of the eyes, skin rash, depression, cracks at the corners of the mouth, discoloration of tongue (deep red)

Reported Interactions

Drug/Nutrient Interactions: Drugs which can cause depletion of riboflavin: Oral contraceptives, tricyclic antidepressants, phenothiazines, antibiotics

Nutrient/Nutrient Interactions: Riboflavin is intimately involved with other B vitamins in many biochemical activities. Therefore, many health professionals suggest that vitamin B₂ be taken along with other B vitamins.

References

Carney MW, Ravindran A, Rinsler MG, et al, "Thiamine, Riboflavin and Pyridoxine Deficiency in Psychiatric Inpatients," *Br J Psychiatry*, 1982, 141:271-2.

Leske MC, Wu SY, Hyman L, et al, "Biochemical Factors in the Lens Opacities. Case-Control Study. The Lens Opacities Case-Control Study Group," *Arch Ophthalmol*, 1995, 113(9):1113-9.

Schoenen J, Jacquy J, and Lenaerts, M. "Effectiveness of High-Dose Riboflavin in Migraine Prophylaxis. A Randomized Controlled Trial," *Neurology*, 1998, 50(2):466-70.

Vitamin B₃

Related Information

Drug-Induced Nutrient Depletions *on page 625*
Pregnancy & Lactation Nutritional Chart *on page 657*
Vitamins/Minerals/Trace Elements/Amino Acids Chart *on page 604*

Natural Product Category Vitamin

Dosage Oral:

Niacin: RDI: 20 mg/day; ODA: 25-100 mg/day

Inositol hexaniacinate: RDI: None established; ODA: 600 mg/day

Active Forms Niacin (nicotinic acid), niacinamide (nicotinamide), inositol hexaniacinate (inositol hexanicotinate)

Reported Uses

Acne vulgaris (4% niacinamide topical gel) (Schlaita, 1995)

Cataracts (Sperduto, 1993)

Hyperlipidemia: Hypercholesterolemia, hypertriglyceridemia (Alderman, 1989; Franceschini, 1993)

Impaired glucose tolerance (Urberg, 1987)

Intermittent claudication (O'Hara, 1988)

Osteoarthritis (Jonas, 1996)

Prevention of myocardial infarction (Canner, 1986)

Raynaud's syndrome (Sunderland, 1988)

Rheumatoid arthritis (Hoffer, 1959)

Schizophrenia (Osmond, 1962)

Type 1 diabetes of recent onset (Pozzilli, 1996)

Type 2 diabetes (Polo, 1998)

Summary
Niacin (nicotinic acid) is a water-soluble B vitamin which lowers elevated blood lipids and may reduce cardiovascular mortality. In addition to being used alone, it has also been used in combination with other cholesterol-lowering drugs. In the past, a high percentage of people discontinued niacin therapy for hyperlipidemia due to the unpleasant "flushing" side effect. Inositol hexaniacinate has been claimed to provide the benefits of niacin without the vasodilatory side effects. Niacin has also been claimed to be beneficial in peripheral vascular disorders. Niacinamide has been used in individuals newly diagnosed with type 1 diabetes, type 2 diabetes, and arthritis.

Pharmacology
Niacin functions as a component of two important coenzymes: Nicotinamide adenine dinucleotide (NAD) and nicotinamide adenine dinucleotide phosphate (NADP). These play an important role in many oxidation-reduction reactions, including those involved in lipid metabolism and carbohydrate metabolism via the Krebs cycle. It also is a component of glucose tolerance factor, augmenting control of blood glucose levels. Niacin appears to support the nervous system, skin, and gastrointestinal function. It is also involved in synthetic pathways, including the synthesis of sex hormones. It may influence the course of coronary artery disease by increasing HDL cholesterol while lowering LDL cholesterol and triglyceride levels. It also lowers lipoprotein (a) and fibrinogen concentrations. Its vasodilating activity has been used in peripheral vascular disorders such as intermittent claudication and Raynaud's syndrome.

Toxicities, Warnings, and Interactions

Toxic dose: Niacin/niacinamide: 300-600 mg; doses >2.5 g/day over time can cause liver damage and glucose intolerance

Toxicity symptoms: Headache, nausea, skin flushing and tingling, sweating

Symptoms of Deficiency

Niacin/niacinamide: Fatigue, irritability, insomnia, emotional lability, blood glucose fluctuations, arthritis, diarrhea, black smooth tongue, mental confusion

Inositol hexaniacinate: There are no known deficiency symptoms associated with inositol hexaniacinate.

Reported Interactions

Drug/Nutrient Interactions: Drugs which can cause depletion of niacin: Estrogen-containing medications, antibiotics, isoniazid

(Continued)

521

Vitamin B₃ *(Continued)*

Nutrient/Nutrient Interactions: Niacin is involved with other B vitamins in numerous biochemical activities and for this reason, many health professionals suggest taking niacin along with other B vitamins in nutritional supplement formulations.

References

Alderman JD, Pasternak RC, Sacks FM, et al, "Effect of a Modified, Well-Tolerated Niacin Regimen on Serum Total Cholesterol, High Density Lipoprotein Cholesterol and the Cholesterol to High Density Lipoprotein Ratio," *Am J Cardiol,* 1989, 64(12):725-9.

Canner PL, Berge KG, Wenger NK, et al, "Fifteen-Year Mortality in Coronary Drug Project Patients: Long-Term Benefit With Niacin," *J Am Coll Cardiol,* 1986, 8(6):1245-55.

Franceschini G and Paoletti R, "Pharmacological Control of Hypertriglyceridemia," *Cardiovasc Drugs Ther,* 1993, 7(3):297-302.

Hoffer A, "Treatment of Arthritis by Nicotinic Acid and Nicotinamide," *Can Med Assoc J,* 1959, 81:235-9.

Jonas WB, Rapoza CP, and Blair WF, "The Effect of Niacinamide on Osteoarthritis: A Pilot Study," *Inflamm Res,* 1996, 45(7):330-4.

O'Hara J, Jolly PN, and Nicol CG, "The Therapeutic Efficacy of Inositol Nicotinate (Hexopal) in Intermittent Claudication: A Controlled Trial," *Br J Clin Pract,* 1988, 42(9):377-83.

Osmond H and Hoffer A, "Massive Niacin Treatment in Schizophrenia: Review of a Nine-Year Study," *Lancet,* 1962, 1:316-20.

Polo V, Saibene A, and Pontiroli AE, "Nicotinamide Improves Insulin Secretion and Metabolic Control in Lean Type 2 Diabetic Patients With Secondary Failure to Sulfonylureas," *Acta Diabetol,* 1998, 35(1):61-4.

Pozzilli P, Browne PD, and Kolb H, "Meta-Analysis of Nicotinamide Treatment in Patients With Recent-Onset IDDM. The Nicotinamide Trialists," *Diabetes Care,* 1996, 19(12):1357-63.

Shalita AR, Smith JG, Parish LC, et al, "Topical Nicotinamide Compared With Clindamycin Gel in the Treatment of Inflammatory Acne Vulgaris," *Int J Dermatol,* 1995, 34(6):434-7.

Sperduto RD, Hut S, Milton RC, et al, "The Linxian Cataract Studies. Two Nutrition Intervention Trials," *Arch Ophthalmol,* 1993, 111(9):1246-53.

Sunderland GT, Belch JJ, Sturrock RD, et al, "A Double-Blind Randomized Placebo Controlled Trial of Hexopal in Primary Raynaud's Disease," *Clin Rheumatol,* 1988, 7(1):46-9.

Urberg M and Zemel MB, "Evidence for Synergism Between Chromium and Nicotinic Acid in the Control of Glucose Tolerance in Elderly Humans," *Metabolism,* 1987, 36(9):896-9.

Vitamin B₅ (Pantothenic Acid)

Related Information

Pregnancy & Lactation Nutritional Chart *on page 657*

Vitamins/Minerals/Trace Elements/Amino Acids Chart *on page 604*

Natural Product Category   Vitamin

Dosage   Oral: RDI: 10 mg/day; ODA: 10-50 mg/day

Active Forms   Calcium pantothenate, pantethine (the stable disulfide form of pantetheine, which is the biologically active form of pantothenic acid and the direct precursor to coenzyme A [CoA]), dexpanthenol (which is the alcohol of pantothenic acid)

Reported Uses

Adrenal support (Tarasov, 1985)

Allergies (Martin, 1991)

Arthritis (Report from GP Research Group, 1980)

Constipation (Guillard, 1979)

Hyperlipidemia (pantethine, but not pantothenic acid, lowers cholesterol and triglycerides) (Arsenio, 1986)

Rheumatoid arthritis (Report from GP Research Group, 1980)

Surgery and wound healing (Lacroix, 1988)

Summary Vitamin B₅ (pantothenic acid) plays a number of essential metabolic roles including the production of steroid hormones and neurotransmitters. It is involved in the metabolism of all carbohydrates, fats, and proteins. Supplementation with pantethine has been claimed to reduce serum lipids, and this effect has been reported to be particularly significant in individuals with diabetes. In addition, supplementation with vitamin B₅ has been claimed to be beneficial in allergies and arthritis. It may also facilitate wound healing and postsurgical recovery.

Pharmacology Physiologically, pantothenic acid is converted to a sulfur-containing compound called pantetheine. Pantetheine is then converted into coenzyme A, which is the only known biologically active form of pantothenic acid. Coenzyme A facilitates the transfer of two-carbon units (acetyl groups) in a wide variety of biochemical reactions. It is involved in the metabolism of lipids and carbohydrates, including activity in the Krebs cycle. In addition, pantothenic acid is required for the synthesis of steroid hormones, augmenting adrenal function. It is required in the synthesis of phospholipids, bile acids, and porphyrin. Synthesis of the neurotransmitter acetylcholine also requires this cofactor. Pantethine, which is the stable and most active form of pantetheine, reportedly lowers elevated triglycerides and LDL cholesterol while raising levels of HDL cholesterol. Due to its involvement in many metabolic pathways, pantothenic acid facilitates the use of many other vitamins.

Toxicities, Warnings, and Interactions Generally safe at high doses

Symptoms of Deficiency None known for isolated vitamin B_5 deficiency, however deficiency of any single B vitamin usually correlates to deficiency of others.

Reported Interactions

Drug/Nutrient Interactions: None known

Nutrient/Nutrient Interactions: There are no known adverse nutrient/nutrient interactions between pantothenic acid and other nutrients. However, pantothenic acid is involved with other B vitamins in many biochemical activities and therefore, many health professionals suggest that vitamin B_5 be taken along with other B vitamins.

References

Arsenio L, Bodria P, Magnati G, et al, "Effectiveness of Long-Term Treatment With Pantethine in Patients With Dyslipidemia," *Clin Ther*, 1986, 8(5):537-45.

"Calcium Pantothenate in Arthritic Conditions. A Report From the General Practitioner Research Group," *Practitioner*, 1980, 224(1340):208-11.

Guillard O, Delmotte JS, Filoche B, et al, "Treatment of Constipation With Vitamin B_5 or Dexpanthenol," *Med Chir Dig*, 1979, 8(7):671-4.

Lacroix B, Didier E, and Grenier JF, "Role of Pantothenic and Ascorbic Acid in Wound Healing Processes: In Vitro Study on Fibroblasts," *Int J Vitam Nutr Res*, 1988, 58(4):407-13.

Martin W, "On Treating Allergic Disorders," *Townsend Letter for Doctors*, 1991, 670-1.

Tarasov IuA, Sheibak VM, and Moiseenok AG, "Adrenal Cortex Functional Activity in Pantothenate Deficiency and the Administration of the Vitamin or Its Derivatives," *Vopr Pitan*, 1985, (4):51-4.

Vitamin B_6 (Pyridoxine)

Related Information

Drug-Induced Nutrient Depletions *on page 625*
Pregnancy & Lactation Nutritional Chart *on page 657*
Vitamins/Minerals/Trace Elements/Amino Acids Chart *on page 604*

Natural Product Category Vitamin

Dosage Oral: RDI: 2 mg/day; ODA: 10-20 mg/day

Active Forms Pyridoxine, pyridoxine hydrochloride, pyridoxal hydrochloride, pyridoxal-5'-phosphate

Reported Uses

Arthritis (Kremer, 1996)
Asthma (Reynolds, 1985)
Autism (Reynolds, 1985)
Cardiovascular disease (Reynolds, 1985)
Carpal tunnel syndrome (Spooner, 1993)
Depression associated with oral contraceptives (Adams, 1973)
Diabetic neuropathy (Jones, 1978)
Epilepsy, B_6-dependant (Crowell, 1983)
Kidney stones (Mitwalli, 1988)
MSG sensitivity (Folkers, 1984)
Nausea and vomiting in pregnancy (Vutyavanich, 1995)
Peptic ulcers (Henrotte, 1992)
PMS (Brush, 1988)

Summary Pyridoxine is a water-soluble B vitamin that functions as a cofactor in more than 100 enzyme reactions. Many of its activities are related to the metabolism of amino acids and other proteins. Because of its effects on the synthesis of neurotransmitters, it may be useful in a variety of neurologic disorders. In addition, supplementation has been claimed to reduce the symptoms of PMS, asthma, and diabetes. Pyridoxine may be of benefit in (Continued)

Vitamin B$_6$ (Pyridoxine) *(Continued)*

pregnancy-associated nausea. It also may reduce homocysteine levels (which may contribute to the development of coronary artery disease in some individuals).

Pharmacology Vitamin B$_6$ is phosphorylated by intracellular enzymes to its active form, pyridoxal-5'-phosphate (PLP). Its metabolic activities include facilitation of transamination, deamination, desulfuration, and decarboxylation reactions. Pyridoxine is necessary for the formation of hemoglobin and the growth of red blood cells. It participates in the conversion of tryptophan to niacin and is required for the synthesis of a variety of neurotransmitters, including serotonin, gamma amino butyric acid (GABA), norepinephrine, acetylcholine, and histamine. Pyridoxine is involved in the metabolism of glycogen to glucose, and facilitates the metabolism of homocysteine, a risk factor for coronary artery disease in some individuals.

Toxicities, Warnings, and Interactions

Toxic dose: 250-1000 mg/day

Toxicity symptoms: Prolonged excesses can cause reversible nerve damage

Symptoms of Deficiency Anemia, irritability, depression, nausea, vomiting, depressed immunity, kidney stones, smooth tongue, premenstrual tension (females)

Reported Interactions

Drug/Nutrient Interactions: Drugs which can cause depletion of vitamin B$_6$: Estrogen-containing medications (oral contraceptives and estrogen replacement therapy), hydralazine, loop diuretics, antibiotics, isoniazid, theophylline, penicillamine

Nutrient/Nutrient Interactions: There are no known adverse nutrient/nutrient interactions between pyridoxine and other nutrients. However, pyridoxine is involved with other B vitamins in many biochemical activities and therefore, many health professionals suggest that vitamin B$_6$ be taken along with other B vitamins. A deficiency of vitamin B$_6$ inhibits the synthesis of melatonin.

References

Adams PW, Rose DP, Folkard J, et al, "Effect of Pyridoxine Hydrochloride (Vitamin B$_6$) Upon Depression Associated With Oral Contraception," *Lancet*, 1973, 1(7809):899-904.

Brush MG, Bennett T, and Hansen K, "Pyridoxine in the Treatment of Premenstrual Syndrome: A Retrospective Survey in 630 Patients," *Br J Clin Pract*, 1988, 42(11):448-52.

Crowell GF and Roach ES, "Pyridoxine-Dependent Seizures," *Am Fam Physician*, 1983, 27(3):183-7.

Folkers K, Shizu Kuishi S, Willis R, et al, "The Biochemistry of Vitamin B$_6$ Is Basic to the Cause of the Chinese Restaurant Syndrome," *Hoppe Seylers Z Physiol Chem*, 1984, 365(3):405-14.

Henrotte JG, Franck G, Santarromana M, et al, "Effect of Pyridoxine on Mice Gastric Ulcers and Brain Catecholamines After an Immobilization Stress," *Ann Nutr Metab*, 1992, 35(5-6):313-7.

Jones CL and Gonzalez V, "Pyridoxine Deficiency: A New Factor in Diabetic Neuropathy," *J Am Podiatry Assoc*, 1978, 68(9):646-53.

Kremer JM and Bigaouette J, "Nutrient Intake of Patients With Rheumatoid Arthritis Is Deficient in Pyridoxine, Zinc, Copper, and Magnesium," *J Rheumatol*, 1996, 23(6):990-4.

Mitwalli A, Ayiomamitis A, Grass L, et al, "Control of Hyperoxaluria With Large Doses of Pyridoxine in Patients With Kidney Stones," *Int Urol Nephrol*, 1988, 20(4):353-9.

Reynolds RD and Natta CL, "Depressed Plasma Pyridoxal Phosphate Concentrations in Adult Asthmatics," *Am J Clin Nutr*, 1985, 41(4):684-8.

Spooner GR, Desai HB, Angel JF, et al, "Using Pyridoxine to Treat Carpal Tunnel Syndrome. Randomized Control Trial," *Can Fam Physician*, 1993, 39:2122-7.

Vutyavanich T, Wongtra-Ngan S, and Ruangsri R, "Pyridoxine for Nausea and Vomiting of Pregnancy: A Randomized, Double-Blind, Placebo-Controlled Trial," *Am J Obstet Gynecol*, 1995, 173(3 Pt 1):881-4.

Vitamin B$_{12}$ (Cobalamin)

Related Information

Drug-Induced Nutrient Depletions *on page 625*

Pregnancy & Lactation Nutritional Chart *on page 657*

Vitamins/Minerals/Trace Elements/Amino Acids Chart *on page 604*

Natural Product Category Vitamin

Dosage Oral: RDI: 4 mcg/day; ODA: 10-500 mcg/day

Active Forms Cyanocobalamin, methylcobalamin

Reported Uses

AIDS (Weinberg, 1998)
Atherosclerosis (due to homocysteine elevation) (Siri, 1998)
Bronchial asthma (Simon, 1951)
Crohn's disease (Simon, 1951)
Depression (Joosten, 1993)
Diabetic neuropathy (Khan, 1969)
Male infertility (Nagai, 1988)
Memory loss (Hector, 1988)
Multiple sclerosis (Sandyk, 1993)
Pernicious anemia (Lederle, 1998)
Sulfite sensitivity (Anibarro, 1992)

Summary Vitamin B_{12} is a water-soluble B vitamin. It serves as a cofactor in cellular enzymatic processes, and is particularly important in the metabolism of cells within the gastrointestinal tract, bone marrow, and nervous system. Supplementation has been claimed to be of benefit in a wide variety of disorders, ranging from atherosclerosis to depression. Absorption from the gastrointestinal tract is dependent on the gastric secretion of intrinsic factor. This factor is absent in individuals with pernicious anemia.

Pharmacology Vitamin B_{12} functions as a cofactor in a number of enzymatic reactions. In particular it is involved in methyl group and hydrogen transfer reactions. Vitamin B_{12} participates in the demethylation of methyltetrahydrofolate to tetrahydrofolate, a step in DNA synthesis and cellular replication. It is required for synthesis of myelin, and is important to maintain the function of nerve cells. In addition, vitamin B_{12} is necessary for the maturation of red blood cells and is required for the metabolism of homocysteine. Vitamin B_{12} is involved in the metabolism of protein, fat, and carbohydrates.

Toxicities, Warnings, and Interactions No known toxicity or serious side effects

Symptoms of Deficiency Megaloblastic anemia, irritability, loss of coordination, fatigue, insomnia, hypersensitivity, sprue

Reported Interactions

Drug/Nutrient Interactions: Drugs which can cause depletion of vitamin B_{12}: Oral contraceptives, phenytoin, colchicine, antibiotics, biguanides (metformin), H_2-receptor antagonists, proton pump inhibitors, timed-release potassium chloride medications

Nutrient/Nutrient Interactions: There are no known adverse nutrient/nutrient interactions between vitamin B_{12} and other nutrients. However, vitamin B_{12} participates with other B vitamins in many biochemical activities, and many health professionals suggest that vitamin B_{12} be taken along with other B vitamins.

References

Anibarro B, Caballero T, Garcia-Ara C, et al, "Asthma With Sulfite Intolerance in Children: A Blocking Study With Cyanocobalamin," *J Allergy Clin Immunol,* 1992, 90(1):103-9.

Hector M and Burton JR, "What are the Psychiatric Manifestations of Vitamin B_{12} Deficiency?," *J Am Geriatr Soc,* 1988, 36(12):1105-12.

Joosten E, van den Berg A, Riezler R, et al, "Metabolic Evidence That Deficiencies of Vitamin B-12 (Cobalamin), Folate, and Vitamin B-6 Occur Commonly in Elderly People," *Am J Clin Nutr,* 1993, 58(4):468-76.

Khan MA, Wakefield GS, and Pugh DW, "Vitamin-B_{12} Deficiency and Diabetic Neuropathy," *Lancet,* 1969, 2(7624):768-70.

Lederle FA, "Oral Cobalamin for Pernicious Anemia: Back From the Verge of Extinction," *J Am Geriatr Soc,* 1998, 46(9):1125-7.

Nagai N, Katayama Y, Iguchi M, et al, "Treatment in Male Infertile Clinic of Kaizuka Municipal Hospital," *Hinyokika Kiyo,* 1988, 34(5):839-46.

Sandyk R and Awerbuch GI, "Vitamin B_{12} and Its Relationship to Age of Onset of Multiple Sclerosis," *Int J Neurosci,* 1993, 71(1-4):93-9.

Simon SW, "Vitamin B_{12} Therapy in Allergy and Chronic Dermatoses," *J Allergy,* 1951, 22:183-5.

Siri PW, Verhoef P, and Kok FJ, "Vitamins B_6, B_{12}, and Folate: Association With Plasma Total Homocysteine and Risk of Coronary Atherosclerosis," *J Am Coll Nutr,* 1998, 17(5):435-41.

Weinberg JB, Shugars DC, Sherman PA, et al, "Cobalamin Inhibition of HIV-1 Integrase and Integration of HIV-1 DNA Into Cellular DNA," *Biochem Biophys Res Commun,* 1998, 246(2):393-7.

Vitamin B Complex-25

Related Information
Organ System Support Using Natural Products *on page 660*
Vitamins/Minerals/Trace Elements/Amino Acids Chart *on page 604*

Natural Product Category Vitamin

Dosage Oral: RDI: None established; ODA: 25-100 mg of vitamins B_1, B_2, B_3, B_5, and B_6 and may also contain B_{12}, folic acid, and biotin

Reported Uses See individual B vitamins

Summary Vitamin B complex-25 is a term that refers to a nutritional supplement that contains many or all of the B vitamins. Taking a vitamin B complex-25 product is an easy and efficient way to ensure that an adequate amount of all the B vitamins are obtained on a daily basis. For example, each tablet in a B complex product might contain 50 mg of vitamins B_1, B_2, B_3, B_5, B_6, inositol, and choline, as well as 50 mcg of folic acid, biotin, and vitamin B_{12}. Keep in mind that many multivitamin products contain adequate levels of the B vitamins. Therefore, anyone taking a high-potency multivitamin usually does not need to take an additional B complex product.

Broad range of support for a wide range of biological activities involving the B vitamins; found in brewer's yeast, organ meats, fish, eggs, milk, nuts, vegetables, and whole grains

Pharmacology A vitamin B complex product provides support for a wide range of pharmacological activities. In general, B vitamins are necessary for the proper metabolism of fats, proteins, and carbohydrates. They are also essential for energy production, functioning of the nervous system, and the synthesis and activity of hormones, neurotransmitters, and enzymes throughout the body. In addition, B vitamins are required for proper growth and development, as well as proper functioning of the heart, muscles, adrenal glands, and mucous membranes.

Toxicities, Warnings, and Interactions
Toxic dose: No side effects at the RDI or ODA doses
Toxic symptoms: Side effects could result from high dose of vitamin B_3 and vitamin B_6

Symptoms of Deficiency A deficiency of the B-Complex vitamins would result in numerous health problems

Vitamin C

Related Information
Organ System Support Using Natural Products *on page 660*
Pregnancy & Lactation Nutritional Chart *on page 657*
Vitamins/Minerals/Trace Elements/Amino Acids Chart *on page 604*

Natural Product Category Vitamin

Dosage Oral: RDI: 60 mg/day; ODA: 250-1000 mg/day

Active Forms Ascorbic acid, calcium ascorbate, magnesium ascorbate, sodium ascorbate, ester C, ascorbyl palmitate

Reported Uses
AIDS (Cathcart, 1984)
Allergies (Johnston, 1996)
Asthma (Bielory, 1994)
Atherosclerosis (Willis, 1954; Jialal, 1990)
Cancer (Block, 1991)
Cataracts (Jacques, 1997)
Cervical dysplasia (Romney, 1985)
Common cold (Pauling, 1986)
Crohn's disease (Linaker, 1979)
Diabetes (Sinclair, 1994)
Gingivitis (Nakamoto, 1984)
Immune enhancement (Pauling, 1986)
Parkinson's disease (Yapa, 1992)
Peptic ulcer (Jarosz, 1998)
Sunburn (Darr, 1992)
Wound healing (Ringsdorf, 1982)

Summary Vitamin C (ascorbic acid) is a water-soluble vitamin which cannot be manufactured in humans. Supplementation has been claimed to augment immune function, increase healing of traumatized tissues, limit allergic reactions or asthma symptoms, and suppress the activity of some carcinogens. Ascorbic acid may be beneficial in lipid management and atherosclerosis. It has also been claimed to have antiviral activity in AIDS and the common cold.

Pharmacology Vitamin C is involved in a variety of oxidation-reduction reactions, energy production, tyrosine metabolism, the reduction and storage of iron, and the activation of folic acid. It plays a role in the synthesis of collagen and elastin, the major structural components of connective tissue (tendons, bone matrix, dentin, blood vessels). Vitamin C is an antioxidant, capable of neutralizing free radicals and assisting in the regeneration of vitamin E. Vitamin C is required for the synthesis of several neurotransmitters and adrenal hormones, which are critical to mediate the physiologic adaptation to stress. In addition, it may prevent the formation of nitrosamines, which are carcinogenic.

Ascorbic acid has multiple activities which may slow atherogenesis. It aids in the biliary excretion of cholesterol, decreases oxidation of cholesterol, and decreases levels of lipoprotein(a) or Lp(a). In addition, it may assist in solubilizing calcium, phospholipids, and cholesterol from atherosclerotic plaques.

Within the immune system, ascorbic acid facilitates production of white blood cells (neutrophils, lymphocytes, and natural killer cells), as well as levels of IgA, IgG, and IgM. It also allows production of interferon and modulates prostaglandin synthesis. Vitamin C functions as a histamine and phosphodiesterase inhibitor. It has been reported to have antiviral activity and aids in the detoxification of heavy metal toxins such as mercury, lead, cadmium, and nickel.

Toxicities, Warnings, and Interactions

Toxic dose: Risk for toxicity is low. Chronic consumption of doses >1000 mg/day may contribute to kidney stone formation, usually in individuals with pre-existing kidney dysfunction.

Toxicity symptoms: Most common side effect of large doses is diarrhea. Excess intake in diabetics may give falsely elevated blood glucose readings.

Symptoms of Deficiency
Slow wound healing, bleeding gums, recurrent infections, allergies, atherosclerotic plaques, bone fragility, joint pain, anemia

Reported Interactions

Drug/Nutrient Interactions: Drugs which can cause depletion of vitamin C: Oral contraceptives, indomethacin, tetracyclines, aspirin and other salicylates

Nutrient/Nutrient Interactions: Elevated levels of vitamin C can cause a depletion of copper and an increased absorption of iron. Vitamin C also regenerates vitamin E back to its active antioxidant status. If vitamin C is taken beyond bowel tolerance, the resulting diarrhea may result in the depletion of many nutrients.

References

Bielory L and Gandhi R, "Asthma and Vitamin C," *Ann Allergy*, 1994, 73(2):89-96.

Block G, "Epidemiologic Evidence Regarding Vitamin C and Cancer," *Am J Clin Nutr*, 1991, 54(6 Supp):1310S-4S.

Cathcart RF 3d, "Vitamin C in the Treatment of Acquired Immune Deficiency Syndrome (AIDS)," *Med Hypotheses*, 1984, 14(4):423-33.

Darr D, Combs S, Dunston S, et al, "Topical Vitamin C Protects Porcine Skin From Ultraviolet Radiation-Induced Damage," *Br J Dermatol*, 1992, 127(3):247-53.

Jacques PF, Taylor A, Hankinson SE, et al, "Long-Term Vitamin C Supplement Use and Prevalence of Early Age-Related Lens Opacities," *Am J Clin Nutr*, 1997, 66(4):911-61.

Jarosz M, Dzieniszewski J, Dabrowska-Ufniarz E, et al, "Effects of High Dose Vitamin C Treatment on *Helicobacter pylori* Infection and Total Vitamin C Concentration in Gastric Juice," *Eur J Cancer Prev*, 1998, 7(6):449-54.

Jialal I, Vega GL, and Grundy SM, "Physiologic Levels of Ascorbate Inhibit the Oxidative Modification of Low Density Lipoprotein," *Atherosclerosis*, 1990, 82(3):185-91.

(Continued)

ALPHABETICAL LISTING OF NATURAL PRODUCTS

Vitamin C (Continued)

Johnston CS, "The Antihistamine Action of Ascorbic Acid," *Subcell Biochem*, 1996, 25:189-213.

Linaker BD, "Scurvy and Vitamin C Deficiency in Crohn's Disease," *Postgrad Med J*, 1979, 55(639):26-9.

Nakamoto T, McCroskey M, and Mallek HM, "The Role of Ascorbic Acid Deficiency in Human Gingivitis-A New Hypothesis," *J Theor Biol*, 1984, 108(2):163-71.

Pauling L, *How to Live Longer and Feel Better*, New York, NY: WH Freeman and Company, 1986, 118-21.

Ringsdorf WM Jr and Cheraskin E, "Vitamin C and Human Wound Healing," *Oral Surg Oral Med Oral Pathol*, 1982, 53(3):231-6.

Romney SL, Duttagupta C, Basu J, et al, "Plasma Vitamin C and Uterine Cervical Dysplasia," *Am J Obstet Gynecol*, 1985, 151(7):976-80.

Sinclair AJ, Taylor PB, Luner J, et al, "Low Plasma Ascorbate Levels in Patients With Type 2 Diabetes Mellitus Consuming Adequate Dietary Vitamin C," *Diabet Med*, 1994, 11(9):893-8.

Willis GC, "Serial Arteriography in Atherosclerosis," *Can Med Assoc J*, 1954, 71:562-68.

Yapa SC, "Detection of Subclinical Ascorbate Deficiency in Early Parkinson's Disease," *Public Health*, 1992, 106(5):393-5.

Vitamin D

Related Information
Drug-Induced Nutrient Depletions *on page 625*
Pregnancy & Lactation Nutritional Chart *on page 657*
Vitamins/Minerals/Trace Elements/Amino Acids Chart *on page 604*

Natural Product Category Vitamin

Dosage Oral: RDI: 400 int. units/day; ODA: 400 int. units/day

Active Forms Vitamin D_2 (ergocalciferol), vitamin D_3 (cholecalciferol), calcitriol (1,25 dihydroxy cholecalciferol)

Reported Uses
Crohn's disease (Andreassen, 1998)
Epilepsy during anticonvulsant therapy (Shafer, 1975)
Hearing loss (Brookes, 1985)
Osteoporosis (Lau, 1999; Matsunaga, 1999)
Psoriasis (Morimoto, 1990)
Rickets (Takeda, 1997)
Scleroderma (Humbert, 1993)

Summary Vitamin D is a fat-soluble vitamin that was isolated in 1930 and named calciferol. Since then more metabolites have been found, and the two major forms of this vitamin are now known to be vitamin D_2 (ergocalciferol) and vitamin D_3 (cholecalciferol). Vitamin D is actually a hormone precursor which can be manufactured by the body. Therefore, in a classical sense, it is not actually an essential nutrient. However, since the disease rickets is related to vitamin D deficiency, it has been traditionally classified as a vitamin.

Pharmacology Vitamin D is activated by a series of physiologic reactions. In the skin, the sun's ultraviolet rays convert 7-dehydroergosterol into vitamin D_3. Vitamin D_3 is hydroxylated in the liver to 25-hydroxycholecalciferol, and undergoes a second hydroxylation in the kidney to form 1,25-dihydroxycholecalciferol (calcitriol), which is the most active form of vitamin D. Calcitriol mediates the intestinal absorption of calcium, phosphorus, magnesium, and zinc. It also modulates bone mineralization and demineralization. In addition, vitamin D is important to maintain normal thyroid function.

Toxicities, Warnings, and Interactions
Toxic dose: Because vitamin D is potentially toxic, it is generally recommended to avoid doses ≥1000 int. units daily. However, some reports indicate that most cases of toxicity involve an intake of 25,000-60,000 int. units daily for 1-4 months.

Toxicity symptoms: Excessive thirst, dehydration, anorexia, nausea, vomiting, headache, constipation, weakness, weight loss, hypercalcemia, kidney stones, arterial calcium deposits

Symptoms of Deficiency Bone and tooth disorders, rickets, osteomalacia

Reported Interactions

Drug/Nutrient Interactions: Drugs which can cause depletion of vitamin D: Cholestyramine, anticonvulsants, corticosteroids, isoniazid, rifampin, H_2-receptor antagonists, mineral oil

Nutrient/Nutrient Interactions: Vitamin D can cause an increase in the absorption of calcium and phosphorus. Vitamin A antagonizes some of the activity of vitamin D.

References

Andreassen H, Rix M, Brot C, et al, "Regulators of Calcium Homeostasis and Bone Mineral Density in Patients With Crohn's Disease," *Scand J Gastroenterol*, 1998, 33(10):1087-93.

Brookes GB, "Vitamin D Deficiency and Deafness: 1984 Update," *Am J Otol*, 1985, 6(1):102-7.

Humbert P, Dupond JL, Agache P, et al, "Treatment of Scleroderma With Oral 1,25-Dihydroxyvitamin D3: Evaluation of Skin Involvement Using Non-invasive Techniques. Results of an Open Prospective Trial," *Acta Derm Venereol*, 1993, 73(6):449-51.

Lau KH and Baylink DJ, "Vitamin D Therapy of Osteoporosis: Plain Vitamin D Therapy Versus Active Vitamin D Analog (D-Hormone) Therapy," *Calcif Tissue Int*, 1999, 65(4):295-306.

Matsunaga S, Ito H, and Sakou T, "The Effect of Vitamin K and D Supplementation on Ovariectomy-Induced Bone Loss," *Calcif Tissue Int*, 1999, 65(4):285-9.

Morimoto S, Yoshikawa K, Fukuo K, et al, "Inverse Relation Between Severity of Psoriasis and Serum 1,25-Dihydroxy-Vitamin D Level," *J Dermatol Sci*, 1990, 1(4):277-82.

Shafer RB and Nuttall FQ, "Calcium and Folic Acid Absorption in Patients Taking Anticonvulsant Drugs," *J Clin Endocrinol Metab*, 1975, 41(06):1125-9.

Takeda E, Yamamoto H, Taketani Y, et al, "Vitamin D-Dependent Rickets Type I and Type II," *Acta Paediatr Jpn*, 1997, 39(4):508-13.

Vitamin E

Related Information

Drug-Induced Nutrient Depletions *on page 625*
Organ System Support Using Natural Products *on page 660*
Pregnancy & Lactation Nutritional Chart *on page 657*
Vitamins/Minerals/Trace Elements/Amino Acids Chart *on page 604*

Natural Product Category Vitamin

Dosage Oral: RDI: Males: 10 int. units/day, females: 8 int. units/day; ODA: 400 int. units/day

Active Forms Natural vitamin E (*d*-alpha tocopherol) and synthetic vitamin E (*dl*-alpha tocopherol), which is a mixture of the d and l isomers. Natural vitamin E is more bioavailable and is retained in the body longer than synthetic vitamin E (Burton, 1998). In most cases, vitamin E is bound to either acetate or succinate in order to increase stability.

Reported Uses

Alzheimer's disease (Sano, 1997)
Atherosclerosis (Chan, 1998)
Benign Prostatic Hypertrophy (BPH) (Thomas, 1999)
Cancer prevention (Das, 1994)
Cataracts (Robertson, 1989)
Cervical dysplasia (Palan, 1991)
Diabetes (Paolisso, 1993)
Dyslipidemias (Porkkala-Sarataho, 1996)
Lupus (Ayres, 1979)
Osteoarthritis (Scherak, 1990)
Peptic ulcer (Suzuki, 1998)
Peripheral circulation (Haeger, 1982)
PMS (London, 1987)
Prevention of myocardial infarction (Stephens, 1996)
Rheumatoid arthritis (Edmonds, 1997)
Sunburn (Ritter, 1997)

Summary Vitamin E is the body's most important fat-soluble antioxidant. It may protect against coronary artery disease and myocardial infarction. In addition, it is claimed to be useful in inflammatory diseases such as arthritis, and in the prevention of some forms of cancer. Supplementation has also been claimed to be of benefit in limiting PMS symptoms and blocking degenerative changes in the brain (Alzheimer's) and eyes (cataracts).

Pharmacology Vitamin E includes eight compounds, including four tocopherols (alpha, beta, gamma, and delta) and four additional tocotrienol derivatives. Alpha tocopherol is the most common and the most potent form of (Continued)

Vitamin E *(Continued)*

vitamin E. Its primary physiologic function is to prevent free radical oxidative damage, including lipid peroxidation. This activity protects normal cellular structure and function, as well as aiding in tissue healing. Cardiovascular benefit may be related to its ability to decrease platelet aggregation, prevent the oxidation of LDL cholesterol, and slow atherogenesis. It is also believed to block the oxidative changes of the lens which may result in cataracts. Blocking oxidation is believed to protect against environmental pollutants and carcinogens, and may slow the aging process.

Toxicities, Warnings, and Interactions

Toxic dose: Relatively nontoxic; because vitamin E can result in an impairment in hemostasis, dosages should be reduced or interrupted 1 week prior to surgical and/or dental procedures

Toxicity symptoms: Use with caution when taking anticoagulants (vitamin E ≥200 int. units can prolong prothrombin time (increase blood thinning)

Amprenavir contains Vitamin E. The manufacturer warns against the use of additional supplementation in individuals receiving this medication.

Symptoms of Deficiency Dry skin, dry hair, dermatologic problems (eczema, psoriasis), cataracts, impaired wound healing, and (in women) PMS or hot flashes

Reported Interactions

Drug/Nutrient Interactions: Drugs that interfere with the absorption of vitamin E include: Cholestyramine, colestipol, orlistat, and mineral oil. Vitamin E may potentiate the anticoagulant effect of warfarin in individuals who are vitamin K deficient (this does not appear to be clinically relevant at doses ≤400 int. units/day). Gemfibrozil depletes vitamin E by an unknown mechanism.

Nutrient/Nutrient Interactions: Iron can bind and inactivate vitamin E. Large doses of vitamin E can interfere with the absorption of vitamin A. Vitamin C regenerates vitamin E back to its active antioxidant status.

References

Ayres S Jr and Mihan R, "Lupus Erythematosus and Vitamin E: An Effective and Nontoxic Therapy," *Cutis*, 1979, 23(1):49-52,54.

Chan AC, "Vitamin E and Atherosclerosis," *J Nutr*, 1998, 128(10):1593-6.

Das S, "Vitamin E in the Genesis and Prevention of Cancer. A Review," *Acta Oncol*, 1994, 33(6):615-9.

Edmonds SE, Winyard PG, Guo R, et al, "Putative Analgesic Activity of Repeated Oral Doses of Vitamin E in the Treatment of Rheumatoid Arthritis. Results of a Prospective Placebo Controlled Double-Blind Trial," *Ann Rheum Dis*, 1997, 56(11):649-55.

Haeger K, "Long Term Study of Alpha-Tocopherol in Intermittent Claudication," *Ann NY Acad Sci*, 1982, 393:369-75.

London RS, Murphy L, Kitlowski KE, et al, "Efficacy of Alpha-Tocopherol in the Treatment of the Premenstrual Syndrome," *J Reprod Med*, 1987, 32(6):400-4.

Palan PR, Mikhail MS, Basu J, et al, "Plasma Levels of Antioxidant Beta-Carotene and Alpha-Tocopherol in Uterine Cervix Dysplasias and Cancer," *Nutr Cancer*, 1991, 15(1):13-20.

Paolisso G, D'Amore A, Giugliano D, et al, "Pharmacologic Doses of Vitamin E Improve Insulin Action in Healthy Subjects and Non-insulin-Dependent Diabetic Patients," *Am J Clin Nutr*, 1993, 57(5):650-6.

Porkkala-Sarataho E, Nyyssonen K, and Salonen JT, "Increased Oxidation Resistance of Atherogenic Plasma Lipoproteins at High Vitamin E Levels in Non-vitamin E Supplemented Men," *Atherosclerosis*, 1996, 124(1):83-94.

Ritter EF, Axelrod M, Minn KW, et al, "Modulation of Ultraviolet Light-Induced Epidermal Damage: Beneficial Effects of Tocopherol," *Plast Reconstr Surg*, 1997, 100(4):973-80.

Robertson JM, Donner AP, and Trevithick JR, "Vitamin E Intake and Risk of Cataracts in Humans," *Ann N Y Acad Sci*, 1989, 570:372-82.

Sano M, Ernesto C, Thomas RG, et al, "A Controlled Trial of Selegiline, Alpha-Tocopherol, or Both as Treatment for Alzheimer's Disease. The Alzheimer's Disease Cooperative Study," *N Engl J Med*, 1997, 336(17):1216-22.

Scherak O, Kolarz G, Schodl C, et al, "High Dosage Vitamin E Therapy in Patients with Activated Arthrosis," *Z Rheumatol*, 1990, 49(6):369-73.

Stephens NG, Parsons A, Schofield PM, et al, "Randomised Controlled Trial of Vitamin E in Patients With Coronary Disease: Cambridge Heart Antioxidant Study," *Lancet*, 1996, 347(9004): 781-6.

Suzuki Y, Ishihara M, Segami T, et al, "Anti-ulcer Effects of Antioxidants, Quercetin, Alpha-Tocopherol, Nifedipine, and Tetracycline in Rats," *Jpn J Pharmacol*, 1998, 78(4):435-41.

Thomas JA, "Diet, Micronutrients, and the Prostate Gland," *Nutr Rev*, 1999, 57(4):95-103.

Vitamin K
Related Information
Drug-Induced Nutrient Depletions *on page 625*
Pregnancy & Lactation Nutritional Chart *on page 657*
Vitamins/Minerals/Trace Elements/Amino Acids Chart *on page 604*

Natural Product Category Vitamin

Dosage Oral: RDI: None established; ODA: Males: 65 mcg/day, females: 55 mcg/day

Active Forms Vitamin K_1 (phylloquinone, derived from plants), vitamin K_2 (menaquinone, derived from animals), vitamin K_3 (menadione, a water-soluble manufactured synthetically)

Reported Uses
Osteoporosis (Kanai, 1997)
Synthesis of blood clotting factors (Igarashi, 1993)

Summary Vitamin K derives its name from a Danish scientist, who named it "Koagulationsvitamin," a reference to its importance in blood coagulation. Vitamin K is synthesized normally by colonic microflora, and stores may be reduced following exposure to some medications, particularly after broad-spectrum antibiotics. In addition to effects on clotting factors, it is required for normal bone calcification, and supplementation has been claimed to be of benefit osteoporosis.

Pharmacology Vitamin K refers to a group of three fat-soluble vitamins called the quinones. Phylloquinone (K_1) occurs in green plants, mena-quinone (K_2) is synthesized by intestinal bacteria, and menadione (K3) is manufactured synthetically. Vitamin K is necessary for the post-translational modification of a number of clotting factors and other proteins. Factors II, VII, IX, and X are all considered vitamin-K dependent. In addition, the anticoagulant proteins, protein C and protein S, are also dependent on vitamin K for production. It is also necessary for the synthesis of osteo-calcin, an important mediator of calcium deposition into the bone matrix.

Toxicities, Warnings, and Interactions Toxic dose: Large doses of Vitamin K_3 (synthetic form) can cause hemolytic anemia in animals and jaundice in infants. Vitamin K_1, derived from alfalfa leaves, is claimed to have a wider range of safety.

Symptoms of Deficiency Slow blood clotting, hemorrhaging
Reported Interactions
Drug/Nutrient Interactions: Drugs which can cause depletion of vitamin K include: Antibiotics, anticonvulsants (barbiturates and phenytoin), antico-agulants, cholestyramine, mineral oil, aspirin and salicylates.
Caution in individuals taking warfarin: Should not change vitamin K intake without physician supervision

Nutrient/Nutrient Interactions: None known

References
Igarashi O, "Vitamin K," *Nippon Rinsho*, 1993, 51(4):910-8.
Kanai T, Takagi T, Masuhiro K, et al, "Serum Vitamin K Level and Bone Mineral Density in Post-menopausal Women," *Int J Gynaecol Obstet*, 1997, 56(1):25-30.

♦ **Vitamins/Minerals/Trace Elements/Amino Acids Chart** *see page 604*
♦ ***Vitex agnus-castus*** *see* Chasteberry (Vitex agnus-castus) *on page 408*
♦ ***Vitis vinifera*** *see* Grape Seed (Vitis vinifera) *on page 451*
♦ **Weight Management** *see page 374*

White Oak *(Quercus alba)*
Related Information
Herb Quick Reference Chart *on page 538*

Natural Product Category Herb
Plant Part Bark
Dosage and Standardization Oral rinse: Use 3 times/day, gargle and expectorate

Reported Uses Used as a soothing agent in mild inflammation of the throat and mouth (Wichtl, 1994)

(Continued)

White Oak *(Quercus alba)* (Continued)

Summary White oak bark is traditionally used as an astringent. It is used as a soothing agent in mild inflammation of the throat and mouth.

Pharmacology White oak bark is used for its tannin content. Used as a gargle, white oak bark is beneficial for inflammation of the oral cavity.

Theoretical Cautions and Contraindications Use caution in individuals with renal or hepatic dysfunction (only if ingested).

General Warnings Caution should be used in individuals having known allergies to plants.

Theoretical Interactions None known

References

Wichtl M, Bisset N, eds. *Herbal Drugs and Phytopharmaceuticals*, Stuttgart: CRC Press, 1994.

White Willow *(Salix alba)*

Related Information

Herb/Drug Potential Interactions *on page 642*
Herb Quick Reference Chart *on page 538*

Natural Product Category Herb

Plant Part Bark

Dosage and Standardization Oral: 500 mg up to 3 times/day, standardized to contain 7% to 9% salicin per dose

Reported Uses Antipyretic; anti-inflammatory; used in reducing fever and in arthritic complaints (Bradley, 1992)

Summary White willow has been used for many years as an anti-inflammatory, analgesic, and antipyretic

Pharmacology White willow contains a variety of tannins, phenolic glycosides (salcortin, fragilin, tremulacin) and salicin. Salicin in white willow may be converted to saligenin in the gastrointestinal tract and absorbed. Following absorption, it is metabolized to salicylic acid. Most of the pharmacologic activity associated with white willow appears to be related to its salicylate effects. Salicylates are antipyretic, analgesic, and anti-inflammatory. In addition, salicylates may inhibit platelet aggregation. At high dosages, they may demonstrate effects on uric acid excretion and glucose regulation. The tannins in willow bark have astringent properties on the mucosal tissues as well as other systemic activities.

Theoretical Cautions and Contraindications Based on salicylate component, do not use in children due to potential for Reye's syndrome. Avoid in individuals with salicylate allergy. Due to pharmacological activity, use caution in individuals with renal or hepatic dysfunction.

General Warnings Use all herbal supplements with extreme caution in children <2 years of age and in pregnancy or lactation. Some herbs are contraindicated in pregnancy or lactation; make sure to observe warnings. Use with caution in individuals on medication and with pre-existing medical conditions. Always review for potential herb-drug interactions (HDIs) and other warnings. Large and prolonged doses may increase the potential for adverse effects. Herbs may cause transient adverse effects such as nausea, vomiting, and GI distress due to a variety of chemical constituents. Caution should be used in individuals having known allergies to plants.

Theoretical Interactions Aspirin, warfarin, methotrexate, metoclopramide, phenytoin, probenecid, spirolactone, valproic acid

References

Bradley PR, ed, *The British Herbal Compendium, Vol 1*, London, England: British Herbal Medicine Association, 1992, 224-6.6;6R

Newall CA, Anderson LA, and Phillipson JD, *Herbal Medicines: A Guide for Health Care Professionals*, London, England: The Pharmaceutical Press, 1996, 268-9.

Wild Yam *(Dioscorea villosa)*

Related Information

Herb/Drug Potential Interactions *on page 642*
Herb Quick Reference Chart *on page 538*

Natural Product Category Herb

Plant Part Tuber

Dosage and Standardization
Oral: 250 mg 1-3 times/day, standardized to contain 10% diosgenin per dose
Topical: Apply as directed

Reported Uses Contains steroidal precursors and used in female vitality, however, conversion to progesterone in the body is poor (Weiss, 1988)

Summary Wild yam tubers are used in the synthesis of progesterone. Wild yam contains steroidal precursors and is used in female vitality.

Pharmacology Wild yam contains the steroidal saponin diosgenin, which is precursor in the synthesis of progesterone containing pharmaceuticals. However, there is no identified pathway for physiologic conversion of wild yam to progesterone in humans.

Theoretical Cautions and Contraindications Use with caution in individuals taking steroidal medications. Phytoestrogen-containing herbs have not been associated with the negative health effects seen with synthetic estrogen. However, use with caution in individuals on hormone replacement therapy or oral contraceptives, or in those with a history of thromboembolic disease or stroke. Contraindicated in individuals with with a history of estrogen-dependent tumors or endometrial cancer.

General Warnings Use all herbal supplements with extreme caution in children <2 years of age and in pregnancy or lactation. Some herbs are contraindicated in pregnancy or lactation; make sure to observe warnings. Use with caution in individuals on medication and with pre-existing medical conditions. Always review for potential herb-drug interactions (HDIs) and other warnings. Large and prolonged doses may increase the potential for adverse effects. Herbs may cause transient adverse effects such as nausea, vomiting, and GI distress due to a variety of chemical constituents. Caution should be used in individuals having known allergies to plants.

Theoretical Interactions Steroidal agents, estrogens, oral contraceptives, estrogen replacement therapies

References
Weiss RF, *Herbal Medicine*, Beaconsfield, England: Beaconsfield Publishers LTD, 1988, 330.

♦ *Withania somnifera* see Ashwagandha *(Withania somnifera)* on page 387

Yohimbe *(Pausinystalia yohimbe)*

Related Information
Common Herbal Supplements Contraindicated During Pregnancy on page 656
Herb/Drug Potential Interactions on page 642
Herb Quick Reference Chart on page 538

Natural Product Category Herb

Plant Part Bark

Dosage and Standardization Oral: 500-750 mg twice daily

Reported Uses May increase sexual vitality in men and women; used in male erectile dysfunction (Riley, 1994)

Summary Yohimbe bark is traditionally used for increased sexual vitality in men and women. Pharmaceutically, yohimbine is isolated from yohimbe and used in male erectile dysfunction.

Pharmacology The alkaloid yohimbine has central nervous system stimulatory activity. Also, yohimbine has selective alpha$_2$ adrenergic blocking properties, which is the basis for its use in erectile dysfunction. Yohimbine also blocks peripheral 5-HT receptors. Aphrodisiac activity may be due to enlargement of the vasculature in the genitals, increase of nerve impulses to genital tissue, and an increased transmission of reflex excitability in the sacral region of the spinal cord.

Theoretical Cautions and Contraindications Contraindicated in pregnancy. Do not use in individuals taking MAO inhibitors or antihypertensives; do not use in hypertensive individuals (De Smet 1994) or cardiovascular disease. Toxic doses may trigger psychosis, hypotension, and cardiac failure. Based on pharmacological activity, use with caution in individuals receiving alpha$_2$ blockers. Based on pharmacological activity, may cause CNS stimulation (anxiety, insomnia), hypertension, and tachycardia.
(Continued)

Yohimbe *(Pausinystalia yohimbe)* *(Continued)*

General Warnings Use all herbal supplements with extreme caution in children <2 years of age and in pregnancy or lactation. Some herbs are contraindicated in pregnancy or lactation; make sure to observe warnings. Use with caution in individuals on medication and with pre-existing medical conditions. Always review for potential herb-drug interactions (HDIs) and other warnings. Large and prolonged doses may increase the potential for adverse effects. Herbs may cause transient adverse effects such as nausea, vomiting, and GI distress due to a variety of chemical constituents. Caution should be used in individuals having known allergies to plants.

Theoretical Interactions MAO inhibitors, antihypertensives, naloxone, tricyclic antidepressants, alpha$_2$ blockers, sympathomimetics

References

De Smet PA and Smeets OS, "Potential Risks of Health Food Products Containing Yohimbe Extracts," *BMJ,* 1994, 309(6959):958.

Riley AJ, "Yohimbine in the Treatment of Erectile Disorder," *Br J Clin Pract,* 1994, 48(3):133-6.

Zinc

Related Information

Drug-Induced Nutrient Depletions *on page 625*
Organ System Support Using Natural Products *on page 660*
Pregnancy & Lactation Nutritional Chart *on page 657*
Vitamins/Minerals/Trace Elements/Amino Acids Chart *on page 604*

Natural Product Category Mineral

Dosage

Oral: RDI: 15 mg/day; ODA: 15-35 mg/day
Topical: Apply to the affected area as needed

Active Forms Zinc arginate, ascorbate, aspartate, citrate, gluconate, glycinate, histidinate, methionate, oxide, picolinate, sulfate, undecylenate

Reported Uses

Acne (Verma, 1980)
Apthous ulcers (Merchant, 1977)
Benign prostatic hypertrophy (BPH) (Leake, 1984)
Common cold (Mossad, 1996)
Crohn's disease (Hendricks, 1988)
Diabetes (Pidduck, 1970)
Diaper rash (Collipp, 1989)
Gastric ulcer healing (Frommer, 1975)
Immune function (Fraker, 1986)
Macular degeneration (Newsome, 1988)
Male sexual vitality (Tikkiwal, 1987)
Osteoporosis (Angus, 1988)
Skin conditions, eczema (David, 1984)
Wound healing (Okada, 1990)

Summary Zinc is necessary for the functioning of over 300 different enzymes and, as such, it plays a vital role in an enormous number of biological processes. Zinc is widely distributed in microorganisms, plants, and animals. In humans, the highest concentrations of zinc are found in the liver, pancreas, kidneys, bone, and muscles. Zinc is also highly concentrated in parts of the eye, prostate gland, sperm, skin, hair, and nails. Cooking acidic foods in galvanized cookware used to be a possible source of excess zinc intake. The widespread use of stainless steel and plastic materials to prepare and store foods has largely eliminated this problem. Galvanized pipes in older plumbing systems used to leach zinc into drinking water supplies, but modern plumbing has phased out the use of galvanized pipes.

Pharmacology Zinc is a cofactor in a number of enzymatic reactions involved in carbohydrate and protein metabolism. Its immunologic activities include regulation of T lymphocytes, CD4, natural killer cells, and interleukin II. In addition, zinc has been claimed to possess antiviral activity. Zinc is an important cofactor for the antioxidant enzyme superoxide dismutase (SOD). It has been shown to play a role in wound healing, especially following burns or surgical incisions. Zinc is necessary for the maturation of sperm and normal fetal development. It is involved in sensory perception (taste, smell, and vision) and controls the release of stored vitamin A from the liver. Within the endocrine system, zinc has been shown to regulate insulin activity and promote the conversion of thyroxine to triiodothyronine.

Toxicities, Warnings, and Interactions

Toxic dose: Prolonged intake at levels >150 mg/day may be associated with toxicity

Toxicity symptoms: Nausea, vomiting, diarrhea, dizziness, anemia, can interfere with copper absorption, impair immune response, lower HDL

Symptoms of Deficiency White spots on fingernails, stretch marks on skin, loss of sense of smell or taste, joint pain, poor sexual development, slowed growth, menstrual irregularities, slow wound healing, recurrent infections, acne, sterility

Reported Interactions

Drug/Nutrient Interactions: Drugs which can cause depletion of zinc: Oral contraceptives, loop diuretics, thiazide diuretics, H_2-receptor antagonists, zidovudine (AZT), D-penicillamine, and ethambutol

Nutrient/Nutrient Interactions: Copper, calcium, and iron compete with zinc for protein-binding sites that regulate absorption. Due to this competition for absorption sites, elevated copper, calcium and/or iron can cause a depletion of zinc.

References

Angus RM, Sambrook PN, Popcock NA, et al, "Dietary Intake and Bone Mineral Density," *Bone Miner,* 1988, 4(3):265-77.

Collipp PJ, "Effect of Oral Zinc Supplements on Diaper Rash in Normal Infants," *J Med Assoc Ga,* 1989, 78(9):621-3.

David TJ, Wells FE, Sharpe TC, et al, "Low Serum Zinc in Children With Atopic Eczema," *Br J Dermatol,* 1984, 111(5):597-601.

Fraker PJ, Gershwin ME, Good RA, et al, "Interrelationships Between Zinc and Immune Function," *Fed Proc,* 1986, 45(5):1474-9.

Frommer DJ, "The Healing of Gastric Ulcers by Zinc Sulphate," *Med J Aust,* 1975, 2(21):793-6.

Hendricks KM and Walker WA, "Zinc Deficiency in Inflammatory Bowel Disease," *Nutr Rev,* 1988, 46(12):401-8

Leake A, Chisholm GD, and Habib FK, "The Effect of Zinc on the 5 Alpha-Reduction of Testosterone by the Hyperplastic Human Prostate Gland," *J Steroid Biochem,* 1984, 20(2):651-5.

Merchant HW, Gangarosa LP, Glassman AB, et al, "Zinc Sulfate Supplementation for Treatment of Recurring Oral Ulcers," *South Med J,* 1977, 70(5):559-61.

Mossad SB, Macknin ML, Medendorp SV, et al, "Zinc Gluconate Lozenges for Treating the Common Cold. A Randomized, Double-Blind, Placebo-Controlled Study," *Ann Intern Med,* 1996, 125(2):81-8.

Newsome DA, Swartz M, Leone NC, et al, "Oral Zinc in Macular Degeneration," *Arch Ophthalmol,* 1988, 106(2):192-8.

Okada A, Takagi Y, Nezu R, et al, "Zinc in Clinical Surgery-A Research Review," *Jpn J Surg,* 1990, 20(6):635-44.

Pidduck HG, Wren PJ, and Evans DA, "Plasma Zinc and Copper in Diabetes Mellitus," *Diabetes,* 1970, 19(4):234-9.

Tikkiwal M, Ajmera RL, and Mathur NK, "Effect of Zinc Administration on Seminal Zinc and Fertility of Oligospermic Males," *Indian J Physiol Pharmacol,* 1987, 31(1):30-4.

Verma KC, Saini AS, and Dhamija SK, "Oral Zinc Sulphate Therapy in Acne Vulgaris: A Double-Blind Trial," *Acta Derm Venereol,* 1980, 60(4):337-40.

♦ *Zingiber officinale* see Ginger (*Zingiber officinale*) on page 440

PART IV. CHARTS AND LISTS

TABLE OF CONTENTS

Herb Quick Reference Chart... 538

Nutraceutical Chart 573

Homeopathic Quick Reference Chart for Common Complaints 587

Vitamins / Minerals / Trace Elements / Amino Acids 604

Drug-Induced Nutrient Depletions 625

Nutrient Depletion and Cancer Chemotherapy 637

Herbal Medicine Use In Pediatrics 641

Herb/Drug Potential Interactions 642

Unsafe Herbs 654

Common Herbal Supplements Contraindicated
    During Pregnancy 656

Pregnancy & Lactation Nutritional Chart........................... 657

Organ System Support Using Natural Products 660

HERB QUICK REFERENCE CHART

Herb/Plant Part Used	Dosage & Standardization	Reported Uses	Complementary Effect With Drug Therapy	Theoretical Cautions/Contraindications/ Adverse Effects	Theoretical Interactive Drug/Drug Category
Aloe (*Aloe spp*) Leaf	Topical: Apply gel 3-4 times/day to affected area	• Burns and other minor skin • Healing agent in wounds, minor • Irritations	None known	• Some wound healing may be delayed when using topical aloe vera gel (Level 2)	None known
Arabinoxylane (isolated from *Ganoderma lucidum*)	Initial: 12 caps (250 mg ea)/day in divided doses for 5-14 days, then decrease dosage to 500 mg (2 x 250 mg) twice daily	• Decreases chemotherapy-induced leukopenia • HIV therapy • Increases NK cell, B cell, and T killer cell activity	None known	• Caution in individuals with renal impairment; MGN-3 contains high levels of phosphorus. DO NOT USE LOADING DOSE in these individuals (Level 2) • May enhance effects of immune stimulants; may limit effects of immune suppressants (Level 2)	None known
Artichoke (*Cynara scolymus*) Leaf	250 mg 2-3 times/day, standardized to contain 15% chlorogenic acid, or 2% to 5% Cynarin per dose	• Adjunctive agent in hyperlipidemia • Eczema and skin disorders; a hepatoprotectant • Improve the flow of bile (choleretic)	None known	• Do not use if allergic to members of the daisy and chrysanthemum (*Compositae*) family • Do not use if bile obstruction is present (Level 2)	None known
Ashwagandha (*Withania somnifera*) Root	450 mg 1-2 times/day, standardized to contain 1.5% withanolides per dose	• Adaptogen to enhance mental and physical performance, improve learning ability, and decrease stress and fatigue • Chemotherapy and radiation protection and therapeutic enhancement of these agents • General tonic in stressful situations, especially insomnia, overwork, nervousness, and restlessness	• Acts as a radiosensitizer when administered with radiation therapy, with heat reportedly enhancing these effects • Reported to protect against cyclophosphamide-induced leukopenia	• Contraindicated in pregnancy and lactation (may be an abortifacient) (Level 2) • Use with caution in narcotic analgesics (studies report it may decrease tolerance to opiates) (Level 2) • Use with caution in individuals on benzodiazepines (may alter levels) (Level 2)	• Benzodiazepines/ anxiolytics • Cyclophosphamide • Narcotic analgesics
Astragalus (*Astragalus membranaceus*) Root	250-500 mg 4 times/day, standardized to a minimum of 0.4% 4'-hydroxy-3'-methoxyisoflavone-7-glycosides per dose	• Adaptogen to increase stamina and energy • Adjunct support for chemotherapy and radiation • Improves resistance to disease and immune function • Improvement of tissue oxygenation	• May decrease cyclophosphamide-induced immune suppression (contradictory study - Khoo, 1995 - see monograph)	• Use with caution in acute infection, especially with a fever • May enhance effects of immune stimulants and may limit effects of immune suppressants (Level 4)	• Cyclophosphamide
Bacopa (*Bacopa monniera*) Leaf	100 mg 3 times/day, standardized to contain 20% bacosides A and B per dose	• Memory enhancement and improving cognitive function	None known	None known	None known

Herb/Plant Part Used	Dosage & Standardization	Reported Uses	Complementary Effect With Drug Therapy	Theoretical Cautions/Contraindications/ Adverse Effects	Theoretical Interactive Drug/Drug Category
Bilberry (*Vaccinium myrtillus*) Berry	80 mg 2-3 times/day, standardized to contain 25% anthocyanosides (calculated as anthocyanidins) per dose	• Antioxidant; used in eye disorders including myopia, diminished visual acuity, dark adaptation, day and night blindness, diabetic retinopathy, cataracts, macular degeneration • Cardiovascular health to help maintain capillary integrity and reduce hyperpermeability, including varicose veins and phlebitis	None known	• Use with caution in pregnancy and lactation (Level 2) • Use with caution in individuals taking anticoagulants (Level 4) • May be contraindicated in individuals with active bleeding (Level 4) • Use with caution in individuals with a history of bleeding or hemostatic disorders (Level 4) • Discontinue use prior to dental or surgical procedures (generally at least 14 days prior) (Level 4)	• Anticoagulants • Antiplatelets • Aspirin and aspirin-containing products • NSAIDs
Bitter Melon (*Momordica charantia*) Fruit	200 mg 2-3 times/day, standardized to contain 5.1% triterpenes per dose	• Antiviral • Hypoglycemic, impaired glucose tolerance (IGT), and diabetes	None known	• Do not use in pregnancy (emmenagogue and abortifacient) (Level 2) • May alter insulin and/or oral hypoglycemic needs in diabetic individuals (Level 2) • Close monitoring of blood sugar levels is recommended	• Insulin • Oral hypoglycemic agents
Black Cohosh (*Cimicifuga racemosa*) Root/rhizome	20-40 mg twice daily, standardized to contain 1 mg triterpenes (27-deoxyactein) per dose	• Arthritis • Mild depression • Phytoestrogenic action; used in menopausal complaints and PMS • Rheumatic complaints	None known	• Contraindicated in pregnancy and lactation (uterine stimulation reported (Level 2) • Caution if individual is taking hormonal drugs such as estrogen or birth control pills; may alter hormonal therapy (Level 4) • Use with caution in individuals allergic to salicylates (Level 4) • May cause nausea, vomiting, and headache in high doses	• Hormone replacement therapy • Oral contraceptives

Herb/Plant Part Used	Dosage & Standardization	Reported Uses	Complementary Effect With Drug Therapy	Theoretical Cautions/Contraindications/ Adverse Effects	Theoretical Interactive Drug/Drug Category
Bladderwrack (*Fucus vesiculosus*) Fronds	600 mg 1-3 times/day	• Rich source of iodine, potassium, magnesium, calcium, and iron; used in hypothyroidism and fibrocystic breast disease	None known	• Use with caution in individuals taking thyroid agents (Level 4) • Use with caution in hyperthyroidism (Level 4) • Caution for individuals with kidney failure (may alter potassium levels) (Level 4) • Avoid use in individuals with iodine sensitivity (Level 4)	• Thyroid agents • Lithium
Boswellia (*Boswellia serrata*) Gum resin	200-400 mg 3 times/day, standardized to contain 65% boswellic acid per dose	• Anti-inflammatory • Arthritis and other inflammatory conditions such as ulcerative colitis	None known	None known.	None known.
Bromelain (*Anas comosus*) Enzymes extracted from pineapple	**Digestive enzyme:** 1-2 tablets 3 times/day with meals, standardized to contain at least 2000 milk clotting units (mcu)/ g/dose **Inflammation:** 1 tablet 3 times/day between meals (either 1 hour before meals or 2 hours after meals)	• Digestive enzyme • Proteolytic agent; used as an anti-inflammatory agent in arthritis • Sinusitis	None known	• Use with caution if taking anticoagulants (Levels 1 & 2) • Use with caution in GI ulceration (Level 3) • Use with caution in individuals with hypertension or other cardiovascular disorders (Levels 1 & 2) • May be contraindicated in individuals with active bleeding (Level 4) • Use with caution in individuals with a history of bleeding or hemostatic disorders (Level 4) • Discontinue use prior to dental or surgical procedures (generally at least 14 days prior) (Level 4)	• Anticoagulants • Antiplatelet agents • Aspirin or aspirin-containing products • NSAIDs
Bupleurum (*Bupleurum falcatum*) Root	500 mg 3 times/day OR 30-60 drops of liquid extract (1:4 w/v) 3 times/ day	• Chronic inflammatory disease • Beneficial for liver support	None known	• Based on possible adrenal stimulation, use with caution in individuals with hypertension, diabetes, edema, or taking diuretics or corticosteroids (Level 4)	If adrenal stimulation occurs: • Antihypertensives • Corticosteroids • Diuretics

Herb/Plant Part Used	Dosage & Standardization	Reported Uses	Complementary Effect With Drug Therapy	Theoretical Cautions/Contraindications/ Adverse Effects	Theoretical Interactive Drug/Drug Category
Calendula (Calendula officinalis) Flower	Topical: Apply to affected area as needed	Topical uses: • Vulnerary • Antibacterial, antifungal, antiviral, antiprotozoal; wound healing agent • Increases wound healing by stimulating immune system	None known	• None known	• None known
Cascara (Rhamnus persiana) Aged bark	100 mg as needed, not to exceed 3 capsules/ day or >2 days, standardized to contain 25% to 30% hydroxyanthracene derivatives per dose	• Anthraquinone laxative	None known	• Avoid in children <12 years of age • May decrease absorption of susceptible oral medications by decreasing bowel transit time (Level 4) • Excessive use may lead to potassium loss and other electrolyte disturbances and may potentiate the effects of various pharmaceutical drugs with narrow therapeutic windows (Level 4) • Use with caution in bowel obstruction, diarrhea, or dehydration (Level 4) • Use with caution in bowel disorders (ulcerative colitis, Crohn's) and appendicitis (Level 4) • Use with caution in cardiovascular disease (overuse may cause electrolyte imbalances) (Level 4)	• Absorption of oral medications could be altered • Antiarrhythmics • Digoxin • Laxatives • Lithium • Phenytoin • Potassium-depleting diuretics • Theophylline

HERB QUICK REFERENCE CHART *(Continued)*

Herb/Plant Part Used	Dosage & Standardization	Reported Uses	Complementary Effect With Drug Therapy	Theoretical Cautions/Contraindications/ Adverse Effects	Theoretical Interactive Drug/Drug Category

Cat's Claw (*Uncaria tomentosa*) Root (bark)	250-1000 mg 3 times/day, standardized to contain not less than 3% pentacyclic oxindole alkaloids and not more than 0.06% tetracyclic oxindole alkaloids per dose	• Antibacterial, antifungal, and antiviral
		• Anti-inflammatory
		• Antioxidant
		• Improve immunity
			None known	• Use with caution in transplant patients (Level 4) or individuals on immunosuppressant therapy (Level 3)
				• Do not use during pregnancy (Level 2)
				• Use with caution in individuals on the following medications:
				  – Anticoagulants (may increase the chance of bleeding due to PAF inhibition) (Level 4)
				  – Nonsteroidal anti-inflammatory drugs (NSAIDs) (may increase the chance of GI bleeding) (Level 4)
				• May be contraindicated in individuals with active bleeding (Level 4)
				• Use with caution in individuals with a history of bleeding or hemostatic disorders (Level 4)
				• Discontinue use prior to dental or surgical procedures (generally at least 14 days prior) (Level 4)
					• Anticoagulants
					• Antiplatelet agents
					• Aspirin or aspirin-containing products
					• Immunosuppressant therapy
					• NSAIDs

Cayenne (*Capsicum annuum*) (*Capsicum frutescens*) Fruit	400 mg 3 times/day, standardized to contain ≥0.25% capsaicin content per dose; may also be standardized to heat units, with 150,000 Scoville heat units being average Topical: Apply as directed by manufacturer	• May stimulate digestion • Circulatory support for cardio-vascular system • Topically in inflammation and pain	None known	• Do not use with GI ulceration (Level 3) • May interfere with monoamine oxidase (MAO) inhibitors and antihypertensive therapies due to increased catecholamine secretion (Level 4) • May decrease bioavailability of salicylates (Level 1)	• Antihypertensives • Aspirin or aspirin-containing products • MAO inhibitors

Herb/Plant Part Used	Dosage & Standardization	Reported Uses	Complementary Effect With Drug Therapy	Theoretical Cautions/Contraindications/Adverse Effects	Theoretical Interactive Drug/Drug Category
Chamomile, German (*Matricaria chamomilla, Matricaria recutita*) Flower	400-1600 mg/day in divided doses, standardized to contain 1% apigenin and 0.5% essential oil per dose Tea: 1 heaping tsp dried flowers in hot water - steep 10 minutes, drink up to 3 times/day Oral rinse: Gargle 2-3 times/day as needed Topical: Apply to affected area as needed	• Carminative, antispasmodic, mild sedative, anxiolytic • Topically for mild inflammation and other skin disorders • Mouth rinse and gargle in oral health	None known	• Use with caution in individuals with severe ragweed allergy or allergy to members of the daisy and chrysanthemum (*Compositae*) family or ragweed pollens (Level 2) • Do not use in pregnancy and lactation (Level 2) • Use with caution in individuals taking sedative medications (effects may be additive with CNS depressants) (Level 4)	• Anxiolytic agents • Sedatives
Chasteberry/Vitex (*Vitex agnus-castus*) Berry	400 mg/day (in the morning, preferably on an empty stomach), standardized to contain 0.5% agnuside and 0.6% aucubin per dose	• Acne • Insufficient lactation and hyperprolactinemia • Progesterone-like action with uses in PMS, menopause, corpus luteum insufficiency, and other menstrual irregularities	None known	• Do not use in pregnancy and lactation due to potential uterine stimulation and emmenagogue effects (Level 3) • May alter hormonal therapy such as birth control and hormone replacement therapy (HRT) (due to potential endocrinologic effect) (Level 4) • May interact with medications that increase dopaminergic activity (metoclopramide, levodopa) or antipsychotics (Level 4)	• Antipsychotics • Hormone replacement therapy • Levodopa • Metoclopramide • Oral contraceptives
Clove (*Syzygium aromaticum*) Oil	Topical: Apply as needed to affected area	• Antiseptic; used in the symptomatic relief of toothaches and teething problems	None known	• NOT FOR INTERNAL USE • Do not use for >48 hours (may cause gingival damage) (Level 3)	None known

HERB QUICK REFERENCE CHART *(Continued)*

Herb/Plant Part Used	Dosage & Standardization	Reported Uses	Complementary Effect With Drug Therapy	Theoretical Cautions/Contraindications/ Adverse Effects	Theoretical Interactive Drug/Drug Category

Coleus (*Coleus forskohlii*) Root	250 mg 1-3 times/day, standardized to contain 1% forskolin per dose OR 50 mg 1-2 times/day, standardized to contain 18% forskolin per dose	• Increases intracellular cAMP; used in asthma, hypertension, congestive heart failure, allergies, eczema
		• Psoriasis
			None known	• Use with caution in hypotension (Level 4)
				• Avoid in peptic ulcer disease (Level 2)
				• Use with caution in individuals taking the following (may increase the effects of these drugs):
				  - Antihypertensives (Level 4)
				  - Antihistamines (Level 4)
				• Use with caution in individuals taking anticoagulants (due to platelet aggregating inhibition) (Level 4)
				• May be contraindicated in individuals with active bleeding (Level 4)
				• Use with caution in individuals with a history of bleeding or hemostatic disorders (Level 4)
				• Discontinue use prior to dental or surgical procedures (generally at least 14 days prior) (Level 4)
					• Anticoagulants
					• Antiplatelet agents
					• Antihistamines
					• Antihypertensives
					• Aspirin or aspirin-containing products
					• Decongestants
					• NSAIDs

Cordyceps (*Cordyceps sinensis*) Fungus	1050 mg 2-3 times/day, standardized to contain 0.14% adenosine and 5% mannitol per dose	• Adaptogenic/tonic to support wellness, longevity, and general health • Adjunct support for chemotherapy and radiation • Antioxidant • Hepatoprotective • Improves sexual vitality • Increases cellular oxygenation; useful during times of stress; reduces tiredness and fatigue; has immunomodulatory effects • Increases stamina and endurance • Supports healthy lung, liver, and kidney function	• Has been reported to decrease the renal toxicity of aminoglycosides and cyclosporine • Increases sex hormone-binding capacity • Protects stem cells and red blood cells during chemotherapy and radiation	• Do not take if allergic to fungus or molds • Use with caution in individuals taking anticoagulants (due to platelet-aggregating inhibition) (Level 4) • Use with caution if taking monoamine oxidase (MAO) inhibitors (Level 4) • May be contraindicated in individuals with active bleeding (Level 4) • Use with caution in individuals with a history of bleeding or hemostatic disorders (Level 4) • Discontinue use prior to dental or surgical procedures (generally at least 14 days prior) (Level 4)	• Aminoglycosides • Anticoagulants • Antiplatelet agents • Aspirin and aspirin-containing products • Chemotherapeutic agents • Cyclosporine • MAO inhibitors • NSAIDs

Herb/Plant Part Used	Dosage & Standardization	Reported Uses	Complementary Effect With Drug Therapy	Theoretical Cautions/Contraindications/ Adverse Effects	Theoretical Interactive Drug/Drug Category
Cranberry (*Vaccinium macrocarpon*) Berry	300-400 mg twice daily, standardized to contain 11% to 12% quinic acid per dose OR 8-16 oz of cranberry juice daily	• Urinary tract infections • May prevent kidney stone nephrolithiasis	None known	None known	None known
Dandelion (*Taraxacum officinale*) Root/leaf	Root: 250-500 mg 3 times/day, standardized to contain 20% taraxasterol per dose OR 5-10 mL 3 times/day of liquid extract (1:1 w/v fresh root or 1:4 w/v dried root) in water or juice Leaf: 250-500 mg, 2-3 times/day OR 5-10 mL 2-3 times/day of liquid extract (1:1 w/v fresh leaf or 1:4 w/v dried leaf) in water or juice	• Disorders of bile secretion (choleretic); appetite stimulation; dyspeptic complaints (root) • Diuretic (leaf)	None known	• Do not use if biliary obstruction or gallstones are present (root) (Level 4) • Use with caution if on diuretics, lithium, digoxin (leaf) (Level 4) • Allergic reaction may develop from contact with plant • Excessive use may lead to electrolyte imbalances (leaf) (Level 4)	• Digoxin • Diuretics • Lithium
Devil's Claw (*Harpagophytum procumbens*) Tuber	100-200 mg 1-2 times/ day, standardized to contain 5% harpagosides (iridoid glycoside) per dose	• Anti-inflammatory • Osteoarthritis, gout, and other inflammatory conditions • Back pain	None known	• Do not use in pregnancy and lactation due to stimulation of the uterine muscle (Level 2) • Do not use in GI disorders (Level 4) • Use with caution if taking antiarrhythmic medications (Level 4) • May be contraindicated in individuals with active bleeding (Level 4) • Use with caution in individuals with a history of bleeding or hemostatic disorders (Level 4) • Discontinue use prior to dental or surgical procedures (generally at least 14 days prior) (Level 4) • Use with caution in individuals taking anticoagulants and cardiac glycosides	• Anticoagulants • Antiarrhythmic medications • Antiplatelets • Aspirin and aspirin-containing products • Cardiac glycosides • NSAIDs • Warfarin

HERB QUICK REFERENCE CHART (Continued)

Herb/Plant Part Used	Dosage & Standardization	Reported Uses	Complementary Effect With Drug Therapy	Theoretical Cautions/Contraindications/ Adverse Effects	Theoretical Interactive Drug/Drug Category
Dong Quai (Angelica sinensis) Root	200 mg twice daily, standardized to contain 0.8% to 1.1% ligustilide per dose	• Phytoestrogenic • Female disorders including PMS, menopause, and irregular menstruation • Blood pressure regulation; energy (especially in females); anemia and blood building properties	None known	• Use with caution if currently taking hormonal therapies such as birth control or hormone replacement therapy (Level 4) • Use with caution in pregnancy and lactation (Level 4) • Use with caution if taking anticoagulants (Levels 2 & 3) • Use with caution if sunbathing or using a tanning booth while taking dong quai; use caution when taking prescription drugs that cause sensitivity to sunlight (Level 4) • Use with caution if hypotensive (Level 4) • Use with caution if taking antihypertensive medications • May be contraindicated in individuals with active bleeding (Level 4) • Use with caution in individuals with a history of bleeding or hemostatic disorders (Level 4) • Discontinue use prior to dental or surgical procedures (generally at least 14 days prior) (Level 4)	• Anticoagulants • Antihypertensives • Antiplatelet agents • Aspirin and aspirin-containing products • Hormone replacement therapy • NSAIDs • Oral contraceptives • Photosensitizing medications

Herb/Plant Part Used	Dosage & Standardization	Reported Uses	Complementary Effect With Drug Therapy	Theoretical Cautions/Contraindications/ Adverse Effects	Theoretical Interactive Drug/Drug Category
Echinacea (*Echinacea purpurea*) Flower, whole plant (*Echinacea angustifolia*) Root	500 mg 3 times/day for 1 day, then 250 mg 4 times/day, standardized to contain 4% echinacosides (*E. angustifolia*) or 4% sesquiterpene esters (*E. purpurea*) per dose. **Plant Juice:** Freshly expressed (*E. purpurea*): Use 60 drops 3 times/day with food for 1 day, then 40 drops 3 times/day with food for up to 10 days, standardized to contain not less than 2.4% soluble beta-1,2 D-fructofuranosides per dose **Topical:** Apply to affected areas as needed	• Arthritis (*angustifolia*) • As an antiviral agent • Increases nonspecific immunity; used in prevention and treatment of colds, flu, minor infections, tonsillitis, sore throat; used in chronic skin complaints (contradictory study for colds and respiratory infections - Grimm, 1999 - see monograph) • Topically as an antibacterial, wound healing agent	None known	• Recommended for not more than 10 days of therapy in treatment of acute infections or by immunsuppressed individuals (Level 4) • Use with caution in individuals with kidney disorders (Level 4) • If used for prophylaxis, cycle 3 weeks on, 1 week off • Use with caution if allergic to plants of the *Asteraceae* family (ragweed, daisy, aster, chrysanthemum); rare but severe reactions have been reported (Level 3)	• Corticosteroids • Immunosuppressants

HERB QUICK REFERENCE CHART *(Continued)*

Herb/Plant Part Used	Dosage & Standardization	Reported Uses	Complementary Effect With Drug Therapy	Theoretical Cautions/Contraindications/ Adverse Effects	Theoretical Interactive Drug/Drug Category
Elder (*Sambucus nigra*, *Sambucus canadensis*) Flower and berry	**Flower:** 500 mg 2-3 times/day, standardized to contain 5% bioflavonoids per dose **Berry:** 500 mg 2-3 times/day standardized to contain 30% anthocyanins with 8% total acids and 7% total phenols per dose OR 15 mL of liquid extract, 2-3 times/day for 3-4 days (*Sambucus canadensis*)	• Anti-inflammatory (flower) • Antiviral, antioxidant; used in influenza (berry) • Colds and influenza (flower) • Diaphoretic (flower) • Diuretic (flower)	None known	• Theoretically, long-term use and/or high doses of elder flowers may alter digoxin and lithium levels (Level 4) • Use with caution if on diuretics (flower) (Level 4)	• Digoxin • Diuretics • Lithium
Ephedra (*Ephedra sinica*) Stem	No more than 8 mg of total ephedra alkaloids per dose or more than 24 mg of total ephedra alkaloids in 24 hours	• Asthma, allergies, and hay fever • Weight loss aid (thermogenic)	None known	• Use caution in individuals with renal impairment including nephrolithiasis (Level 2) • Use with extreme caution in individuals with hypertension, heart disease, thyroid disease, diabetes, or prostate problems (Level 2) • Use with extreme caution when taking other stimulant medications and OTC stimulants (Level 2) • Do not use if taking MAO inhibitors (Level 2) • Do not use in pregnancy and lactation (Level 2)	• Antiarrhythmics • Beta-blockers • Calcium channel blockers • Cardiac glycosides • Insulin • MAO inhibitors • Oral hypoglycemics • OTC stimulants • Sympathomimetic medications • Thyroid medications

Herb/Plant Part Used	Dosage & Standardization	Reported Uses	Complementary Effect With Drug Therapy	Theoretical Cautions/Contraindications/ Adverse Effects	Theoretical Interactive Drug/Drug Category

Evening Primrose (*Oenothera biennis*) Seed oil	500 mg to 8 g/day (depending on severity of condition) standardized to contain 8% to 9% gamma-linolenic acid (GLA) and at least 72% linoleic acid (LA) per dose	• Atopic eczema
		• Attention deficit disorder (ADD) / Attention deficit-hyperactivity disorder (ADHD)
		• Diabetic neuropathy
		• Endometriosis
		• Hyperglycemia
		• Irritable bowel
		• Multiple sclerosis
		• Omega-6 essential fatty acid supplementation
		• PMS, menopause
		• Psoriasis
		• Rheumatoid arthritis
			None known	• Do not use in individuals currently on phenothiazine antipsychotics or diagnosed with schizophrenia; contra-indicated in epilepsy (Levels 1 & 2)
				• Use with caution in individuals on the following:
				  - Anticoagulants (may reduce platelet aggregation) (Level 4)
				  - With seizures and/or on seizure medication (may lower seizure threshold) (Level 2)
				• May be contraindicated in individuals with active bleeding (Level 4)
				• Use with caution in individuals with a history of bleeding or hemostatic disorders (Level 4)
				• Discontinue use prior to dental or surgical procedures (generally at least 14 days prior) (Level 4)
					• Anticoagulants
					• Anticonvulsant agents
					• Antiplatelet agents
					• Antiseizure agents
					• Aspirin and aspirin-containing products
					• NSAIDs
					• Phenothiazines

Eyebright (*Euphrasia officinalis*) Whole plant	250 mg twice daily Infusion: Infuse 1-2 tsp of dried whole plant; apply as warm compress to eyes 2-3 times/day	• Eye fatigue and catarrh of the eyes	None known	• In rare instances, may cause itching and redness of eyes with increased lacrimation level (Level 4) • If condition does not improve within 24-48 hours, seek medical attention	None known
Fenugreek (*Trigonella foenum-graecum*) Seed	250-500 mg 2-3 times/day	• Beneficial in supporting blood sugar regulation	None known	• May alter insulin and/or oral hypogly-cemic needs in diabetic individuals (Level 4) • Close monitoring of blood sugar levels is recommended	• Insulin • Oral hypoglycemic agents

HERB QUICK REFERENCE CHART *(Continued)*

Herb/Plant Part Used	Dosage & Standardization	Reported Uses	Complementary Effect With Drug Therapy	Theoretical Cautions/Contraindications/ Adverse Effects	Theoretical Interactive Drug/Drug Category
Feverfew *(Tanacetum parthenium)* Leaf	100-250 mg/day standardized to contain 0.2% parthenolide per dose 250 mg 3 times/day for inflammation and rheumatoid arthritis	• Preventative treatment of migraine headaches • Anti-inflammatory and rheumatoid arthritis	None known	• Do not use in pregnancy due to emmenagogue effect (Level 2) • Do not use if the individual is allergic to the daisy and chrysanthemum *(Compositae)* family • Use with caution in individuals on anticoagulant therapy (Level 4) • Abrupt discontinuation may increase migraine frequency • May be contraindicated in individuals with active bleeding (Level 4) • Use with caution in individuals with a history of bleeding or hemostatic disorders (Level 4) • Discontinue use prior to dental or surgical procedures (generally at least 14 days prior) (Level 4)	• Anticoagulants • Antiplatelet agents • Aspirin and aspirin-containing products • NSAIDs
Garcinia *(Garcinia cambogia)* Fruit	500-1000 mg 3 times/ day on an empty stomach, either 30 minutes before meals or 1 hour after eating, standardized to 50% (-)-hydroxy citric acid [(-)-HCA] per dose	• May be effective in weight reduction protocols • May be effective in controlling sugar levels and supporting pancreas function	None known	• Use with caution if taking hypoglycemic medications (may further lower blood sugar levels) (Level 4) • Use with caution if taking hypolipidemic agents (Level 4)	• Hypolipidemic agents • Insulin • Oral hypoglycemics

Herb/Plant Part Used	Dosage & Standardization	Reported Uses	Complementary Effect With Drug Therapy	Theoretical Cautions/Contraindications/ Adverse Effects	Theoretical Interactive Drug/Drug Category

Garlic (*Allium sativum*) Bulb	400 mg 2-3 times/day, equivalent to 1200 mg of fresh garlic or 10 mg of alliin standardized to provide 4 mg of total allicin potential (TAP) per dose OR 600 mg of aged extract 1-3 times/day, standardized to contain 1 mg/g S-allyl cysteine (SAC) per dose	• Aged garlic extracts improve antioxidant benefits
		• Beneficial to the immune system
		• Has antibiotic effect, especially against bacteria and fungi
		• Hypertension
		• May lower cholesterol and blood fats
		• Mild PAF inhibitor
			• Reported to increase the fungicidal, amphotericin B, against *Cryptococcus neoformans*	• May cause GI distress in sensitive individuals
				• Use with caution in individuals on the following medications:
				  - Anticoagulants (Levels 3 & 4)
				  - Hypoglycemic agents (Level 4)
				  - Antihypertensives (Level 4)
				• May be contraindicated in individuals with active bleeding (Level 4)
				• Use with caution in individuals with a history of bleeding or hemostatic disorders (Level 4)
				• Discontinue use prior to dental or surgical procedures (generally at least 14 days prior) (Level 4)
					• Amphotericin B
					• Anticoagulants
					• Antihypertensives
					• Antiplatelet agents
					• Aspirin and aspirin-containing products
					• Hypoglycemic agents
					• Insulin
					• NSAIDs

Ginger (*Zingiber officinalis*) Root	250 mg 3 times/day with food, standardized to contain 4% volatile oils or 5% total pungent compounds, most prominently 6-gingerol and 6-shogaol per dose	• Antiemetic • GI distress and dyspepsia • Anti-inflammatory properties	• May decrease nausea associated with radiation and chemotherapy • Decreases gastric emptying delays associated with cisplatin	• Use with caution in individuals on anticoagulants (may increase chances of bleeding due to PAF inhibition) (Level 4) • May be contraindicated in individuals with active bleeding (Level 4) • Use with caution in individuals with a history of bleeding or hemostatic disorders (Level 4) • Discontinue use prior to dental or surgical procedures (generally at least 14 days prior) (Level 4)	• Anticoagulants • Antiplatelet agents • Aspirin and aspirin-containing products • Cardiac glycosides • Chemotherapy agents • Cisplatin • NSAIDs

HERB QUICK REFERENCE CHART *(Continued)*

Herb/Plant Part Used	Dosage & Standardization	Reported Uses	Complementary Effect With Drug Therapy	Theoretical Cautions/Contraindications/ Adverse Effects	Theoretical Interactive Drug/Drug Category
Ginkgo (*Ginkgo biloba*) Leaf	40-80 mg 3 times/day, standardized to contain 24% to 27% ginkgo flavone glycosides and 6% to 7% triterpenes per dose	• Alzheimer's disease • Asthma • Cerebral vascular insufficiency • Dementia • Impotence / sexual dysfunction • Intermittent claudication • Macular degeneration • Memory enhancement • Peripheral vascular insufficiency • Reported to increase peripheral blood flow • Resistant depression • Tinnitus	None known	• Use with caution in individuals on anti-coagulants (may increase chances of bleeding due to PAF inhibition (Levels 3 & 4) • Use with caution in individuals on monoamine oxidase (MAO) inhibitors as ginkgo may enhance the effects of these medications (Level 4) • May be contraindicated in individuals with active bleeding (Level 4) • Use with caution in individuals with a history of bleeding or hemostatic disorders (Level 4) • Discontinue use prior to dental or surgical procedures (generally at least 14 days prior) (Level 4)	• Anticoagulants • Antiplatelet agents • Aspirin and aspirin-containing products • MAO inhibitors • NSAIDs

Herb/Plant Part Used	Dosage & Standardization	Reported Uses	Complementary Effect With Drug Therapy	Theoretical Cautions/Contraindications/ Adverse Effects	Theoretical Interactive Drug/Drug Category

Ginseng (Panax) (Panax ginseng) Root	100–600 mg/day in divided doses, standardized to contain a minimum of 5% ginsenosides per dose A regimen of 4 weeks on 2 weeks off is recommended for maximum benefits	• Adrenal tonic
		• Enhances mental and physical performance; increases energy, decreases stress; improves immune function; adjunct support for chemotherapy and radiation
			• Helps the body adapt to stresses caused by chemo-therapy and radiation	• Do not use in acute infections, kidney failure
				• Use with caution if taking stimulants (eg, caffeine, decongestants) (Level 4)
				• May cause vaginal breakthrough bleeding (Level 3) and interfere with hormonal therapy (Level 4)
				• Use with caution in:
				  – Hypertension and hypertensive agents (Level 4)
				  – Anticoagulant therapy (Levels 3 & 4)
				  – MAO inhibitors (primarily phenelzine) (Levels 3 & 4)
				• May cause mastalgia in prolonged and high doses (Level 3)
				• Ginseng abuse syndrome (GAS) may occur in prolonged, high doses (diarrhea, hypertension, palpitations, tachycardia, nervousness, skin eruptions, insomnia) (Level 3)
				• May be contraindicated in individuals with active bleeding (Level 4)
				• Use with caution in individuals with a history of bleeding or hemostatic disorders (Level 4)
				• Discontinue use prior to dental or surgical procedures (generally at least 14 days prior) (Level 4)
					• Anticoagulants
					• Antihypertensives
					• Antiplatelet agents
					• Aspirin and aspirin-containing products
					• Chemotherapeutic agents
					• CNS stimulants
					• Digoxin
					• Hormonal replacement therapy
					• MAO Inhibitors
					• NSAIDs
					• Oral contraceptives
					• Sympathomimetics

553

HERB QUICK REFERENCE CHART *(Continued)*

Herb/Plant Part Used	Dosage & Standardization	Reported Uses	Complementary Effect With Drug Therapy	Theoretical Cautions/Contraindications/ Adverse Effects	Theoretical Interactive Drug/Drug Category
Ginseng (Siberian) (*Eleutherococcus senticosus*) Root	100–200 mg twice daily standardized to contain 0.8% eleutherosides B and E per dose A regimen of 4 weeks on 2 weeks off is recommended for maximum benefits	• Adaptogen • Beneficial in athletic performance, decreasing stress and fatigue; reported to increase immune system function	None known	• Use with caution when taking stimulants (caffeine, decongestants) (Level 4) • Use with caution in cardiovascular disease (Level 4) • Use with caution if on antihypertensive (Level 3) OR anticoagulant medications (Level 4) • Should not be taken in high doses during acute phases of infection, especially when accompanied by a high fever • Extensive or prolonged use may heighten estrogenic activity (Level 4) • Use with caution in the following: - Concurrent with digoxin therapy (Level 3) - May increase effects of hexobarbital (Level 2) • Use with caution if on hypoglycemic medications or insulin • May be contraindicated in individuals with active bleeding (Level 4) • Use with caution in individuals with a history of bleeding or hemostatic disorders (Level 4) • Discontinue use prior to dental or surgical procedures (generally at least 14 days prior) (Level 4)	• Anticoagulants • Antihypertensives • Antiplatelet agents • Aspirin and aspirin-containing products • Barbiturates • Insulin • NSAIDs • Oral hypoglycemics • OTC stimulants

Herb/Plant Part Used	Dosage & Standardization	Reported Uses	Complementary Effect With Drug Therapy	Theoretical Cautions/Contraindications/ Adverse Effects	Theoretical Interactive Drug/Drug Category
Golden Seal (*Hydrastis canadensis*) Root, rhizome	250 mg 2-4 times/day, standardized to contain 10% alkaloids or 2.5% berberine and 1.5% to 5% hydrastine per dose	• Mucous membrane tonifying; antibacterial, antifungal; used in inflammation of the mucosal membranes; treatment of gastritis, bronchitis, cystitis, infectious diarrhea	None known	• Contraindicated in pregnancy (Level 2) • High doses (2-3 g) may cause hypotension (Level 2) or GI distress (Level 3) • Doses of 18 g (toxic dose) have been reported to induce CNS depression (Level 3) • Overdose associated with myocardial damage, respiratory failure (Level 3) • Extended use of high doses associated with neuroexcitation, hallucinations, delirium, and GI disorders (Level 3) • High-dose hydrastine has been associated with hypertension, hyperreflexia, and seizures • Use with caution in individuals with cardiovascular disorder	None known
Gotu Kola (*Centella asiatica*) Leaf	50-250 mg 2-3 times/day, standardized to contain 10% to 30% asiaticosides and 2% to 4% triterpenes per dose Topical: Apply a 0.2% to 0.4% preparation topically to wound areas, 2-3 times/day	• Topically in wound healing and other tissue damage such as hemorrhoids • Regulation of connective tissue; modulates connective tissue synthesis; supports memory function • Venous insufficiency	None known	• Contraindicated in pregnancy (Level 2) • May cause contact dermatitis (Level 3) • Use with caution in individuals taking sedative medications (effects may be additive with other CNS depressants) (Level 3) • In high doses, may elevate cholesterol (Level 2) • Large doses may be sedating	• Anxiolytics • Sedative medications

HERB QUICK REFERENCE CHART (Continued)

Herb/Plant Part Used	Dosage & Standardization	Reported Uses	Complementary Effect With Drug Therapy	Theoretical Cautions/Contraindications/ Adverse Effects	Theoretical Interactive Drug/Drug Category
Grape Seed (*Vitis vinifera*) Seed/skin	25-100 mg 1-3 times/day, standardized to contain 40% to 80% proanthocyanidins or a procyanidolic value >95% per dose	• Antioxidant • Treatment of allergies, asthma; improves peripheral circulation; decreases platelet aggregation, capillary fragility; improves general circulation; inflammation	None known	• Use with caution in individuals on anticoagulant therapy due to platelet inhibition (Level 4) • Use with caution (may inhibit xanthine oxidase) (Level 2) • May increase toxicity of methotrexate • May be contraindicated in individuals with active bleeding (Level 4) • Use with caution in individuals with a history of bleeding or hemostatic disorders (Level 4) • Discontinue use prior to dental or surgical procedures (generally at least 14 days prior) (Level 4)	• Anticoagulants • Antiplatelet agents • Aspirin and aspirin-containing products • NSAIDs • Xanthine oxidase inhibitors
Grapefruit Seed (*Citrus paradisi*) Seed extract	100 mg 1-3 times/day with meals Drops: 5-10 drops 2-3 times/day Oral rinse: 5-10 drops diluted in water 2-3 times/day; swish and expectorate	• Antifungal, antibacterial, antiparasitic agent	None known	• Until further information is available, avoid concurrent use with nonsedating antihistamines	• Nonsedating antihistamines

Herb/Plant Part Used	Dosage & Standardization	Reported Uses	Complementary Effect With Drug Therapy	Theoretical Cautions/Contraindications/ Adverse Effects	Theoretical Interactive Drug/Drug Category
Green Tea (Camellia sinensis) Leaf	250-500 mg/day, standardized to contain 50% to 97% polyphenols/dose, containing at least 50% (-)epigallocatechin-3-gallate (EGCG) **Caffeine-free products are recommended**	• Antioxidant to aid in cancer prevention, cardiovascular disease • Adjunct support for chemotherapy and radiation • May lower cholesterol • Platelet-inhibiting action • Anticariogenic activity	• Reported to enhance the inhibitory effects of doxorubicin (Adriamycin®) on tumor growth	• Use caution if taking anticoagulants (Level 2); if taking other stimulants such as caffeine and decongestants, unless a caffeine-free product is used (Level 4) • If product is not decaffeinated, may cause gastric irritation, decreased appetite, insomnia, decreased nervousness (Level 4) • If product is not decaffeinated, use caution in peptic ulcer and cardiovascular disease (Level 4); high doses may potentially interact with: - Aspirin/acetaminophen (increase effect of caffeine) (Level 4) - Barbiturates (decrease effect of caffeine) (Level 4) - Fluconazole, quinidine, verapamil, oral contraceptives (inhibit caffeine metabolism) (Level 4) - MAOIs (may elevate blood pressure) (Level 4) - Quinolones (may decrease caffeine clearance) (Level 4) - Theophylline (may increase toxicity) (Level 4) - Phenytoin (may increase metabolism of caffeine) (Level 4) • Addition of milk to green tea may significantly lower the antioxidant potential of this agent • May be contraindicated in individuals with active bleeding (Level 4) • Use caution with a history of bleeding or hemostatic disorders (Level 4) • Discontinue use prior to dental or surgical procedures (generally at least 14 days prior) (Level 4)	• Anticoagulants • Antiplatelet agents • Aspirin and aspirin-containing products • Doxorubicin (Adriamycin®) • Iron • Magnesium • NSAIDs • Radiation With high doses of caffeinated product: • Acetaminophen • Acid inhibitors (H₂/proton pump inhibitors) • Adenosine • Aspirin • Barbiturates • Benzodiazepines • Beta-blockers • Clozapine • CNS stimulators • Fluconazole • MAOIs • Oral contraceptives • Phenobarbital • Phenytoin • Quinidine • Quinolones • Sympathomimetics • Theophylline • Verapamil • Warfarin

HERB QUICK REFERENCE CHART *(Continued)*

Herb/Plant Part Used	Dosage & Standardization	Reported Uses	Complementary Effect With Drug Therapy	Theoretical Cautions/Contraindications/ Adverse Effects	Theoretical Interactive Drug/Drug Category
Ground Ivy (*Hedera helix*) Leaf	50 mg 3 times/day of a 5-7.5:1 w/v tablet	• Mucolytic action; used in upper respiratory congestion and coughs	None known	• Contraindicated in epilepsy (Level 4)	None known

Guggul (*Commiphora mukul*) Resin	500 mg 3 times/day, standardized to contain 5% guggulsterones per dose	• Hypercholesterolemic agent; used in lowering blood cholesterol levels	None known	• Use with caution in pregnancy and lactation due to thyroid-stimulating properties (Level 4)
				• Use with caution in individuals on the following:
				  - Thyroid agents (Level 4)
				  - Anticoagulants (Level 4)
				• Reported to decrease metabolism of diltiazem and propranolol, so caution should be used in calcium channel blocker and beta-blocker medications (Level 1)
				• May be contraindicated in individuals with active bleeding (Level 4)
				• Use with caution in individuals with a history of bleeding or hemostatic disorders (Level 4)
				• Discontinue use prior to dental or surgical procedures (generally at least 14 days prior) (Level 4)
					• Anticoagulants
					• Antihypertensives
					• Antiplatelet agents
					• Aspirin and aspirin-containing products
					• Beta-blockers (specifically propranolol)
					• Calcium channel blockers (specifically diltiazem)
					• NSAIDs
					• Thyroid agents

Gymnema (*Gymnema sylvestre*) Leaf	250-500 mg 1-3 times/day, standardized to contain 25% gymnemic acids per dose	• Regulation of blood sugar levels, diabetes	None known	• Use with caution in hypoglycemic agents and insulin (Level 4)	• Hypoglycemic agents • Insulin

Hawthorn (*Crataegus oxyacantha*) Flower/leaf/berry	250 mg 1-3 times/day, standardized to contain at least 2% vitexin-2-O-rhamnoside and/or a minimum of 10% to 20% procyanidins per dose	• Congestive heart failure
		• Treatment of angina, hypotension/hypertension, peripheral vascular diseases, tachycardia; used as a cardiotonic
			• Used synergistically with digoxin in Europe	• Contraindicated in pregnancy (Levels 2 & 3)
				• Use with caution in individuals on the following:
				  - Antihypertensives (Level 4)
				  - Angiotensin-converting enzyme (ACE) inhibitors (Level 4)
					• ACE inhibitors
					• Antiarrhythmics
					• Antihypertensives (vasodilators, angiotensin receptor blockers)
					• Cardiac glycosides (digoxin)

Herb/Plant Part Used	Dosage & Standardization	Reported Uses	Complementary Effect With Drug Therapy	Theoretical Cautions/Contraindications/ Adverse Effects	Theoretical Interactive Drug/Drug Category
Hops (*Humulus lupulus*) Strobiles	100 mg twice daily as needed, standardized to contain 5.2% bitter acids and 4% flavonoids per dose	• Mild sedative and hypnotic	None known	• Use with caution in individuals on the following (action may be potentiated): - Hypnotics (Level 4) - Antianxiety medications (Level 4) - Antipsychotics (Level 4) - Antidepressants (Level 4) - Alcohol (Level 4) • Use caution when driving an automobile or operating heavy machinery • Use with caution while taking sedative medications (reported to increase sleeping time induced by pentobarbital) (Levels 2 & 4)	• Antianxiety agents • Antidepressants • Antipsychotics • Ethanol • Hypnotics • Pentobarbital • Sedatives
Horse Chestnut (*Aesculus hippocastanum*) Seed	300 mg 1-2 times/day, standardized to contain 50 mg escin (16%) per dose Topical: Apply 2% escin gel, 1-2 times/day to affected area	• Varicose veins, hemorrhoids, other venous insufficiencies; deep venous thrombosis; lower extremity edema • Topically in the same conditions	None known	• Use with caution in individuals on anticoagulants (may increase chances of bleeding due to PAF inhibition) (Level 4) • Use with caution in individuals with renal and/or hepatic impairment (Level 4) • May be contraindicated in individuals with active bleeding (Level 4) • Use with caution in individuals with a history of bleeding or hemostatic disorders (Level 4) • Discontinue use prior to dental or surgical procedures (generally at least 14 days prior) (Level 4)	• Anticoagulants • Antiplatelet agents • Aspirin and aspirin-containing products • NSAIDs
Horsetail (*Equisetum arvense*) Shoots	300 mg 3 times/day as needed, standardized to contain 10% silica per dose	• Diuretic • High mineral content (including silicic acid); used in bone and connective tissue strengthening, including osteoporosis	None known	• Diuretic effect may cause electrolyte disturbances and may potentiate certain pharmaceutical drugs with narrow therapeutic windows (Level 4) • May deplete thiamine (vitamin B₁) from the body due to thiaminase activity (Levels 2 & 4)	• Antiarrhythmics • Digoxin • Diuretics • Lithium • Phenytoin • Theophylline • Vitamin B₁

HERB QUICK REFERENCE CHART *(Continued)*

Herb/Plant Part Used	Dosage & Standardization	Reported Uses	Complementary Effect With Drug Therapy	Theoretical Cautions/Contraindications/ Adverse Effects	Theoretical Interactive Drug/Drug Category
HuperzineA (isolated from *Huperzia serrata* - Chinese club moss)	50 mcg 1-3 times/day	• As an AChE inhibitor in senile dementia and Alzheimer's disease	None known	• Use with caution if taking AChE inhibitors, tacrine, donepezil (Level 4)	• AChE inhibitors • Donepezil • Tacrine

Kava Kava (*Piper methysticum*) Root, rhizome	100-250 mg 1-3 times/day as needed, standardized to contain 30% kavalactones per dose
	
	Sedation: 250-500 mg at bedtime, standardized to contain 30% kavalactones per dose
		• Anxiety; sedation; skeletal muscle relaxation; postischemic episodes	None known	• Do not use during pregnancy (Level 3)
				• Do not use in Parkinson's disease (has been reported to cause dopamine antagonism) (Level 4)
				• Use with caution if taking the following:
				  - Alprazolam (may increase sedative effects) (Level 3)
				  - Ethanol (may increase ethanol toxicity) (Level 4);
				• May cause drowsiness or sedation in higher doses (Level 2)
				• Use caution when driving an automobile or operating heavy machinery
				• Long-term use of high doses has resulted in rash (Level 3)
				• Use with caution in individuals on the following (action may be potentiated):
				  - Sedatives (Level 4)
				  - Antianxiety medications (Level 4)
				  - Hypnotics (Level 4)
				  - Antipsychotics (Level 4)
				  - Antidepressants (Level 4)
					• Antianxiety agents (Alprazolam)
					• Antidepressants
					• Antipsychotics
					• Ethanol
					• Hypnotics
					• Levodopa
					• Sedatives

Lavender (*Lavendula officinalis*) Oil	**Topical:** Apply to affected area, either diluted or undiluted, 2-4 times/day	• Topically as a wound healing agent and on minor burns	None known	• Topical or inhalation use only	None known

Herb/Plant Part Used	Dosage & Standardization	Reported Uses	Complementary Effect With Drug Therapy	Theoretical Cautions/Contraindications/ Adverse Effects	Theoretical Interactive Drug/Drug Category
Lemon Balm/ Melissa (Melissa officinalis) Whole plant	Topical: Apply (a 70:1 w/v concentrated product) to affected area 2-4 times/day at the first sign of a cold sore or fever blister (burning, itching, tingling) Internal: For teething, use 2-5 drops of a (1:1 w/v) fresh plant or a (1:4 w/v) dried plant extract diluted in liquid 3 times/ day as needed	• Antiviral agent in relieving herpes virus • Sedative agent in pediatrics	None known	None known	None known

HERB QUICK REFERENCE CHART *(Continued)*

Herb/Plant Part Used	Dosage & Standardization	Reported Uses	Complementary Effect With Drug Therapy	Theoretical Cautions/Contraindications/ Adverse Effects	Theoretical Interactive Drug/Drug Category

Licorice (*Glycyrrhiza glabra*) Root	250–500 mg 3 times/day, standardized to contain 20% glycyrrhizinic acid OR 15–30 drops of liquid extract (1:4 w/v) dried root 3 times/day in juice or other beverage
	
	DGL (deglycyrrhizinated) Licorice: 250 mg 3 times/day chewed either 1 hour before or 2 hours after meals and at bedtime, standardized to contain no more than 2% glycyrrhizin per dose
		• Adrenal insufficiency
		• Chewable DGL products used in GI ulceration
		• Licorice extract beneficial as an expectorant and antitussive
			None known	• Use with caution in individuals with hepatic or renal problems (Level 4)
				• Use with caution in individuals on the following (licorice may deplete potassium):
				  - Thiazide diuretics (Level 4)
				  - Potassium-sparing diuretics (Level 4)
				• Use with caution in individuals on laxatives (Level 4), cardiac glycosides (Level 4), and corticosteroids (Level 4)
				• Use with caution in individuals on nitrofurantoin (Level 1) (DGL licorice may increase excretion of nitrofurantoin in individuals with UTI)
				• Recommend potassium supplementation when using licorice
				• Use with caution if on oral contraceptives or hormone replacement therapy (Level 4)
				• Do not use in hypertension, hepatic problems, renal problems, or obesity due to possible mineralocorticoid effects of licorice (glycyrrhizin content) (Levels 1 & 3)
				• Do not use in arrhythmias, congestive heart failure, or edematous states
				• May be contraindicated in individuals with active bleeding (Level 4)
				• Use with caution in individuals with a history of bleeding or hemostatic disorders (Level 4)
				• Discontinue use prior to dental or surgical procedures (generally at least 14 days prior) (Level 4)
					• Anticoagulants
					• Antihypertensives
					• Antiplatelet agents
					• Aspirin and aspirin-containing products
					• Cardiac glycosides
					• Corticosteroids
					• Diuretics
					• Hormonal therapy
					• Laxatives
					• Nitrofurantoin
					• NSAIDs
					• Oral contraceptives
					• Potassium-depleting medications

Herb/Plant Part Used	Dosage & Standardization	Reported Uses	Complementary Effect With Drug Therapy	Theoretical Cautions/Contraindications/ Adverse Effects	Theoretical Interactive Drug/Drug Category
Marshmallow (*Althaea officinalis*) Root	500 mg 3 times/day or as needed	• Mucilaginous, demulcent; used in cough preparations); peptic ulceration	None known	• Use with caution, may interfere with absorption of other oral medications (Level 4) • Use with caution if taking hypoglycemic medications (may further lower blood sugar levels) (Level 4)	• Insulin • Oral hypoglycemics
Mastic (*Pistacia lentiscus*) Resin	1000-2000 mg/day in divided doses	• Reported to inhibit *H. pylori*; used in peptic ulcer disease	None known	None known	None known
Milk Thistle (*Silybum marianum*) Seed	80-200 mg 1-3 times/day, standardized to contain 80% silymarin per dose	• Antidote for Death Cup mushroom poisoning • Antioxidant activity specifically for hepatic cells; used in liver diseases; acute/chronic hepatitis; jaundice; as a cholagogue • Hepatoprotective against pharmaceutical drug toxicities including psychotropics (such as phenothiazines, butyrophenones), ethanol, and acetaminophen	• Hepatoprotective against psychotropics (such as phenothiazines, butyrophenones), ethanol, acetaminophen and other drugs potentially toxic to the liver	None known	
Muira Puama (*Ptychopetalum olacoides*) Bark/root	125-250 mg twice daily	• Athletic performance enhancement • Increased sexual vitality of males	None known	• Use with caution in individuals taking steroidal medications	• Steroidal medications
Olive Leaf (*Olea europaea*) Leaf	250-500 mg 1-3 times/day, standardized to contain 15% to 23% oleuropein per dose	• Antibiotic • Antifungal • Antiviral Has hypoglycemic and antihypertensive activity	None known	• Do not use in individuals with gallstones due to cholagogue effect (Level 4) • Use with caution in individuals on insulin, hypoglycemic, and antihypertensive agents (Level 4)	• Antihypertensive agents • Hypoglycemic agents • Insulin
Parsley (*Petroselinum crispum*) Leaf (oil)	Dilute a few drops of parsley oil in a cup of water, gargle, and expectorate Oral: 1-2 pearls 1-3 times/day as needed	• Antibacterial • Antifungal • Halitosis	None known	For encapsulated parsley products: • Use with caution if on MAO inhibitors • Extremely large doses of constituents (apiole and myristicin) have been associated with hematologic, renal, and hepatic toxicity (Level 2)	• MAO inhibitors

HERB QUICK REFERENCE CHART *(Continued)*

Herb/Plant Part Used	Dosage & Standardization	Reported Uses	Complementary Effect With Drug Therapy	Theoretical Cautions/Contraindications/ Adverse Effects	Theoretical Interactive Drug/Drug Category

Passion Flower *(Passiflora spp)* Whole plant	**Anxiety:** 100 mg 2-3 times/day, standardized to contain 3.5% isovitexin per dose
	
	Insomnia: 200 mg at bedtime, standardized to contain 3.5% isovitexin per dose
		• Sedative agent	None known	• May cause drowsiness; use caution when driving an automobile or operating heavy machinery
				• Use with caution in individuals on the following (action may be potentiated):
				  - Antianxiety medications (Level 4)
				  - Hypnotics (Level 4)
				  - Antipsychotics (Level 4)
				  - Antidepressants (Level 4)
				• Use with caution while taking sedative medications (reported to increase sleeping time induced by pentobarbital) (Level 2)
					• Antidepressants
					• Anxiolytics
					• Barbiturates
					• Sedatives

Peppermint *(Mentha piperita)* Leaf/oil	1 tablet (enteric coated) 2-3 times/day, containing 0.2 mL oil per tablet; the oil should contain: • not less than 4.5% w/w and not more than 10% w/w of esters calculated as methyl acetate • not less than 44% w/w calculated as menthol and not more than 15% w/w and not more than 32% w/w ketones calculated as menthone **Children <8 years of age:** Infuse 1 tsp of dried leaf; cool before using; give 1-2 tsp 1-3 times/ day as needed	• Digestive complaints as a carminative and spasmolytic • Irritable bowel syndrome	None known	• Do not use in individuals with biliary tract obstruction, cholecystitis, gallstones, hiatal hernia, or severe liver damage (Level 4) • Use with caution in individuals on calcium channel blockers (Level 2)	• Calcium channel blockers

Herb/Plant Part Used	Dosage & Standardization	Reported Uses	Complementary Effect With Drug Therapy	Theoretical Cautions/Contraindications/ Adverse Effects	Theoretical Interactive Drug/Drug Category
Psyllium (*Plantago ovata, Plantago ispaghula*) Seed	1-3 tsp with 6-8 oz water in the morning and evening	• Bulk-forming laxative containing 10% to 30% mucilage	None known	• Avoid in bowel obstruction (Level 4) • May cause abdominal cramps, diarrhea, constipation	None known
Pygeum (*Pygeum africanum, Prunus africana*) Bark	50-100 mg twice daily, standardized to contain 12% to 13% phytosicrols (ß-sitosterol) per dose	• Benign prostatic hypertrophy	None known	• Use with caution in individuals taking finasteride (Level 4) • Use with caution in individuals receiving treatment for benign prostatic hyperplasia (BPH) (alpha-adrenergic blockers, finasteride)	• Alpha-adrenergic blockers • Finasteride
Red Clover (*Trifolium pratense*) Tops	500 mg/day, standardized to contain 40 mg isoflavones per dose OR 30-60 drops 2-3 times/day of a liquid extract (1:1 w/v) in juice or other beverage	• Management of menopausal symptoms (contains 4 phytoestrogens) • Liquid extract used for liver detoxification and kidney detoxification	None known	• Contraindicated in pregnancy and lactation (proprietary extract) (Level 4) • Use with caution in individuals using birth control and hormone replacement therapy (HRT) (may alter hormonal therapy) (Level 4) • Use with caution while taking anticoagulants (Level 4) • May be contraindicated in individuals with active bleeding (Level 4) • Use with caution in individuals with a history of bleeding or hemostatic disorders (Level 4) • Discontinue use prior to dental or surgical procedures (generally at least 14 days prior) (Level 4)	• Anticoagulants • Antiplatelet agents • Aspirin and aspirin-containing products • Hormonal replacement therapy • NSAIDs • Oral contraceptives

Herb/Plant Part Used	Dosage & Standardization	Reported Uses	Complementary Effect With Drug Therapy	Theoretical Cautions/Contraindications/ Adverse Effects	Theoretical Interactive Drug/Drug Category
Red Yeast Rice (*Monascus purpureus*)	1200 mg twice daily, standardized to 0.4% total HMG-CoA reductase inhibitors per dose	• Hypercholesterolemic agent; may lower triglycerides and raise HDL cholesterol	None known	• Contraindicated in pregnancy or lactation (or if trying to become pregnant) (Level 4) • Contraindicated in individuals with a known hypersensitivity to rice or yeast (Level 4) • Contraindicated in individuals with a history of liver disease or at risk for liver disease; with active liver disease, serious infections, organ transplantation, or recent major surgery (Level 4) • Use with caution in individuals currently on pharmaceutical cholesterol-lowering drugs (Level 4) • Keep out of reach of children; do not use if <20 years of age • HMG-CoA reductase inhibitors have been associated with rare but serious adverse effects, including hepatic and skeletal muscle disorders (myopathy, rhabdomyolysis); although these effects have not been specifically reported for red yeast rice (Level 4) • Do not use in individuals who consume >1-2 alcohol-containing drinks per day (Level 4) • Discontinue use at first sign of hepatic dysfunction • Use with caution in individuals taking anticoagulant medications (Level 4) • May be contraindicated in individuals with active bleeding (Level 4) • Use with caution in individuals with a history of bleeding or hemostatic disorders (Level 4) • Discontinue use prior to dental or surgical procedures (generally at least 14 days prior) (Level 4)	• Anticoagulants • Antiplatelet agents • Aspirin and aspirin-containing products • Cyclosporine • Erythromycin • Gemfibrozil • HMG-CoA reductase inhibitors • Hypercholesterolemic agents • Itraconazole • Niacin • NSAIDs

Herb/Plant Part Used	Dosage & Standardization	Reported Uses	Complementary Effect With Drug Therapy	Theoretical Cautions/Contraindications/ Adverse Effects	Theoretical Interactive Drug/Drug Category
Rehmannia (*Rehmannia glutinosa*) Root (cured)	250 mg 1-3 times/day, standardized to contain 1% glutannic acid per dose	• Immunosuppressive agent in rheumatoid arthritis	• Decreases toxicity of cyclophosphamide	• Use with caution in individuals on immunosuppressant agents (increased effect possible) (Level 4)	• Cyclophosphamide • Immunosuppressants
Reishi (*Ganoderma lucidum*) Mushroom	150-300 mg 3-4 times/day, standardized 4% triterpenes and 10% to 12.5% polysaccharides and 4% triterpenes per dose	• Immunomodulation, fatigue, chemo- and radioprotection, antihypertensive, anticonvulsive	• Chemoprotective • May increase the effectiveness of cefazolin as an antimicrobial agent	• Use with caution if taking anticoagulant medications (Levels 3 & 4) • Use with caution if taking antihypertensive medications (Level 4) • May be contraindicated in individuals with active bleeding (Level 4) • Use with caution in individuals with a history of bleeding or hemostatic disorders (Level 4) • Discontinue use prior to dental or surgical procedures (generally at least 14 days prior) (Level 4)	• Anticoagulants • Antihypertensives • Antiplatelet agents • Aspirin and aspirin-containing products • Cefazolin • Chemotherapeutic agents • NSAIDs
Saw Palmetto (*Serenoa repens*) Berry	160 mg twice daily, standardized to contain at least 80% to 90% fatty acids and sterols per dose	• Treatment of benign prostatic hypertrophy (BPH)	• Finasteride	• Use with caution in individuals on alpha-adrenergic blocking agents (Level 4)	• Alpha-adrenergic blocking agents • Finasteride
Schisandra (*Schizandra chinensis*) Berry	100 mg twice daily, standardized to contain at least 9% schisandrins per dose	• Adaptogen/health tonic; hepatic protection and detoxification • Adjunct support for chemotherapy and radiation • Increases endurance, stamina, work performance	• Cardioprotective action during administration of doxorubicin (Adriamycin®)	• Do not use in pregnancy due to uterine stimulation (Level 2) • Theoretically, enzyme enhancement may alter metabolism of many drugs (Level 4) • Use with caution in individuals on calcium channel blockers (Level 2)	• Calcium channel blockers • Chemotherapeutic agents (doxorubicin)

HERB QUICK REFERENCE CHART *(Continued)*

Herb/Plant Part Used	Dosage & Standardization	Reported Uses	Complementary Effect With Drug Therapy	Theoretical Cautions/Contraindications/ Adverse Effects	Theoretical Interactive Drug/Drug Category
Senna (*Cassia senna*) Seed	15-30 mg of sennosides per dose at bedtime	• Anthraquinone laxative	None known	• May decrease absorption of oral medications by decreasing bowel transit time (Level 4) • Use with caution in bowel obstruction, diarrhea, or dehydration (Level 4) • Use with caution in bowel disorders (ulcerative colitis, Crohn's) and appendicitis (Level 4) • Use with caution in cardiovascular disease (overuse may cause electrolyte imbalances) (Level 4) • Excessive use may lead to potassium loss and other electrolyte disturbances and may potentiate the effects of various pharmaceutical drugs with narrow therapeutic windows (Level 4) • Avoid in children <12 years of age	• Absorption of oral medications could be altered • Antiarrhythmics • Digoxin • Lithium • Laxatives • Phenytoin • Potassium-depleting diuretics • Theophylline
Stinging Nettle (*Urtica dioica*) Leaf, root	**Leaf:** 300-1200 mg 2-4 times/day as needed of freeze-dried leaf **Root:** 250 mg 1-3 times/day standardized to contain 1% to 2% plant silica per dose	• Allergic rhinitis (leaf) • Benign prostatic hyperplasia (root) • Gout (leaf) • Increases uric acid excretion (leaf)	None known	• Use with caution in individuals with renal insufficiency or disease due to silica content (Level 4) • Do not use in pregnancy due to potential uterine stimulation (Level 2)	None known

Herb/Plant Part Used	Dosage & Standardization	Reported Uses	Complementary Effect With Drug Therapy	Theoretical Cautions/Contraindications/ Adverse Effects	Theoretical Interactive Drug/Drug Category
St John's Wort (Hypericum perforatum) Flowering buds	300 mg 3 times/day, standardized to contain 0.3% to 0.5% hypericin and/or 3% to 5% hyperforin per dose A minimum of 4-6 weeks of therapy is recommended Topical: Apply oil extract as needed to affected area	• Mild to moderate depression, melancholia, anxiety • Antiviral activity in increased doses • Antibacterial, anti-inflammatory; used topically for minor wounds and infections • May be used topically for bruises, muscle soreness, and sprains	None known	• Do not use in pregnancy (Level 2) • Use with caution in individuals currently on antidepressant therapy (Level 4); not for use in severe depression • May elevate reversible liver enzyme function in high doses (Level 2) • Use with caution in individuals taking digoxin (may alter levels of this medication) (Level 1) • May alter the actions of monoamine oxidase (MAO) inhibitors and select serotonin reuptake inhibitors (SSRIs) (Level 1) • May cause photosensitivity in susceptible individuals (Levels 1 & 2) • Use with caution in individuals on reserpine, as the effects of reserpine may be antagonized by concurrent use with St John's wort (Level 2) • Use with caution in individuals on narcotic medications, may enhance the sleeping time induced by these drugs (Level 2)	• Antidepressants (SSRIs and tricyclics) • CNS depressants • Digoxin • MAO inhibitors • Narcotic medications • Photosensitizing agents • Reserpine • Sedatives
Tea Tree (Melaleuca alternifolia) Volatile oils	Topical: Apply oil (preferably diluted) to affected area as needed Oral rinse: Dilute a few drops of tea tree oil in a cup of water, gargle, and expectorate	• Antibacterial • Antifungal • Used in mouthwash for dental and oral health • Used topically for burns, cuts, scrapes, insect bites	None known	• May cause allergic dermatitis in sensitive individuals (Level 3) • Not for ingestion	None known
Thyme (Thymus vulgaris) Leaf	20-40 drops 3 times/day in juice or beverage, of a liquid extract (1:1 w/v fresh leaf to 1:4 w/v dried leaf)	• Antifungal • Coughs and upper respiratory congestion	None known	• Use with caution in urinary tract or GI inflammation (Level 4) • Use with caution in individuals with sensitivity or allergy to oregano (Labiatae spp) (Level 4)	None known

HERB QUICK REFERENCE CHART (Continued)

Herb/Plant Part Used	Dosage & Standardization	Reported Uses	Complementary Effect With Drug Therapy	Theoretical Cautions/Contraindications/ Adverse Effects	Theoretical Interactive Drug/Drug Category
Tribulus (*Tribulus terrestris*) Whole plant	250-500 mg 3 times/day, standardized to contain 20% steroidal saponins per dose	• Steroidal properties, used for enhanced athletic performance and increased sexual vitality	None known	• Use with caution if taking steroidal medications (Level 4)	• Androgens • Estrogens • Hormone replacement therapy • Oral contraceptives • Steroidal agents
Turmeric (*Curcuma longa*) Root	300 mg 3 times/day with meals, standardized to contain 95% curcuminoids per dose	• Anti-inflammatory • Antioxidant • Antirheumatic; used in arthritic problems • May lower blood lipid levels	None known	• Use with caution in individuals with GI disorders or if peptic ulceration is present (Level 4) • Use with caution if currently taking anticoagulant medications (Levels 1 & 4) • Do not use if biliary obstruction is present (Level 4) • May be contraindicated in individuals with active bleeding (Level 4) • Use with caution in individuals with a history of bleeding or hemostatic disorders (Level 4) • Discontinue use prior to dental or surgical procedures (generally at least 14 days prior) (Level 4)	• Anticoagulants • Antiplatelets • Aspirin and aspirin-containing products • NSAIDs
Tylophora (*Tylophora asthmatica*) Leaf	250 mg 1-3 times/day, standardized to contain 0.1% tylophorine per dose	• Allergies • Asthma	None known	• Use with caution if taking asthma medications (effects may be increased) (Level 4) • Use with caution in individuals with diabetes, fluid retention edema, congestive heart failure (CHF), and cardiovascular disease (arrhythmia, hypertension) (Level 4)	• Antiarrhythmics • Beta-blockers • Bronchodilators • Hypertensives • Insulin • Oral hypoglycemics

Herb/Plant Part Used	Dosage & Standardization	Reported Uses	Complementary Effect With Drug Therapy	Theoretical Cautions/Contraindications/ Adverse Effects	Theoretical Interactive Drug/Drug Category
Uva Ursi (*Arctostaphylos uva-ursi*) Leaf	100–200 mg/day, standardized to contain 10% to 25% arbutin per dose	• Urinary tract infections and kidney stone prevention	None known	• Decreased effect in acidic urine; best if urine is base pH (drink 1 tsp of baking soda in water prior to use) • May cause green brown discoloration of urine • Contraindicated in pregnancy and lactation (Level 2) • Contraindicated in renal failure (Level 4)	None known
Valerian (*Valeriana officinalis*) Root	200 mg 1–4 times/day, standardized to contain 0.8% to 1% valerenic acids per dose Sedative dose: 200–400 mg at bedtime	• Sedative or hypnotic; used in nervous tension during PMS, menopause; used in restless motor syndromes and muscle spasms	None known	• May cause drowsiness or sedation; use with caution when driving a car or operating heavy machinery (Level 2) • Do not use in children <3 years of age • Use only valepotriate and baldrinal-free supplements in children <12 years of age due to potential to mutagenic properties (Level 2) • Use with caution in individuals on the following (action may be potentiated): - Antianxiety medications (Level 4) - Hypnotics (Level 4) - Antipsychotics (Level 4) - Antidepressants (Level 4) - Histamines • Reported to increase sleeping time induced by pentobarbital (Level 2)	• Antidepressants • Antihistamines • Anxiolytics • Barbiturates • CNS depressants • Hypnotics • Sedatives
Vinpocetine isolated from (*Vinca minor*)	10–40 mg twice daily	• Memory enhancement; increased brain function as a cerebral metabolic enhancing agent	None known	None known	None known
White Oak (*Quercus alba*) Bark	Oral rinse: Gargle and expectorate 3 times/day	• Soothing agent in mild inflammation of the throat and mouth	None known	• Caution in renal or hepatic dysfunction if ingested (Level 4)	None known

HERB QUICK REFERENCE CHART *(Continued)*

Herb/Plant Part Used	Dosage & Standardization	Reported Uses	Complementary Effect With Drug Therapy	Theoretical Cautions/Contraindications/ Adverse Effects	Theoretical Interactive Drug/Drug Category
White Willow (*Salix alba*) Bark	500 mg up to 3 times/day, standardized to contain 7% to 9% salicin per dose	• Antipyretic; anti-inflammatory; used in reducing fever and in arthritic complaints	None known	• Do not use in children due to potential for Reye's syndrome (Level 4) • Use with caution in renal or hepatic dysfunction (Level 4)	• Aspirin • Methotrexate • Metoclopramide • Phenytoin • Probenecid • Spironolactone • Valproic acid
Wild Yam (*Dioscorea villosa*) Tuber	250 mg 1-3 times/day, standardized to contain 10% diosgenin per dose Topical: Apply as directed	• Contains steroidal precursors and used in female vitality; however, conversion to progesterone in the body is reportedly poor	None known	• Use with caution if taking steroidal medications (Level 4) • Use with caution if taking oral contraceptives or hormone replacement therapy (Level 4) • Contraindicated in individuals with a history of estrogen-dependent tumors, endometrial cancer (Level 4)	• Androgens • Estrogens • Hormone replacement therapy • Oral contraceptives • Steroidal medications
Yohimbe (*Pausinystalia yohimbe*) Bark	500-750 mg twice daily	• May increase sexual vitality in men and women; used in male erectile dysfunction	None known	• Do not use if taking MAO inhibitors (Level 4) • Do not use if hypertensive or on antihypertensive medications (Levels 3 & 4) • Use with caution if taking alpha-blocking agents (Level 4) • Contraindicated in pregnancy • Toxic doses may trigger psychosis, hypotension, and cardiac failure	• Alpha-blocking agents • Antihypertensives • MAO inhibitors • Sympathomimetics • Tricyclic antidepressants

Level 1: Interaction reported in human studies
Level 2: Interaction reported in animal studies
Level 3: Interaction reported in case reports
Level 4: Potential interaction based on the pharmacological activity of the herb

572

NUTRACEUTICAL CHART

Nutrient	Dosage Range	Reported Uses	Functions in the Body	Deficiency Symptoms	Toxicities/Warnings/Interactions
Acetyl-L-Carnitine (ALC)	500-2000 mg/day in divided doses	• Alzheimer's disease • Depression • Improves peripheral nerve function in diabetes	• Enhances energy production in the mitochondria • Enhances cellular oxygenation, helps prevent damage from hypoxia or lack of oxygen • Promotes the synthesis and release of acetylcholine in the brain • Protects and enhances the activity of acetylcholine and dopamine neurons in the brain • Increases the number of nerve growth hormone (NGH) receptors and the amount of nerve growth hormone that is produced	• Deficiency studies in humans have not been conducted • Deficiency may cause age-related memory loss	• No known toxicity or serious side effects • Occasional reports of mild abdominal discomfort, restlessness, vertigo, and headache
Adrenal Extract	100-200 mg 1-3 times/day	• Fatigue and stress	• Supports adrenal function • Promotes energy production • Enhances immune function	• Deficiency studies in humans have not been conducted	• May cause excitability in large doses
Alpha-Lipoic Acid / Lipoic Acid / Thioctic Acid	25-600 mg/day	• Improves nerve blood flow, reduces oxidative stress and improves nerve conduction in diabetic neuropathy • Prevention of cataracts • Protection against stroke and other brain disorders • Glaucoma	• Antioxidant against water-soluble and fat-soluble free radicals • Provides antioxidant protection both inside and outside of cells • As a cofactor that plays a role in the production of cellular energy (ATP) • Prevents the symptoms that accompany vitamin E deficiency • Increases insulin receptor sensitivity	• Lipoic acid deficiency in humans has not been reported • Deficiency would likely result in higher levels of lactic acid which could cause muscle fatigue	• Diabetics should monitor blood sugar levels if using lipoic acid to improve glucose regulation • Rashes have been reported infrequently

573

NUTRACEUTICAL CHART *(Continued)*

Nutrient	Dosage Range	Reported Uses	Functions in the Body	Deficiency Symptoms	Toxicities/Warnings/Interactions
Androstenedione	50-100 mg/day, usually about 1 hour before exercising	• Increases strength and muscle mass	• Precursor to testosterone; converted in the body to testosterone, which does the following: - Regulates the development and function of reproductive organs, the development of sperm, secondary sexual characteristics and sexual function - Enhances muscle mass and bone tissue - Helps increase energy levels and strength, and faster recovery and growth after exercise • Does not convert to estrogen	• Deficiency studies in humans have not been conducted	• Whether toxicity and side effects are possible is controversial - Some experts state that if they occur, they would be similar to excess testosterone - Others claim that most of the androstenedione taken by mouth is destroyed in the liver and the amount that reaches the bloodstream is insufficient to cause toxicity • At this time, some sports organizations (Olympics, NFL) ban its use, while others (Major League Baseball) permit it • Caution should be used in prostate conditions and hormone-sensitive tumors • Use with caution in individuals with congestive heart failure • Contraindicated in individuals with hypertension
Aortic Extract	100 mg/day	• Enhances function, structure, and integrity of arteries and veins • Protects against various forms of vascular disease	• Improves arterial function and blood flow • Prevents damage to arteries • Reduces formation of blood clots • Lowers total cholesterol while raising HDL-cholesterol	• Since the components in aortic extract are not essential nutrients for humans, no deficiency condition exists	• Safe and nontoxic; no side effects have been reported
Betaine Hydrochloride	325-650 mg with meals that contain protein	• Aids in digestion (hypochlorhydria and achlorhydria)	• Digestive aid	• Hypochlorhydria and achlorhydria are common digestive problems	• High dosages can cause gastric irritation • Not to be taken by individuals with ulcers

Nutrient	Dosage Range	Reported Uses	Functions in the Body	Deficiency Symptoms	Toxicities/Warnings/Interactions
Bifidobacterium bifidum (bifidus)	5-10 billion CFU/day (dairy-free) Refrigerate to maintain optimum potency	• Crohn's disease • Diarrhea • Irritable bowel syndrome • Maintains healthy anaerobic microflora in the colon • Ulcerative colitis	• Produce short-chain fatty acids (SCFAs) in the colon, which create a slightly acidic environment that is unfavorable for the growth of pathological bacteria, yeasts, and molds • Short-chain fatty acids formed by bifidobacteria are the main source of energy for the cells that form the inner surface of the colon	• Gas, bloating, diarrhea or constipation, bad breath, chronic vaginal yeast infections	• No known toxicity or serious side effects
Bismuth	120 mg 4 times/day, 20 min before meals for ulcer therapy	• Treatment of ulcers	• Protective coating for inflamed surfaces such as ulcers • May suppress growth of bacteria such as *Campylobacter pylori* and *Helicobacter pylori*	• Bismuth is not considered to be a nutrient and there is no deficiency condition associated with it	• Possible neurological toxicity with long-term use • Treatment should not last longer than 6-8 wks
Caprylic Acid	300 mg 1-4 times/ day, preferably 30 min before meals	• Antifungal, antiyeast agent • Dysbiosis	• Antifungal/antiyeast activity	• Deficiency studies in humans have not been conducted	• No known toxicity or serious side effects
Chitosan	750-1500 mg (of a 90% deacetylation product), 2-3 times/ day 30 min before meals	• May be useful in weight reduction	• Potentially inhibits intestinal absorption of dietary fat • May chelate heavy metals	• Deficiency studies in humans have not been conducted	• May inhibit absorption of fat-soluble dietary supplements (vitamins, fatty acids, and lipid-containing herbs), so do not take at the same time lipid-soluble or lipid-dispersible dietary supplements are taken
Chlorophyll	Tablets: 2-3 tabs/day Liquid: 1 tsp/day in water or juice	• Absorbs odors; bad breath • Bacteriostatic • Protects against toxins • Anti-inflammatory, wound healing, antioxidant properties	• Supportive antioxidant • Protects against toxins	• Since chlorophyll is not an essential nutrient for humans, no deficiency condition exists	• No known toxicity or serious side effects

NUTRACEUTICAL CHART *(Continued)*

Nutrient	Dosage Range	Reported Uses	Functions in the Body	Deficiency Symptoms	Toxicities/Warnings/Interactions
Chondroitin Sulfate	300-1500 mg/day	• Osteoarthritis	• Aids in improving cartilage function • Used as nutritional support in sports injury, acute traumatic injury, and other connective tissue injuries • Supports joint and connective tissue health in combination with glucosamine	• Deficiency studies in humans have not been conducted	• No known toxicity or serious side effects
Coenzyme Q₁₀	30-200 mg/day	• Adjunct cancer therapy • Angina • Chronic fatigue • Congestive heart failure • Diabetes • Hypertension • Mitral valve prolapse • Muscular dystrophy • Obesity • Periodontal disease	• Involved in the manufacture of ATP, the primary source of energy for humans • Functions as an antioxidant • Has the ability to enter mitochondria (the area of a cell where energy is produced) and provides protection against free radical damage	• Cardiovascular problems are the most frequent sign of deficiency, including elevated blood pressure, congestive heart failure, mitral valve prolapse, and angina pectoris • Deficiency increases the incidence of periodontal disease	• May decrease response to warfarin

Collagen (Type II)	200-400 mg 3 times/day
	
	Topical: Apply as needed
		• Arthritis
		• Topical application for wound healing
		  - Pressure ulcers
		  - Venous stasis ulcers
		  - Diabetic ulcers
		  - Ulcers resulting from arterial insufficiencies
		  - Surgical wounds
		  - Traumatic wounds
		  - First and second degree burns
			• Supports collagen production
			• Functions as an anti-inflammatory
			• Improves joint flexibility
			• Reduces destruction of collagen
				• Deficiency studies in humans have not been conducted	• No known toxicity or serious side effects

Colostrum	500-1000 mg 1-3 times/day	• Antidiarrheal • Antiviral properties • Immune system support	• Supports immune function • Aids energy production	• Deficiency studies in humans have not been conducted	• No known toxicity or serious side effects • Use with caution in individuals allergic to dairy products

Nutrient	Dosage Range	Reported Uses	Functions in the Body	Deficiency Symptoms	Toxicities/Warnings/Interactions
Conjugated Linoleic Acid (CLA)	1000-2000 mg 3 times/day in divided doses	• Increases metabolism and decreases body fat	• Helps transport glucose and reduce body fat • Antioxidant • Enhances the immune system	• Deficiency studies in humans have not been conducted, but weight gain would be a result of deficiency	• No known toxicity or serious side effects
Creatine	10-20 g/day in divided doses, for 1 week during the loading phase, then 5 g/day during the maintenance phase	• Athletic performance: enhances energy production and protein synthesis for muscle building	• Enhances the production of energy and muscle building • An immediately available source of energy for muscle contraction • Promotes protein synthesis	• Deficiency studies in humans have not been conducted	• May cause elevation of serum creatinine (not a reflection of renal dysfunction) • Use with caution in renal or hepatic disease • No known toxicity or serious side effects
Cyclo-Hispro	200-300 mg of powdered prostate extract containing cyclo-hispro, 2-4 times/day	• Type 2 diabetes	• Helps control glucose metabolism in individuals with noninsulin-dependent diabetes • Stimulates intestinal absorption of zinc	• Deficiency studies in humans have not been conducted	• May alter glucose regulation • Diabetics should carefully monitor blood sugar levels
Dehydro-epiandrosterone (DHEA)	5-50 mg/day; doses of 100 mg/day are sometimes prescribed for elderly individuals	• Anti-aging • Depression • Diabetes • Fatigue • Lupus	• Precursor for the synthesis of over 50 other hormones in the human body • Estrogen and testosterone are two of the main hormones that are made from DHEA • Stimulates the production of insulin growth factor-1 (IGF-1), which stimulates anabolic metabolism, accelerates muscle growth and maintenance, improves insulin sensitivity, and enhances energy production • Has been reported to decrease the need for insulin doses	• Low blood levels may be associated with an increased risk for many of the common diseases of aging • Low levels are associated with high blood pressure, elevated cholesterol levels, and increased platelet aggregation (blood clot formation)	• No known toxicity or serious side effects (long-term human studies have not yet been conducted) • Should not be used by individuals with a history of prostate or breast cancer • May alter glucose regulation • Diabetics should carefully monitor blood sugar levels • Use with caution in individuals with hepatic dysfunction

577

NUTRACEUTICAL CHART (Continued)

Nutrient	Dosage Range	Reported Uses	Functions in the Body	Deficiency Symptoms	Toxicities/Warnings/Interactions
Docosahexaenoic Acid (DHA)	125-500 mg 1-2 times/day	• Alzheimer's disease • Attention-deficit disorder (ADD) and attention-deficit hyperactivity disorder (ADHD) • Crohn's disease • Diabetes • Eczema • Elevated blood pressure • Elevated triglycerides • Psoriasis • Rheumatoid arthritis	• Important for eye and brain development in infants • Lowers serum triglycerides • Most abundant fat in brain cells • May play a role in cellular electrical communication	• Vision problems • Lower IQ • Slower rate of learning	• Contraindicated in individuals with active bleeding • Use with caution in individuals with a history of bleeding or hemostatic disorders • Use with caution in individuals taking anticoagulant medications, NSAIDs, or antiplatelet medications • Discontinue use prior to dental or surgical procedures (generally at least 14 days prior)
Fish Oils (EPA & DHA)	750 mg 2-3 times/day	• Crohn's disease • Diabetes • Dysmenorrhea • Eczema • Elevated blood pressure • Elevated triglycerides • Memory • Psoriasis • Rheumatoid arthritis	• Mediates inflammatory response • Source of essential fatty acids necessary for nerve tissue, hormone, and cell membranes • Protection against high blood pressure, elevated cholesterol and triglycerides, plaque formation, arthritis, eczema, psoriasis	• increased risk of cardiovascular disease • Inflammatory problems	• High doses may cause GI upset, loose stools, and nausea • May alter glucose regulation • Diabetics should carefully monitor blood sugar levels • Contraindicated in individuals with active bleeding • Use with caution in individuals with a history of bleeding or hemostatic disorders • Use with caution in individuals taking anticoagulant medications, NSAIDs, or antiplatelet medications

Nutrient	Dosage Range	Reported Uses	Functions in the Body	Deficiency Symptoms	Toxicities/Warnings/Interactions
Flaxseed Oil	1 Tbsp/day, which contains ~58% to 60% omega-3	• Source of omega-3 essential fatty acid, also known as alpha-linolenic acid or ALA: - An integral part of the structure of cell walls and cellular membranes - Necessary for the transport and oxidation of cholesterol; - Precursors for an important group of chemicals called the prostaglandins	• Omega-3 is a primary structural component of cellular membranes throughout the body • Omega-3 is converted into longer-chain fatty acids, which are precursors for prostaglandins (regulatory chemicals) that control a variety of body functions including pain, inflammation, swelling, blood pressure, cholesterol levels, digestive processes, synthesis of sex hormones, smooth muscle activity, fluid retention, blood clotting, nerve transmission, and the immune system	• Symptoms may include cardiovascular problems, elevated blood pressure, increased platelet stickiness, increased inflammation, asthma, allergies, problems with skin and hair • Other problems can develop from a deficiency because it upsets the synthesis of prostaglandins	• No known toxicity or serious side effects
Glucosamine (Sulfate or Hydrochloride)	500 mg 3-4 times/day	• Osteoarthritis • Rheumatoid arthritis and other inflammatory conditions	• Protective effect against joint damage and to improve joint mobility • Building block to connective tissues like cartilage and collagen • Component to the natural lubricant found in joints	• Deficiency studies in humans have not been conducted	• No known toxicity or serious side effects • Occasional reports of mild stomach discomfort • Based on animal studies, may alter glucose regulation

579

NUTRACEUTICAL CHART (Continued)

Nutrient	Dosage Range	Reported Uses	Functions in the Body	Deficiency Symptoms	Toxicities/Warnings/Interactions
Glutathione	500-3000 mg/day in divided doses	• May protect against alcohol-induced liver damage • Strengthen immune system • Ulcers	• Detoxifies many compounds in the body, especially in the liver • Helps protect the body against toxins from cigarette smoke, excess alcohol, overdoses of aspirin, and exposure to radiation • Helps support the immune system • Helps transport certain amino acids across cellular membranes • Involved in the synthesis of fatty acids	• Decreased macrophage activity and a weakened immune system • Increase in free radical damage throughout the body, especially in the membranes of red blood cells and mitochondria • Decreases the body's ability to detoxify many compounds in the liver • Could result in hair loss and baldness	• No known toxicity or serious side effects
Hydroxymethyl Butyrate (HMB)	500-1000 mg 3 times/day	• Increases muscle mass during intense exercise	• Anticatabolic agent that may reduce protein/muscle breakdown by shifting protein turnover in favor of new muscle growth resulting in greater gains in muscle size and strength • Increases the body's ability to build muscle and burn fat with intense exercise • Increases endurance	• Deficiency studies in humans have not been conducted	• No known toxicity or serious side effects

Nutrient	Dosage Range	Reported Uses	Functions in the Body	Deficiency Symptoms	Toxicities/Warnings/Interactions
5-Hydroxytryptophan (5-HTP)	50-100 mg 1-3 times/day	• Anxiety • Depression (comparable to fluvoxamine and tricyclic antidepressants) • Fibromyalgia • Headaches • Migraines • Obesity • Sleep disorders, insomnia (stimulates the production of melatonin)	• Precursor to serotonin • Influences the synthesis of melatonin • Reported to increase levels of brain dopamine and norepinephrine • Influences activities controlled by serotonin, which include mood regulation (anxiety and depression), impulse control (aggression and obsessive behavior), appetite, pain control and sleep	• Deficiency studies in humans have not been conducted • Symptoms may include anxiety, depression, sleep disturbances	• May have additive effects with tryptophan, St John's wort, and SAMe • 5-HTP should not be taken concurrently with anti-depressants, such as tricyclics; select serotonin reuptake inhibitors (SSRIs); and mono-amine oxidase inhibitors (MAOI) except under the supervision of a physician, because 5-HTP increases the activity of these drugs • 5-HTP has been reported to occasionally cause gastrointestinal upset
Inositol Hexaphosphate (IP-6)	600-800 mg 3-4 times/day, taken together with 200-250 mg of inositol	• Anticancer agent	• Decreases cellular proliferation • Causes differentiation of malignant cells	• Not an essential nutrient for humans, so no deficiency condition exists	• No known toxicity or serious side effects
Ipriflavone	200 mg 3 times/day	• Prevention and treatment of osteoporosis	• Inhibits bone resorption • Stimulates new bone growth	• Not an essential nutrient for humans, so no deficiency condition exists	• No known toxicity or serious side effects; however, until further research is done, women with a history of estrogen-positive breast cancer should consult a physician before use
Isoflavones	500-1000 mg of soy extract daily (13% to 17% genistein) containing a minimum of 100 mg of total isoflavones per 1000 mg	• Cancer prevention • Chemotherapy • Decrease bone loss • Lower elevated cholesterol • Menopausal symptoms	• Phytoestrogenic • Lowers LDL and raises HDL • Stimulates bone remodeling	• Deficiency studies in humans have not been conducted	• Women who are on estrogen medications should consult their physician • Estrogen-positive breast cancer patients should use with caution

NUTRACEUTICAL CHART (Continued)

Nutrient	Dosage Range	Reported Uses	Functions in the Body	Deficiency Symptoms	Toxicities/Warnings/Interactions
Lactobacillus acidophilus	5–20 billion CFU/day (dairy-free) Refrigerate to maintain optimum potency	• Recolonize the gastrointestinal (GI) tract with beneficial bacteria during and after antibiotics • Constipation • Enhance immunity • Infant diarrhea • Lower elevated cholesterol • Lactose intolerance • Vaginal infections	• Act as a barrier against infection by producing natural antibiotics in the gastrointestinal (GI) tract • Produce a wide range of B-vitamins and vitamin K in the intestinal tract	• Gas, bloating, diarrhea or constipation, bad breath, and chronic vaginal yeast infections	• No known toxicity or serious side effects
Liver Extract	500 mg 1–3 times/day	• Liver tonic	• Useful in fat utilization • Promotion of liver tissue regeneration and prevention of liver damage • Detoxification • Antioxidant effects (high in SOD) • Rich in heme	• Deficiency studies in humans have not been conducted	• Do not use in iron storage disorders such as hemochromatosis
Lutein	2–6 mg/day	• Cataracts • Macular degeneration	• Antioxidant and a member of the carotenoids • Strengthens capillaries • Concentrates in the eye, filters out blue light and prevents macular degeneration	• Development of cataracts and macular degeneration • Weak capillaries and easy bruising	• No known toxicity or serious side effects
Lycopene	5 mg 1–3 times/day	• Atherosclerosis • Cancer prevention (especially prostate) • Macular degeneration	• Antioxidant and a member of the carotenoids • Reported to protect against macular degeneration, atherosclerosis and several types of cancer, especially prostate cancer	• Deficiency studies in humans have not been conducted • Low levels have been correlated to an increased risk of atherosclerosis and some forms of cancer (prostate)	• No known toxicity or serious side effects
Malic Acid	500 mg 3–4 times/day with food	• Fibromyalgia • Aluminum toxicity	• Promotes cellular production of energy • Decreases lactic acid stage by improving delivery to Krebs cycle	• Deficiency studies in humans have not been conducted	• No known toxicity or serious side effects • Occasionally produces gastrointestinal (GI) disturbance

Nutrient	Dosage Range	Reported Uses	Functions in the Body	Deficiency Symptoms	Toxicities/Warnings/Interactions
Melatonin	0.5-6 mg nightly	• Insomnia • Jet lag	• Functions as a hormone that regulates on 24-hour circadian rhythm • Regulates the sleep/wake cycle • Possesses antioxidant activity • Controls the output of growth hormone and sex hormones	• Insomnia and other sleep disturbances	• No known toxicity or serious side effect (long-term human studies have not been conducted) • Taking too much can cause morning grogginess and undesired drowsiness
Methyl Sulfonyl Methane	2000-6000 mg/day	• Pain relief • Interstitial cystitis • Lupus • Osteoarthritis	• Anti-inflammatory agent • Influences inflammatory mediators	• Deficiency studies in humans have not been conducted	• No known toxicity or serious side effects
Modified Citrus Pectin	8-15 g/day Take 5-10 capsules (500 mg each) 3 times/day or dissolve 1/2-1 rounded tsp in water or juice 3 times/day	• Elevated cholesterol • Anticancer activity	• Helps to lower cholesterol • Active against several forms of cancer	• Not an essential nutrient for humans, so no deficiency condition exists	• Do not use if allergic to citrus • Use with caution in renal failure
N-Acetyl Cysteine	200-500 mg up to 3 times/day	• Acetaminophen toxicity • AIDS • Asthma; functions as a mucolytic agent and an antioxidant • Bronchitis • Cardioprotective during chemotherapy • Fatigue • Heavy metal detoxification • Increases glutathione production	• A sulfhydryl compound that is a powerful detoxifying agent capable of detoxifying heavy metals such as mercury, cadmium, and lead • Increase the body's stores of glutathione • Functions as an antioxidant in two ways: - Neutralizes hydrogen peroxide, hypochlorous acid, and the hydroxyl radical; and - Enhances glutathione formation • Functions as an antiviral agent	• Deficiency would compromise the immune system by decreasing liver detoxification capabilities, reducing antioxidant activity, and lowering the body's ability to eliminate heavy metal toxins	• No known toxicity or serious side effects • Large doses (5-6 g/day) have been reported to cause diarrhea • Some antibiotics may become inactivated if taken in conjunction with N-acetyl-L-cysteine

NUTRACEUTICAL CHART *(Continued)*

Nutrient	Dosage Range	Reported Uses	Functions in the Body	Deficiency Symptoms	Toxicities/Warnings/Interactions
Nicotinamide Adenine Dinucleotide (NADH)	2.5-5 mg 1-4 times/day	• Parkinson's disease • Stamina and energy • Chronic fatigue syndrome	• Essential coenzyme in the production of cellular energy • Facilitates DNA-repair mechanisms • Antioxidant • Stimulates the production of dopamine and adrenaline	• Deficiency studies in humans have not been conducted	• No known toxicity or serious side effects
Pancreatic Extract	500-1000 mg 3 times/day before meals to aid digestion or 10-20 min before meals or on an empty stomach for anti-inflammatory effects	• Adjunct support for anti-inflammatory activity • Adjunct support for cancer therapy • Autoimmune diseases • Digestive aid • Food allergies • Celiac disease	• Improves digestion and absorption of nutrients • Supports pancreatic function	• Gas, abdominal bloating and discomfort, indigestion	• No known toxicity or serious side effects
Para-Aminobenzoic Acid (PABA)	100-400 mg/day	• Peyronie's disease • Scleroderma • Vitiligo	• Facilitates the breakdown and utilization of proteins • Aids in the production of red blood cells • Promotes skin health, hair pigmentation, and health of the intestines	• PABA deficiency has not been reported in humans	• No known toxicity or serious side effects at doses below 400 mg/day • Can cause low blood sugar, rash, fever, and liver damage in large doses
Phosphatidyl Choline	500-1000 mg 2-3 times/day	• Alcohol-induced liver damage • Alzheimer's disease; may be helpful for some patients • Gallstones • Hepatitis	• Necessary for cell membrane integrity and the breakdown of fats • Enhances the synthesis of acetylcholine	• Deficiency studies in humans have not been conducted	• No known toxicity or serious side effects

584

Nutrient	Dosage Range	Reported Uses	Functions in the Body	Deficiency Symptoms	Toxicities/Warnings/Interactions
Phosphatidylserine	100 mg 1-3 times/day	• Alzheimer's disease • Depression • Memory enhancement	• Helps provide cell membranes with their fluidity, flexibility, and permeability • Stimulates the release of various neurotransmitters, such as acetylcholine and dopamine • Enhances ion transport and increases the number of certain neurotransmitter receptor sites in the brain • May reduce cortisol levels and have an antistress effect	• Depression, loss of memory, and cognitive decline	• No known toxicity or serious side effects
Pregnenolone	5-30 mg/day depending on age and gender	• Natural precursor for the production of DHEA, cortisol, progesterone, estrogens, and testosterone in the body • Arthritis • Improved mental performance	• Precursor for DHEA and steroid and sex hormones	• Deficiency studies in humans have not been conducted	• No known toxicity or serious side effects, but caution is advised because pregnenolone can stimulate the synthesis of many hormones
Progesterone (Natural Topical)	Dosage for topical progesterone depends on the strength of the extract; follow manufacturer's directions	• Breast cancer prevention • Endometriosis • Menopause symptoms • Osteoporosis • PMS symptoms	• Hormone replacement • Aids bone remodeling	• Increased symptoms of PMS or menopause with edema weight gain, emotional problems • Possible increased risk of breast cancer	• No known toxicity or serious side effects • Hormonal regulation may be disrupted • Women taking hormone medication should check with their physician
Pyruvate	250-750 mg 3 times/day, preferably with meals; dosages from 2500-5000 mg/day have been used for weight loss	• Improving athletic performance • Obesity and weight loss	• Facilitates the transport of glucose into muscle cells, increasing energy available for the muscles	• Pyruvate is not an essential nutrient. There are no studies reporting a deficiency state associated with pyruvate or pyruvic acid.	• Large doses of pyruvate can cause gastrointestinal disturbances, such as gas, bloating, and diarrhea
Quercetin	300-500 mg 1-3 times/day	• Allergies • Atherosclerosis • Cataracts • Peptic ulcers	• Antioxidant • Antihistamine • Anti-inflammatory agent • Strengthens capillaries	• Easy bruising, frequent nosebleeds, or other signs of weak capillaries	• No known toxicity or serious side effects

NUTRACEUTICAL CHART *(Continued)*

Nutrient	Dosage Range	Reported Uses	Functions in the Body	Deficiency Symptoms	Toxicities/Warnings/Interactions
S-Adenosylmethionine (SAMe)	400–1600 mg/day	• Cardiovascular disease • Depression • Fibromyalgia • Insomnia • Liver disease • Rheumatoid arthritis • Osteoarthritis	• Antidepressant • Antioxidant • Necessary for methylation, trans-sulphurating reactions, and polyamine synthesis • Necessary for synthesis of glutathione • Liver detoxification • Synthesis of melatonin	• Deficiency studies have not been conducted. However, a deficiency would probably result in decreased antioxidant activity and weaken liver detoxification capability	• No known toxicity or serious side effects • Occasional dry mouth, nausea, and restlessness • Use caution when combining SAMe with other antidepressants, tryptophan, 5-HTP, St John's wort. SAMe is not effective for depressive symptoms associated with bipolar disorder.
Shark Cartilage	3000 mg 3 times/day taken 20 min before meals Retention enema: 15–20 g/day	• Cancer therapy • Osteoarthritis • Rheumatoid arthritis	• Contains antiangiogenesis factors that prevent tumor growth • Anti-inflammatory	• Deficiency studies in humans have not been conducted	• Nausea is the most frequent side effect.
Spleen Extract	150–300 mg 2-3 times/day	• Support after removal of the spleen or in people with low spleen function	• Provides splenic factors which support immune function	• People with low spleen activity or spleen removal or who have compromised immune function	• No known toxicity or serious side effects
Thymus Extract	250–500 mg 3 times/day	• Immune support	• Immunomodulator	• Deficiency studies in humans have not been conducted	• No known toxicity or serious side effects
Thyroid Extract	60 mg 1-3 times/day	• Fatigue, immune support	• Regulates metabolism • Reportedly supports thyroid metabolism	• Deficiency studies in humans have not been conducted	• Caution if on thyroid medication • Use with caution in individuals with cardiovascular disease • Use with caution in individuals with CNS disorders
Tocotrienols	60–220 mg/day	• Elevated cholesterol • Cancer prevention • Ultraviolet light protection	• Fat-soluble antioxidants	• Weakened immune system with increased risks of cancer and cardiovascular disease	• No known toxicity or serious side effects

HOMEOPATHIC QUICK REFERENCE CHART FOR COMMON COMPLAINTS

Common Complaint	Name of Remedy	Typical Dosage	Symptoms
Acne Vulgaris	Baptisia tinctoria	6X or 6C 30X or 30C	Drainage support
	Hepar sulphuris calcareum		Pimples on forehead and face that are painful to touch, promotes suppuration
	Kali bromatum		Adolescent pustular acne on face, chest, and back
	Pulsatilla		Pimples filled with yellowish discharge, generally used for shy, emotional females
	Sulphur		Red, infected, and sore pimples; skin feels itchy
Allergies / Hayfever	Allium cepa	6X or 6C 30X or 30C	Burning nasal discharge, worse indoors, eye sensitive to light, sneezing, sensation of hook sticking in throat, worse by warm food or drinks
	Ambrosia		General improvement of ragweed response including sneezing, burning eyes, and runny nose
	Arsenicum album		Feel worn out, sneezing, eyes sensitive to light
	Arundo mauritanica		Itching, burning eyes and runny nose, ears, and roof of mouth itch
	Drosera rotundifolia		Profuse, fluid discharge with sneezing
	Histaminum		May counteract histaminic release in body
	Kali bichromicum		Nasal congestion with thick, yellow discharge, crusts in nose, headaches centered in the eyes
	Sabadilla		Violent sneezing, watery eyes, puffy red eyelids, headache, better from warm drinks
Alzheimer's Disease / Senility	Alumina	6X or 6C 30X or 30C	Weak memory, absence of ideas, distracted
	Hyoscyamus niger		Confusion, loss of memory, delirium
Amenorrhea	Ferrum metallicum	6X or 6C 30X or 30C	Weak, tired women with flushed face and rapid pulse
	Pulsatilla		Late periods, insufficient pale menstruation, tires easily
Arthritis (Osteoarthritis)	Arnica montana	6X or 6C 30X or 30C	Pain and inflammation, joints feel bruised, pain in back and shoulders, worse with movement
	Bryonia alba		Joints are swollen, red, and hot; every muscle aches, pain in back and limbs, slightest movement aggravates
	Calcarea phosphorica		Joints feel cold, pain and stiffness worse with change in weather, pain in shoulder and arms, weakness climbing stairs
	Dulcamara		Joint pain when weather is humid, somewhat better from motion
	Rhus toxicodendron		Joint stiffness especially in the morning, better by walking and moving around, pain relieved by heat but aggravated by cold and dampness

HOMEOPATHIC QUICK REFERENCE CHART FOR COMMON COMPLAINTS *(Continued)*

Common Complaint	Name of Remedy	Typical Dosage	Symptoms
Arthritis (Rheumatoid)	Arnica montana	6X or 6C 30X or 30C	Pain and inflammation, joints feel bruised, pain in back and shoulders, worse with movement
	Apis mellifica		Burning, sting pains; sudden swelling, better from cold applications, worse from heat
	Causticum		Stiff neck, dull ache in hands and arms, drawing pains in hands, stiffness of legs and feet
	Colchicum autumnale		Red painful swelling, especially of smaller joints, fingers, toes, wrists and ankles; worse from slightest motion
	Ledum palustre		Painful small joints, especially toes that pop and crack; better from cold applications
	Rhus toxicodendron		Joint stiffness especially in the morning, better by walking and moving around; pain relieved by heat but aggravated by cold and dampness
Asthma	Antimonium tartaricum	6X or 6C 30X or 30C	Chest full of phlegm but unable to expectorate it
	Aralia racemosa		Spasmodic irritation of respiratory tract in the evening or upon lying down
	Arsenicum album		Very restless and anxious with perspiration, worse at night; chronic asthma
	Ipecacuanha		Sudden wheezing, weight in chest, dyspnea, constant, gagging cough; rose by motion, worse from cold air
	Natrum sulphuricum		Worse in damp weather, rattling in the chest, sneezing, worse early in the morning
Athlete's Foot (Tinea Pedis) / Jock Itch (Tinea Cruris)	Agaricus muscarius	6X or 6C 30X or 30C	Itchy, red skin that feels as if it is being pricked by ice-cold needles
	Arsenicum iodatum		Inflammatory scale eruption with powdery appearance
	Borax		Skin looks unhealthy, patchy, whitish eruptions that are surrounded by red
	Lycopodium clavatum		Itching and burning with excoriation of skin
Attention Deficit Disorder (ADD) / Attention Deficit Hyperactivity Disorder (ADHD)	Agaricus muscarius	6X or 6C 30X or 30C	Difficulty in learning, nervous children; aversion to mental tasks
	Baryta carbonica		Physically and intellectually backward children, anxiousness, aversion to play, poor memory, inattention to studies
	Hyoscyamus niger		Insomnia and nightmares, fearful, very talkative
	Stramonium		Very restless, impulsive, talkative, sometimes hysterical, obstinate, uncontrolled fury
	Tarentula hispana	12C	Irritable and moody, constantly moving, headaches, indifference, anger, poor memory
Benign Prostatic Hypertrophy (BPH)	Apis mellifica	6X or 6C 30X or 30C	Frequent urination with stinging and burning, worse from heat
	Sabal serrulata		Frequent nocturnal urination, painful urination
	Thuja occidentalis		Chronic genitourinary tract disorders

Common Complaint	Name of Remedy	Typical Dosage	Symptoms
Breast-feeding	Cinchona officinalis (China)	6X or 6C 30X or 30C	Weakness and anemia during breast-feeding
	Pulsatilla		Overabundant milk supply
Bruises	Arnica montana	6X or 6C 30X or 30C	Bruises and black and blue marks
	Hypericum perforatum		Nerve pain from bruising
	Ruta graveolens		Bruises of the periosteum and pain from bruising the shin, kneecap, or elbow
Burns (Minor)	Apis mellifica	6X or 6C 30X or 30C	Minor burns with pinkish swelling
	Belladonna		Minor burns with red swelling
	Calendula officinalis (topical)	N/A	Topically for minor burns, relieves pain and protects the wound
	Cantharis	6X or 6C 30X or 30C	Minor burns with large painful blister
	Hypericum perforatum		Minor burns with nerve pain
	Rhus toxicodendron		Minor burns with small blister
	Urtica urens		Minor burns with burning, stinging pain
Candidiasis	Agaricus muscarius	6X or 6C 30X or 30C	Leucorrhoea with itching and irritation
	Arsenicum album		Acrid leucorrhoea, thick discharge
	Borax		Leucorrhoea, vaginal itching and burning
	Zincum metallicum		Leucorrhoea with much itching, pruritus vulvae
Cataracts	Calcarea carbonica	6X or 6C 30X or 30C	Opacity and ulceration of the cornea, eyes sensitive to light
	Cineraria maritima	6X or 6C 30X or 30C (external and topical)	Internally and externally for cataracts and corneal
	Phosphorus	30X or 30C	Cloudy vision
	Silicea	6X or 6C 30X or 30C	Cloudiness of lens, cloudy sight, photophobia
Chemotherapy and Radiation	Cadmium sulphuricum	6X or 6C 30X or 30C	Very chilly, intense nausea and vomiting, debilitating exhaustion
	Conium maculatum		Extreme nausea, painful stomach spasms, painful liver, constipation, dizziness, photophobia
	Ipecacuanha		Continuous nausea and vomiting with no relief after vomiting, clean tongue, worse lying down
	Phytolacca decandra		Vertigo, abdominal pain, constipation, pressure over eyes and in temples
	Solanum nigrum		Nausea, loss of appetite
Chronic Fatigue Syndrome (CFS)	Arsenicum album	6X or 6C 30X or 30C	Weak, pale, sensitive to cold, burning sensations, restless, worse at night between 1:00-3:00 AM, better from heat
	Gelsemium sempervirens		General weakness, lethargy, sleepiness, stiffness in body, limbs feel heavy
	Phosphoricum acidum		Prostration and severe fatigue, nervous exhaustion, better from heat and rest, worse from any physical or mental effort

HOMEOPATHIC QUICK REFERENCE CHART FOR COMMON COMPLAINTS *(Continued)*

Common Complaint	Name of Remedy	Typical Dosage	Symptoms
Circulation (Peripheral) / Problems	Cactus grandiflorus	6X or 6C 30X or 30C	Bruise easily, constricting sensation around the heart
	Dulcamara	6X or 6C 30X or 30C	Rheumatic pains, worse from damp cold weather and better with movement
	Lachesis mutus	6C	Cold feet, palpitations, varicose veins
	Secale cornutum	6X or 6C	Leg cramps, cold extremities, skin is cold to the touch, relived by exposure to cold
Cold / Flu	Aconitum napellus	6X or 6C	Sudden onset, especially after exposure to cold wind, sneezing, burning throat, worse at night
	Anas barbariae (hepatis et cordis extractum)	200C	Onset of flu symptoms including fever, chills, muscle aches, headache
	Belladonna		Sudden onset, high temperature, eyes sensitive to light, red, hot face, burning, sore throat worse on right side
	Bryonia alba		Flu-like symptoms with fever, intense thirst, muscle aches, fatigue, headache, worse from slightest movement
	Ferrum phosphoricum	6X or 6C 30X or 30C	Cold comes on slowly, mild fever, prone to nosebleeds
	Gelsemium sempervirens		Fever and flu-like symptoms, sluggish and achy with chills
	Mercurius vivus		Sweating, sneezing, excessive salivation, thick yellowish-green mucus, bad breath
	Natrum muriaticum		Cold in early stages, repeated sneezing, thin clear mucus, stuffy nose, cold sores
Colic	Chamomilla		Very irritable, appears to be in severe pain, but seems to improve when carried around, clingy, sweaty head, diarrhea
	Colocynthis .		Sharp, cramp-like pains relieved by pressure on abdomen or bending over
	Magnesia phosphorica	6X or 6C 30X or 30C	Cramp-like pains relieved by gentle pressure on abdomen and warmth
	Nux vomica		Spasms in the gut, stomachache after eating, constipation
	Veratrum album		Weakness, body feels cold, copious excretions (perspiration, diarrhea, or vomit), better from heat, worse in humid weather

Common Complaint	Name of Remedy	Typical Dosage	Symptoms
Constipation	Graphites	6X or 6C 30X or 30C	No urge to defecate, large stools that are painful to pass, itching and burning of the anus after evacuation, constipation during menstrual periods
	Hydrastis canadensis		No urge to defecate, sinking feeling in the upper abdomen, constipation during pregnancy or after childbirth
	Nux vomica		Sedentary individuals, urge to defecate but unable to do so, when stool occurs there is a feeling of incomplete stool
	Plumbum metallicum		Abdominal cramping and pain, stool is passed with great difficulty and is dry and hard
	Veratrum album		Much straining in an effort to evacuate the bowels, often breaking out in a sweat
Cough	Aconitum napellus	6X or 6C 30X or 30C	Constant short, dry cough, stuffy nose, dry mucous membranes, sudden onset, worse from cold air
	Bryonia alba		Dry, hard, painful hacking cough with painful chest, dry mouth, thirst for cold drinks, better from pressure on the chest, worse at night and from movement
	Grindelia		Dry cough, roughness in the chest, nocturnal cough
	Phosphorus	30X or 30C	Dry, hard, tickling cough from tickling in the throat (especially when talking), tightness in chest, hoarseness or loss of voice, bronchitis, chest feels heavy, worse from talking and activity, worse at night
Cough / Croup	Spongia tosta	6X or 6C 30X or 30C	Dry, barking, hard cough, croup, laryngitis, dryness of mucous membranes, worse from swallowing and talking, better from eating and drinking (especially warm drinks)
Crohn's Disease	Aloe socotrina	6X or 6C 30X or 30C	Burning diarrhea with much mucus, sensation of fullness in the abdomen, poor anal sphincter control
	Cinchona officinalis (China)		Painless foul-smelling diarrhea that leaves individual feeling weak, bloating, indigestion, worse at night and after eating
Croup	Cuprum metallicum	6X or 6C 30X or 30C	Spasmodic ringing cough relieved by drinking cold water
	Drosera rotundifolia		Tickle in larynx brings on deep spasmodic nonstop coughing, laryngitis and hoarse voice, worse from lying down
	Rumex crispus		Spasmodic dry cough, hoarseness, worse breathing in cold air, better from covering head with bedcovers
	Sticta pulmonaria		Dry, racking, spasmodic incessant cough, worse at night

HOMEOPATHIC QUICK REFERENCE CHART FOR COMMON COMPLAINTS *(Continued)*

Common Complaint	Name of Remedy	Typical Dosage	Symptoms
Depression	Aurum metallicum	6X or 6C 30X or 30C	Sadness, despair, disgusted with life, constant self-reproach, intolerant to noise, better from music, tendency to be irritable and angry
	Kali bromatum		Sadness with an uncontrollable desire to cry, restlessness (especially of the hands), insomnia with nightmares, memory loss, indifference to life
	Sepia		Pessimistic, indifferent to everything and everyone, afraid of being alone, sadness, aversion to sex
Diaper Rash	Calcarea carbonica	6X or 6C 30X or 30C	Burning, chapped and itching skin
	Calendula officinalis (topical)	N/A	Has antalgic and antiseptic action when used topically on skin irritations and ulcers
	Mercurius corrosivus	6X or 6C 30X or 30C	Burning and redness of skin
	Sulphur		Red, burning, itchy rash, worse from water
Diarrhea	Arsenicum album	6X or 6C 30X or 30C	Watery, offensive diarrhea, often with burning pain, exhaustion, thirst for small sips of water, anxious and restless, diarrhea from food poisoning
	Colocynthis		Painful diarrhea relieved by bending forward
	Natrum sulphuricum		Watery stools early in the morning or after breakfast, flatulence
	Podophyllum peltatum		Profuse, gushing, watery diarrhea, abdomen rumbles and gurgles, diarrhea immediately after eating, worse in the morning
	Veratrum album		Profuse watery stool, pain in the abdomen before stool, cold sweat, exhaustion, thirst for large amounts of cold water
Diverticulitis	Argentum nitricum	6X or 6C 30X or 30C	Cutting pains in the abdomen, flatulence
	Arsenicum album		Watery, offensive diarrhea, often with burning pain, exhaustion, anxious and restless
	Colocynthis		Intense abdominal discomfort and pain, inflammation of the abdomen, cramping, relief obtained by motion
Dyslipidemia	Carduus marianus	6X or 6C 30X or 30C	Disturbed sugar metabolism, hepatic complaints, enlarged liver, drainage remedy for liver
	Chelidonium majus	6X or 6C	Lethargy, abdominal distention, enlarged liver, sluggish bowels, liver disorders, dull ache or liver pain that radiates to right shoulder
	Cholesterinum	6X or 6C 30X or 30C	Enlarged liver, burning pain in side, jaundice, gallstones
	Petroleum		Heartburn, abdominal distention, aversion to meat and fatty foods, gastralgia when stomach is empty

Common Complaint	Name of Remedy	Typical Dosage	Symptoms
Dysmenorrhea	Chamomilla	6X or 6C 30X or 30C	Intolerable pain, excessive flow, irritable
	Cimicifuga racemosa		Pain in pelvic region that moves from one side to the other, premenstrual headache, sharp abdominal pains that are relieved from doubling up, profuse flow with clots
	Magnesia phosphorica		Crampy, spasmodic pains preceding menstrual flow, better from warmth, worse from motion
Eczema	Calcarea carbonica	6X or 6C 30X or 30C	Skin hot and burning, chapped, red and raised eruptions, worse from cold applications
	Cantharis		Large, burning, itching blisters on the skin, relieved by cold compresses
	Croton tiglium		Extremely itchy, vesicular eruptions, scratching makes skin very painful, often on face or genital area
	Graphites		Scabby, dry, scaly skin
	Mezereum		Scabby pus-filled eruptions covered by thick whitish crusts, usually on face, chin, scalp, back of hands
	Sulphur		Red, burning, itchy rash, worse from water
Endometriosis	Apis mellifica	6X or 6C 30X or 30C	Burning, stinging pains, ovaritis (predominately right-sided)
	Belladonna		Abdomen swollen and sensitive to touch, stitching pain
	Kali iodatum		Pressure in the uterus when walking, griping pain in abdomen
	Lachesis mutus	6C	Left-sided ovarian pain, cannot bear pressure
Epilepsy	Bufo rana	6X or 6C 30X or 30C	Clonic spasms, confusion and loss of memory
	Calcarea carbonica		Petit mal, loss of consciousness without convulsion
	Causticum		Petit mal, sudden loss of consciousness
	Cicuta virosa		Fixed, staring gaze, frothing at the mouth, violent convulsions
	Cuprum metallicum		Muscle cramps and violent muscle spasms
	Hyoscyamus niger		Delirium and convulsions, phobias, muscle spasms
Fatigue	Arsenicum album	6X or 6C 30X or 30C	Restlessness despite extreme exhaustion, minor depression, anxiety
	Carbo vegetabilis		Stagnation of blood circulation, exhaustion, general weakness, pale appearance, tendency to faint
	Natrum muriaticum		Minor depression, weakness, mental tiredness, difficulty concentrating, absentmindedness

HOMEOPATHIC QUICK REFERENCE CHART FOR COMMON COMPLAINTS *(Continued)*

Common Complaint	Name of Remedy	Typical Dosage	Symptoms
Fever	Aconitum napellus	6X or 6C 30X or 30C	Sudden onset of fever, worse about midnight, pale face, sweaty, restless and thirsty
	Belladonna		Sudden, violent fever, hot, red skin, pounding pulse
	Bryonia alba		Feverish, irritable, very thirsty, feels worse from moving
	Ferrum phosphoricum		Fever comes on gradually, flushed cheeks, throbbing headache, chilly, better from cold applications
	Gelsemium sempervirens		Fever with lethargy or dullness, aching muscles, lack of thirsty, headache made worse by movement
	Phosphorus	30X or 30C	Fever, wants sympathy, intense thirst for cold drinks that are vomited when they become warm in the stomach
Fibrocystic Breast Disease (FBD)	Graphites	6X or 6C 30X or 30C	Swollen mammary glands, sore nipples
	Phytolacca decandra		Multiple hard, painful nodules, cracked nipples, breasts are painful before and during menstrual periods
Fibromyalgia	Lacticum acidum	6X or 6C 30X or 30C	Disturbed cell respiration, rheumatic complaints
	Magnesia phosphorica		Sudden, intense, spasmodic pains that are cramp-like or neuralgic, erratic, better from heat and pressure
	Rhus toxicodendron		Stiff joints, swollen painful joints, better from motion, better from heat and hot applications, worse in cold, damp weather
Gallbladder / Gallstones	Berberis vulgaris	6X or 6C 30X or 30C	Cramp-like pains in the hepatic region, shooting pains
	Cinchona officinalis (China)		Much flatulence, distended abdomen, shooting, pressing pains in hepatic region, very tender to touch
	Lycopodium clavatum		Poor digestion, abdominal bloating, colic, sharp pain, cramping (especially after meal)
Gingivitis	Kreosotum	6X or 6C 30X or 30C	Painful, swollen, dark red gums that bleed when touched, offensive breath, decayed teeth
	Phosphorus	30X or 30C	Bleeding gums, inflammation of the gingiva
Glaucoma	Aconitum napellus	6X or 6C 30X or 30C	Pain extending down face, worse by motion or touch
	Belladonna		Pain, throbbing headache, sensitive to light
	Cineraria maritima		Intense pressure, pain
Halitosis	Mercurius solubilis	6X or 6C 30X or 30C	Bad breath, excess salivation, tongue retains teeth marks, bleeding gums
	Nux vomica		Yellowish-white coating on back of tongue, indigestion

Common Complaint	Name of Remedy	Typical Dosage	Symptoms
Headache	Apis mellifica	6X or 6C 30X or 30C	Stinging, stabbing, burning headache, body feels tender, worse in hot, stuffy room
	Belladonna		Throbbing, drumming ache in temples, right side of head as if band is tightening around head, flushed face, noise/light sensitivity, worse in hot sun
	Bryonia alba		Bursting, splitting headache, sharp, stabbing pain (especially forehead or eyes), thirst, constipation, worse by slightest movement
	Gelsemium sempervirens		Dull, heavy, aching head, feels like band around head, affects temples, above eyes, neck, and shoulders
	Glonoinum		Throbbing, congestive headache, exploding sensation in head; head feels enlarged, stiff neck
	Ignatia amara		Feels like nail being driven through side of head
	Nux vomica		Dull, dizzy headache, irritable, worse in morning, headaches caused by overindulgence of food, coffee, tobacco, or alcohol
	Theridion	6C or 30C	Dizziness with nausea, intolerance to any noise, worse from closing eyes
Headache (Migraine)	Iris versicolor	6X or 6C 30X or 30C	Headache starts with blurred vision, sharp, throbbing pain mostly located above the eyes, especially on the right side
	Lachesis mutus	6C	Congestive headaches, especially left-sided, menopausal headaches, worse from heat and alcohol
	Natrum muriaticum	6X or 6C 30X or 30C	Pounding in the head, especially in the morning, worse from moving the eyes or head
	Spigelia anthelmia		Intense, neuralgic pain above left eye or left side of head, worse from noise and in the morning
	Thuja occidentalis		Boring, pressing pain, especially left-sided
Hemorrhoids	Aesculus hippocastanum	6X or 6C 30X or 30C	Shooting pains in the rectum and back, purplish hemorrhoids that burn and itch
	Carduus marianus		Constipation, varicose veins
	Hamamelis virginiana		Sore, bruised feeling in the rectum, bleeding hemorrhoids, lower back ache, worse from warmth and any contact
	Podophyllum peltatum		Hemorrhoids and rectal prolapse, better from lying on the stomach, worse in the early morning
	Sulphur		Constipation, hemorrhoids that burn and itch, worse at night

HOMEOPATHIC QUICK REFERENCE CHART FOR COMMON COMPLAINTS *(Continued)*

Common Complaint	Name of Remedy	Typical Dosage	Symptoms
Herpes Simplex 1	Baptisia tinctoria	6X or 6C 30X or 30C	Mouth sores on lip, red and shiny
	Croton tiglium		Burning vesicular eruptions
	Muriaticum acidum		Scaly eruptions
	Rhus toxicodendron		Small vesicles filled with clear liquid that itch and burn, not relieved by scratching, better from hot applications
Herpes Simplex 2	Capsicum annuum	6X or 6C 30X or 30C	Sensitive inflammations that burn intensely
	Natrum muriaticum		Recurrent genital eruptions
	Rhus toxicodendron		Small vesicles filled with clear liquid that itch and burn, not relived by scratching, better from hot applications
Hyperglycemia / Diabetes / Insulin Resistance	Lycopodium clavatum	6X or 6C 30X or 30C	Craving for sugar and sweets, intolerance to onions and starchy foods, feeling of fullness after a few bites of food, flatulence, distended abdomen
	Phaseolus		Diabetes mellitus
	Phosphoricum acidum		Excessive urination, nervous exhaustion
	Syzygium jambolanum		Excessive thirst, weakness
	Uranium nitricum	6C	Glycosuria, nocturnal enuresis
Hypertension (High Blood Pressure)	Cactus grandiflorus	6X or 6C 30X or 30C	Constricting sensation, pain radiates to the left arm
	Glonoinum		Sudden palpitations, feels as if blood rushes to the head, throbbing headache
	Natrum muriaticum		Pains in chest, shortness of breath
Hyperthyroidism	Iodium	30C	Loss of weight despite good appetite, trembling, anxiety and depression, better from eating
	Lycopus virginicus	6X or 6C 30X or 30C	Hyperthyroidal syndromes, heart palpitations
	Natrum muriaticum		Loss of weight despite good appetite, very thirsty, moody
Hypoglycemia	Lycopodium clavatum	6X or 6C 30X or 30C	Headache if hunger is not immediately appeased
	Phosphorus	30X or 30C	Weakness from not eating
	Sulphur	6X or 6C 30X or 30C	Weakness from not eating
Hypothyroidism	Arsenicum album	6X or 6C 30X or 30C	Weakness, nervous restlessness, cold sensitive
	Fucus vesiculosus		Coldness of hands and feet, lowered metabolism
	Thyroidinum	6X	Sarcode support

Common Complaint	Name of Remedy	Typical Dosage	Symptoms
Indigestion / Heartburn	Argentum nitricum	6X or 6C 30X or 30C	Gastralgia, poor digestion, excessive belching, stomach pains and bloating, hiatal hernia
	Carbo vegetabilis		Weak digestion, sour belching brings temporary relief, bloating, foul flatulence, difficulty digesting fats, better in open air
	Lycopodium clavatum		Sense of fullness after eating a small amount, rumbling gas in the lower abdomen, sluggish digestion, sleepiness after meals, worse lying down, better after belching
	Nux vomica		Stomach feels bloated after eating, coated tongue, worse from alcohol and heavy meals, better after a short nap
Insect Bites / Stings	Apis mellifica	6X or 6C 30X or 30C	Burning stinging pains, pinkish swelling, puffiness, worse from heat
	Calendula officinalis (topical)	N/A	Relieves pain and swelling when applied topically
	Ledum palustre	6X or 6C 30X or 30C	Edematous swelling, hot, tearing pain, itching and burning, very sensitive to touch, better from cold application
	Tarentula hispana	12C	Itching, pricking pain with redness
Insomnia	Coffea cruda	6X or 6C 30X or 30C	Nervous excitement that keeps the mind active, often awaken about 3:00 AM and cannot go back to sleep
	Ignatia amara		Intellectual strain
	Lycopodium clavatum		Cannot stop mind from thinking about day's events
	Nux vomica		Light, disturbed sleep with bad dreams, often due to overexertion or overindulgence in food and drink, always feel as if more sleep is needed
Irritable Bowel Syndrome (IBS)	Argentum nitricum	6X or 6C 30X or 30C	Inflammation and ulceration of the stomach and intestines, diarrhea, anticipation anxiety, desire for sugar and sweets even though these are difficult to digest
	Colchicum autumnale		Hypersensitivity to odors, smell of food brings nausea, copious diarrhea and flatulence
	Colocynthis.		Intense, spasmodic pain in the digestive tract, better from doubling up, painful diarrhea
Macular Degeneration	Carbo vegetabilis	6X or 6C 30X or 30C	Circulatory debility
	Secale cornutum		Poor circulation
Memory Problems	Anacardium orientale	6X or 6C 30X or 30C	Depression, loss of memory, indecisiveness, irritability, mental effort is difficult
	Baryta carbonica		Difficulty remembering, forgetfulness
	Cocculus indicus		Forgetfulness

HOMEOPATHIC QUICK REFERENCE CHART FOR COMMON COMPLAINTS *(Continued)*

Common Complaint	Name of Remedy	Typical Dosage	Symptoms
Menopause	Kali carbonicum	6X or 6C 30X or 30C	Weary, anxious, weakness in the legs, stabbing, burning pains with perspiration
	Lachesis mutus	6C	Hot flashes and left-sided ovarian discomfort, symptoms worse in morning, tender breasts, morning headache
	Sepia	6X or 6C 30X or 30C	Dysmenorrhea, irritability, cold, weepy, craving sweet or salty foods, sallow patches, flooding during period
Menorrhagia	Calcarea carbonica		General paleness, cramping pain in abdomen and small of back, profuse menstrual flow
	Sabina	6X or 6C 30X or 30C	Periods are early, heavy and prolonged, discharge consists of red, clotted blood and is aggravated by any movement
	Sanguinaria canadensis		Profuse menses with headache
	Secale cornutum		Heavy flow, great debility
Motion Sickness	Ambra grisea		Attack of dizziness, sensation of weakness in the stomach, loss of balance
	Cocculus indicus		Severe nausea, dizziness, vomiting, mere thought of food brings wave of nausea
	Ipecacuanha	6X or 6C 30X or 30C	Constant nausea, diarrhea, vomiting does not relieve the nausea, a great deal of saliva in the mouth
	Nux vomica		Constant nausea, splitting headache, vomiting
	Petroleum		Dizziness and nausea from riding in car or boat, cold sweat, empty feeling in stomach relieved by eating
	Tabacum		Severe nausea, cold sweat, violent retching and vomiting with every movement, better in open air and when eyes are closed
Multiple Sclerosis (MS)	Carboneum sulphuratum.		Numbness of fingers, inability to hold small objects, weakness in upper limbs
	Causticum	6X or 6C 30X or 30C	Severe general weakness, joint stiffness, chronic, progressive paralysis
	Lathyrus sativus		Paralytic sensation in the limbs, heavy legs with vague pain, uncertain gait, staggering
	Phosphorus	30X or 30C	Rigidity in limbs, weakness and heaviness in limbs

Common Complaint	Name of Remedy	Typical Dosage	Symptoms
Muscle Soreness / Stiffness	Arnica montana (internal and topical)	6X or 6C 30X or 30C	Sharp stabbing pain in a muscle, muscle strain and overexertion
	Rhododendron chrysanthemum		Joint pains, lumbago, burning rheumatic pains, worse before a storm and from humidity
	Rhus toxicodendron		Swollen, painful joints, tendinitis, muscle fatigue, joint stiffness, worse at the start of motion, but improves with continuing movement, worse in damp cold
	Ruta graveolens		Bone and tendon pain, feel bruised all over, stiff limbs and joints, tendinitis, wrist pain, sciatica, muscle strain and sprains
Nausea / Vomiting	Ipecacuanha	6X or 6C 30X or 30C	Constant nausea, diarrhea, vomiting does not relieve the nausea, a great deal of saliva in the mouth
	Nux vomica		Constant nausea, splitting headache, vomiting, nausea during menstrual period
	Pulsatilla		Nausea from pastry, ice cream, and greasy food, eructation tastes like food eaten
	Tabacum		Severe nausea, cold sweat, violent retching and vomiting with every movement, better in open air and when eyes are closed
Osteoporosis	Calcarea carbonica	6X or 6C 30X or 30C	Weak ankles and swollen joints, sensitive to cold
	Calcarea fluorica		Tendency to bony knots, induration of the bones
	Calcarea phosphorica		Rheumatic pains with weakness in the hips, fragile bones, white spots on the nails
	Hekla lava		Supports calcium metabolism
Otitis Media	Belladonna	6X or 6C 30X or 30C	Sudden onset, intense, throbbing pain, fever, hot, red face, especially right ear, worse at night, relieved by warmth
	Chamomilla		Violent pain with much suffering, red cheeks, very restless, worse from warmth and at night
	Mercurius solubilis		Soreness of internal ear, tearing, shooting, drawing pains in the ear, ear and auditory tube inflamed, discharge
Parkinson's Disease	Cuprum metallicum	6X or 6C 30X or 30C	Periodic spasmodic pains, muscle cramps and spasms, violent cramps in the calves and feet especially at night
	Mercurius solubilis		Tremor in hands with weakness, jerking of arms, great weakness, knees give out, sensation of rigidity, torpor and cramping in thighs and legs, cramps in toes
	Thuja occidentalis		Severe neuralgia with muscle tremors, tearing pain in muscles and joints, worse from humidity and cold, better from heat
	Zincum metallicum		Continual restlessness, especially of the feet and legs, prickling sensations
Performance Enhancement	Arnica montana	6X or 6C 30X or 30C	Sharp stabbing pain in muscles, muscle strain and overexertion
	Lacticum acidum		Muscle soreness and recovery from exercise

HOMEOPATHIC QUICK REFERENCE CHART FOR COMMON COMPLAINTS *(Continued)*

Common Complaint	Name of Remedy	Typical Dosage	Symptoms
Poison Ivy / Poison Oak	Apis mellifica	6X or 6C 30X or 30C	Patches of red, swollen skin that stings or burns, very sensitive to touch, relieved by cold applications
	Cantharis		Itching, burning skin
	Croton tiglium		Itching, burning skin, vesicular inflammation
	Mezereum		Redness, inflammation and itching, fluid filled vesicles, burning and stinging
	Rhus toxicodendron		Small vesicles filled with clear liquid that itch and burn, not relieved by scratching, better from hot applications
	Sulphur		Weepy rash that itches and burns, temporary relief from scratching, which then increases the itching or burning, worse from warm applications
Premenstrual Syndrome (PMS)	Apis mellifica	6X or 6C 30X or 30C	Right-sided ovarian discomfort, burning, stinging pains, better from cold, worse from heat
	Lachesis mutus	6C	Left-sided ovarian discomfort, hot flashes, nervousness and anxiety, improvement when menstrual period starts
	Lycopodium clavatum	6X or 6C 30X or 30C	Irritability, depression, craves sweets, right-sided ovarian pain
	Natrum muriaticum		Fluid retention, swollen breasts, sadness, irritability
	Pulsatilla		PMS symptoms, mood swings and crying, painful breasts, hot flashes, irregular periods
	Sepia		Profuse menses, melancholy, weakness
Psoriasis	Arsenicum album	6X or 6C 30X or 30C	Dry scaly skin, shiny, inflamed
	Graphites		Obstinate dryness, red spots, itching, vesicles ooze honey-like discharge when cracked
	Sulphur		Rough, chapped skin, skin cracks easily
Rosacea	Belladonna	6X or 6C 30X or 30C	Bright red, blotchy face
	Lachesis mutus	6C	Hypertrophy of the nose accompanied by reddish acne, symptoms appear during menopause
	Sanguinaria canadensis	6X or 6C 30X or 30C	Reddish cheeks, lesions that burn and sting, worse from heat, symptoms appear during menopause
	Sepia		Itchy eruptions by mouth and nose, rash heals from the center outward
	Thuja occidentalis		Heat in the face, burning, red cheeks
Scleroderma	Rhododendron chrysanthemum	6X or 6C 30X or 30C	Wrenching pain and soreness in joints and thighs, swelling of legs and feet, drawing and tearing pains, weakness in limbs
	Sulphur		Red, burning, itchy rashes, worse from getting wet, better from cold applications
	Thuja occidentalis		Edema about the joints that affects epithelia, tearing, pulsing pains

Common Complaint	Name of Remedy	Typical Dosage	Symptoms
Sexual Vitality (Females)	Agnus castus	6X or 6C 30X or 30C	Frigidity without sexual desire
	Conium maculatum		Impotence due to abstinence
	Natrum muriaticum		Disappointment in love, fatigued and distracted
	Sepia		Total lack of interest in sex
Sexual Vitality (Males)	Graphites	6X or 6C 30X or 30C	Sad, melancholic, sexual weakness that makes ejaculation difficult
	Lycopodium clavatum		Difficulty having an erection, enlarged prostate, lack of self-confidence
	Phosphoricum acidum		Improves energy
	Sabal serrulata		Improves sexual vitality
Sinusitis	Hepar sulphuris calcareum	6X or 6C 30X or 30C	Painful throbbing sinuses, worse from touch, aggravated by draft of air, better from heat applications
	Hydrastis canadensis		Thick, yellow, sticky, stringy nasal discharge, burning pains in the nose and sinuses
	Kali bichromicum		Yellow or greenish-yellow nasal discharge with crusts in the nose, pain and pressure at the base of the nose
	Silicea		Chronic sinusitis, sensitive to cold
Sore Throat	Apis mellifica	6X or 6C 30X or 30C	Stinging, burning pain in the throat, relieved by drinking cold liquids or sucking on ice, high fever
	Belladonna		Sudden onset, dry, red throat that is very sore, worse on right side, swollen tonsils, constant desire to swallow, but an aversion to drinking
	Crotalus horridus		Swollen glands, sensation as if a plug is being swallowed
	Mercurius corrosivus		Intense burning in throat, worse from pressure, throat feels constricted, very swollen glands
	Phosphorus	30X or 30C	Fever, aching, scraping, burning throat, swollen tonsils, very thirsty for cold water
Sprains / Strains	Arnica montana	6X or 6C 30X or 30C	Swelling and pain, sore muscles
	Bellis perennis		Deep muscle injuries and injuries to joints
	Bryonia alba		Swollen, painful joint, worse from movement
	Rhus toxicodendron		Hot, swollen joints and sore muscles, better after motion
	Ruta graveolens		Minor injuries to tendons or ligaments
Stress / Anxiety	Aconitum napellus	6X or 6C 30X or 30C	Sudden onset, restlessness, anxiety, fears, sometimes fear of death
	Ignatia amara		Effects of emotions, especially sad events, lump in the throat, nervous yawning, moodiness, keeps emotions bottled up inside and constantly goes over them
	Phosphoricum acidum		Mental or emotional strain, physical exhaustion, tightness in chest, hair loss

601

HOMEOPATHIC QUICK REFERENCE CHART FOR COMMON COMPLAINTS *(Continued)*

Common Complaint	Name of Remedy	Typical Dosage	Symptoms
Sunburn	Apis mellifica	6X or 6C 30X or 30C	Burning, stinging skin, hives that develop from exposure to the sun, relieved by cold compresses, feverish
	Belladonna		Red, hot, painful skin, intense thirst, fever
	Calendula officinalis (topical)	N/A	Topically for relief of minor skin irritations
	Hypericum	6X or 6C 30X or 30C	Tingling, burning pain, pain involving the nerve endings
Systemic Lupus Erythematosus (SLE)	Apis mellifica	6X or 6C 30X or 30C	Swollen joints, allergic reactions, extreme sensitivity
	Arsenicum album		Sensation of weakness, rapid failure of strength, burning pains, edema
	Causticum		General weakness, burning sensation in connective tissue
	Rhus toxicodendron		Swelling, stiffness on first moving, trembling sensation in limbs
	Ruta graveolens		Dull, tearing pains, feeling as if falling from side to side while walking, heaviness of legs
	Thuja occidentalis		Global fatigue and prostration, great weakness in legs (especially when going upstairs), swelling in ends of toes
Teething	Calcarea fluorica	6X or 6C 30X or 30C	Small, crooked teeth, poor quality tooth enamel
	Calcarea phosphorica		Slow dentition, cold hands and feet, cranky child
	Chamomilla		Very painful teething, child is very irritable and wants to be held
	Mercurius corrosivus		Drooling and excessive salivation associated with teething, gums are red and sore, diarrhea
Ulcerative Colitis	Aloe socotrina	6X or 6C 30X or 30C	Mucus in stools, alternating constipation and diarrhea, flatulence
	Antimonium crudum		Diarrhea alternating with constipation, half-solid, half-liquid stools, belching
	Cinchona officinalis (China)		Much foul-smelling flatulence, painless diarrhea that contains undigested food, diarrhea especially after meals
	Colocynthis		Cramping abdominal pain, painful diarrhea, better from pressure and bending double
Ulcer (Aphthous)	Borax	6X or 6C 30X or 30C	Very painful sores in the mouth, on the tongue, and inside the cheek that tend to bleed, sores start out red and are very painful to contact (especially acidic or salty foods), mouth feels hot
	Kali muriaticum		Mouth ulcers that look whitish, thick saliva
	Natrum muriaticum		Exanthema on mouth and lips, cold sores
Ulcer (Duodenal or Peptic)	Bismuthum oxydatum	6X or 6C 30X or 30C	Nausea after eating, pain in stomach, strong inclination to vomit, burning in the stomach
	Hydrastis canadensis		Chronic gastritis, dull stomach pains, emptiness in the pit of the stomach, faintness
	Nux vomica		Gastrointestinal dyspepsia

Common Complaint	Name of Remedy	Typical Dosage	Symptoms
Urinary Tract Infection (UTI)	Benzoicum acidum	6X or 6C 30X or 30C	Irritation of the bladder, dark-colored urine that has a very strong odor
	Cantharis		Strong, persistent painful urge to urinate, sudden onset, urine is passed in drops that burn intensely, small of back may ache
	Mercurius corrosivus		Intense straining that produces scant, dark-colored urine, burning when urinating
	Nitricum acidum		Prickly pains, frequent but scanty urination, prickly, burning in urethra upon urination
	Staphysagria		Burning pains in the urethra that are relieved by urinating, "honeymooner's" cystitis, irritable
	Sulphur		Pain in kidney region, scanty urine, frequency and urgency of urination
Weight Management	Calcarea carbonica	6X or 6C 30X or 30C	Short, stocky individuals who tend to be overweight and inactive, sensitive to cold
	Graphites		Poor oxygenation, always cold, slow metabolism
	Growth hormone	30C	Regulation of endocrine system
	Picricum acidum	6X or 6C 30X or 30C	Reduced metabolism, lack of energy
	Thyroidinum	6X	Regulation and support of thyroid function
Wounds (Minor) / Cuts / Scrapes	Apis mellifica	6X or 6C 30X or 30C	Puncture wounds that are swollen and hot with stinging pains, better from cold applications
	Calendula officinalis (topical)	N/A	Topically for minor skin irritations from cuts and scrapes
	Hepar sulphuris calcareum	6X or 6C 30X or 30C	Red, swollen, painful wounds
	Hypericum perforatum		Nerve pain from cuts and scrapes
	Ledum palustre		Puncture wounds associated with redness, swelling and throbbing pain

Note: The most common dosages for the majority of single homeopathic remedies are 6X or 6C and 30X or 30C, unless otherwise designated by the Homeopathic Pharmacopoeia of the United States (HPUS). Combination homeopathic remedies often contain various dilutions, all of which may be beneficial for a given condition.

603

VITAMINS / MINERALS / TRACE ELEMENTS / AMINO ACIDS

Vitamins/ Minerals/Trace Elements/Amino Acids	RDI / ODA*	Reported Uses	Functions in the Body	Food Sources	Deficiency Symptoms	Toxic Dose/ Toxicity Symptoms
L-Arginine	RDI: None established ODA: 3000–6000 mg/day	• Helps lower elevated cholesterol • Increases lean body mass • Inflammatory bowel disease • Male infertility • Surgery and wound healing	• Detoxification or urea • Supports immune function • Helps protect against liver toxins such as alcohol and carbon tetrachloride	Meat, nuts, eggs, milk, cheeses	• Rash, hair loss, poor wound healing, constipation, fatty liver, cirrhosis	Toxicity Symptoms: • Diarrhea • Can provoke an outbreak of herpes simplex if lysine levels are low
Beta-carotene (known as Provitamin A)	RDI: None established ODA: 10,000–30,000 int. units daily	• Cancer prevention • Immune enhancement • Photo-protection	• Antioxidant • Precursor to vitamin A	Dark green leafy vegetables, yellow and orange fruits and vegetables	• Low dietary intake of beta-carotene has been correlated to some forms of cancer • Increased free radical activity and weakened immune system	• No known toxicity
Biotin	RDI:30 mcg/day ODA: 30–300 mcg/day	• Brittle nails • Diabetes • Diabetic neuropathy • Seborrheic dermatitis • Uncombable hair syndrome	• Involved in metabolism of fatty acids, carbohydrates, and protein • Involved in maintaining the health of skin, hair, sweat glands, nerves, and bone marrow	Liver, kidney, egg yolks, milk, yeast, whole grains, nuts, cauliflower, legumes	• High cholesterol • Skin problems • Muscle weakness • Hair loss	• No known toxicity
Boron	RDI: None established ODA: None established	• Osteoarthritis • Osteoporosis • Rheumatoid arthritis	• Needed for normal calcium and bone metabolism • Plays a role in mental alertness and motor activity • Plays an important role in the metabolism of magnesium • Has a regulatory effect on the production of estrogens and testosterone	Fresh fruits and vegetables, nuts	• Decreased blood • Ionized calcium and calcitonin • Calcium loss and bone demineralization	Toxic Dose: • 150 mg/liter of water Toxicity Symptoms: • Nausea, diarrhea, skin rashes, fatigue

604

Vitamins/ Minerals/Trace Elements/Amino Acids	RDI / ODA*	Reported Uses	Functions in the Body	Food Sources	Deficiency Symptoms	Toxic Dose/ Toxicity Symptoms
Branched-Chain Amino Acids (BCAAs) / including Leucine / L-Leucine / Isoleucine / Valine / L-Valine	RDI: None established ODA: Isoleucine: 900 mg/day Leucine: 1200 mg/day Valine: 1050 mg/day	• Assist in building muscle and lean body mass	• Serve as a direct source of energy for skeletal muscles • Promote protein synthesis in muscle and they regulate protein metabolism throughout the body • Reportedly play a role in helping to regulate insulin secretion • Decrease the rate of protein catabolism under stressful conditions	Protein foods from animals including meats, cheeses, and eggs	• Human deficiencies are rare • Severe valine deficiency is reported to cause neurological defects in the brain • Isoleucine deficiency may cause muscle tremors • There are no reports of leucine deficiencies	• No known toxicity or serious side effects; however, ingesting large doses of BCAAs may result in a decline of brain levels of serotonin and dopamine
Calcium	RDI: 1000 mg/day ODA: 1000-1500 mg/day	• Blood pressure regulation • Cancer prevention • Elevated cholesterol • Hypertension • Kidney stones • Osteoporosis • PMS • Pregnancy	• Plays a role in bone and tooth formation • Involved in blood clotting, heart rhythm • Plays a role in nerve transmission • Involved in muscle growth and contraction • Supports proper functioning of cell membranes	Collards, turnip greens, broccoli, kale, yogurt, milk and dairy products, tempeh, tofu, salmon with bones, sardines	• Muscle cramps • Irritability • Insomnia • Osteoporosis • Hypertension • Tetany • Poor growth in children	**Toxic Dose:** • Large doses normally show no toxic effects **Toxicity Symptoms:** • With parathyroid imbalances, magnesium deficiency, or vitamin D overdoses, calcium can result in soft tissue calcification • Some calcium supplements may contain lead, check for manufacturers who certify low lead levels

VITAMINS / MINERALS / TRACE ELEMENTS / AMINO ACIDS *(Continued)*

Vitamins/ Minerals/Trace Elements/Amino Acids	RDI / ODA*	Reported Uses	Functions in the Body	Food Sources	Deficiency Symptoms	Toxic Dose/ Toxicity Symptoms
L-Carnitine	RDI: None established ODA: 500–2000 mg/day in divided doses	• Congestive heart failure • Enhances athletic performance • Lowers elevated cholesterol and triglycerides • Male infertility • Weight loss	• Supports heart function (affects the production of energy in muscle tissue) • Regulates fat metabolism by facilitating the transport of fats across cell membranes into the mitochondria for energy production • Helps the body oxidize amino acids to produce energy when necessary • Helps metabolize ketones • Increases energy and endurance • Increases the oxidation of fats	Meat, nuts, eggs, milk, cheeses	• Deficiencies are rare because the body produces carnitine relatively easily • Symptoms include elevated blood lipids, abnormal liver function, muscle weakness, reduced energy, and impaired glucose control	• No known toxicity or serious side effects
Chromium	RDI: None established ODA: 200–600 mcg/day	• Atherosclerosis • Elevated cholesterol • Elevated triglycerides • Glaucoma • Hypoglycemia • Type 1 diabetes • Type 2 diabetes • Weight loss	• A component of glucose tolerance factor, which reportedly enhances the blood sugar lowering effects of insulin by facilitating the uptake of glucose into cells • May help insulin bind to its receptors, thereby increasing the activity of insulin and reducing the amount of insulin required to control blood sugar • Influences the metabolism of carbohydrates and fats	Brewer's yeast, liver, cheese, legumes, peas, whole grains, black pepper, molasses	• Blood sugar fluctuations • High cholesterol and triglyceride levels • Glucose intolerance	**Toxicity Symptoms:** • Excess intake can result in tissue accumulation and can inhibit rather than enhance insulin activity • Extreme excesses may be carcinogenic

Vitamins/ Minerals/Trace Elements/Amino Acids	RDI / ODA*	Reported Uses	Functions in the Body	Food Sources	Deficiency Symptoms	Toxic Dose/ Toxicity Symptoms
Copper	RDI: 2 mg/day ODA: 2-3 mg/day	• Anemia • Osteoporosis • Rheumatoid arthritis	• Plays a role in bone and collagen formation, nerve tissue, prostaglandins, hair and skin color, healing processes, red blood cell production • Plays a role in mental and emotional processes • Component of superoxide dismutase and other antioxidant enzymes	Shellfish, liver, poultry, cherries, nuts, cocoa, gelatin, whole grains, eggs, legumes, peas, avocados, dark green leafy vegetables	• Anemia • Inflammation • Arthritis • Low white blood cells • Fragile connective tissue • Cardiovascular damage • Bone demineralization • Diminished pigmentation	Toxicity Symptoms: • Hemolytic anemia, hemoglobinuria, jaundice, nausea, vomiting, epigastric pain, headache, dizziness, weakness, diarrhea, hemochromatosis
Folic Acid	RDI: 400 mcg/day ODA: 400-1000 mcg/day	• Alcoholism • Anemia • Atherosclerosis • Birth defects • Crohn's disease • Depression • Gingivitis • Osteoporosis • Pregnancy and lactation • Prevention of cervical dysplasia, colon and breast cancer	• Involved in growth, development, and reproduction • Involved in the production of red blood cells • Supports healthy functioning of the nervous system • Supports hair and skin	Liver, salmon, eggs, asparagus, green leafy vegetables, broccoli, sweet potatoes, beans, whole wheat	• Anemia • Heartburn • Fatigue • Diarrhea • Constipation • Depression • Frequent infections • Mental confusion	Toxic Symptoms: • Large doses can mask symptoms of B_{12} deficiency

VITAMINS / MINERALS /
TRACE ELEMENTS / AMINO ACIDS (Continued)

Vitamins/ Minerals/Trace Elements/Amino Acids	RDI / ODA*	Reported Uses	Functions In the Body	Food Sources	Deficiency Symptoms	Toxic Dose/ Toxicity Symptoms
L-Glutamine	RDI: None established ODA: 500-4000 mg 3 times/day	• Adjunct therapy for HIV and cancer • Alcoholism • Catabolic; wasting processes • Immunosupportive • Peptic ulcers • Performance enhancement • Postsurgical healing • Ulcerative colitis and other forms of inflammatory bowel disease	• Source of energy for cells of the GI tract • Promotes protein synthesis and muscle growth • Alternative brain fuel • Blocks cortisol-induced protein catabolism • May be conditionally essential in GI disorders and tissue-wasting phenomena	Yogurt, granola, meats, nuts, eggs, milk, cheeses	• Deficiency studies in humans have not been conducted	• No known toxicity or serious side effects
Iodine	RDI: 150 mcg/day ODA: 250 mcg/day	• Fibrocystic breast disease • Goiter prevention • Mucolytic agent	• Structural component of thyroid hormone • Regulation of cellular oxidation	Iodized salt, seafood, saltwater shellfish, kelp	• Goiter • Cretinism	Toxic Dose: • Iodine toxicity is rare except in cases of existing hyperthyroidism where doses as small as 1 mg can result in cessation of thyroid hormone production and thyrotoxicosis Toxicity Symptoms: • Rashes, nausea, headaches • Extensive long-term intake can result in thyroid goiter

Vitamins/ Minerals/Trace Elements/Amino Acids	RDI / ODA*	Reported Uses	Functions in the Body	Food Sources	Deficiency Symptoms	Toxic Dose/ Toxicity Symptoms
Iron	RDI: Males and Post-menopausal females: 10 mg/day Premenopausal females 15 mg/day ODA: Specific for each individual	• Anemia • Menorrhagia • Pregnancy • Restless leg syndrome	• Supports growth and development in children • Involved in the production of hemoglobin • Helps build resistance to disease • Necessary for energy production	Blackstrap molasses, liver, lean beef, eggs, fish, spinach, asparagus, prunes, raisins, sea vegetables, oysters, sardines, lima beans, legumes, dark green leafy vegetables	• Fatigue • Anemia • Intolerance to cold • Intellectual impairment • Reduced resistance to colds and infections • Spoon shaped nails • Pica	**Toxicity Symptoms:** • Early signs of toxicity: Bloody diarrhea, severe nausea, abdominal pain, vomiting with blood • Late signs of toxicity: Weakness, collapse, pallor, blue lips, blue hands, blue fingernails, shallow breathing, convulsions, coma, weak, rapid heartbeat • Iron is the most common cause of pediatric poisonings. Iron-containing products must be packaged in child-resistant safety packaging.
L-Lysine	RDI: None established ODA: 500-1000 mg/day	• Angina pectoris • Herpes simplex • Osteoporosis	• Essential amino acid involved in synthesis of connective tissue, neurotransmitters, and carbohydrate metabolism	Yogurt, granola, meats, nuts, eggs, milk, cheeses	• Human deficiency has not been defined	**Toxicity Symptoms:** • Rare association with interstitial nephritis • No known toxicity or serious side effects at normal doses

609

VITAMINS / MINERALS / TRACE ELEMENTS / AMINO ACIDS (Continued)

Vitamins/ Minerals/Trace Elements/Amino Acids	RDI / ODA*	Reported Uses	Functions in the Body	Food Sources	Deficiency Symptoms	Toxic Dose/ Toxicity Symptoms
Magnesium	RDI: 400 mg/day ODA: 400–800 mg/day	• ADD/ADHD • Asthma • Cardiovascular disease • Congestive heart failure • Diabetes • Epilepsy • Fatigue • High blood pressure • Kidney stones • Migraine headaches • Mitral valve prolapse • Muscle cramps • Nervousness • Osteoporosis • PMS	• Required for the metabolism of carbohydrates and proteins • Necessary for muscle contraction-relaxation and the conduction of nerve impulses • Essential for the production and transfer of energy and for protein and lipid synthesis • Decreases platelet stickiness, helps thin the blood, blocks calcium uptake, and relaxes blood vessels • Involved in calcium metabolism, synthesis of vitamin D, and the integrity of skeletal bone-crystal formation • Helps bind calcium to tooth enamel, creating an effective barrier to tooth decay	Soybeans, whole grains, shellfish, salmon, liver, almonds, cashews, molasses, bananas, potatoes, milk, green vegetables, honey, cocoa	• Muscle cramps and weakness • Insomnia • Loss of appetite and gastrointestinal disorders • Kidney stones • Osteoporosis • Cardiac problems • Personality changes, nervousness, fear restlessness, anxiety, irritability, confusion, depression	• Generally not toxic in healthy adults • Patients with kidney disease should consult their physician before using magnesium supplements, antacids, or laxatives **Toxicity Symptoms:** • Doses over 1000 mg can cause diarrhea, drowsiness, weakness, lethargy

Vitamins/ Minerals/Trace Elements/Amino Acids	RDI / ODA*	Reported Uses	Functions in the Body	Food Sources	Deficiency Symptoms	Toxic Dose/ Toxicity Symptoms
Manganese	**RDI:** None established **ODA:** None established	• Diabetes • Epilepsy • Osteoporosis	• Participates in formation of connective tissue, fats, cholesterol, bones, blood clotting factors, proteins, and glucose transport • Functions as an antioxidant cofactor for enzymes • Component of mitochondrial superoxide dismutase (SOD) • Needed for protein digestion and synthesis of mucopolysaccharides • May be useful as part of therapy for osteoporosis	Green leafy vegetables, nuts, whole grains, wheat bran, wheat germ	• Seldom deficient in humans	• Toxicity is rare • Industrial exposure can be toxic **Toxicity Symptoms:** • Excessive doses can cause nausea • Long-term toxicity can produce dementia, psychiatric disorders resembling schizo-phrenia, and neurologic disorders resembling Parkinson's disease

VITAMINS / MINERALS / TRACE ELEMENTS / AMINO ACIDS (Continued)

Vitamins/Minerals/Trace Elements/Amino Acids	RDI / ODA*	Reported Uses	Functions in the Body	Food Sources	Deficiency Symptoms	Toxic Dose/Toxicity Symptoms
L-Methionine	**RDI:** None established **ODA:** 500-3000 mg/day	• Liver detoxification	• Precursor for the synthesis of cysteine, cysteine, and taurine • Enzymatically converted into S-adenosyl methionine (SAMe) or 'active methionine,' which participates in many biochemical reactions • Involved in the detoxification of organochlorines and many other toxic substances in the liver • Precursor for the synthesis of glutathione, which plays a role in maintaining proper levels of the antioxidant enzyme glutathione peroxidase • Helps metabolize homocysteine • One of three amino acids needed by the body to manufacture creatine monohydrate, which is essential for energy production and muscle building	Tuna, salmon, wild game, cheeses, meats, fowl, eggs, milk, nuts, chocolate	• Symptoms of deficiency include hair loss, poor skin tone, toxic elevation of metabolic waste products, and liver malfunction	• Supplementation without adequate intake of folic acid, vitamin B$_6$, and vitamin B$_{12}$ can increase the conversion of methionine to homocysteine and increase risk for cardiovascular disease **Toxic Dose:** • Toxicity is rare (generally only observed in excessive dosages) • Extremely high doses may increase urinary excretion of calcium and induce hallucinations **Toxicity Symptoms:** • May include ataxia, hyperactivity, hemosiderosis, reduced growth, loss of appetite, suppressed hematocrit

Vitamins/Trace Minerals/Amino Acids	RDI / ODA*	Reported Uses	Functions in the Body	Food Sources	Deficiency Symptoms	Toxic Dose/ Toxicity Symptoms
L-Phenylalanine D-Phenylalanine	RDI: None established ODA: 1500 mg/day	• Addiction (reward deficiency syndrome) • Depression • Pain relief • Vitiligo	• Precursor for tyrosine, epinephrine, norepinephrine, dopamine, thyroxine, and melanin • Influences the synthesis of many important brain neuropeptides including vasopressin, ACTH, somatostatin, enkephalin, angiotensin II, and cholecystokinin • Converted to phenyl-ethylamine, a chemical that occurs naturally in the brain and appears to elevate mood • Inhibits the breakdown and extends the activity of enkephalins and endorphins, which are the body's natural analgesics • Stimulates the release in the stomach of cholecystokinin (CCK), a hormone that seems to induce a feeling of fullness that may reduce the desire for food	Meats, fowl, wild game, ricotta and cottage cheese, wheat germ	• Deficiency rarely occurs in humans • Symptoms include behavioral changes, eye disorders, poor vascular health, increase in appetite, and weight gain	• Hyperactive children and individuals that suffer from migraine headaches have been found to have elevated plasma phenylalanine • Phenylketonuria (PKU) a genetic abnormality causing toxicity from elevated phenylalanine results in severe mental retardation • Ingestion of the artificial sweetener aspartame causes a rapid increase in brain levels of phenylalanine

613

VITAMINS / MINERALS / TRACE ELEMENTS / AMINO ACIDS *(Continued)*

Vitamins/Minerals/Trace Elements/Amino Acids	RDI / ODA*	Reported Uses	Functions in the Body	Food Sources	Deficiency Symptoms	Toxic Dose/Toxicity Symptoms
Phosphorus	RDI: None established ODA: 800-1200 mg/day	• No reported therapeutic uses	• Involved in bone and tooth formation • Plays a role in cell growth and repair • Assists in energy maintenance • Involved in heart contraction • Supports kidney function • Involved in the healthy activity of nerves and muscles • Involved in the body's use of vitamins • Component of cell membranes	Fish, poultry, eggs, whole grains, legumes, nuts, milk and dairy products	• Deficiency is uncommon • Muscle cramps • Dizziness • Bone problems • Anorexia • Weakness • Stiff joints • Fragile bones	Toxic Dose: • Over-consumption is possible on the typical American diet that is high in meats, dairy products, soda pop Toxicity Symptoms: • This diet may influence calcium absorption and utilization
Potassium	RDI: None established ODA: None established Experts recommend keeping potassium intake to under 3500 mg/day	• Cardiac arrhythmias • Congestive heart failure • Hypertension • Kidney stones	• Involved in healthy, steady functioning of the nervous system • Supports the heart, muscles, kidneys, blood • Involved in acid-base balance • Important for fluid balance	Dried apricots, cantaloupe, bananas, citrus fruit, lima beans, potatoes, avocados, broccoli, liver, milk, peanut butter	• Muscle fatigue • General fatigue • Swelling in extremities • Confusion • Irregular heart beat	Toxic Dose: • If potassium excretion is impaired and potassium chloride or potassium tablets are taken in high dosages, blood levels of potassium can become dangerously high • Use with extreme caution in individuals with renal disease Toxicity Symptoms: • High blood levels of potassium may cause muscular weakness, vomiting, and cardiac disturbances

Vitamins/Trace Elements/Amino Acids	RDI / ODA*	Reported Uses	Functions in the Body	Food Sources	Deficiency Symptoms	Toxic Dose/ Toxicity Symptoms
Selenium	**RDI:** Males: 70 mcg/day Females: 55 mcg/day ODA: 200 mcg/day	• AIDS • Atherosclerosis • Bronchial asthma • Cancer prevention • Cardiomyopathy • Cataracts • Chemotherapy / Radiation support • Eczema	• Cofactor in glutathione peroxidase • Detoxification of heavy metals • Part of glutathione peroxidase • Part of the deiodinase enzyme that converts thyroxine (T_4) to triiodothyronine (T_3) • Potentiates vitamin E • Reported to have antiviral activity, increase T lymphocytes and enhance natural killer cell activity	Whole grains, soybeans, tuna, seafood, Brazil nuts, brown rice, lean meat, pineapples, chicken	• Sore muscles • Increased red blood cell fragility • Destructive changes to the heart and pancreas • Weakens the immune system	**Toxic Dose:** • Can be toxic • Intake should be restricted to no more than 700 mcg/day unless supervised by a physician **Toxicity Symptoms:** • Loss of hair and nails, skin lesions, nervous system abnormalities, digestive dysfunction and a garlic-like breath odor • Although deaths from toxicity have been reported in livestock, no deaths have occurred in humans
Sodium	**RDI:** None established **ODA:** None established Experts recommend keeping sodium intake to under 3000 mg/day	• No reported therapeutic uses	• Helps maintain normal fluid levels in the body • Involved in healthy muscle functioning • Supports blood and lymph system • Needed for nerve impulse transmission	Most foods, especially salted foods, soy sauce, cheese, milk, seafood, water	• Deficiency is uncommon and usually induced by excessive vomiting, diarrhea, or profuse sweating • Fainting • Intolerance to heat • Muscle cramps • Swelling in extremities	**Toxicity Symptoms:** • Excess sodium intake is associated with high blood pressure and edema

VITAMINS / MINERALS /
TRACE ELEMENTS / AMINO ACIDS (Continued)

Vitamins/ Minerals/Trace Elements/Amino Acids	RDI / ODA*	Reported Uses	Functions in the Body	Food Sources	Deficiency Symptoms	Toxic Dose/ Toxicity Symptoms
L-Taurine	RDI: None established ODA: 1500-3000 mg/day	• Congestive heart failure • Diabetes • Epilepsy • Hypertension	• As an amino acid (protein-building block) • Inhibitory neurotransmitter that helps to stabilize nerve cell membranes • As a component of bile acids to help regulate the absorption of fats and fat-soluble vitamins • Regulates the volume of fluid in cells, especially in the kidneys and central nervous system • Helps regulate the contraction and pumping action of the heart muscle and may provide a cardio-protective effect • Protects the photoreceptors in the retina of the eye from damage	Meats, fish, organ meats (especially brains)	• In preterm and term infants, taurine insufficiency results in impaired fat absorption, bile acid secretion, vision disturbances, and liver malfunction, all of which can be reversed by taurine supplementation	• No known toxicity or serious side effects
L-Tyrosine	RDI: None established ODA: 1000-5000 mg/day	• Alzheimer's disease • Depression • Hypothyroidism • Phenylketonuria (PKU) • Substance abuse	• Precursor for dopamine, norepinephrine, epinephrine, and cholecystokinin (CCK) • Necessary for synthesis of melanin and thyroid hormones	Pork, fowl, wild game, ricotta and cottage cheese, wheat germ	• Depression and emotional disturbances • Underactive thyroid and disturbed metabolism	• No known toxicity or serious side effects • Not to be taken by individuals on MAO-inhibiting antidepressants

Vitamins/Trace Elements/Amino Acids	RDI / ODA*	Reported Uses	Functions in the Body	Food Sources	Deficiency Symptoms	Toxic Dose/ Toxicity Symptoms
Vanadium (as **Vanadium Pentoxide** or **Vanadyl Sulfate**)	**RDI:** None established **ODA:** 250 mcg 1-3 times/ day	• Type 1 diabetes • Type 2 diabetes	• Functions as a cofactor, which enhances or inhibits various enzymes • Stimulates glucose metabolism and improves glucose control • Reported to be involved in nicotinamide adenine dinucleotide phosphate (NADPH) oxidation reactions, lipoprotein lipase activity, amino acid transport, and the growth of red blood cells • At higher dosage levels, reported to assist in lowering elevated serum cholesterol and triglyceride levels • Promotes tissue anabolism	Fats, vegetable oils, grains, meats, fish, nuts, dill seeds, parsley, black pepper, mushrooms	• Deficiency studies in humans have not been conducted	• No dietary toxicity or serious side effects have been reported • Industrial exposure has resulted in toxicity • Caution for diabetics (may increase the need to regulate blood sugar)

VITAMINS / MINERALS /
TRACE ELEMENTS / AMINO ACIDS (Continued)

Vitamins/ Minerals/Trace Elements/Amino Acids	RDI / ODA*	Reported Uses	Functions in the Body	Food Sources	Deficiency Symptoms	Toxic Dose/ Toxicity Symptoms
Vitamin A (Retinol)	**RDI:** Males: 5000 int. units/day Females: 4000 int. units/day **ODA:** 5000 int. units/day (unless pregnant or planning pregnancy)	• Acne • AIDS • Cancer prevention • Cervical dysplasia • Crohn's disease • Measles • Menorrhagia • Night blindness • PMS • Ulcerative colitis	• Strengthens mucous membranes, the immune system, adrenal glands, eyes, skin • Needed for bone and tooth growth • Needed for hormone synthesis and regulation, reproduction • Antioxidant • Cancer protection	• Liver, fish liver oil, vitamin A-fortified milk, butter, egg yolks, cheese	• Night blindness • Eye problems • Increased susceptibility to infections • Faulty tooth and bone formation • Reduced steroid synthesis	**Toxic Dose:** • Doses >60,000 int. units/day have resulted in toxicity • Pregnant women should not exceed 4000 int. units/day due to risk of birth defects **Toxicity Symptoms:** • Headache, nausea, vomiting, fatigue, weakness, anorexia, weight loss, nosebleeds, blurred vision, bone pain, joint pain, dry skin, rashes, hair loss, amenorrhea, liver and spleen enlargement, transient hydrocephalus, stunted growth
Vitamin B-Complex	• See individual B-vitamins	• See individual B-vitamins	• Broad range of support for a wide range of biological activities involving the B vitamins	• Brewer's yeast, organ meats, fish, eggs, milk, nuts, vegetables, whole grains	• A deficiency of the B-complex vitamins would result in numerous health problems	**Toxic Dose:** • None known **Toxicity Symptoms:** • Side effects could result from high doses of vitamin B_3 and vitamin B_6
Vitamin B₁ (Thiamin)	**RDI:** 1.5 mg/day **ODA:** 5-10 mg/day	• Alcoholism • Alzheimer's disease • Anemia • Congestive heart failure • Diabetes • Insomnia • Neurological conditions • Psychiatric patients	• Supports healthy functioning of the heart, muscles, and nerves • Plays a role in the breakdown of carbohydrates for energy • Helps maintain normal enzyme function	• Brewer's yeast, kidney, liver, wheat germ, peas, peanuts, whole grains, nuts, rice bran, brown rice	• Fatigue • Memory loss • Irritability • Depression • Loss of reflexes • Wasting • Weakness • Edema • Abnormal heart rhythm • Enlarged heart • Heart failure	• No known toxic effects from oral intake

618

Vitamins/Minerals/Trace Elements/Amino Acids	RDI / ODA*	Reported Uses	Functions in the Body	Food Sources	Deficiency Symptoms	Toxic Dose/Toxicity Symptoms
Vitamin B₂ (Riboflavin)	RDI: 1.7 mg/day ODA: 5-10 mg/day	• Cataracts • Depression • Migraines	• Plays a role in the breakdown and use of carbohydrates, fats, and proteins • Involved in cell energy production • Supports the production of adrenal hormones • Helps the body utilize other vitamins • Supports the eyes	Brewer's yeast, kidney, liver, heart, milk, broccoli, Brussels sprouts, asparagus, green leafy vegetables, wheat germ, almonds, cottage cheese, yogurt, eggs, tuna, salmon	• Light-sensitivity • Reddening of the eyes • Skin rash • Depression • Cracks at the corners of the mouth • Deep red tongue	• No known toxicity
Vitamin B₃ (Niacin) (Niacinamide) (Inositol-Hexaniacinate) [non-flushing niacin]	RDI: 20 mg/day ODA: 25-100 mg/day Inositol Hexaniacinate: RDI: None established ODA: 600 mg/day	• Acne vulgaris (4% niacinamide topical gel) • Cataracts • Cholesterol (elevated) • Circulation • Diabetes - Type 1 (recent onset) • Diabetes - Type 2 • Elevated triglycerides • Glucose intolerance • Heart attack prevention • Intermittent claudication • Osteoarthritis • Raynaud's disease • Rheumatoid arthritis • Schizophrenia	• Involved in the breakdown of carbohydrates and fats • Supports healthy functioning of the nervous and digestive systems • Involved in the production of sex hormones • Helps maintain healthy skin	Brewer's yeast, liver, poultry, fish, peanuts, eggs, milk, whole grains Inositol hexaniacinate: Does not occur naturally in nature	Niacin/Niacinamide • Fatigue • Irritability • Insomnia • Emotional stability • Blood sugar fluctuations • Arthritis • Diarrhea • Black smooth tongue • Mental confusion Inositol hexaniacinate: There are no known deficiency symptoms associated with inositol hexaniacinate	Toxic Dose: • Niacin/Niacinamide: 300-600 mg; doses greater than 2.5 g/day can cause liver damage and glucose intolerance • Inositol hexaniacinate: No known toxicity Toxicity Symptoms: • Headache, nausea, skin flushing and tingling, sweating

VITAMINS / MINERALS / TRACE ELEMENTS / AMINO ACIDS *(Continued)*

Vitamins/ Minerals/Trace Elements/Amino Acids	RDI / ODA*	Reported Uses	Functions in the Body	Food Sources	Deficiency Symptoms	Toxic Dose/ Toxicity Symptoms
Vitamin B₅ (Pantothenic Acid)	**RDI:** 10 mg/day **ODA:** 10–50 mg/day	• Adrenal support • Allergies • Arthritis • Constipation • Hyperlipidemia (pantethine, but not pantothenic acid, lowers cholesterol and triglycerides) • Surgery and wound healing	• Involved in the breakdown and use of carbohydrates and fats • Supports normal growth and development • Involved in the production of adrenal and sex hormones • Helps the body use other vitamins • Supports the sinuses	Liver, kidney, heart, fish, egg yolks, cheese, bran, whole grain cereals, sweet cauliflower, sweet potatoes, beans, nuts, brewer's yeast	• None known for vitamin B₅ alone, but deficiency of any B vitamin usually means deficiency of others	• Generally safe at high doses
Vitamin B₆ (Pyridoxine)	**RDI:** 2 mg/day **ODA:** 10–20 mg/day	• Arthritis • Asthma • Autism • Cardiovascular disease • Carpal tunnel syndrome • Depression • Diabetes • Epilepsy (B₆-dependent) • Kidney stones • MSG sensitivity • Nausea and vomiting in pregnancy • Peptic ulcer • PMS	• Involved in the breakdown of proteins, carbohydrates, and fats • Involved in healthy functioning of the nervous and digestive systems • Involved in the production of red blood cells and antibodies • Helps maintain healthy skin	Soybeans, liver, kidney, poultry, tuna, fish, bananas, legumes, potatoes, oatmeal, wheat germ	• Premenstrual tension • Anemia • Irritability • Depression • Nausea • Vomiting • Depressed immunity • Kidney stones • Smooth tongue	**Toxic Dose:** • 250–1000 mg/day **Toxicity Symptoms:** • Prolonged excesses can cause reversible nerve damage

Vitamins/Trace Elements/Amino Acids	RDI / ODA*	Reported Uses	Functions in the Body	Food Sources	Deficiency Symptoms	Toxic Dose/ Toxicity Symptoms
Vitamin B₁₂ (Cobalamin)	RDI: 4 mcg/day ODA: 10–500 mcg/day	• AIDS • Atherosclerosis • Bronchial asthma • Crohn's disease • Depression • Diabetes. • Male infertility • Memory loss • Multiple sclerosis • Pernicious anemia • Sulfite sensitivity	• Involved in growth and development • Involved in production of red blood cells • Helps the body use folic acid • Supports healthy functioning of the nervous system	Liver, oysters, poultry, fish, clams, eggs, dairy products	• Megaloblastic anemia • Irritability • Loss of coordination • Fatigue • Insomnia • Hypersensitivity • Sprue	• No known toxicity
Vitamin C	RDI: 60 mg/day ODA: 250–1000 mg/day	• AIDS • Allergies • Asthma • Atherosclerosis • Cancer • Cataracts • Cervical dysplasia • Crohn's disease • Diabetes • Elevated cholesterol • Gingivitis • Immunity • Parkinson's disease • Peptic ulcer • Sunburn • Wound healing	• Plays a major role in collagen formation, which is important for healthy intervertebral discs, teeth, bones, gums, ligaments, and blood vessels • Involved in the production of neurotransmitters and adrenal gland hormones • Plays an important role in immune response to infection and in supporting wound healing • Helps in absorption of iron from the digestive tract	Rose hips, sweet peppers, broccoli, cauliflower, kale, asparagus, spinach, tomatoes, lemons, strawberries, papayas, cantaloupe, oranges, grapefruit, kiwis, liver	• Slow wound healing • Bleeding gums • Recurrent infections • Allergies • Atherosclerotic plaques • Bone fragility • Joint pain • Anemia	Toxic Dose: • Excesses are excreted in urine, therefore risk for toxicity is small • Some research shows no toxic effects in doses up to 10,000 mg • When doses >1000 mg/day are consumed regularly, kidney stone formation can occur in patients with existing kidney disease Toxicity Symptoms: • Most common side effect of large doses is diarrhea • Excess intake in diabetics may give false high blood glucose readings

VITAMINS / MINERALS / TRACE ELEMENTS / AMINO ACIDS *(Continued)*

Vitamins/ Minerals/Trace Elements/Amino Acids	RDI / ODA*	Reported Uses	Functions in the Body	Food Sources	Deficiency Symptoms	Toxic Dose/ Toxicity Symptoms
Vitamin D	RDI: 400 int. units/day ODA: 400 int. units/day	• Crohn's disease • Epilepsy • Hearing Loss • Osteoporosis • Psoriasis • Rickets • Scleroderma	• Supports bone and tooth formation and muscle function • Necessary for proper absorption of calcium, phosphorus, magnesium, and zinc • Supports healthy functioning of the thyroid gland	Fish liver oil, fortified milk, salmon, herring, sardines, liver, butter, eggs, sunshine is the best source	• Bone and tooth problems • Rickets • Osteomalacia	**Toxic Dose:** • Because vitamin D is potentially toxic, it is generally recommended to avoid doses >1000 int. units/day. However, some reports indicate that most cases of toxicity involve the intake of 25,000-60,000 int. units/day for 1-4 months • Adults should consume no more than 3 times the RDA for prolonged periods of time **Toxicity Symptoms:** • Excessive thirst, loss of appetite, nausea, vomiting, headache, constipation, weakness, weight loss, raised blood calcium, kidney stones, calcium deposits in arteries

Vitamins/ Minerals/Trace Elements/Amino Acids	RDI / ODA*	Reported Uses	Functions in the Body	Food Sources	Deficiency Symptoms	Toxic Dose/ Toxicity Symptoms
Vitamin E	**RDI:** Males: 10 int. units/day Females: 8 int. units/day **ODA:** 400 int. units/day	• Alzheimer's disease • Atherosclerosis • Benign prostatic hypertrophy (BPH) • Cataracts • Cancer • Cervical dysplasia • Diabetes • Dyslipidemia • Heart attacks • Increases immune function • Lupus • Osteoarthritis • Peptic ulcer • Peripheral circulation • PMS • Rheumatoid arthritis • Sunburn	• Aids in tissue healing • Essential for normal cell structure • Helps maintain normal enzyme function • Involved in the formation of red blood cells • Believed to slow aging of cells • Helps protect tissues from damage by pollutants	Wheat germ oil, wheat germ, egg yolks, butter, most vegetable oils, liver, nuts, whole wheat flour, green leafy vegetables	• Dry skin • Dull dry hair • PMS • Hot flashes • Eczema • Psoriasis • Cataracts • Poor wound healing	• Relatively nontoxic • Caution when taking anti-coagulants; vitamin E can increase blood thinning

VITAMINS / MINERALS / TRACE ELEMENTS / AMINO ACIDS *(Continued)*

Vitamins/ Minerals/Trace Elements/Amino Acids	RDI / ODA*	Reported Uses	Functions in the Body	Food Sources	Deficiency Symptoms	Toxic Dose/ Toxicity Symptoms
Vitamin K	**RDI:** None established **ODA:** Males: 65 mcg/day Females: 55 mcg/day	• Blood clotting • Osteoporosis	• Essential for blood-clotting • Necessary for bone formation	Liver, dark green leafy vegetables, cabbage-type vegetables	• Blood clotting difficulty • Hemorrhaging	**Toxic Dose:** • Large doses of Vitamin K₃ (the synthetic form) can cause hemolytic anemia in animals and jaundice in infants • Vitamin K, derived from alfalfa leaves has a wider range of safety
Zinc	**RDI:** 15 mg/day **ODA:** 15-35 mg/day **Topical:** Apply to affected area as needed	• Acne • Aphthous ulcers • Athlete's foot • Benign prostatic hypertrophy (BPH) • Common cold • Crohn's disease • Diabetes • Diaper rash • Immune function • Macular degeneration • Male sexual vitality • Osteoporosis • Skin conditions • Ulcers • Wound healing	• Needed for protein production • Promotes burn and wound healing • Supports the immune system • Involved in carbohydrate and protein digestion • Needed for sperm production, normal fetal growth and development • Needed for proper functioning of insulin • Involved in many enzymes • Needed for vitamin A transport	Brewer's yeast, liver, seafood, wheat germ, bran, oatmeal, nuts, peas, carrots, spinach, sunflower seeds	• White spots on fingernails • Stretch marks on skin • Loss of sense of smell or taste • Joint pain • Poor sexual development • Slowed growth • Menstrual irregularities • Slow wound healing • Recurrent infections • Acne • Sterility	**Toxic Dose:** • Some individuals may experience toxic effects from zinc with prolonged intake at levels >150 mg/day **Toxicity Symptoms:** • Nausea, vomiting, diarrhea, dizziness, anemia, can interfere with copper absorption, impair immune response, and lower HDL

RDI: Recommended Dietary Intake
ODA: Optimum Daily Allowance

DRUG-INDUCED NUTRIENT DEPLETIONS

PRESCRIPTION AND NONPRESCRIPTION PRODUCTS

Drug	Brand Names	Nutrient Depletions	Potential Depletion Problems
ANTACIDS			
Magnesium and Aluminum Antacids			
Aluminum Hydroxide, Magnesium Hydroxide, Magnesium Oxide, Magnesium Sulfate, Aluminum Hydroxide and Magnesium Hydroxide, Aluminum Hydroxide and Magnesium Carbonate, Aluminum Hydroxide and Magnesium Trisilicate, Aluminum Hydroxide, Magnesium Hydroxide, and Simethicone	Various products	Calcium on page 400, Phosphorus on page 489	See individual nutrient monographs
Sodium Bicarbonate	Various products	Potassium on page 490	See individual nutrient monographs
ANTIBIOTICS			
General Antibiotics			
Penicillins, Cephalosporins, Fluoroquinolones, Macrolides, Aminoglycosides, Sulfonamides	Various products	Lactobacillus acidophilus on page 467, Bifidobacteria bifidum (bifidus) on page 391, Vitamin B₁ on page 519, Vitamin B₂ on page 520, Vitamin B₃ on page 521, Vitamin B₆ on page 523, Vitamin B₁₂ on page 524, Biotin on page 393, Inositol on page 521, Vitamin K on page 531	Short-term nutrient depletion effects are minimal; however, alteration of gut microflora can allow dysbiosis to develop, which can further inhibit the digestion and absorption of nutrients and cause a weakening of the immune system.
Penicillins	Various products	Potassium on page 490	Irregular heartbeat, muscle weakness, fatigue, edema

DRUG-INDUCED NUTRIENT DEPLETIONS *(Continued)*

PRESCRIPTION AND NONPRESCRIPTION PRODUCTS *(continued)*

Drug	Brand Names	Nutrient Depletions	Potential Depletion Problems
Tetracyclines	Achromycin®; Sumycin®; Topicycline®; Various products	Calcium on page 400	Osteoporosis, heart/blood pressure irregularities, tooth decay
		Magnesium on page 473	Cardiovascular problems, asthma, osteoporosis, cramps, PMS
		Iron on page 464	Anemia, weakness, fatigue, hair loss, brittle nails
		Bifidobacteria bifidum (bifidus) on page 391, Lactobacillus acidophilus on page 467, Vitamin B₁ on page 519, Vitamin B₂ on page 520, Vitamin B₃ on page 521, Vitamin B₆ on page 523, Vitamin B₁₂ on page 524, Vitamin K on page 531, Biotin on page 393, Inositol on page 521	Short-term depletion effects are minimal
Aminoglycosides			
Neomycin	Mycifradin®; Neofradin®; Neo-Tabs®	Beta-Carotene on page 390, Iron on page 464, Vitamin A on page 518, Vitamin B₁₂ on page 524, Calcium on page 400, Magnesium on page 473, Potassium on page 490	Minimal problems with short-term use
Sulfonamides			
Co-Trimoxazole	Bactrim®, Cotrim®; Septra®; Sulfatrim®	Bifidobacteria bifidum (bifidus) on page 391, Folic Acid on page 435, Lactobacillus acidophilus on page 467	
Pentamidine	NebuPent™; Pentacarinat®; Pentam-300®	Magnesium on page 473	Cardiovascular problems, asthma, osteoporosis, cramps, PMS
Tuberculosis Drugs			
Isoniazid, INH	Laniazid®; Nydrazid®	Vitamin B₆ on page 523	Anemia, tiredness, weakness, increased cardiovascular disease risk
		Vitamin B₃ on page 521	Skin, gastrointestinal, nervous system problems
		Vitamin D on page 528	Osteoporosis, muscle weakness, hearing loss

626

PRESCRIPTION AND NONPRESCRIPTION PRODUCTS (continued)

Drug	Brand Names	Nutrient Depletions	Potential Depletion Problems
Rifampin	Rifadin®, Rimactane®	Vitamin D on page 528	Osteoporosis, muscle weakness, hearing loss
Ethambutol	Myambutol®	Zinc on page 534	Slow wound healing, loss of sense of smell and taste, lower immunity
		Copper on page 416	Anemia, fatigue, cardiovascular and connective tissue problems
ANTICONVULSANTS			
Barbiturates	Amytal®, Tuinal®, Butalan®, Buticaps®, Butisol Sodium®, Mebaral®, Brevital® Barbita®, Nembutal®, Luminal®, Solfoton®, Seconal™, Pentothal®	Vitamin D on page 528	Osteoporosis, muscle weakness, hearing loss
		Calcium on page 400	Osteoporosis, heart/blood pressure irregularities, tooth decay
		Folic Acid on page 435	Birth defects, cervical dysplasia, anemia, cardiovascular disease
		Vitamin K on page 531	Blood clotting and skeletal problems
		Biotin on page 393	Hair loss, depression, cardiac irregularities, dermatitis
Phenytoin	Dilantin®	Vitamin D on page 528	Osteoporosis, muscle weakness, hearing loss
		Calcium on page 400	Osteoporosis, heart/blood pressure irregularities, tooth decay
		Folic Acid on page 435	Birth defects, cervical dysplasia, anemia, cardiovascular disease
		Vitamin K on page 531	Blood coagulation and skeletal problems
		Vitamin B₁₂ on page 524	Anemia, tiredness, weakness, increased cardiovascular disease risk
		Vitamin B₁ on page 519	Depression, irritability, memory loss, muscle weakness, edema
Carbamazepine	Carbatrol®, Epitol®, Tegretol®	Folic Acid on page 435	Birth defects, cervical dysplasia, anemia, cardiovascular disease risk
		Vitamin D on page 528	Osteoporosis, muscle weakness, hearing loss
		Biotin on page 393	Hair loss, depression, cardiac irregularities, dermatitis
Primidone	Mysoline®	Folic Acid on page 435	Birth defects, cervical dysplasia, anemia, cardiovascular disease
		Biotin on page 393	Hair loss, depression, cardiac irregularities, dermatitis
Valproic Acid	Depacon®, Depakene®, Depakote®	Folic Acid on page 435	Birth defects, cervical dysplasia, anemia, cardiovascular disease
		Carnitine on page 403	Muscle weakness, cramps, fatigue

PART IV. CHARTS AND LISTS

DRUG-INDUCED NUTRIENT DEPLETIONS *(Continued)*

PRESCRIPTION AND NONPRESCRIPTION PRODUCTS *(continued)*

Drug	Brand Names	Nutrient Depletions	Potential Depletion Problems
ANTIDIABETICS			
Sulfonylureas			
Acetohexamide	Dymelor®		
Glyburide	DiaBeta® Glynase®; PresTab™, Micronase®	Coenzyme Q₁₀ *on page 412*	High blood pressure, congestive heart failure, low energy
Tolazamide	Tolinase®		
Biguanides			
Metformin	Glucophage®	Vitamin B₁₂ *on page 524*	Anemia, tiredness, weakness, increased cardiovascular disease risk
		Coenzyme Q₁₀ *on page 412*	High blood pressure, congestive heart failure, low energy
		Folic Acid *on page 435*	Birth defects, cervical dysplasia, anemia, cardiovascular disease
ANTIFUNGALS			
Amphotericin B	Various products	Calcium *on page 400*	Osteoporosis, heart/blood pressure irregularities, tooth decay
		Magnesium *on page 473*	Cardiovascular problems, asthma, osteoporosis, cramps, PMS
		Potassium *on page 490*	Irregular heartbeat, muscle weakness, fatigue, edema
ANTIHISTAMINES			
Hydroxyzine	Various products	Melatonin *on page 477*	Insomnia; increased free radical activity which reportedly weakens the immune system and may increase cancer risks
ANTI-INFLAMMATORIES			
Salicylates			
Aspirin, Choline Magnesium Trisalicylate, Choline Salicylate	Various products	Vitamin C *on page 526*	Lowered immune system, easy bruising, poor wound healing
		Folic Acid *on page 435*	Birth defects, cervical dysplasia, anemia, cardiovascular disease
		Iron *on page 464*	Anemia, weakness, fatigue, hair loss, brittle nails
		Potassium *on page 490*	Irregular heartbeat, muscle weakness, fatigue, edema
		Sodium *on page 504*	Muscle weakness, dehydration, loss of appetite, poor concentration
Salsalate	Various products	Folic Acid *on page 435*	Birth defects, cervical dysplasia, anemia, cardiovascular disease

PRESCRIPTION AND NONPRESCRIPTION PRODUCTS (continued)

Drug	Brand Names	Nutrient Depletions	Potential Depletion Problems
Nonsteroidal Anti-Inflammatory Drugs			
Ibuprofen, Naproxen, Sulindac, Piroxicam, Diclofenac, Diflunisal, Etodolac, Fenoprofen, Ketoprofen, Ketorolac, Meclofenamate, Nabumetone, Tolmetin, Mefenamic Acid	Aleve®, Anaprox®, Naprelan®, Naprosyn®, Clinoril®, Feldene®, Ponstel®, Cataflam®, Motrin® Voltaren®, Dolobid®, Lodine®, Nalfon®, Actron®, Orudis®, Oruvail®, Acular®, Toradol®, Meclomen®, Relafen®; Tolectin®	Folic Acid *on page 435*	Birth defects, cervical dysplasia, anemia, cardiovascular disease
Indomethacin	Indochron E-R®; Indocin®	Folic Acid *on page 435*	Birth defects, cervical dysplasia, anemia, cardiovascular disease
		Iron *on page 464*	Anemia, weakness, fatigue, hair loss, brittle nails
Corticosteroids			
Betamethasone, Budesonide, Cortisone, Dexamethasone, Flunisolide, Fluticasone, Hydrocortisone, Mometasone, Methylprednisolone, Prednisone, Prednisolone, Triamcinolone	Various products	Calcium *on page 400*	Osteoporosis, heart/blood pressure irregularities, tooth decay
		Vitamin D *on page 528*	Osteoporosis, muscle weakness, hearing loss
		Potassium *on page 490*	Irregular heartbeat, muscle weakness, fatigue, edema
		Zinc *on page 534*	Slow wound healing, loss of sense of smell and taste, lower immunity
		Vitamin C *on page 526*	Lowered immune system, easy bruising, poor wound healing
		Magnesium *on page 473*	Cardiovascular problems, asthma, osteoporosis, cramps, PMS
		Folic Acid *on page 435*	Birth defects, cervical dysplasia, anemia, cardiovascular disease
		Selenium *on page 502*	Lower immunity, reduced antioxidant protection
		Vitamin B₁₂ *on page 524*	Anemia, tiredness, weakness, increased cardiovascular disease risk
		Chromium *on page 410*	Glucose tolerance which results in elevated blood sugar and insulin levels; elevated cholesterol and triglycerides
Sulfasalazine	Azulfidine®	Folic Acid *on page 435*	Birth defects, cervical dysplasia, anemia, cardiovascular disease

DRUG-INDUCED NUTRIENT DEPLETIONS *(Continued)*

PRESCRIPTION AND NONPRESCRIPTION PRODUCTS *(continued)*

Drug	Brand Names	Nutrient Depletions	Potential Depletion Problems
ANTIVIRALS			
Reverse Transcriptase Inhibitors			
Didanosine, Lamivudine, Stavudine, Zalcitabine, Zidovudine	Various products	Copper *on page 416*	Anemia, fatigue, cardiovascular and connective tissue problems
		Zinc *on page 534*	Slow wound healing, loss of sense of smell and taste, lower immunity
		Vitamin B₁₂ *on page 524*	Anemia, tiredness, weakness, increased cardiovascular disease risk
		Carnitine *on page 403*	Muscle weakness, cramps, fatigue
Non-Nucleosides			
Delavirdine, Nevirapine		Potassium *on page 490*	Irregular heartbeat, muscle weakness, fatigue, edema
Foscarnet		Calcium *on page 400*	Osteoporosis, heart/blood pressure irregularities, tooth decay
		Magnesium *on page 473*	Cardiovascular problems, asthma, osteoporosis, cramps, PMS
ANXIOLYTICS / BENZODIAZEPINES			
Alprazolam	Various products	Melatonin *on page 477*	Insomnia; increased free radical activity which reportedly weakens the immune system and may increase cancer risks
Diazepam			
BRONCHODILATORS			
Theophylline	Various products	Vitamin B₆ *on page 523*	Depression, sleep disturbance, increased cardiovascular disease risk
		Vitamin B₁ *on page 519*	Depression, irritability, memory loss, muscle weakness, edema
Beta₂-Adrenergic Agonists			
Albuterol	Various products	Potassium *on page 490*	Irregular heartbeat, muscle weakness, fatigue, edema
Terbutaline			
CANCER CHEMOTHERAPY			
	See Special Section on Nutrient Depletion and Cancer Chemotherapy *on page 637*		
CARDIOVASCULAR DRUGS			
Vasodilators			
Hydralazine	Apresoline®	Vitamin B₆ *on page 523*	Anemia, tiredness, weakness, increased cardiovascular disease risk
		Coenzyme Q₁₀ *on page 412*	High blood pressure, congestive heart failure, low energy

PRESCRIPTION AND NONPRESCRIPTION PRODUCTS (continued)

Drug	Brand Names	Nutrient Depletions	Potential Depletion Problems
Loop Diuretics			
Furosemide, Bumetanide, Ethacrynic Acid	Lasix®; Bumex®; Edecrin®	Calcium on page 400	Osteoporosis, heart/blood pressure irregularities, tooth decay
		Magnesium on page 473	Cardiovascular problems, asthma, osteoporosis, cramps, PMS
		Vitamin B₁ on page 519	Depression, irritability, memory loss, muscle weakness, edema
		Vitamin B₆ on page 523	Depression, sleep disturbance, increased cardiovascular disease risk
		Vitamin C on page 526	Lowered immune system, easy bruising, poor wound healing
		Potassium on page 490	Irregular heartbeat, muscle weakness, fatigue, edema
		Zinc on page 534	Slow wound healing, loss of sense of smell and taste, lower immunity
Thiazide Diuretics			
Hydrochlorothiazide, Methyclothiazide, Indapamide, Metolazone	Aquatensen®; Enduron® Esidrix®; Ezide®; HydroDIURIL®; Hydro-Par®; Microzide®; Oretic®; Lozol®; Mykrox®; Zaroxolyn®	Magnesium on page 473	Cardiovascular problems, asthma, osteoporosis, cramps, PMS
		Potassium on page 490	Irregular heartbeat, muscle weakness, fatigue, edema
		Zinc on page 534	Lowered immune system, slow wound healing
		Coenzyme Q₁₀ on page 412	High blood pressure, congestive heart failure, low energy
		Sodium on page 504	Muscle weakness, dehydration, loss of appetite, poor concentration
		Phosphorus on page 489	Stunted growth, skeletal problems, increased tooth decay
Potassium-sparing Diuretics			
Triamterene	Dyrenium®	Calcium on page 400	Osteoporosis, heart/blood pressure irregularities, tooth decay
		Folic Acid on page 435	Birth defects, cervical dysplasia, anemia, cardiovascular disease
		Zinc on page 534	Slow wound healing, loss of sense of smell and taste, lower immunity
Hydrochlorothiazide and Triamterene	Dyazide®, Maxzide®	Calcium on page 400	Osteoporosis, heart/blood pressure irregularities, tooth decay
		Folic Acid on page 435	Birth defects, cervical dysplasia, anemia, cardiovascular disease
		Vitamin B₆ on page 523	Depression, sleep disturbances, increased cardiovascular disease risk
ACE Inhibitors			
Captopril, Enalapril	Capoten®, Vasotec®	Zinc on page 534	Slow wound healing, loss of sense of smell and taste, lower immunity
Centrally-Acting Antihypertensives			
Clonidine	Catapres®, Duraclon®		
Methyldopa	Aldomet®	Coenzyme Q₁₀ on page 412	High blood pressure, congestive heart failure, low energy

DRUG-INDUCED NUTRIENT DEPLETIONS (Continued)

PRESCRIPTION AND NONPRESCRIPTION PRODUCTS (continued)

Drug	Brand Names	Nutrient Depletions	Potential Depletion Problems
Chlorthalidone	Hygroton®; Thalitone®	Zinc on page 534	Slow wound healing, loss of sense of smell and taste, lower immunity
Cardiac Glycosides			
Digoxin	Lanoxin®	Calcium on page 400	Osteoporosis, heart/blood pressure irregularities, tooth decay
		Magnesium on page 473	Cardiovascular problems, asthma, osteoporosis, cramps, PMS
		Phosphorus on page 489	Stunted growth, skeletal problems, increased tooth decay
		Vitamin B₁ on page 519	Depression, irritability, memory loss, muscle weakness, edema
Beta-Blockers			
Propranolol, Metoprolol, Atenolol, Pindolol, Acebutolol, Betaxolol, Bisoprolol, Carteolol, Carvedilol, Esmolol, Labetalol, Nadolol, Sotalol, Timolol	Betachron E-R®, Inderal®; Lopressor®, Toprol XL®; Tenormin®; Visken®; Sectral®; Betoptic®, Kerlone®, Zebeta®; Cartrol®, Ocupress®; Coreg®; Brevibloc®; Normodyne®, Trandate®; Corgard®; Betapace®; Betimol®; Blocadren®, Timoptic®	Coenzyme Q₁₀ on page 412	High blood pressure, congestive heart failure, low energy
Calcium Channel Blockers			
Nifedipine	Adalat®; Procardia®		
Verapamil	Calan®; Covera-HS®; Isopto®; Verelan®	Potassium on page 490	Irregular heartbeat, muscle weakness, fatigue, edema
CHOLESTEROL LOWERING DRUGS			
HMG-CoA Reductase Inhibitors			
Atorvastatin	Lipitor®		
Cerivastatin	Baycol®		
Lovastatin	Mevacor®	Coenzyme Q₁₀ on page 412	High blood pressure, congestive heart failure, low energy
Fluvastatin	Lescol®		
Pravastatin	Pravachol®		
Simvastatin	Zocor®		

PRESCRIPTION AND NONPRESCRIPTION PRODUCTS (continued)

Drug	Brand Names	Nutrient Depletions	Potential Depletion Problems
Bile Acid Sequestrants			
Cholestyramine	Prevalite®; Questran®	Vitamin A on page 518, Beta-Carotene on page 390, Vitamin D on page 528, Vitamin E on page 529, Vitamin K on page 531, Vitamin B₁₂ on page 524, Folic Acid on page 435, Iron on page 464, Calcium on page 400, Magnesium on page 473, Phosphorus on page 489, Zinc on page 534	See individual nutrient monographs
Colestipol	Colestid®	Vitamin A on page 518, Beta-Carotene on page 390, Vitamin D on page 528, Vitamin E on page 529, Vitamin B₁₂ on page 524, Folic Acid on page 435, Iron on page 464	See individual nutrient monographs
Miscellaneous			
Gemfibrozil	Gemcor®; Lopid®	Coenzyme Q₁₀ on page 412	High blood pressure, congestive heart failure, low energy
		Vitamin E on page 529	Greater free radical activity which weakens the immune system, increases the risk to conditions such as cardiovascular disease and cancer; accelerates the aging process
ELECTROLYTE REPLACEMENT			
Potassium Chloride (Timed Release)	Various products	Vitamin B₁₂ on page 524	Anemia, tiredness, weakness, increased cardiovascular disease risk

DRUG-INDUCED NUTRIENT DEPLETIONS (Continued)

PRESCRIPTION AND NONPRESCRIPTION PRODUCTS (continued)

Drug	Brand Names	Nutrient Depletions	Potential Depletion Problems
FEMALE HORMONES			
Oral Contraceptives			
		Folic acid on page 435	Birth defects, cervical dysplasia, anemia, cardiovascular disease
		Vitamin B$_6$ on page 523	Depression, sleep disturbances, increased cardiovascular disease risk
		Vitamin B$_2$ on page 520	Problems with skin, eyes, mucous membranes, nerves
		Vitamin B$_{12}$ on page 524	Anemia, tiredness, weakness, increased cardiovascular disease risk
Oral Contraceptives	Various products	Vitamin C on page 526	Lowered immune system, easy bruising, poor wound healing
		Magnesium on page 473	Cardiovascular problems, asthma, osteoporosis, cramps, PMS
		Zinc on page 534	Slow wound healing, loss of sense of smell and taste, lower immunity
		Vitamin B$_3$ on page 521	Skin, gastrointestinal, nervous system problems
		Melatonin on page 477	Insomnia; increased free radical activity which reportedly weakens the immune system and may increase cancer risks
Estrogen Replacement (ERT) and Hormone Replacement (HRT) Therapies			
Estrogens, Conjugated, Estrogen and Medroxyprogesterone, Raloxifene, Estrogens, Esterified	Various products	Vitamin B$_6$ on page 523	Depression, sleep disturbances, increased cardiovascular disease risk
		Magnesium on page 473	Cardiovascular problems, asthma, osteoporosis, cramps, PMS
		Melatonin on page 477	Insomnia; increased free radical activity which reportedly weakens the immune system and may increase cancer risks
GOUT MEDICATIONS			
		Vitamin B$_{12}$ on page 524	Anemia, tiredness, weakness, increased cardiovascular disease risk
		Sodium on page 504	Muscle weakness, dehydration, loss of appetite, poor concentration
Colchicine		Potassium on page 490	Irregular heartbeat, muscle weakness, fatigue, edema
		Beta-Carotene on page 390	Lower immunity, reduced antioxidant protection
		Calcium on page 400	Osteoporosis, heart/blood pressure irregularities, tooth decay
		Phosphorus on page 489	Stunted growth, skeletal problems, increased tooth decay

PRESCRIPTION AND NONPRESCRIPTION PRODUCTS *(continued)*

Drug	Brand Names	Nutrient Depletions	Potential Depletion Problems
LAXATIVES			
Mineral Oil	Various products	Vitamin A *on page 518*, Beta-Carotene *on page 390*, Vitamin D *on page 528*, Vitamin E *on page 529*, Vitamin K *on page 531*, Calcium *on page 400*, Phosphorus *on page 489*	See individual nutrient monographs
Bisacodyl	Various products	Potassium *on page 490*	Irregular heartbeat, muscle weakness, fatigue, edema
Phosphate Enema			
Fleet® phosphate enema		Calcium *on page 400*	Osteoporosis, heart/blood pressure irregularities, tooth decay
		Magnesium *on page 473*	Cardiovascular problems, asthma, osteoporosis, cramps, PMS
PSYCHOTHERAPEUTICS			
Tricyclic Antidepressants			
Amitriptyline	Elavil®		
Desipramine	Norpramin®; Pertofrane®		
Nortriptyline	Aventyl®; Pamelor®	Vitamin B₂ *on page 520*, Coenzyme Q₁₀ *on page 412*	Problems with skin, eyes, mucous membranes, nerves
Doxepin	Adapin®; Sinequan®; Zonalon®		High blood pressure, congestive heart failure, low energy
Imipramine	Janimine®; Tofranil®		
Phenothiazines			
Chlorpromazine	Ormazine®; Thorazine®	Vitamin B₂ *on page 520*,	Problems with skin, eyes, mucous membranes, nerves
Thioridazine	Mellaril®	Coenzyme Q₁₀ *on page 412*,	High blood pressure, congestive heart failure, low energy
Fluphenazine	Permitil®; Prolixin®	Melatonin *on page 477*	Insomnia; increased free radical activity which reportedly weakens the immune system and may increase cancer risks
Butyrophenones			
Haloperidol	Haldol®	Coenzyme Q₁₀ *on page 412*	High blood pressure, congestive heart failure, low energy
		Melatonin *on page 477*	Insomnia; increased free radical activity which reportedly weakens the immune system and may increase cancer risks

635

DRUG-INDUCED NUTRIENT DEPLETIONS *(Continued)*

PRESCRIPTION AND NONPRESCRIPTION PRODUCTS *(continued)*

Drug	Brand Names	Nutrient Depletions	Potential Depletion Problems
H₂-Receptor Antagonists			
		ULCER MEDICATIONS	
Cimetidine	Tagamet®	Vitamin B₁₂ on *page 524*	Anemia, tiredness, weakness, increased cardiovascular disease risk
Famotidine	Pepcid®	Folic Acid on *page 435*	Birth defects, cervical dysplasia, anemia, cardiovascular disease
Nizatadine	Axid®	Vitamin D on *page 528*	Osteoporosis, muscle weakness, hearing loss
Ranitidine	Tritec® Zantac®	Calcium on *page 400*	Osteoporosis, heart/blood pressure irregularities, tooth decay
		Iron on *page 464*	Anemia, weakness, fatigue, hair loss, brittle nails
		Zinc on *page 534*	Slow wound healing, loss of sense of smell and taste, lower immunity
Proton Pump Inhibitors			
Lansoprazole	Prevacid®	Vitamin B₁₂ on *page 524*	Anemia, tiredness, weakness, increased cardiovascular disease risk
Omeprazole	Prilosec®		
		MISCELLANEOUS	
Levodopa	Dopar®; Larodopa®	Potassium on *page 490*	Irregular heartbeat, muscle weakness, fatigue, edema
Methotrexate	Folex®, Rheumatrex®	Folic Acid on *page 435*	Birth defects, cervical dysplasia, anemia, cardiovascular disease
		Vitamin B₆ on *page 523*	Depression, sleep disturbances, increased cardiovascular disease risk
		Magnesium on *page 473*	Cardiovascular problems, asthma, osteoporosis, cramps, PMS
Penicillamine	Cuprimine®; Depen®	Zinc on *page 534*	Slow wound healing, loss of sense of smell and taste, lower immunity
		Copper on *page 416*	Anemia, fatigue, cardiovascular and connective tissue problems

NUTRIENT DEPLETION AND CANCER CHEMOTHERAPY

The agents used in cancer chemotherapy may have potent effects on an individual's nutritional status. Many questions with respect to nutrient depletion have not been specifically addressed in this population; however, the impact on general nutritional status may be profound. Nutritional compromise results from two major effects of chemotherapy. Nutrient intake may be decreased by chemotherapy-induced nausea and vomiting. Chemotherapy can also cause varying degrees of toxicity to the cells that line the gastrointestinal tract which can limit the absorption of nutrients. There is a wide variability between individual chemotherapeutic agents and their relative potential to cause these two effects.

Decreased nutrient intake caused by chemotherapy-induced nausea, vomiting, and anorexia may be mediated through the central nervous system or by local gastrointestinal factors. The emetogenic effects of most agents are limited to the first few hours following administration, but occasionally may be persistent. An extreme case is represented by cisplatin, which may induce severe nausea and vomiting for up to a week following administration. Widespread general nutritional compromise may be anticipated only in persistent cases. In particular, the absorption of all nutrients including vitamins, minerals, amino acids, and fatty acids may be compromised in the patient who is experiencing prolonged nausea and vomiting and/or anorexia.

A second distinct process may compromise nutrition during chemotherapy. This results from a direct toxic effect on cells lining the gastrointestinal tract, and is often evidenced by the development of inflammatory changes in the mucous membranes (mucositis), which are particularly notable in the oral cavity (stomatitis). In many cases, a side effect of chemotherapy drugs that exert cytotoxic effects is the actual destruction of the microvilli in the lining of the gastrointestinal tract. This has several consequences. It may result in diarrhea and destroy the cells that are involved in the absorption of nutrients. At the same time, it creates raw, inflamed intestinal tissue. Eating causes food and digestive juices to come into contact with the raw tissue, which can result in a great deal of pain. Many patients substantially reduce their food intake to avoid pain. Since this form of compromise may require a longer period for recovery, agents which result in mucotoxicity and cytotoxicity may have a more significant nutritional impact. These conditions can hinder the absorption of all nutrients including vitamins, minerals, amino acids, and fatty acids.

In addition to these primary mechanisms, select agents may be associated with unique gastrointestinal effects. As examples, asparaginase may cause pancreatitis and malabsorption, while vincristine may result in severe constipation and/or functional bowel obstruction due to a neurotoxic mechanism. Whether individual chemotherapeutic agents deplete nutrients by means other than diminished absorption has not been thoroughly evaluated. However, depletion secondary to cytotoxic effects, inflammatory responses, and effects on major organ function may be expected.

CHEMOTHERAPY TABLES

For convenience, chemotherapeutic agents may be grouped into five general classes. These include alkylating agents, antineoplastic antibiotics, antimetabolites, natural source derivatives, and a miscellaneous grouping. Although there is some variability within groups, agents within these classes often demonstrate a characteristic gastrointestinal toxicity profile.

Alkylating agents: These agents are associated with moderate to high potential for nausea and vomiting but do not usually cause severe toxicity to the gastrointestinal mucosa.

NUTRIENT DEPLETION AND CANCER CHEMOTHERAPY
(Continued)

Antineoplastic antibiotics: These agents are associated with moderate potential for nausea and vomiting but often cause severe toxicity to the gastrointestinal mucosa.

Antimetabolites: These agents are associated with low to moderate potential for nausea and vomiting but may cause severe toxicity to the gastrointestinal mucosa.

Natural source derivatives: These agents are associated with low to moderate potential for nausea and vomiting and may cause severe toxicity to the gastrointestinal mucosa.

A final category of agents used in cancer chemotherapy are the biological response modifiers. These chemotherapy agents do not have specific gastrointestinal effects. They are generally hormonal antagonists or cytokines/immune response modifying agents. Included in this category are aldesleukin, anastrozole, bicalutamide, interferon alfa, leuprolide, megestrol, nilutamide, and tamoxifen.

The following tables list agents according to these broad classifications. Although studies of specific nutrient depletion in the setting of cancer chemotherapy are limited, the following tables may be used to identify the primary mechanism of nutritional impact an agent may have. The number in the second column corresponds to the potential of an agent to cause nausea, vomiting, and anorexia. On this scale, 1 corresponds to the lowest potential, while a rating of 5 indicates the greatest potential to cause this effect. The third column provides additional detail and highlights the extent of mucosal toxicity noted with an individual agent.

ALKYLATING AGENTS

Drug Name	Emetogenic Rating	Mucosal Effects and Notes
Busulfan	2	Mucosal effects rare
Carboplatin	3	Emetogenic, but little mucocutaneous effect
Carmustine	4-5	Nausea and vomiting persist for 4-6 hours; few mucosal effects
Chlorambucil	1	Infrequent nausea, vomiting, diarrhea, or oral ulceration
Cisplatin	4-5	Highly emetogenic, persisting for up to 1 week; mucosal effects <1%
Cyclophosphamide	1-4	Nausea/vomiting increase with dose; stomatitis/mucositis may occur
Dacarbazine	4-5	Highly emetogenic, duration 2-4 hours; rare mucosal effects
Ifosfamide	3-4	Significant nausea and vomiting, up to 3 days; limited mucosal effects
Lomustine	4-5	Nausea and vomiting common, stomatitis and diarrhea in 1% to 10%
Mechlorethamine	5	Highly emetogenic, duration 2-8 hours; diarrhea in 1% to 10%
Melphalan	1-5	Emetogenic only at high doses; infrequent stomatitis and diarrhea
Procarbazine	4	Significant nausea/vomiting; infrequent stomatitis (1% to 2%)
Streptozocin	5	Highly emetogenic, duration 1-12 hours
Thiotepa	2-5	Mucositis frequent at doses used in bone marrow transplant (BMT)

ANTINEOPLASTIC ANTIBIOTICS

Drug Name	Emetogenic Rating	Mucosal Effects and Notes
Bleomycin	2	High mucosal toxicity
Dactinomycin	5	Highly emetogenic, duration 4-24 hours; high mucocutaneous toxicity
Daunorubicin	3	High mucosal toxicity
Doxorubicin	3-4	High mucosal toxicity
Idarubicin	3	High mucosal toxicity; GI hemorrhage up to 30%
Mitomycin	3	High mucosal toxicity
Mitoxantrone	3	Severe diarrhea and mucosal toxicity
Pentostatin	2	Diarrhea in >10%; stomatitis ~5%
Plicamycin	2	Moderate to high incidence of stomatitis (1% to 10%)

NUTRIENT DEPLETION AND CANCER CHEMOTHERAPY
(Continued)

ANTIMETABOLITES

Drug Name	Emetogenic Rating	Mucosal Effects and Notes
Cladribine	1	Low nausea/vomiting; little mucosal toxicity
Cytarabine	2-4	High mucosal toxicity
Floxuridine	1	High mucosal toxicity
Fludarabine	1	Mild nausea/vomiting; stomatitis and GI bleeding may occur
Fluorouracil	2-3	Anorexia and stomatitis; mucocutaneous toxicity may be severe
Gemcitabine	1	Stomatitis 10% to 14%
Hydroxyurea	2	Anorexia and stomatitis may be severe
Mercaptopurine	1	Moderate to high stomatitis 1% to 10%; pancreatitis
Methotrexate	2-4	High incidence of mucosal damage, also pancreatitis
Thioguanine	1	High mucosal toxicity

NATURAL SOURCE (Plant) DERIVATIVES

Drug Name	Emetogenic Rating	Mucosal Effects and Notes
Docetaxel	1	High mucosal toxicity; diarrhea in ~25%
Etoposide	2	Some mucosal 1% to 6%; diarrhea in 1% to 13%
Irinotecan	3	Very high incidence of diarrhea*
Paclitaxel	1	High mucositis incidence, severe at higher doses
Teniposide	3	High mucositis incidence; diarrhea up to 75%
Topotecan	2	Nausea in up to 70%, emesis <30%, diarrhea in up to 42%
Vinblastine	1	Stomatitis and diarrhea are common
Vincristine	1	High mucosal toxicity; common constipation and adynamic ileus
Vinorelbine	1	High mucositis in >44%; constipation 35%

*Two forms: Early (within 30 minutes) due to cholinergic mechansim and late (after 6-10 days) due to direct cellular toxicity.

MISCELLANEOUS

Drug Name	Emetogenic Rating	Mucosal Effects and Notes
Asparaginase	1	May cause pancreatitis/malabsorption but little direct mucotoxicity
Mitotane	4	May cause severe nausea, vomiting, diarrhea (occurs in ~20%)

HERBAL MEDICINE USE IN PEDIATRICS

Herbal or phytomedicines can be used in the pediatric population, but their preparation, method of administration, and dosage adjustments should be done with extreme care. Proprietary preparations are available for most herbal products. However, pharmacists can compound specific products for pediatric needs. Always use a quality herbal product that has substantial quality assurance standards supporting its manufacturing. Typical methods of administration in children include oral (liquid extracts and teas) and topical (creams, gels, and ointments). Natural supplements may help expedite healing and decrease the symptoms of various common complaints in pediatrics. Keep in mind that the rate of spontaneous recovery from many acute conditions is much higher in children than adults.[1] Allowing the natural course of healing is important in the overall scheme of treatment for such common childhood illnesses as diarrhea, colds, flu, and other viruses. Use the following empirical formulas based on age and weight when dosing herbal medicines in the form of liquid extracts:

Young's Rule:
$$\frac{Age}{Age + 12} \times Adult\ dose = Dose\ for\ child$$

Clarke's Rule:
$$\frac{Weight\ (in\ lbs) \times Adult\ dose}{150} = Dose\ for\ child$$

Fried's Rule (for infants):
$$\frac{Age\ (in\ mos) \times Adult\ dose}{150} = Dose\ for\ infant$$

Consider the following guidelines when recommending herbal medicines for childhood illnesses:

- Limit the number of natural medicines given to a child for an illness
- Always follow the manufacturer's suggested dosages
- Use the lowest possible dose to alleviate symptoms and stimulate healing
- Be aware of contraindications and potential adverse reactions for any dietary supplement
- If symptoms do not improve within 24 hours, consult a physician
- Use of herbal supplements in infants should be supervised by a qualified health provider
- Use homeopathic medicines for infants because of their safety and lack of side effects, whenever possible

---

1. Schilcher H, *Phytotherapy in Paediatric,* Stuttgart, Germany: Medpharm Scientific Publishers, 1997, 15.

HERB/DRUG POTENTIAL INTERACTIONS

This section contains a classification of specific herbs whose constituents or actions (proven or reputed) may potentially interact with conventional pharmaceutical drugs. The botanical classifications are based upon the known chemical constituents of each herb, the pharmacological properties, and the side effects of each classification according to scientific principles and accepted theory. The **potential interactions** listed are based upon the chemical constituent properties of the herbs and most of the interactions are theorized. See the Herb Quick Reference Chart *on page 538* for a detailed interaction profile. Remember that many plants have constituents that may balance any potential adverse effect. Throughout this section, the most commonly used herbs are in **bold print**.

CARDIOACTIVE HERBS

A qualified healthcare provider should use these herbs with caution, especially in cardiac patients and those on cardioactive medications.

Cardioactive Herbs	Bioactive Constituent(s) With Potential Adverse Effect
Broom (*Cytisus scoparius*) tops	Alkaloid content has cardio-depressant activity
Kola (*Cola* spp.) nut	Caffeine content
Coltsfoot (*Tussilago farfara*) leaf	Calcium channel-blocking ability; SHOULD NOT BE TAKEN INTERNALLY due to pyrrolizidine alkaloids
Devil's Claw (*Harpagophytum procumbens*) tubers	May have chronotropic and inotropic effects; cardiotonic
Dogbane (*Apocynum cannabinum*) root	Contains cardiac glycosides
Figwort (*Scrophularia nodosa*) whole plant	Contains cardiac glycosides
Foxglove (*Digitalis purpurea*) whole plant	Contains cardiac glycosides
Fumitory (*Fumaria officinalis*) whole plant	Contains cardiotonic alkaloids
Ginger (*Zingiber officinalis*) root	Cardioactive constituents; avoid large and prolonged doses
Ginseng, Panax (*Panax ginseng*) root	Cardiotonic activity
Golden seal (*Hydrastis canadensis*) rhizome	Cardioactive alkaloid (berberine)
Hawthorn (*Crataegus oxyacantha*) leaf/flower/berry	Cardiotonic activity
Immortal (*Asclepias asperula*) root	Contains cardiac glycosides
Lily-of-the-Valley (*Convallaria majalis*) whole plant	Contains cardiac glycosides
Lime, Linden (*Tilia* spp) flower	Cardiotoxic in large doses
Mistletoe (*Viscum* spp) leaf	Contains viscotoxin (may have a negative inotropic effect)
Motherwort (*Leonurus cardiaca*) whole plant	Contains cardiac glycosides
Night-blooming Cereus (**Cactus grandiflorus**) fruit	Cardiotonic amines and tyramine; not for use with MAO inhibitors
Pleurisy (*Asclepias tuberosa*) root	Contains cardiac glycosides
Prickly Ash (*Zanthoxylum* spp) bark	May interfere with sodium, potassium, ATPase
Quassia, Jamaican (*Picrasma excelsa*) stem wood	Quinine-like properties; larger doses may interfere with cardiac medications

LIVER METABOLISM

The liver metabolizes many pharmaceutical drugs, and any alteration of this metabolism can cause either an increase or decrease in the drug's pharmacological effects. Some herbs also tend to increase liver metabolism by stimulating the liver directly or indirectly. Patients taking the following pharmaceuticals along with the listed herbs should be advised to use caution with herbs that may potentially alter liver function.

Drug Category	Herbs That May Alter Liver Enzymes	Herbs That May Cause Hepatotoxicity Due to Pyrrolizidine Alkaloids
ACE inhibitors Antiasthmatics Anticoagulants Anticonvulsants Antidepressants (Tricyclic) Glucocorticoids Oral contraceptives	American Mandrake (*Podophyllum peltatum*) Balmony (*Chelone glabra*) Barberry (*Berberis vulgaris*) Blue Flag (*Iris versicolor*) Button Bush (*Cephalanthus* spp) Fringetree (*Chionanthus virginicus*) **Golden Seal** (*Hydrastis canadensis*) Greater Celandine (*Chelidonium majus*) Leptandra (*Veronicastrum virginicum*) Oregon Grape (*Berberis aquifolium*) Sagebrush (*Artemisia tridentata*) Virginia Snakeroot, Serpentaria (*Aristolochia serpentaria*) Wahoo, Burning Bush (*Euonymus atropurpureus*)	Coltsfoot (*Tussilago farfara*) Comfrey (*Symphytum officinale*) Hound's Tongue (*Cynoglossum officinalis*) Life Root, Squaw Weed (*Senecio aureus*)

MINERAL ABSORPTION

Herbs that contain tannins may alter the absorption of iron, calcium, copper, zinc, and magnesium contained in supplements and foods. These bivalent minerals may possibly form an insoluble complex with the tannin phytochemicals found in the herbs, thereby rendering them unusable by the body in varying percentages (depending on factors such as total tannin content in the herbs and individual biochemical susceptibility). Dose vitamin and mineral suplements separately from tannin-containing herbs, if possible.

Herbs That May Alter Absorption Due to Tannin Content
Artichoke (*Cynara scolymus*)
Bayberry (*Myrica cerifera*)
Bilberry (*Vaccinium myrtillus*)
Cascara (*Rhamnus purshiana*)
Corn silk (*Zea mays*)
Elder (*Sambucus canadensis, Sambucus nigra*)
Feverfew (*Tanacetum parthenium*)
Grape Seed (*Vitis vinifera*)
Green Tea (*Camellia sinensis*)
Ground Ivy (*Nepeta hederacea*)
Hops (*Humulus lupulus*)
Horse Chestnut (*Aesculus hippocastanum*)
Juniper (*Juniperus communis*)
Mistletoe (*Viscum* spp)
St. John's Wort (*Hypericum perforatum*)
Uva Ursi (*Arctostaphylos uva-ursi*)
White Willow (*Salix alba*)
Yarrow (*Achillea millefolium*)

HERB/DRUG POTENTIAL INTERACTIONS *(Continued)*

GI ABSORPTION

These herbal agents may alter the absorption of other herbs and pharmaceutical drugs by direct or indirect inhibition or alteration of digestion and absorption.

Herbs That May Alter GI Absorption
Aloe (*Aloe* spp)
Buckeye, California (*Aesculus californica*)
Buckeye, Ohio (*Aesculus glabra*)
Buckthorn (*Rhamnus frangula*)
Buckthorn, California (*Rhamnus californica*)
Cascara (*Rhamnus purshiana*)
Cayenne (*Capsicum* spp)
Coffee (*Caffea* spp)
Horse Chestnut (*Aesculus hippocastanum*)
Ephedra, Ma Huang, Chinese Ephedra (*Ephedra sinica*)
Marshmallow (*Althea officinalis*)
Mormon Tea, American Ephedra (*Ephedra nevadensis*)
Senna (*Cassia angustifolia*)
Spanish Bayonet (*Yucca* spp)
Uva Ursi, Manzanita, Bearberry (*Arctostaphylos Uva-Ursi*)
Wafer Ash, Hop Tree (*Ptelea* spp)

MAO INHIBITION

Tyramine-containing foods can be the causative agents in precipitating a hypertensive crisis while on MAOI therapy. Similarly, herbs that contain even trace amounts of tyramine should not be used in patients taking MAOI medications.

Herbs That May Interact With MAOI Due to Tyramine Content
Mistletoe (*Viscum album, Viscum flavescens*)
Night Blooming Cereus (*Cactus grandiflorus*)
Shepherd's Purse (*Capsella bursa-pastoris*)

SYMPATHOMIMETIC HERBS

The potential effects of sympathomimetic herbs are listed below with the primary constituent noted. Always use caution in appropriate patients when using herbs with sympathomimetic activity.

Sympathomimetic Herbs	Biochemical Constituent(s)
Calamus, Sweet Flag (*Acorus calamus*)	beta-asarone
Cayenne (*Capsicum annum*)	amines
Coffee (*Caffea arabica*)	caffeine
Fu-tse, Fo-tzu (*Aconitum carmichaelii*)	amines
Guarana (*Paullinia cupana*)	caffeine, hypoxanthines
Kola nut (*Cola sp*)	caffeine
Ephedra, Ma Huang, Chinese Ephedra (*Ephedra sinica*)	ephedrine and its alkaloids
Mescal Buttons, Peyote (*Lophophora* spp)	mescaline
Mormon Tea (*Ephedra nevadensis*)	ephedrine and its alkaloids
Night Blooming Cereus (*Cactus grandiflorus*)	cardiac glycosides
Scotch Broom Tops (*Cytisus scoparius*)	cytisine, sparteine

Sympathomimetic Herbs	Biochemical Constituent(s)
Syrian Rue (*Peganum harmala*)	harmine alkaloids
Yellow Jasmine (*Gelsemium sempervirens*)	gelsemine
Yohimbe (*Corynanthe yohimbe*)	yohimbine

Potential Pharmacological Effects of Sympathomimetic Herbs	Contraindications of Sympathomimetic Herbs	Potential Side Effects of Sympathomimetic Herb Overdosage
Increase blood pressure; vasoconstriction; increase respiration CNS effects; decongestant effects Increase blood glucose Appetite suppression; sleep disturbances Increase heart rate Bronchial relaxation	Concurrent use with MAO inhibitors; diabetes Concurrent use with OTC decongestants Glaucoma Heart problems such as arrhythmias Hypertension Concurrent use with anticoagulants Pregnancy Hyperthyroidism Patients with pre-existing psychiatric disorders	Restlessness; tremor; hyperactivity Dizziness; irritability Headache Anorexia, dry mouth

PARASYMPATHOMIMETIC (CHOLINERGIC) HERBS

Bittersweet (*Solanum dulcamara*)
Blood Root (*Sanguinaria canadensis*)
Blue Flag (*Iris versicolor*)
Bryony (*Bryonia alba*)
Buckeye, California (*Aesculus californica*)
Buckeye, Ohio (*Aesculus glabra*)
Dogbane, Canadian Hemp (*Apocynum cannabinum*)
Dogwood, Jamaican (*Piscidia erythrina*)
False or Green Hellebore (*Veratrum alba*)
Horse Chestnut (*Aesculus hippocastanum*)
HuperzineA, Qian Cengta (isolated from *Huperiza serrata*)
Immortal (*Asclepias asperula*)
Indian Tobacco (*Lobelia inflata*)
Jaborandi (*Pilocarpus jaborandi*)
Leptandra (*Veronicastrum virginicus*)
Death Cup Mushroom (*Amanita muscaria*)
Pasque Flower (*Anemone pulsatilla*)
Pink Root (*Spigelia*)
Pleurisy Root (*Asclepias tuberosa*)
Pokeweed (*Phytolacca* spp)
Senega Snakeroot (*Polygala senega*)
Tobacco (*Nicotiana tabacum*)
Wahoo (*Euonymus atropurpureus*)
Yohimbe (*Corynanthe yohimbe*)

The potential effects of parasympathomimetic herbs, especially in high and prolonged doses, are listed below. Always use caution in appropriate patients when using herbs with parasympathomimetic activity.

HERB/DRUG POTENTIAL INTERACTIONS *(Continued)*

Potential Pharmacological Effects of Parasympathomimetic Herbs	Contraindications of Parasympathomimetic Herbs	Potential Side Effects of Parasympathomimetic Herb Overdosage
Vasodilation Chronotropic (decrease heart rate) Stimulation of secretions Bronchoconstriction Stimulation of urinary tract Increase GI tone Increase peristalsis	Asthma Concurrent use with the following: Pilocarpine, metoclopramide (Reglan®), bethanechol, carbachol Hyperthyroidism Coronary insufficiency Peptic ulcer Concurrent use with OTC antihistamines	Flushing Sweating Headache Asthmatic attack precipitation Hypotension Decrease visual acuity Epigastric distress Increase salivation

PARASYMPATHOLYTIC (ANTICHOLINERGIC) HERBS

> Belladonna (*Atropa belladonna*)
> Bittersweet (*Solanum dulcamara*)
> Henbane (*Hyoscyamus niger*)
> Jimson Weed (*Datura stramonium*)

The potential effects of parasympatholytic herbs, especially in high and prolonged doses, are listed below. Always use caution in appropriate patients when using herbs with parasympatholytic activity.

Potential Pharmacological Effects of Anticholinergic Herbs	Contraindications of Anticholinergic Herbs	Potential Side Effects of Anticholinergic Herb Overdosage
Decrease GI motility Decrease heart rate Cycloplegia Decrease glandular secretions (sweating) Decrease gastric secretions	Concurrent use with phenothiazines (ie, chlorpromazine (Thorazine®) Concurrent use with tricyclic antidepressants (ie, amitriptyline (Elavil®) Concurrent use with H_2 blockers (ie, cimetidine (Tagamet®), ranitidine (Zantac®), famotidine (Pepcid®) Concurrent use with antiparkinsonian agents Concurrent use with antifungal agents (ie, ketoconazole (Nizoral®) Glaucoma	Dry mouth Constipation Hypotension Arrhythmia Urinary retention Pupil dilation

VASOPRESSOMIMETIC HERBS

These herbs may alter blood pressure.

> Goat's Head (*Tribulis* spp)
> Mescal, Peyote (*Lophophora*)
> **Yohimbe** (*Corynanthe yohimbe*)

THYROID FUNCTION

Increase Function

These herbs may potentially stimulate the thyroid gland and alter the levels of thyroid medications. They should be used with caution in individuals with hyperthyroidism or in individuals taking thyroid medications.

Herbs That May Stimulate the Thyroid Gland	Pharmacological Effects of Thyroid-Stimulating Herbs
Bladderwrack (*Fucus vesiculosus*) Fu-tse, Fo-tzu (*Aconitum carmichaeli*) **Gotu Kola** (*Centella asiatica*) **Ephedra**, Ma Huang (*Ephedra sinica*) Mustard (*Brassica* spp) **Yohimbe** (*Corynanthe yohimbe*)	Increase heart rate Increase basal metabolism Increase metabolism of bile acids and cholesterol Increase absorption of glucose, thermogenic Osteoporosis Insomnia Increase bowel movements

Decrease Function

These herbs may potentially decrease thyroid function and should be used with caution in patients with hypothyroidism or on thyroid medications.

Herbs That May Depress the Thyroid Gland
Bugleweed (*Lycopus virginica*)
Garlic (*Allium sativa*)
Motherwort (*Leonurus cardiaca*)

ALDOSTERONE-ENHANCING HERBS

Use with caution in patients on diuretics and in patients with hypertension.

Herbs That May Be Aldosterone Synergistic	Potential Pharmacological Effects of Aldosterone Synergistic Herbs	Contraindications of Aldosterone Synergistic Herbs	Side Effects of Aldosterone Synergistic Herbs
Licorice (*Glycyrrhiza glabra*) Horehound (*Marrubium vulgare*)	Loss of potassium; distal sodium Reabsorption	Hypertension; hypernatremia Use of laxatives, hypokalemia Nausea/vomiting Renal problems Concurrent use of diuretics Concurrent use of penicillin Edema	Muscular weakness Edema, intestinal dilatation (ileus)

HERB/DRUG POTENTIAL INTERACTIONS *(Continued)*

ANABOLIC HERBS

These herbs have been reported to contain steroidal or steroidal-precursor constituents that may be active *in vivo*. Use these herbs with caution in patients on steroidal drug or in patients with contraindications for steroidal drugs.

> Devil's Club (*Oplopanax horridum*)
> **Dong Quai** (*Angelica sinensis*)
> Ginseng, American (*Panax quinquifolium*)
> **Ginseng, Asian** (*Panax Ginseng*)
> **Ginseng, Siberian** (*Eleutherococcus senticosus*)
> **Muira puama** (*Ptychopetalum spp*)
> Sarsaparilla (*Smilax spp*)
> Suma (*Pfaffia paniculata*)
> **Tribulus** (*Tribulus terrestris*)
> **Wild Yam** (*Dioscorea villosa*)

PHYTOESTROGENIC HERBS

These herbs contain phytoestrogenic compounds that mimic the body's natural estrogen. Phytoestrogen-containing herbs have not been associated with the negative health effects seen with synthetic estrogen. However, use with caution in individuals on hormone replacement therapy or oral contraceptives or with a history of estrogen-dependent tumors, endometrial cancer, thromboembolic disease, or stroke.

Phytoestrogenic Herbs	Bioactive Component(s)
Alfalfa (*Medicago sativa*)	Coumestans
Black Cohosh (*Cimicifuga racemosa*)	Isoflavones, estrogens
Bloodroot (*Sanguinaria canadensis*)	Unnamed steroidals
Hops (*Humulus lupulus*)	Estriol, estradiol
Kudzu (*Pueraria lobata*)	Isoflavones
Licorice (*Glycyrrhiza glabra*)	Estriol
Pomegranate (*Punica granatum*)	Estrone, estradiol
Red Clover (*Trifolium pratense*)	Coumestans, isoflavones
Soybean (*Glycine Max*)	Isoflavones
Thyme (*Thymus vulgaris*)	Saponins
Yucca (*Yucca spp*)	Sarsasapogenin

PHYTOPROGESTOGENIC HERBS

These herbs contain compounds that have been reported to contain progestogenic action. Use these herbs with caution when taking hormonal supplementation, including birth control pills and hormone replacement therapy (HRT).

> **Chasteberry** (*Vitex agnus-castus*)
> Bloodroot (*Sanguinaria canadensis*)
> Oregano (*Oregano spp*)
> Damiana (*Turnera spp*)
> Yucca (*Yucca spp*)

COAGULANT HERBS

These herbs should be used with caution in individuals with bleeding disorders.

> Agrimony (*Agrimonia eupatoria*)
> **Golden Seal** (*Hydrastis canadensis*)
> Mistletoe (*Viscum* spp)
> Yarrow (*Achillea millefolium*)

ANTICOAGULANT HERBS

These herbs are contraindicated in individuals with active bleeding (eg, peptic ulcer, intracranial bleeding). Use with caution in individuals with a history of bleeding, hemostatic disorders, or drug-related hemostatic problems. Use with caution in individuals taking anticoagulant medications, including warfarin, aspirin, aspirin-containing products, NSAIDs, antiplatelet agents (eg, ticlopidine, clopidogrel, dipyridamole), or herbs with antiplatelet activity (eg, garlic, ginkgo, ginseng), and vitamin E. Discontinue use prior to dental or surgical procedures (generally at least 14 days prior). Listed below are some of the most commonly recognized anticoagulant botanical constituents. It should be noted that there might be unidentified constituents in these botanicals that may have anticoagulant activity.

Anticoagulant Herbs	Bioactive Constituents
Alfalfa (*Medicago sativa*)	Coumarin constituents
Angelica (*Angelica archangelica*)	Coumarin constituents
Anise (*Pimpinella anisum*)	Coumarin constituents
Arnica, Leopard's Bane (*Arnica montana*) NOT FOR INTERNAL USE	Hispidulin
Asafetida (*Ferula asafetida*)	Coumarin constituents
Bilberry (*Vaccinium myrtillus*)	Proanthocyanidins
Birch (*Betula barosma*)	Salicylate constituents
Bladderwrack (*Fucus vesiculosis*)	Unknown constituents
Bromelain (*Anas comosus*)	Bromelain enzyme
Cat's Claw (*Uncaria tomentosa*)	Proanthocyanidins
Celery (*Apium graveolens*)	Coumarin constituents
Coleus (*Coleus forskohlii*)	Forskohlin
Cordyceps (*Cordyceps sinensis*)	Adenosine
Dong Quai (*Angelica sinensis*)	Furocumarins
Evening Primrose (*Oenothera biennis*)	Gamma-linolenic acid
Fenugreek (*Trigonella foenum-graecum*)	Coumarin constituents
Feverfew (*Tanacetum parthenium*)	Parthenolides
Garlic (*Allium sativum*)	Ajoene, allicin, alliin
Ginger (*Zingiber officinalis*)	Kaempferol, coumarin constituents
Ginkgo (*Ginkgo biloba*)	Catechin, ginkgolides, kaempferol
Ginseng, American (*Panax quinquifolium*)	Ginsenosides
Ginseng, Panax (*Panax ginseng*)	Ginsenosides
Ginseng, Siberian (*Eleutherococcus senticosus*)	Eleutherosides
Grape Seed (*Vitis vinifera*)	Proanthocyanidins
Green Tea (*Camellia sinensis*)	Catechins
Guggul (*Commiphora mukul*)	Guggulsterones
Horse Chestnut (*Aesculus hippocastanum*)	Coumarin constituents
Horseradish (*Radicula armoracia*)	Kaempferol
Prickly Ash (*Zanthoxylum* spp)	Coumarin constituents
Quassia (*Picrasma excelsa*)	Coumarin constituents
Red Clover (*Trifolium pratense*)	Coumarin constituents
Reishi (*Ganoderma lucidum*)	Adenosine
Turmeric (*Curcuma longa*)	Curcuminoids
Sweet Clover (*Melilotus* spp)	Coumarin constituents
White Willow (*Salix alba*)	Salicylate constituents

HERB/DRUG POTENTIAL INTERACTIONS *(Continued)*

TOPICAL ALLERGENIC HERBS

These herbs have been reported to be allergenic in susceptible individuals. Use these herbs with caution in predisposed individuals.

> Bittersweet (*Solanum dulcamara*)
> **Chamomile, German** (*Matricaria chamomilla*)
> Coffee (*Caffea arabica*)
> Devil's Dung (*Ferula asafetida*)
> **Echinacea** (*Echinacea* spp)
> **Feverfew** (*Tanacetum parthenium*) May cause aphthous ulcers if chewed
> Flax (*Linum* spp)
> **Garlic** (*Allium sativum*)
> Ginseng, American (*Panax quinquifolium*)
> **Gotu Kola** (*Centella asiatica*)
> Male Fern (*Dryopteris filix-mas*)
> Propolis
> Spanish Bayonet (*Yucca* spp)

BLOOD SUGAR

Hyperglycemic Herbs

These herbs have been reported to potentially increase blood sugar levels. Use these herbs with caution in hyperglycemic individuals.

> Elecampane (*Inula helenium*)
> Ginseng, American (*Panax quinquifolium*)
> **Gotu Kola** (*Centella asiatica*)

Hypoglycemic Herbs

These herbs have been reported to lower blood sugar levels *in vivo* or *in vitro*. Use these herbs with caution in hypoglycemic individuals. Monitor blood sugar levels appropriately. As these herbs tend to lower blood sugar levels to varying degrees, use with caution in individuals taking insulin and/or oral hypoglycemic medications, because these herbs may lower blood sugar even further.

> Alfalfa (*Medicago sativa*)
> **Aloe** (*Aloe* spp)
> **Bilberry** (*Vaccinium myrtillus*)
> **Bitter Melon** (*Momordica charantia*)
> Burdock (*Arctium lappa*)
> Celery (*Apium graveolens*)
> Corn silk (*Zea mays*)
> Damiana (*Turnera* spp)
> Elecampane (*Inula helenium*)
> Eucalyptus (*Eucalyptus globulus*)
> **Fenugreek** (*Trigonella foenum-graecum*)
> **Garcinia** (*Garcinia cambogia*)
> **Garlic** (*Allium sativum*)
> **Ginger** (*Zingiber officinale*)
> **Ginseng, American** (*Panax quinquifolium*)
> **Gymnema** (*Gymnema sylvestre*)
> Juniper (*Juniperus communis*)
> **Marshmallow** (*Althaea officinalis*)
> Myrrh (*Commiphora* spp)
> Sage (*Salvia* spp)
> **Stinging Nettle** (*Urtica dioica*)
> Tansy (*Tanacetum vulgare*)

BLOOD PRESSURE

Hypertensive Herbs

These herbs have been reported to increase blood pressure and should not be used in individuals who are hypertensive or susceptible to hypertension.

Hypertensive Herb	Biological Effects
Bayberry (*Myrica cerifera*)	Myricitrin mineralocorticoid effects
Blue Cohosh (*Caulophyllum thalictroides*)	Nicotinic action due to methyl-cytisine; alkaloidal effect
Broom (*Sarothamnus scoparius*)	Alkaloidal effect
Cayenne (*Capsicum annum*)	Increased catecholamine secretion
Coltsfoot (*Tussilago farfara*)	Pressor activity; NOT FOR INTERNAL USE
Ephedra (*Ephedra sinica*)	Sympathomimetic; elevated heart rate
Ginger (*Zingiber officinalis*)	Increased catecholamine secretion
Ginseng, American (*Panax quinquifolium*)	Ginsenosides (Rg-1) may increase blood pressure in high doses or long-term use
Kola (*Cola* spp)	Vasoconstriction due to caffeine content
Licorice (*Glycyrrhiza glabra*)	Mineralocorticoid effect
Mate (*Ilex paraguariensis*)	Vasoconstriction due to caffeine content

Hypotensive Herbs

These herbs have been reported to lower blood pressure. Use with caution in hypotensive individuals. Use with caution in individuals on antihypertensive medications, as these herbs may lower blood pressure even further.

> Aconite, Monkshood (*Aconitum columbianum*)
> Arnica, Leopard's Bane (*Arnica montana*)
> Baneberry (*Actaea* spp)
> **Black Cohosh** (*Cimicifuga racemosa*)
> Bryony (*Bryonia alba*)
> California Poppy (*Eschscholzia californica*)
> Choke Cherry, Wild Cherry (*Prunus serotina*)
> **Coleus** (*Coleus forskohlii*)
> **Golden Seal** (*Hydrastis canadensis*) [in high doses]
> Green or False Hellebore (*Veratrum alba*)
> **Hawthorn** (*Crataegus oxyacantha*)
> Immortal (*Asclepias asperula*)
> Indian Tobacco (*Lobelia inflata*)
> Jaborandi (*Pilocarpus jaborandi*)
> Mistletoe, European (*Viscum album*)
> Night Blooming Cereus (*Cactus grandiflorus*)
> Pasque Flower (*Anemone pulsatilla*)
> Periwinkle (*Vinca major*)
> Pleurisy Root (*Asclepias tuberosa*)
> Quinine (*Cinchona* spp)
> Shepherd's Purse (*Capsella bursa-pastoris*)

CHOLESTEROL

Hypolipidemic Herbs

These herbs have been reported to lower blood cholesterol levels. Use with caution in individuals on hypolipidemic medications, as these herbs may lower the blood cholesterol levels even further.

HERB/DRUG POTENTIAL INTERACTIONS *(Continued)*

> Alfalfa (*Medicago sativa*)
> **Artichoke** (*Cynara scolymus*)
> Blue Cohosh (*Caulophyllum thalictroides*)
> **Fenugreek** (*Trigonella foenum-graecum*)
> **Garlic** (*Allium sativum*)
> **Ginger** (*Zingiber officinale*)
> **Guggul** (*Commiphora mukul*)
> **Gymnema** (*Gymnema sylvestre*)
> Plantain (*Plantago spp*)
> Skullcap (*Scutellaria laterifolia*)
> Myrrh (*Commiphora spp*)
> Tansy (*Tanacetum vulgare*)
> **Red Yeast Rice** (*Monascus purpureus*)

Hyperlipidemic Herbs

Gotu Kola (Centella asiatica) has been reported to potentially raise blood cholesterol levels in large doses and in prolonged doses.

DIURETIC HERBS

As with many pharmaceutical agents used for increasing diuresis, herbs with phytochemical constituents that are used as diuretic agents may potentially cause electrolyte imbalances in the body. Use these herbs with caution in individuals currently taking the following medications:

- Antiarrhythmics
- Digoxin
- Dilantin
- Lithium
- Potassium-depleting diuretics
- Theophylline

> **Artichoke** (*Cynara scolymus*)
> Celery (*Apium graveolens*) seed
> Corn (*Zea mays*) silk
> Couchgrass (*Agropyron repens*) rhizome
> **Dandelion** (*Taraxacum officinale*) leaf
> **Elder** (*Sambucus nigra/ Sambucus canadensis*) flower
> **Horsetail** (*Equisetum arvense*) shoots
> Juniper (*Juniperus communis*) berry
> **Kava kava** (*Piper methysticum*) root
> Shepherd's purse (*Capsella bursa-pastoris*) whole plant
> **Uva ursi** (*Arctostaphylos uva-ursi*) leaf
> Yarrow (*Achillea millefolium*) flower

LAXATIVE HERBS

Laxative herbs can negatively affect nutrients, drugs, and other dietary supplements by altering their absorption, metabolism, and excretion. Whether anthraquinone-containing herbs (stimulant) or bulk-forming laxative herbs, there could be alterations in drug levels such as digitalis and lithium. Also, there can be a potential decrease in the absorption of and an increase in the excretion of vitamins, minerals, and other nutrients when using laxative herbs.

Aloe (*Aloe* spp) leaf
Cascara (*Rhamnus persiana*) bark
Eyebright (*Euphrasia* spp) herb
Plantain (*Plantago lanceolata*) leaf
Psyllium (*Plantago psyllium*) husks
Rhubarb (*Rheum palmatum*) root
Senna (*Cassia senna*) fruit
Yellow Dock (*Rumex crispus*) root

References

These references, along with current published scientific literature, are the basis for the information in this document. It is to be noted that all of the interactions and adverse drug reactions (ADRs) are potential in susceptible individuals and cannot be one hundred percent predictable. Use sound professional judgment when recommending herbal medicines in individuals.

C. A. Newall, et al, Herbal Medicines: *A Guide for Health Care Professionals*, London, England: The Pharmaceutical Press, 1996.

F Brinker, *Herb Contraindications and Drug Interactions*, Sandy, Oregon: Eclectic Institute, 1997.

M McGuffin, et al, *Botanical Safety Handbook*, Boca Raton, FL: CRC Press, 1997.

PR Bradley, ed, *British Herbal Compendium*, Vol. 1, Bournemouth, England: British Herbal Medicine Association, 1992.

A Leung, et al, *Encyclopedia of Common Natural Ingredients Used in Foods, Drugs, and Cosmetics*, New York, NY: A Wiley-Interscience Publication, 1996.

P DeSmet, et al, *Adverse Effects of Herbal Drugs*, vols 1, 2, and 3, Berlin, Germany: Springer Verlag, 1993.

V Schulz, et al, *Rational Phytotherapy*, Berlin, Germany: Springer Verlag, 1998.

UNSAFE HERBS

Herbs are generally safe when taken in recommended doses and when potential side effects and contraindications are noted. However, some herbs that have been reported to be toxic in laboratory animals and human subjects, and toxic effects of certain plant species can be seen in even small doses. Toxic effects are a function of many factors including:

- **Patient status** - geriatric, pediatric, and health-compromised individuals should only use herbal therapies with professional advice

- **Dosage amount** - the safety of an herb is dependent upon using it in the correct dosage and form

- **Length of therapy** - kava taken in appropriate amounts can be an excellent herb for anxiety, but taken in prolonged and large amounts kava has been associated with a "yellowing" of the skin

- **Absorption, metabolism, elimination, and other kinetic principles**

Toxic effects can also be seen if the herbal product does not contain the correct species or if proper manufacturing controls are not followed. Always use reputable companies with appropriate quality control procedures in place.

The following chart lists selected plant species that are considered to contain toxic constituents and should therefore not be recommended as herbal medicines.

Plant Species	Toxic Effect	Comments
Arnica (*Arnica montana*)	Internal use of full strength arnica has resulted in mucous membrane irritation and may result in fatal gastroenteritis, muscle paralysis, increased or decreased pulse rate, palpitations, shortness of breath, and even death	Safe to use in homeopathic preparations
Butterbur (*Petasites* spp)	Potentially hepatotoxic due to presence of pyrrolizidine alkaloids[1]	
Chaparral, Creosote bush (*Larrea tridentata*)	Contains potentially hepatotoxic constituents[2]	
Coltsfoot (*Tussilago farfara*)	Potentially hepatotoxic due to presence of pyrrolizidine alkaloids[3]	
Comfrey (*Symphytum officinale*)	Root is potentially hepatotoxic due to presence of pyrrolizidine alkaloids[4]	Leaf is used topically as a wound-healing agent in various external preparations. USE EXTERNALLY ONLY.
Indian tobacco (*Lobelia inflata*)	Contains toxic nicotinic alkaloid lobeline that causes nausea vomiting, headache, tremors, and dizziness in small doses. In larger doses may cause diaphoresis, paresis, convulsions, tachycardia, hypotension, Cheyne-Stokes respiration, hypothermia, and even death[5]	Use only under the supervision of a qualified healthcare provider
Jimson weed (*Datura stramonium*)	Contains toxic tropane alkaloids that cause hallucinations and have potent anticholinergic properties[6]	Use only under the supervision of a qualified healthcare provider for symptoms of Parkinson's disease.
Pennyroyal oil (from *Mentha pulegium* or *Hedeoma pulegioides*)	Reported to be an abortifacient that causes nausea, vomiting, seizures, hallucinations, renal, and hepatotoxicity[7]	

Plant Species	Toxic Effect	Comments
Pokeweed root (*Phytolacca decandra* or *Phytolacca americana*)	May cause severe gastrointestinal symptoms such as cramps, nausea, and vomiting in sensitive individuals and in large and repeated doses. The berry and the leaf may be toxic even in small doses[8]	Use only under the supervision of a qualified healthcare provider.
Rauwolfia (*Rauwolfia* spp)	Contains numerous alkaloids that are hypotensive and may cause CNS disturbances[9,10]	Use only under the supervision of a qualified healthcare provider.
Sassafras (*Sassafras albidum*)	Root contains 1% to 2% volatile oil, consisting mainly of the toxin saffrole, which is reported to be hepatotoxic[11]	

1. Hirono I, et al, "Carcinogenic Activity of Petasitenine, A New Pyrrolizidine Alkaloid Isolated from Petasites Japonicus Maxim," *J Natl Cancer Inst*, 1977, 58(4):1155-7.
2. Sheikh NM, et al, "Chaparral-Associated Hepatotoxicity," *Arch Intern Med*, 1997, 157(8):913-9.
3. Hirono I, et al, "Carcinogenic Activity of Coltsfoot, Tussilago Farfara L," *Gann*, 1976, 67(1):125-9.
4. Ridker PM, et al, "Hepatic Venocclusive Disease Associated With the Consumption of Pyrrolizidine-Containing Dietary Supplements," *Gastroenterology*, 1985, 88(4):1050-4.
5. Kim HL, "Effects of SKF 525-A, Phenobarbital and 3-Methylcholanthrene on the Toxicity of Lobeline Sulfate," *Vet Human Toxicol*, 1985, 27(1):1-2.
6. Fodor G, et al, "Tropane Alkaloids," *Nat Prod Rep*, 1991, 8(6):603-12.
7. Anderson IB, et al, "Pennyroyal Toxicity: Measurement of Toxic Metabolite Levels in Two Cases and Review of the Literature," *Ann Intern Med*, 1996, 124(8):726-34.
8. Lewis WH, et al, "Poke Root Herbal Tea Poisoning," *JAMA*, 1979, 242(25):2759-60.
9. Pfeifer HJ, et al, "Clinical Toxicity of Reserpine in Hospitalized Patients: A Report From the Boson Collaborative Drug Surveillance Program," *Am J Med Sci*, 271(3):269-76.
10. La Barre J, "Hypotensive Effects of the Completely De-reserpinised Extract of *Rauwolfia vomitoria*," *Arzneim-forsch/Drug Res*, 1973, 23(4):600-5.
11. Kapadia GJ, et al, "Carcinogenicity of Some Folk Medicinal Herbs in Rats," *J Natl Cancer Inst*, 1978, 60(3):683-6.

COMMON HERBAL SUPPLEMENTS CONTRAINDICATED DURING PREGNANCY

Ashwagandha (*Withania somnifera*)
Bitter Melon (*Momordica charantia*)
Black Cohosh (*Cimicifuga racemosa*)
Burdock (*Arctium lappa*)
Cats Claw (*Uncaria tomentosa*)
Celery (*Apium graveolens*)
Chamomile, German (*Matricaria chamomilla*)
Chamomile, Roman (*Anthemis nobilis*)
Chasteberry/Vitex (*Vitex agnus castus*)
Devil's Claw (*Harpagophytum procumbens*)
Feverfew (*Tanacetum parthenium*)
Ginseng, Panax (*Panax ginseng*)
Golden Seal (*Hydrastis canadensis*)
Gotu Kola (*Centella asiatica*)
Kava Kava (*Piper methysticum*)
Licorice (*Glycyrrhiza glabra*)
Red Clover (*Trifolium pratense*) [as Promensil]
Rosemary (*Rosmarinus officinalis*)
Schisandra (*Schizandra chinensis*)
St John's Wort (*Hypericum perforatum*)
Stinging Nettle (*Urtica dioica*)
Uva Ursi (*Arctostaphylos uva-ursi*)
Yohimbe (*Pausinystalia yohimbe*)

PREGNANCY & LACTATION NUTRITIONAL CHART

Vitamin/ Mineral/Trace Element	Pregnancy Dosage RDI*	Lactation Dosage RDI*	Function in the Body	Cautions/Contraindications
Beta-carotene (Provitamin A)	None established	None established	• Antioxidant • Precursor to vitamin A	Nontoxic
Biotin	None established	None established	• Important for healthy hair and skin • Aids in producing energy from fats and carbohydrates	Nontoxic
Calcium	1200 mg/day	1200 mg/day	• Essential for healthy bone and tooth formation • Aids muscle growth and contraction	• Body excretes excess from large doses
Chromium	None established	None established	• Enhances insulin receptor binding • Aids insulin sensitivity	• May be toxic in large doses, so do not exceed 200-600 mcg/day • May decrease blood sugar
Folic acid	400 mcg/day	First 6 mos: 280 mcg/day Second 6 mos: 260 mcg/day	• Essential for development of healthy cells • Important for prevention of birth defects	• Nontoxic • Some classes of drugs deplete folic acid • Deficiency is common • Women should have folic acid status evaluated before becoming pregnant
Iodine	175 mcg/day	200 mcg/day	• Thyroid hormone regulation and metabolism	Nontoxic
Iron	30 mg/day	15 mg/day	• Involved in hemoglobin production and oxygen transport • Plays a role in energy production • Important for proper immune function	• Relatively safe • Body absorbs less iron when iron stores are full
Magnesium	320 mg/day	First 6 mos: 355 mg/day Second 6 mos: 340 mg/day	• Necessary for blood sugar metabolism and energy production • Important for proper nerve function • Plays a role in muscle contraction and relaxation	• Nontoxic • Excess is excreted by kidneys

PREGNANCY & LACTATION
NUTRITIONAL CHART *(Continued)*

Vitamin/ Mineral/Trace Element	Pregnancy Dosage RDI*	Lactation Dosage RDI*	Function in the Body	Cautions/Contraindications
Phosphorus	1200 mg/day	1200 mg/day	• Involved in bone and tooth formation • Necessary for energy production • Helps regulate pH balance in bodily fluids	• Excess phosphorus can deplete calcium
Selenium	65 mcg/day	75 mcg/day	• Antioxidant • Important for proper immune function • Has anti-viral effects	• Do not exceed 200 mcg/day due to potential toxicity
Vitamin A (Retinol)	4000 int. units/day	First 6 mos: 6500 int. units/ day Second 6 mos: 6000 int. units/day	• Necessary for normal growth and development • Essential for proper eye function • Important for proper immune function	• Doses >4000 int. units/day can be toxic to the fetus (caution women of childbearing age not to exceed 4000 int. units/day)
Vitamin B₁ (Thiamine)	1.5 mg/day	1.6 mg/day	• Important for energy metabolism • Supports proper nerve, muscle and heart function	Nontoxic
Vitamin B₂ (Riboflavin)	1.6 mg/day	6 mos: 1.8 mg/day Second 6 mos: 1.7 mg/day	• Involved in cell energy production • Plays a role in the breakdown of fats, carbohydrates, and proteins	Nontoxic
Vitamin B₃ (Niacin)	17 mg/day	20 mg/day	• Involved in the breakdown of carbohydrates and fats • Supports healthy functioning of the nervous and digestive systems	• Nontoxic • Do not take sustained release niacin products
Vitamin B₅ (Pantothenic Acid)	None established	None established	• Aids in the breakdown and use of fats • Supports normal growth and development	Nontoxic
Vitamin B₆ (Pyridoxine)	2.2 mg/day	2.1 mg/day	• Helps maintain healthy skin • Involved in the production of red blood cells and antibodies • Involved in the breakdown of carbohydrates, fats, and proteins	Nontoxic

Vitamin/Mineral/Trace Element	Pregnancy Dosage RDI*	Lactation Dosage RDI*	Function in the Body	Cautions/Contraindications
Vitamin B₁₂ (Cobalamin)	2.2 mcg/day	2.6 mcg/day	• Necessary for growth and development • Helps the synthesis of myelin • Supports healthy nervous system activity • Helps the body use folic acid	• Nontoxic
Vitamin C	70 mg/day	First 6 mos: 95 mg/day Second 6 mos: 90 mg	• Supports healthy immune system function • Plays a role in collagen formation	• Nontoxic
Vitamin D	400 int. units/day	400 int. units/day	• Necessary for proper calcium absorption • Supports bone and tooth formation • Supports healthy thyroid gland function	• Excess levels can result in hypercalcemia with calcium deposits in soft tissue
Vitamin E	10 int. units/day	First 6 mos: 12 int. units/day Second 6 mos: 11 int. units/day	• Antioxidant • Enhances immune system function • Aids in tissue healing	• Nontoxic at normal dosages • Natural vitamin E is recommended
Vitamin K	65 mcg/day	65 mcg/day	• Necessary for healthy bone formation • Essential for blood clotting	• Higher dosages are prescription only
Zinc	15 mg/day	6 mos: 19 mg/day Second 6 mos: 16 mg/day	• Important for protein production • Aids normal fetal growth and development • Enhances immune system function • Promotes wound healing	• Can be toxic at very high dosages

RDI: Recommended dietary intake

ORGAN SYSTEM SUPPORT USING NATURAL PRODUCTS

Organ System	Herbal Support*	Nutritional Support	Homeopathic Support
Adrenal Glands	Ashwagandha: 450 mg/day Cordyceps: 1050 mg, 2 times/day Ginseng (Panax): 200 mg/day Ginseng (Siberian): 200 mg/day Licorice: 250 mg, 3 times/day Schisandra: 100 mg, 2 times/day	Adrenal extract†: 200 mg 1-2 times/day B complex: 25 mg/day Vitamin C: 500-1000 mg, 2 times/day	Argentum nitricum 6X or 6C Natrum muriaticum 6X or 6C Silicea 6X or 6C
Brain	Ginkgo: 40 mg, 3 times/day Gotu Kola: 100 mg, 3 times/day HuperzineA: 50 mcg/day Vinpocetine: 10 mg, 2 times/day	Acetyl-L-carnitine: 500 mg, 2-3 times/day Phosphatidyl choline: 500 mg, 2 times/day Phosphatidylserine: 100 mg, 2 times/day	Anacardium orientale 6X or 6C Plumbum metallicum 6X or 6C Sulphur 6X or 6C
Eyes	Bilberry: 80 mg, 2 times/day Eyebright: 250 mg, 2 times/day	Beta carotene: 10,000 int. unit/day Lutein: 2 mg/day Vitamin C: 1000 mg/day	Cineraria 6X or 6C Phosphorus 30X or 30C
Heart	Cayenne: 400 mg 3 times/day Garlic: 400 mg 2 times/day or 600 mg/day aged extract Grape seed: 100 mg/day Green tea: 500 mg/day Hawthorn: 250 mg/day	Aortic extract†: 100 mg/day Coenzyme Q$_{10}$: 30 mg/day Fish oils: 1000 mg/day or Flaxseed oil: 1 Tbsp/day Magnesium: 400 mg/day Vitamin E: 400 int. unit/day	Convallaria majalis 6X or 6C Cactus grandiflorus 6X or 6C Magnesia phosphorica 6X or 6C
Immune System	Astragalus: 250 mg 2 times/day Cordyceps: 1050 mg 2 times/day Echinacea: 250 mg/day - 3 weeks on and 1 week off Ginseng (Siberian): 200 mg/day, 2 weeks on and 1 week off Reishi: 250 mg/day Schisandra: 100 mg/day with food	Vitamin A: 5000 int. unit/day Vitamin C: 1000 mg/day Selenium: 200 mcg/day Thymus extract†: 250 mg/day Zinc: 50 mg/day	Arsenicum album 6X or 6C Baptisia tinctoria 6X or 6C Conium 6X or 6C Pyrogenium 6X or 6C Thuja occidentalis 6X or 6C

Organ System	Herbal Support*	Nutritional Support	Homeopathic Support
Kidneys	Cordyceps: 1050 mg, 2 times/day Cranberry: 300 mg/day Dandelion (leaf): 250 mg/day	Vitamin C: 1000 mg/day Vitamin E: 400 int. unit/day	*Berberis vulgaris* 6X or 6C *Cantharis* 6X or 6C *Rubia tinctoria* 6X or 6C *Staphisagria* 6X or 6C
Liver/ Gallbladder	Artichoke: 250 mg/day Milk thistle: 160 mg/day Schisandra: 100 mg/day	Liver extract†: 500 mg/day L-Carnitine: 250 mg/day N-Acetyl cysteine: 500 mg/day	*Arsenicum album* 6X or 6C *Carduus marianus* 6X or 6C *Chelidonium autumnale* 6X or 6C *Phosphorus* 6X or 6C
Lungs	Cordyceps: 1050 mg, 2 times/day	Vitamin C: 1000 mg/day Fish oils: 750 mg 2-3 times/day or Flaxseed oil: 1 Tbsp/day	*Antimonium tartaricum* 6X or 6C *Carbo vegetabilis* 6X or 6C *Hepar sulphuris calcareum* 6X or 6C
Pancreas	Bitter melon: 200 mg/day Fenugreek: 250 mg/day Green tea: 250 mg/day	Chromium: 200 mcg/day Vanadium pentoxide: 250 mcg/day Zinc: 25 mg/day	*Kali iodatum* 6X or 6C *Lycopodium clavatum* 6X or 6C
Thymus	Astragalus: 250 mg/day Echinacea: 250 mg/day, 3 weeks on and 1 week off	Thymus extract†: 250 mg/day Vitamin C: 1000 mg/day Zinc: 25 mg/day	*Helianthus annuus* 6X or 6C *Cinchona officinalis* 6X or 6C *Calcarea sulphurica* 6X or 6C *Sulphur iodatum* 6X or 6C

* **Note:** Use standardized extracts of herbs whenever possible.
† Use New Zealand glandular extracts for purity.

661

PART V. GLOSSARY OF NATURAL MEDICINE TERMS

Abortifacient – Agent that causes abortion

Adaptogen – Plant substance that strengthens the general or nonspecific resistance of the body to stress

Aerobic – Oxygen dependent

Allopathy – Medicine oriented to the treatment of diseases and suppression of symptoms

Alterative – Herb that gradually restores proper functioning of the body

Amino Acid – Organic compounds marked by an amino group (NH_2) and a carboxylic (COOH) group, the building blocks of proteins

Anaerobic – Nonoxygen dependent

Antibacterial – Agent that destroys or stops the growth of bacteria

Anticatarrhal – Agent that reduces the formation of mucus or promotes its excretion

Antifungal – Agent that destroys or stops growth of fungus

Anti-inflammatory – Agent that reduces inflammation

Antimicrobial – Agent that kills microorganisms or suppresses their multiplication or growth

Antioxidant – Agent that neutralizes free radicals and/or reduces the process of oxidation in the body

Antispasmodic – Agent that prevents or relieves spasms

Antiviral – Agent that destroys or stops the growth of a virus

Arndt-Schulz Law of Pharmacology – Rule that states that small doses increase function, medium doses inhibit function, and large doses block function over time

Astringent – Agent that has a constricting or binding effect on tissues or fluid secretion

Avogadro's Number – 6.02×10^{23} molecules of a substance per gram

B Cell – Type of white blood cell that is produced in the bone marrow and is present in blood, lymph, and connective tissues, which respond when stimulated by certain antigens

Carminative – Agent whose main action is to soothe and relieve gases in the gastrointestinal tract

Carotenoids – One of a group of pigments (as carotene) ranging in color from light yellow to purple, which are widely distributed in plants and animals

Catarrh – Increase in mucus discharge from mucous membranes

Centesimal – Hahnemann's potency scale from 1 to 100

Chemoprotective – Capable of protecting healthy cells against the side effects of chemotherapy

Cholagogue – Substance that stimulates bile flow from the liver into the gallbladder and duodenum

Choleretic – Substance that stimulates bile flow, thus aiding assimilation of fats

Classical Homeopathy – Using a single homeopathic remedy to fit the total symptom picture of an individual

Clinical Homeopathy – Use of a homeopathy remedy for a therapeutic effect on a particular symptom

Coenzyme – Substance that activates enzyme substrates

(Continued)

Collagen – Fibrous insoluble protein (representing about 30% of total body protein) found in the connective tissue including skin, bones, ligaments, and cartilage

Combination Homeopathic Remedy - Medicine that contains more than one homeopathic ingredient

Complex Homeopathy – Using combination homeopathic formulas, usually in low potencies, for specific biological action (ie, motion sickness and sinusitis)

Constitutional Type – Homeopathic term that describes the individual's inherited traits and acquired physical, emotional, and intellectual makeup

Decimal – In homeopathic terms, a potency scale from 1 to 10 (X or D) developed by Samuel Dubs about 1838

Demulcent – Substance rich in mucilage that soothes, softens, and protects irritated or inflamed tissue

Detoxification – Process of eliminating stored toxins from the body through various organs of elimination

Diaphoretic – Agent that increases perspiration

Dietary Supplement – Product that is ingested and intended to supplement the diet by increasing total dietary intake (eg, vitamins, minerals, amino acids, herbs, enzymes, glandulars)

Dietary Supplement Health and Education Act of 1994 (DSHEA) – Federal law that regulates labeling and advertising claims for dietary supplements

Drainage Remedy – Remedy that increases the efficiency of detoxification in an organ of elimination

Drug-Induced Nutrient Depletion - Nutrient(s) that are depleted through the pharmacologic activity of a drug

Dysbiosis – Dysfunction or imbalance in the microflora in the intestines

Electromagnetic – Exhibiting magnetism arising from electric charge in motion

Emmenagogue – Stimulates normal menstrual flow

Endotoxin – Substance produced or formed in the body which may have a deleterious effect on metabolism depending on its concentration

Enzyme – Organic catalyst that induces chemical reactions in living matter without undergoing change itself

Ergogenic – Agent that enhances performance (often used in terms of athletics)

Essential Fatty Acids – Two fats (linoleic acid and alpha-linolenic acid) that are necessary for biological activities that cannot be produced by the body

Exotoxin – Substance in the environment that may have a deleterious effect on the body's metabolism depending on its concentration

Fat-soluble – Capable of being dissolved in fat

Febrifuge – Agent that reduces fever

Fluid Extract – Liquid extract prepared so that 1 mL of product equals 1 g of medicinal herb (1:1 w/v)

Free Radical – Unstable compound with a free electron that damages other molecules from which it steals an electron to regain its own stability

Freeze-dried – Process of taking fresh plant material, freezing it at very low temperatures, then gently heating it to remove the liquid, thereby producing stable herbal products if kept away from light and humidity

Glutathione Peroxidase – Important antioxidant enzyme containing glutathione, which is a tripeptide of glutamic acid, cysteine, and glycine

Good Manufacturing Practices (GMPs) - Quality control procedures that all dietary supplement manufacturers should follow (herbal industry currently follows food service GMPs)

Hair Analysis – Use of hair for tissue biopsy to determine potential, beneficial, and toxic mineral/metal relationships

Hepatoprotective – Substance that protects the liver from damage that could result from alcoholism, oxidative stress, exposure to environmental toxins, medications, and other causes

Herbal Medicine – Use of plant materials to promote amelioration of symptoms or provide a nutritional effect

Homeopathic Dilution – Process of creating a homeopathic remedy of a specified dosage

Homeopathic *Materia Medica* – Book listing homeopathic agents by ingredient with subsequent provings (toxicology data)

Homeopathic Pharmacopoeia of the United States (HPUS) – Official compendium listing homeopathic remedies and their uses

Homeopathic Potency – Number assigned to a remedy that indicates its strength (eg, a 6X remedy would signify a 1/10 dilution)

Homeopathy – Field of medicine based on the science of microdoses and the Law of Similars

Homeostasis – State of equilibrium in the body, characterized by the absence of disease

Hormesis – Use of microdoses that extend or improve function of the body; the small dose effect

Hypercholesterolemia – Elevated blood cholesterol

Immunomodulation – Act of creating homeostatic balance in the immune system

Infinitesimal Dose – Dilution that is generally regarded in homeopathy to be beyond Avogadro's number

Isoflavones – Group of plant-based substances (primarily soybeans and red clover) with weak estrogenic activity

Krebs Cycle – Primary energy production metabolic pathway in the body

Law of Similars (*Similia similibus curantur*) – Principal tenant of homeopathy, which means "likes are cured by likes"; that is a substance that creates a given set of symptoms in its crude dose can be used in a low dose to treat those same symptoms

Leukotrienes – Compounds produced from arachidonic acid in response to mediators of inflammation that result in allergic and inflammatory reactions

Lipophilic Toxin – Substance that is lipid soluble, which may have a deleterious effect in metabolism depending on its concentration

Lutein – Component of the carotenoid family that may have nutraceutical benefit, particularly for the eyes

Lycopene – Nutraceutical found in fruits and vegetables, especially tomatoes and strawberries

Macrophage – Mononuclear cell with phagocytic activity that acts as a sentinel of the immune system by differentiating and destroying abnormal and infected cells

Meta-analysis – Statistical methodology that utilizes data from multiple trials to verify results and to give a stronger statistical outcome

Mother Tincture – Initial starting dilution used as the base for homeopathic potencies

(Continued)

Nature Killer Cells – Cells in the immune system capable of mediating cyto-toxic reactions without prior sensitization against the target

Neurotransmitters – Specific chemical agent released by a presynaptic cell that crosses the synapse upon excitation to react with a postsynaptic cell

Nonsteroidal Anti-Inflammatory Drugs (NSAIDs) – Class of pharmaceutical agents designed to reduce inflammation

Nutraceutical – Agents that are primarily developed from natural sources (plants or animals) that deliver a concentrated amount of a bioactive substance, which offer medical or health benefits

Nutritional Therapy – Use of nutritional agents to support bodily function for therapeutic effect

Optimal Daily Allowance (ODA) - Attempt to define the optimal daily allow-ance of a nutritional substance for maximum health and wellness

Organotherapy – Utilizing small quantities of organ extracts, which are taken from healthy animals, to promote health or alleviate symptoms or condi-tions

Phagocyte – Scavenger cell capable of ingesting particulate matter

Phytoequivalence – Standardization of a botanical agent so as to attain a consistent delivery of active compounds

Phytoestrogen – Plant-based compound with weak estrogenic activity

Phytonutrients – Nutrients that come from plant

Phytotherapy – Therapeutic application of medicinal herbs

Potentize – Act of dilution and succussion of a homeopathic remedy

Prostaglandin – Class of physiologically active substances that regulate a wide variety of biological activities

Proving – Homeopathic process in which a substance is given to a healthy individual and all of the physical, emotional, and psychological changes are noted

Provitamin – Precursor that can be transformed to a vitamin the body

Radioprotective – Capable of protecting healthy cells against the side effects of radiation, including radiation therapy

Recommended Dietary Allowance (RDA) - Set of daily nutritional values established by the U.S. Government that are sufficient to protect the average person from chronic degenerative diseases such as scurvy, beri-beri, and pellagra

Repertory – Index of body systems with related symptoms that includes a listing of the homeopathic remedies specific for each symptom

Standardization or Guaranteed Potency – Means that the botanical extract has been assayed for and contains (within a range of ± 10%) a certain known level of constituents

Submolecular Level Remedy - Remedy diluted out past Avogadro's number

Succussion – Manufacturing process that involves shaking a homeopathic dilution with impact in order to potentize the substance

T Cells – Type of lymphocyte that matures in the thymus that has suppressing or killing activity for the immune system

Thromboxane – Potent inducer of platelet aggregation

Tincture – Liquid prepared from a medicinal plant substance in a ratio from 1:5 w/v (1 part herb to 5 parts solvent) to 1:10 w/v (1 part herb to 10 parts solvent)

Tonic – Remedy that promotes vigor and helps to strengthen or regulate a weakened organ or body function

Trace Minerals – Minerals whose dosages are measured in microgram quantities

Vermifuge – Agent that causes the expelling of worms or parasites

Vulnerary – Herbs that promote healing of wounds by protecting against infection and stimulation of cell growth

Water-soluble – Capable of being dissolved in water

Wild-crafted – Plant or plant part that is gathered in the wild for manufacturing into a herbal supplement

Xenobiotic – Toxin that is pathogenic by nature whose excretion may disrupt metabolism

Xenotoxin – External or internal (xenobiotic) agent that can alter enzyme function or cellular messengers or that has a direct effect on homeostatic control of a biological system

NATURAL PRODUCT CATEGORY INDEX

NATURAL PRODUCT CATEGORY INDEX

AMINO ACID
Arginine 385
Branched-Chain Amino Acids (BCAAs) 398
Carnitine 403
Glutamine 446
Lysine 473
Methionine 478
Phenylalanine 487
Taurine 508
Tyrosine 514

HERB
Aloe (*Aloe* spp) 381
Arabinoxylane 384
Artichoke (*Cynara scolymus*) 386
Ashwagandha (*Withania somnifera*) 387
Astragalus (*Astragalus membranaceus*) [Milk Vetch] 388
Bacopa (*Bacopa monniera*) 389
Bilberry (*Vaccinium myrtillus*) 392
Bitter Melon (*Momordica charantia*) 394
Black Cohosh (*Cimicifuga racemosa*) 395
Bladderwrack (*Fucus vesiculosus*) 396
Boswellia (*Boswellia serrata*) 397
Bromelain (*Anas comosus*) 399
Bupleurum (*Bupleurum falcatum*) 400
Calendula (*Calendula officinalis*) 401
Cascara (*Rhamnus persiana*) 404
Cat's Claw (*Uncaria tomentosa*) 404
Cayenne (*Capsicum annuum, Capsicum frutescens*) 405
Chamomile, German (*Matricaria chamomilla, Matricaria recutita*)
. . . . 407
Chasteberry (*Vitex agnus-castus*) 408
Clove (*Syzygium aromaticum*) 411
Coleus (*Coleus forskohlii*) 413
Cordyceps (*Cordyceps sinensis*) 417
Cranberry (*Vaccinium macrocarpon*) 418
Dandelion (*Taraxacum officinale*) 420
Devil's Claw (*Harpagophytum procumbens*) 422
Dong Quai (*Angelica sinensis*) 425
Echinacea (*Echinacea purpurea, Echinacea angustifolia*) 426
Elder (*Sambucus nigra, Sambucus canadensis*) 428
Ephedra (*Ephedra sinica*) 429
Evening Primrose (*Oenothera biennis*) 430
Eyebright (*Euphrasia officinalis*) 431
Fenugreek (*Trigonella foenum-graecum*) 432
Feverfew (*Tanacetum parthenium*) 432
Garcinia (*Garcinia cambogia*) 437
Garlic (*Allium sativum*) 438
Ginger (*Zingiber officinale*) 440
Ginkgo (*Ginkgo biloba*) 441
Ginseng, Panax (*Panax ginseng*) 442
Ginseng, Siberian (*Eleutherococcus senticosus*) 444
Golden Seal (*Hydrastis canadensis*) 448
Gotu Kola (*Centella asiatica*) 449
Grapefruit Seed (*Citrus paradisi*) 450
Grape Seed (*Vitis vinifera*) 451
Green Tea (*Camellia sinensis*) 452
Ground Ivy (*Hedera helix*) 454
Guggul (*Commiphora mukul*) 454
Gymnema (*Gymnema sylvestre*) 455
Hawthorn (*Crataegus oxyacantha*) 456
Hops (*Humulus lupulus*) 457
Horse Chestnut (*Aesculus hippocastanum*) 458
Horsetail (*Equisetum arvense*) 459
HuperzineA (*Huperzia serrata*) 460
Ipriflavone 464
Kava Kava (*Piper methysticum*) 466
Lavender (*Lavendula officinalis*) 468

Lemon Balm/Melissa *(Melissa officinalis)* 469
Licorice *(Glycyrrhiza glabra)* 470
Marshmallow *(Althaea officinalis)* 476
Mastic *(Pistacia lentiscus)* 477
Milk Thistle *(Silybum marianum)* 479
Muira Puama *(Ptychopetalum olacoides)* 481
Olive Leaf *(Olea europaea)* 483
Parsley *(Petroselinum crispum)* 485
Passion Flower *(Passiflora spp)* 486
Peppermint *(Mentha piperita)* 486
Psyllium *(Plantago ovata, Plantago isphagula)* 492
Pygeum *(Pygeum africanum, Prunus africana)* 493
Red Clover *(Trifolium pratense)* 495
Red Yeast Rice *(Monascus purpureus)* 496
Rehmannia *(Rehmannia glutinosa)* 497
Reishi *(Ganoderma lucidum)* 497
Saw Palmetto *(Serenoa repens)* 500
Schisandra *(Schizandra chinensis)* 501
Senna *(Cassia senna)* 503
Stinging Nettle *(Urtica dioica)* 505
St John's Wort *(Hypericum perforatum)* 506
Tea Tree *(Melaleuca alternifolia)* 509
Thyme *(Thymus vulgaris)* 509
Tribulus *(Tribulus terrestris)* 511
Turmeric *(Curcuma longa)* 512
Tylophora *(Tylophora asthmatica)* 513
Uva Ursi *(Arctostaphylos uva-ursi)* 515
Valerian *(Valeriana officinalis)* 515
Vinpocetine 517
White Oak *(Quercus alba)* 531
White Willow *(Salix alba)* 532
Wild Yam *(Dioscorea villosa)* 532
Yohimbe *(Pausinystalia yohimbe)* 533

MINERAL
Bismuth 393
Boron 397
Calcium 400
Chromium 410
Copper 416
Iodine 463
Iron 464
Magnesium 473
Manganese 475
Phosphorus 489
Potassium 490
Selenium 502
Sodium 504
Vanadium 516
Zinc 534

NUTRACEUTICAL
Acetyl-L-Carnitine (ALC) 380
Alpha-Lipoic Acid 381
Androstenedione 383
Betaine Hydrochloride 391
Bifidobacterium bifidum (bifidus) 391
Caprylic Acid 402
Chitosan 409
Chlorophyll 409
Chondroitin Sulfate 410
Coenzyme Q_{10} 412
Collagen (Type II) 414
Colostrum 415
Conjugated Linoleic Acid (CLA) 415
Creatine 419
Cyclo-Hispro 420
Dehydroepiandrosterone (DHEA) 421
Docosahexaenoic Acid (DHA) 424
(Continued)

NUTRACEUTICAL *(Continued)*

Fish Oils 434
Flaxseed Oil... 435
Glucosamine 446
Glutathione 447
Hydroxymethyl Butyrate (HMB) 461
5-Hydroxytryptophan (5-HTP) 461
Inositol Hexaphosphate (IP-6) 462
Isoflavones (Soy).. 465
Lactobacillus acidophilus 467
Lutein 472
Lycopene 472
Malic Acid 475
Melatonin 477
Methyl Sulfonyl Methane (MSM) 479
Modified Citrus Pectin (MCP) 480
N-Acetyl Cysteine (NAC) 482
Nicotinamide Adenine Dinucleotide (NADH) 483
Para-Aminobenzoic Acid (PABA)........................... 485
Phosphatidyl Choline (PC)................................ 488
Phosphatidyl Serine (PS)................................. 489
Pregnenolone 491
Progesterone 491
Pyruvate 494
Quercetin 494
SAMe (S-adenosyl methionine) 498
Shark Cartilage 503
Spleen Extract 505
Tocotrienols 511

NUTRACEUTICAL, GLANDULAR

Adrenal Extract 380
Aortic Extract 384
Liver Extract.. 471
Pancreatic Extract 484
Thymus Extract 510
Thyroid Extract 510

VITAMIN

Beta-Carotene 390
Biotin 393
Folic Acid... 435
Vitamin A (Retinol)...................................... 518
Vitamin B_1 (Thiamine) 519
Vitamin B_2 520
Vitamin B_3 521
Vitamin B_5 (Pantothenic Acid) 522
Vitamin B_6 (Pyridoxine) 523
Vitamin B_{12} (Cobalamin) 524
Vitamin B Complex-25.................................... 526
Vitamin C 526
Vitamin D... 528
Vitamin E 529
Vitamin K 531

ALPHABETICAL INDEX

ALPHABETICAL INDEX

Acetylcysteine *see* *N*-Acetyl Cysteine (NAC) 482
Acetyl-L-Carnitine (ALC) 380
Acne Vulgaris 44
Adrenal Extract 380
Adrenal Glandular Extract *see* Adrenal Extract 380
Aesculus hippocastanum see Horse Chestnut *(Aesculus hippocastanum)*
. . . . 458
ALA *see* Flaxseed Oil 435
ALC *see* Acetyl-L-Carnitine (ALC) 380
Allergies / Hay Fever 48
Allium sativum see Garlic *(Allium sativum)* 438
Aloe *(Aloe* spp) 381
Aloe spp *see* Aloe *(Aloe* spp) 381
Alpha-linolenic Acid *see* Flaxseed Oil 435
Alpha-lipoate *see* Alpha-Lipoic Acid 381
Alpha-Lipoic Acid 381
Althaea officinalis see Marshmallow *(Althaea officinalis)* 476
Alzheimer's Disease / Senility 52
Amenorrhea 56
American Elder *see* Elder *(Sambucus nigra, Sambucus canadensis)*
. . . . 428
Anas comosus see Bromelain *(Anas comosus)* 399
Androstenedione 383
Angelica sinensis see Dong Quai *(Angelica sinensis)* 425
Aortic Extract 384
Aotic Glandular Extract *see* Aortic Extract 384
Arabinoxylane 384
Arabinoxylane Compound *see* Arabinoxylane 384
Arctostaphylos uva-ursi see Uva Ursi *(Arctostaphylos uva-ursi)* 515
Arginine 385
Arthritis (Osteo) 60
Arthritis (Rheumatoid) 64
Artichoke *(Cynara scolymus)* 386
Ascorbic Acid *see* Vitamin C 526
Ashwagandha *(Withania somnifera)* 387
Asian Ginseng *see* Ginseng, Panax *(Panax ginseng)* 442
Asthma 68
Astragalus *(Astragalus membranaceus)* [Milk Vetch] 388
Astragalus membranaceus see Astragalus *(Astragalus membranaceus)*
[Milk Vetch] 388
Athlete's Foot / Jock Itch 72
Attention Deficit Disorder (ADD) / Attention Deficit Hyperactivity Disorder
(ADHD) 76
Bacopa *(Bacopa monniera)* 389
Bacopa monniera see Bacopa *(Bacopa monniera)* 389
Bearberry *see* Uva Ursi *(Arctostaphylos uva-ursi)* 515
Benign Prostatic Hypertrophy (BPH) 80
Beta-Carotene 390
Betaine Hydrochloride 391
Bifidobacterium bifidum (bifidus) 391
Bilberry *(Vaccinium myrtillus)* 392
Biotin 393
Bismuth 393
Bitter Melon *(Momordica charantia)* 394
Black Cohosh *(Cimicifuga racemosa)* 395
Bladderwrack *(Fucus vesiculosus)* 396
Boron 397
Boswellia *(Boswellia serrata)* 397
Boswellia serrata see Boswellia *(Boswellia serrata)* 397
Branched-Chain Amino Acids (BCAAs) 398
Breast-Feeding 84
Bromelain *(Anas comosus)* 399
Bupleurum *(Bupleurum falcatum)* 400
Bupleurum falcatum see Bupleurum *(Bupleurum falcatum)* 400
Calcium 400
Calendula *(Calendula officinalis)* 401
Calendula officinalis see Calendula *(Calendula officinalis)* 401
Camellia sinensis see Green Tea *(Camellia sinensis)* 452

Candidiasis 88
Caprylic Acid 402
Capsicum annuum see Cayenne (Capsicum annuum, Capsicum
    frutescens) 405
Capsicum frutescens see Cayenne (Capsicum annuum, Capsicum
    frutescens) 405
Carnitine 403
Cascara (Rhamnus persiana) 404
Cassia senna see Senna (Cassia senna) 503
Cataracts 92
Cat's Claw (Uncaria tomentosa) 404
Cayenne (Capsicum annuum, Capsicum frutescens) 405
Centella asiatica see Gotu Kola (Centella asiatica) 449
Cervical Dysplasia 96
Chamomile, German (Matricaria chamomilla, Matricaria recutita) 407
Chasteberry (Vitex agnus-castus) 408
Chastetree see Chasteberry (Vitex agnus-castus) 408
Chemotherapy and Radiation 100
Chinese angelica see Dong Quai (Angelica sinensis) 425
Chitosan 409
Chlorophyll 409
Chondroitin Sulfate 410
Chromium 410
Chronic Fatigue Syndrome (CFS) 106
Cimicifuga racemosa see Black Cohosh (Cimicifuga racemosa) 395
Circulation (Peripheral) Problems 110
Citrus paradisi see Grapefruit Seed (Citrus paradisi) 450
CLA see Conjugated Linoleic Acid (CLA) 415
Clove (Syzygium aromaticum) 411
Cobalamin see Vitamin B_{12} (Cobalamin) 524
Coenzyme 1 see Nicotinamide Adenine Dinucleotide (NADH) 483
Coenzyme Q_{10} 412
Cold / Flu 114
Coleus (Coleus forskohlii) 413
Coleus forskohlii see Coleus (Coleus forskohlii) 413
Colic 118
Collagen (Type II) 414
Colostrum 415
Commiphora mukul see Guggul (Commiphora mukul) 454
Common Herbal Supplements Contraindicated During Pregnancy 656
Conditions/Decision Trees/Considerations 44
Coneflower see Echinacea (Echinacea purpurea, Echinacea angustifolia)
    426
Conjugated Linoleic Acid (CLA) 415
Constipation 122
Copper 416
Cordyceps (Cordyceps sinensis) 417
Cordyceps sinensis see Cordyceps (Cordyceps sinensis) 417
Cough 126
Cranberry (Vaccinium macrocarpon) 418
Crataegus oxyacantha see Hawthorn (Crataegus oxyacantha) 456
Creatine 419
Crohn's Disease 130
Croup 134
Curcuma longa see Turmeric (Curcuma longa) 512
Cyclo-Hispro 420
Cynara scolymus see Artichoke (Cynara scolymus) 386
Dandelion (Taraxacum officinale) 420
Dehydroepiandrosterone (DHEA) 421
Depression 138
Devil's Claw (Harpagophytum procumbens) 422
DHA see Docosahexaenoic Acid (DHA) 424
DHEA see Dehydroepiandrosterone (DHEA) 421
Diaper Rash 142
Diarrhea 146
Dimethyl Sulfone see Methyl Sulfonyl Methane (MSM) 479
Dioscorea villosa see Wild Yam (Dioscorea villosa) 532
Diverticulitis 150

DMSO₂ see Methyl Sulfonyl Methane (MSM) 479
Docosahexaenoic Acid (DHA) 424
Dong Quai (Angelica sinensis) 425
Drug-Induced Nutrient Depletions 625
Dyslipidemia.. 154
Dysmenorrhea 158
Echinacea angustifolia see Echinacea (Echinacea purpurea, Echinacea
    angustifolia) 426
Echinacea (Echinacea purpurea, Echinacea angustifolia) 426
Echinacea purpurea see Echinacea (Echinacea purpurea, Echinacea
    angustifolia) 426
Eczema 162
Elderberry see Elder (Sambucus nigra, Sambucus canadensis)........ 428
Elder (Sambucus nigra, Sambucus canadensis)..................... 428
Eleutherococcus senticosus see Ginseng, Siberian (Eleutherococcus
    senticosus)... 444
Endometriosis 166
Ephedra (Ephedra sinica) 429
Ephedra sinica see Ephedra (Ephedra sinica) 429
Epilepsy 170
Equisetum arvense see Horsetail (Equisetum arvense) 459
Euphrasia officinalis see Eyebright (Euphrasia officinalis)...... 431
European Elder see Elder (Sambucus nigra, Sambucus canadensis)
    428
Evening Primrose (Oenothera biennis) 430
Evening Primrose Oil see Evening Primrose (Oenothera biennis) ... 430
Eyebright (Euphrasia officinalis) 431
Fatigue 174
Fenugreek (Trigonella foenum-graecum)........................... 432
Fever 178
Feverfew (Tanacetum parthenium) 432
Fibrocystic Breast Disease (FBD) 182
Fibromyalgia 186
Field Horsetail see Horsetail (Equisetum arvense) 459
Fish Oils... 434
Flaxseed Oil... 435
Folic Acid 435
Fucus vesiculosus see Bladderwrack (Fucus vesiculosus) 396
Gallbladder / Gallstones 190
Ganoderma lucidum see Reishi (Ganoderma lucidum) 497
Garcinia cambogia see Garcinia (Garcinia cambogia) 437
Garcinia (Garcinia cambogia) 437
Garlic (Allium sativum).. 438
Ginger (Zingiber officinale)................................... 440
Gingivitis 194
Ginkgo biloba see Ginkgo (Ginkgo biloba) 441
Ginkgo (Ginkgo biloba) 441
Ginseng, Panax (Panax ginseng) 442
Ginseng, Siberian (Eleutherococcus senticosus)................. 444
Glaucoma 198
Glossary of Natural Medicine Terms 663
Glucosamine 446
Glucosamine Hydrochloride see Glucosamine 446
Glucosamine Sulfate see Glucosamine 446
Glutamine 446
Glutathione 447
Glycyrrhiza glabra see Licorice (Glycyrrhiza glabra) 470
Golden Seal (Hydrastis canadensis) 448
Gotu Kola (Centella asiatica) 449
Grapefruit Seed (Citrus paradisi) 450
Grape Seed (Vitis vinifera) 451
Green Tea (Camellia sinensis) 452
Ground Ivy (Hedera helix) 454
GSH see Glutathione 447
Guggul (Commiphora mukul)...................................... 454
Gymnema (Gymnema sylvestre) 455
Gymnema sylvestre see Gymnema (Gymnema sylvestre) 455
Halitosis 202

Harpagophytum procumbens see Devil's Claw (Harpagophytum
    procumbens) 422
Hawthorn (Crataegus oxyacantha) 456
Headache / Migraine Headache 206
Hedera helix see Ground Ivy (Hedera helix) 454
Hemorrhoids 210
Herbal Medicine Use In Pediatrics 641
Herb/Drug Potential Interactions 642
Herb Quick Reference Chart 538
Herpes Simplex 1 214
Herpes Simplex 2 218
HMB see Hydroxymethyl Butyrate (HMB) 461
Homeopathic Quick Reference Chart for Common Complaints 587
Hops (Humulus lupulus) 457
Horse Chestnut (Aesculus hippocastanum) 458
Horsetail (Equisetum arvense) 459
5-HTP see 5-Hydroxytryptophan (5-HTP) 461
Humulus lupulus see Hops (Humulus lupulus) 457
Huperzia serrata see HuperzineA (Huperzia serrata) 460
HuperzineA (Huperzia serrata) 460
Hydrastis canadensis see Golden Seal (Hydrastis canadensis) 448
Hydroxymethyl Butyrate (HMB) 461
5-Hydroxytryptophan (5-HTP) 461
Hyperglycemia / Diabetes / Insulin Resistance 222
Hypericum perforatum see St John's Wort (Hypericum perforatum) .. 506
Hypertension (High Blood Pressure) 226
Hyperthyroidism 230
Hypoglycemia 234
Hypothyroidism 238
Indigestion / Heartburn 242
Inositol Hexaphosphate (IP-6) 462
Insomnia 246
Introduction to Conditions 41
Introduction to Glandular Extracts 36
Introduction to Herbs 11
Introduction to Homeopathy 31
Introduction to Natural Medicine 9
Introduction to Nutrition 19
Iodine 463
IP-6 see Inositol Hexaphosphate (IP-6) 462
Ipriflavone 464
Iron 464
Irritable Bowel Syndrome (IBS) 250
Isoflavones (Soy) 465
Kava Kava (Piper methysticum) 466
Lactobacillus acidophilus 467
L-Arginine see Arginine 385
Lavender (Lavendula officinalis) 468
Lavendula officinalis see Lavender (Lavendula officinalis) 468
L-Carnitine see Carnitine 403
Lemon Balm/Melissa (Melissa officinalis) 469
L-Glutamine see Glutamine 446
Licorice (Glycyrrhiza glabra) 470
Lipoic Acid see Alpha-Lipoic Acid 381
Liver Extract 471
L-Lysine see Lysine 473
L-Methionine see Methionine 478
L-Phenylalanine see Phenylalanine 487
L-Taurine see Taurine 508
L-Tyrosine see Tyrosine 514
Lutein 472
Lycopene 472
Lysine 473
Macular Degeneration 254
Magnesium 473
Malic Acid 475
Manganese 475
Marshmallow (Althaea officinalis) 476

Mastic *(Pistacia lentiscus)* 477
Matricaria chamomilla see Chamomile, German *(Matricaria chamomilla, Matricaria recutita)* 407
Matricaria recutita see Chamomile, German *(Matricaria chamomilla, Matricaria recutita)* 407
MCP *see* Modified Citrus Pectin (MCP) 480
Melaleuca alternifolia see Tea Tree *(Melaleuca alternifolia)* 509
Melatonin 477
Melissa see Lemon Balm/Melissa *(Melissa officinalis)* 469
Melissa officinalis see Lemon Balm/Melissa *(Melissa officinalis)* 469
Memory Problems 258
Menopause 262
Menorrhagia 266
Mentha piperita see Peppermint *(Mentha piperita)* 486
Methionine 478
Methyl Sulfonyl Methane (MSM) 479
MGN-3 (Proprietary Extraction) *see* Arabinoxylane 384
Milk Thistle *(Silybum marianum)* 479
Milk Vetch *see* Astragalus *(Astragalus membranaceus)* [Milk Vetch]
. . . . 388
Minor Injury / Wound Healing 270
Modified Citrus Pectin (MCP) 480
Momordica charantia see Bitter Melon *(Momordica charantia)* 394
Monascus purpureus see Red Yeast Rice *(Monascus purpureus)* 496
Motion Sickness 274
MSM *see* Methyl Sulfonyl Methane (MSM) 479
Muira Puama *(Ptychopetalum olacoides)* 481
Multiple Sclerosis (MS) 278
Muscle Soreness / Stiffness 282
NAC *see* N-Acetyl Cysteine (NAC) 482
N-Acetyl Cysteine (NAC) 482
NADH *see* Nicotinamide Adenine Dinucleotide (NADH) 483
Nausea / Vomiting 286
Nettle *see* Stinging Nettle *(Urtica dioica)* 505
Nicotinamide Adenine Dinucleotide (NADH) 483
Nutraceutical Chart 573
Nutrient Depletion and Cancer Chemotherapy 637
Oenothera biennis see Evening Primrose *(Oenothera biennis)* 430
Olea europaea see Olive Leaf *(Olea europaea)* 483
Olive Leaf *(Olea europaea)* 483
Organ System Support Using Natural Products 660
Osteoporosis 290
Otitis Media 294
PABA *see* Para-Aminobenzoic Acid (PABA) 485
Panax ginseng see Ginseng, Panax *(Panax ginseng)* 442
Pancreatic Extract 484
Pancreatic Glandular Extract *see* Pancreatic Extract 484
Pantothenic Acid *see* Vitamin B_5 (Pantothenic Acid) 522
Para-Aminobenzoic Acid (PABA) 485
Parkinson's Disease 298
Parsley *(Petroselinum crispum)* 485
Passiflora spp see Passion Flower *(Passiflora spp)* 486
Passion Flower *(Passiflora spp)* 486
Pausinystalia yohimbe see Yohimbe *(Pausinystalia yohimbe)* 533
PC *see* Phosphatidyl Choline (PC) 488
Peppermint *(Mentha piperita)* 486
Performance Enhancement 302
Petroselinum crispum see Parsley *(Petroselinum crispum)* 485
Phenylalanine 487
Phosphatidylcholine see Phosphatidyl Choline (PC) 488
Phosphatidyl Choline (PC) 488
Phosphatidylserine see Phosphatidyl Serine (PS) 489
Phosphatidyl Serine (PS) 489
Phosphorus 489
Piper methysticum see Kava Kava *(Piper methysticum)* 466
Pistacia lentiscus see Mastic *(Pistacia lentiscus)* 477
Plantago isphagula see Psyllium *(Plantago ovata, Plantago isphagula)*
. . . . 492

Plantago ovata see Psyllium (Plantago ovata, Plantago isphagula) 492
Poison Ivy / Poison Oak 306
Potassium 490
Pregnancy & Lactation Nutritional Chart 657
Pregnenolone 491
Premenstrual Syndrome (PMS) 310
Progesterone 491
PS see Phosphatidyl Serine (PS) 489
Psoriasis 314
Psyllium (Plantago ovata, Plantago isphagula) 492
Ptychopetalum olacoides see Muira Puama (Ptychopetalum olacoides)
    481
Pygeum (Pygeum africanum, Prunus africana) 493
Pyridoxine see Vitamin B$_6$ (Pyridoxine) 523
Pyruvate.. 494
Quercetin 494
Quercus alba see White Oak (Quercus alba) 531
Red Clover (Trifolium pratense)................................... 495
Red Yeast Rice (Monascus purpureus) 496
Rehmannia glutinosa see Rehmannia (Rehmannia glutinosa) 497
Rehmannia (Rehmannia glutinosa) 497
Reishi (Ganoderma lucidum) 497
Retinol see Vitamin A (Retinol) 518
Rhamnus persiana see Cascara (Rhamnus persiana) 404
Riboflavin see Vitamin B$_2$ 520
Rosacea 318
S-adenosylmethionine see SAMe (S-adenosyl methionine) 498
Salix alba see White Willow (Salix alba) 532
Sambucus canadensis (American Elder) see Elder (Sambucus nigra,
    Sambucus canadensis) 428
Sambucus nigra (European Elder) see Elder (Sambucus nigra, Sambucus
    canadensis) 428
SAMe (S-adenosyl methionine) 498
Saw Palmetto (Serenoa repens) 500
Schisandra (Schizandra chinensis) 501
Schizandra chinensis see Schisandra (Schizandra chinensis) 501
Scleroderma... 322
Selenium 502
Senna (Cassia senna) 503
Serenoa repens see Saw Palmetto (Serenoa repens) 500
Sexual Vitality (Females) 326
Sexual Vitality (Males) 330
Shark Cartilage 503
Siberian Ginseng see Ginseng, Siberian (Eleutherococcus senticosus)
    444
Silybum marianum see Milk Thistle (Silybum marianum) 479
Sinusitis 334
Sodium... 504
Sore Throat 338
Soy Isoflavones see Isoflavones (Soy) 465
Spleen Extract 505
Stinging Nettle (Urtica dioica) 505
St John's Wort (Hypericum perforatum) 506
Stress / Anxiety 342
Suggested Daily Intake of Nutritional Supplements.................. 27
Sunburn.. 346
Systemic Lupus Erythematosus (SLE) 350
Syzygium aromaticum see Clove (Syzygium aromaticum) 411
Tanacetum parthenium see Feverfew (Tanacetum parthenium) 432
Taraxacum officinale see Dandelion (Taraxacum officinale) 420
Taurine 508
Tea Tree (Melaleuca alternifolia) 509
Teething.. 354
Thiamin see Vitamin B$_1$ (Thiamine) 519
Thiamine see Vitamin B$_1$ (Thiamine) 519
Thioctic acid see Alpha-Lipoic Acid 381
Thyme (Thymus vulgaris) 509
Thymus Extract 510

Thymus Glandular Extract *see* Thymus Extract 510
Thymus vulgaris see Thyme *(Thymus vulgaris)* 509
Thyroid Extract.. 510
Thyroid Glandular Extract *see* Thyroid Extract 510
Tocotrienols 511
Tribulus terrestris see Tribulus *(Tribulus terrestris)* 511
Tribulus *(Tribulus terrestris)*.................................. 511
Trifolium pratense see Red Clover *(Trifolium pratense)* 495
Trigonella foenum-graecum see Fenugreek *(Trigonella foenum-graecum)*
.... 432
Turmeric *(Curcuma longa)*....................................... 512
Tylophora asthmatica see Tylophora *(Tylophora asthmatica)* 513
Tylophora *(Tylophora asthmatica)* 513
Tyrosine 514
Ubiquinone *see* Coenzyme Q$_{10}$ 412
Ulcer (Aphthous) 358
Ulcerative Colitis 366
Ulcer (Duodenal and Peptic) 362
Uncaria tomentosa see Cat's Claw *(Uncaria tomentosa)* 404
Unsafe Herbs.. 654
Urinary Tract Infection (UTI) 370
Urtica dioica see Stinging Nettle *(Urtica dioica)* 505
Uva Ursi *(Arctostaphylos uva-ursi)* 515
Vaccinium macrocarpon see Cranberry *(Vaccinium macrocarpon)* 418
Vaccinium myrtillus see Bilberry *(Vaccinium myrtillus)* 392
Valeriana officinalis see Valerian *(Valeriana officinalis)*...... 515
Valerian *(Valeriana officinalis)* 515
Vanadium.. 516
Vinca minor see Vinpocetine 517
Vinpocetine 517
Vitamin A (Retinol)... 518
Vitamin B$_1$ (Thiamine) 519
Vitamin B$_2$ 520
Vitamin B$_3$ 521
Vitamin B$_5$ (Pantothenic Acid) 522
Vitamin B$_6$ (Pyridoxine) 523
Vitamin B$_{12}$ (Cobalamin) 524
Vitamin B Complex-25 526
Vitamin C... 526
Vitamin D... 528
Vitamin E... 529
Vitamin K... 531
Vitamins/Minerals/Trace Elements/Amino Acids Chart 604
Vitex agnus-castus see Chasteberry *(Vitex agnus-castus)* 408
Vitis vinifera see Grape Seed *(Vitis vinifera)* 451
Weight Management 374
White Oak *(Quercus alba)*...................................... 531
White Willow *(Salix alba)*..................................... 532
Wild Yam *(Dioscorea villosa)*.................................. 532
Withania somnifera see Ashwagandha *(Withania somnifera)* 387
Yohimbe *(Pausinystalia yohimbe)* 533
Zinc.. 534
Zingiber officinale see Ginger *(Zingiber officinale)*.......... 440

NOTES

NOTES

NOTES

NOTES

NOTES

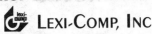
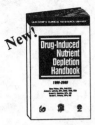
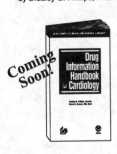
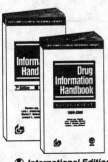

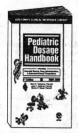
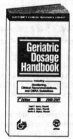
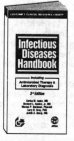

DRUG INFORMATION HANDBOOK FOR ADVANCED PRACTICE NURSING 1999/2000

by Beatrice B. Turkoski, RN, PhD; Brenda R. Lance, RN, MSN; Mark F. Bonfiglio, PharmD

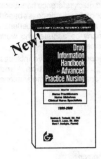

This handbook was designed specifically to meet the needs of Nurse Practitioners, Clinical Nurse Specialists, Nurse Midwives and graduate nursing students. The handbook is a unique resource for detailed, accurate information, which is vital to support the advanced practice nurse's role in patient drug therapy management.

A concise introductory section reviews topics related to Pharmacotherapeutics.

Over 4750 U.S., Canadian, and Mexican medications are covered in the 1055 monographs. Drug data is presented in an easy-to-use, alphabetically organized format covering up to 46 key points of information including Adult, Pediatric and Geriatric Dosing (with adjustments for renal/hepatic impairment), Laboratory Tests used to monitor drug therapy, Pregnancy/Breast-feeding Implications, Physical Assessment/Monitoring Guidelines and Patient Education/Instruction. Monographs are cross-referenced to an Appendix of over 230 pages of valuable comparison tables and additional information. Also included are two indices, Pharmacologic Category and Controlled Substance, which facilitate comparison between agents.

DRUG INFORMATION HANDBOOK FOR NURSING 2nd Edition 1999/2000

by Beatrice B. Turkoski, RN, PhD; Brenda R. Lance, RN, MSN; Mark F. Bonfiglio, PharmD

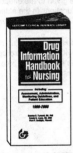

Registered Professional Nurses and upper-division nursing students involved with drug therapy will find this handbook provides quick access to drug data in a concise easy-to-use format.

Over 4750 U.S., Canadian, and Mexican medications are covered with up to 43 key points of information in each monograph. The handbook contains basic pharmacology concepts and nursing issues such as patient factors that influence drug therapy (ie, pregnancy, age, weight, etc) and general nursing issues (ie, assess-ment, administration, monitoring, and patient education). The Appendix contains over 220 pages of valuable information.

DRUG INFORMATION HANDBOOK FOR PHYSICIAN ASSISTANTS
1999-2000 by Michael J. Rudzinski, RPA-C, RPh; J. Fred Bennes, RPA, RPh

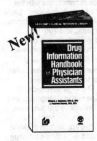

This comprehensive and easy-to-use handbook covers over 3600 drugs and also includes monographs on commonly used herbal products. There are up to 24 key fields of information per monograph, such as Pediatric And Adult Dosing With Adjustments for Renal/hepatic Impairment, Labeled And Unlabeled Uses, Pregnancy & Breast-feeding Precautions, and Special PA issues. Brand (U.S. and Canadian) and generic names are listed alphabetically for rapid access. It is fully cross-referenced by page number and includes alphabetical and pharmacologic indices.

To order call toll free: 1-800-837-LEXI (5394)

ANESTHESIOLOGY & CRITICAL CARE DRUG HANDBOOK
2nd Edition 1999-2000
by Andrew J. Donnelly, PharmD; Francesca E. Cunningham, PharmD; and Verna L. Baughman, MD

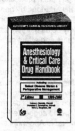

Contains over 512 generic medications with up to 25 fields of information presented in each monograph. It also contains the following Special Issues and Topics: Allergic Reaction, Anesthesia for Cardiac Patients in Noncardiac Surgery, Anesthesia for Obstetric Patients in Nonobstetric Surgery, Anesthesia for Patients With Liver Disease, Chronic Pain Management, Chronic Renal Failure, Conscious Sedation, Perioperative Management of Patients on Antiseizure Medication, Substance Abuse and Anesthesia.

The Appendix includes Abbreviations & Measurements, Anesthesiology Information, Assessment of Liver & Renal Function, Comparative Drug Charts, Infectious Disease-Prophylaxis & Treatment, Laboratory Values, Therapy Recommendation, Toxicology, *and much more . . .*

DRUG INFORMATION HANDBOOK FOR ONCOLOGY 1999-2000
by Dominic A. Solimando, Jr, MA; Linda R. Bressler, PharmD, BCOP; Polly E. Kintzel, PharmD, BCPS, BCOP; Mark C. Geraci, PharmD, BCOP

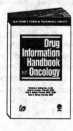

This comprehensive and easy-to-use oncology handbook was designed specifically to meet the needs of anyone who provides, prescribes, or administers therapy to cancer patients.

Presented in a concise and uniform format, this book contains the most comprehensive collection of oncology-related drug information available. Organized like a dictionary for ease of use, drugs can be found by looking up the *brand or generic name*!

This book contains 253 monographs, including over 1100 Antineoplastic Agents and Ancillary Medications.

It also contains up to 33 fields of information per monograph including Use, U.S. Investigational, Bone Marrow/Blood Cell Transplantation, Vesicant, Emetic Potential. A Special Topics Section, Appendix, and Therapeutic Category & Key Word Index are valuable features to this book, as well.

DRUG INFORMATION HANDBOOK FOR THE ALLIED HEALTH
PROFESSIONAL 7th Edition 2000-2001
by Leonard L. Lance, BSPharm; Charles Lacy, PharmD; Lora L. Armstrong, BSPharm, and Morton P. Goldman, PharmD

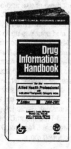

Working with clinical pharmacists, hospital pharmacy and therapeutics committees, and hospital drug information centers, the authors have assisted hundreds of hospitals in developing institution specific formulary reference documentation.

The most current basic drug and medication data from those clinical settings have been reviewed, coalesced, and cross-referenced to create this unique handbook. The handbook offers quick access to abbreviated monographs for 1,573 generic drugs.

This is a great tool for physician assistants, medical records personnel, medical transcriptionists and secretaries, pharmacy technicians, and other allied health professionals.

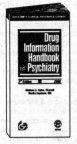
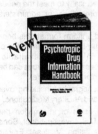
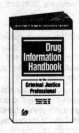

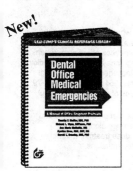
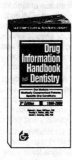
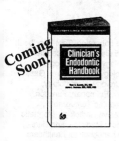
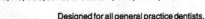

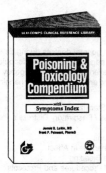
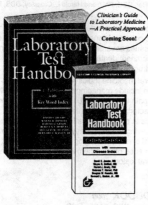
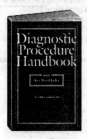

LEXI-COMP, INC

1100 Terex Road · Hudson, OH 44236

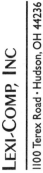

NO POSTAGE
NECESSARY
IF MAILED
IN THE
UNITED STATES

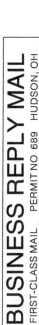

BUSINESS REPLY MAIL

FIRST-CLASS MAIL   PERMIT NO 689   HUDSON, OH

POSTAGE WILL BE PAID BY ADDRESSEE

LEXI-COMP, INC.
Natural Therapeutics Pocket Guide
1100 Terex Road
Hudson, OH 44236-9915

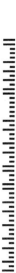

Thank you!

for purchasing Lexi-Comp's *Natural Therapeutics Pocket Guide*

Return this postage-paid card so we can keep you up-to-date on all the latest products, promotions and upgrades.

☐ Please put me on your **"Mailing List"**.

☐ Please put me on your **"Standing Order List"** to automatically receive the new edition each year.

Please print the title of the book here that you would like to receive a new edition of automatically each year.

_____

☐ Please send me information on **quantity discounts.**

Name (First): _____ (Last): _____

Title / Occupation: _____

Institution / Company: _____

Address: _____

City: _____ State/Province: _____

Zip/Postal Code: _____ Country: _____

Telephone: (_____) _____ Fax: (_____) _____

E-Mail Address: _____

OTHER AREAS OF INTEREST (listed alphabetically by topic):

☐ Advanced Practice Nursing Drug Information   ☐ Geriatric Dosage Information

☐ Allied Health Professional Drug Information   ☐ Infectious Diseases

☐ Anesthesiology & Critical Care Drug Information   ☐ Laboratory Tests

☐ Cardiology Drug Information   ☐ Natural Therapeutics

☐ Clinician's Endodontic Handbook   ☐ Nursing Drug Information

☐ Criminal Justice Professional Drug Information   ☐ Oncology Drug Information

☐ Dental Office Medical Emergencies   ☐ Pediatric Dosage

☐ Dentistry Drug Information   ☐ PA's Drug Information

☐ Diagnostic Procedures   ☐ Poisoning & Toxicology

☐ Drug-Induced Nutrient Depletion   ☐ Psychiatry Drug Information

☐ Drug Information   ☐ Psychotropic Drug Information

ALSO INTERESTED IN THE FOLLOWING:

☐ Formulary or Laboratory Custom Publishing Service

☐ Lexi-Comp's CRL™ on CD-ROM   ___ Academic ___ Personal ___ Institutional

☐ Lexi-Comp database on a hand-held device   ___ Palm Pilot   ___ Windows CE™   ___ Other